YONI SHAKTI

PRAISE FOR YONI SHAKTI

"In Yoni Shakti, *Uma Dinsmore-Tuli has done a splendid job of bringing forward her own very original work in yoga and female sexuality, while contextualizing it within a rich synthesis of inspired written work of others who share her passion for the subject. Her direct manner of speaking to the reader communicates both a wealth of knowledge and hands-on practicality, making it a very fresh and smart 'how to' book. I was enthralled!"*

– Vicki Noble is a feminist healer, scholar, artist and wisdom teacher, author of numerous books, including *Motherpeace*, *Shakti Woman*, and *The Double Goddess*

"Uma Dinsmore-Tuli re-interprets the symbology of the Mahavidyas, the sacred circle of tantric Wisdom Goddesses, in the light of the feminine life-cycle. This book is full of practical wisdom and insight. It's a powerful contribution to the feminine approaches to yoga that are being birthed now in the Western yoga world."

– Sally Kempton, spiritual teacher and author of
Awakening Shakti and Meditation for the Love of It

"The modern world is a masculine world and we have lost the sense of the feminine. Uma Dinsmore-Tuli and her husband Nirlipta Tuli's book, Yoni Shakti, *is a great contribution in restoring the balance and discovering the power of divine feminine. It is an inspiring and informative book full of profound wisdom."*

– Satish Kumar, activist, author, environmentalist and
editor of *Resurgence* magazine

"Uma Dinsmore-Tuli joins the revolution for true freedom by bringing her awesome experience into the practice of yoga to help women access innate power."

– Maya Tiwari, world spiritual teacher and author of
Women's Power to Heal through Inner Medicine

"Yoni Shakti *is the pathway to not only loving and celebrating your cunt but also to riding the rhythms of your body, the seasons and the moon."*

– Colette Nolan aka Lady Cunt Love,
founder of Cherish the Cunt campaign, activist, poet and educator

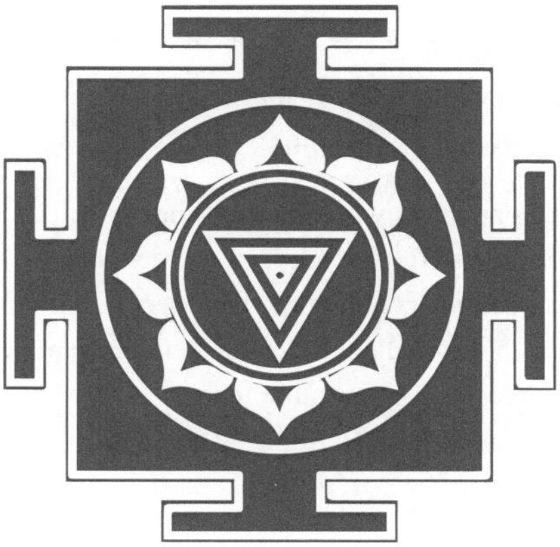

YONI SHAKTI

A WOMAN'S GUIDE TO POWER AND FREEDOM THROUGH YOGA AND TANTRA

A lifetime companion and compendium of blood wisdom, womb yoga, sacred sexuality, positive health and spiritual empowerment

by Uma Dinsmore-Tuli, PhD
Illustrations by Nirlipta Tuli

YOGAWORDS

Dedication

For my daughter Rajakumari Prayaag Eileen Dinsmore-Tuli,
and for my mother Meryl (Muire) Elizabeth Josephine Dinsmore.

In memory of my grandmothers:
Eileen Dinsmore (née Waters) (1907–1979) and
Elizabeth Jessie Moore (née Guy) (1888–1992)

And to all the mothers and daughters who find this work of value,
I share the sincere hope that through this yoga, all our daughters
and their future sisters and daughters and granddaughters will live in freedom,
with no need to contend with the challenges and difficulties experienced by
their mothers, grandmothers and great-grandmothers.

Jagadambe mātāki jai!

Yoni Shakti
A Woman's Guide to Power and Freedom through Yoga and Tantra

First published in 2014 by YogaWords, an imprint of Pinter & Martin Ltd

ISBN 978-1906756-15-4

Reprinted 2015, 2016, 2018

Managing editor: Zoë Blanc
Editorial support: Mark Singleton
Sanskrit editor: Lucy Crisfield
Design concept: Ben Jarlett
Jacket design: Spiral Path Design

British library cataloguing-in-publication data
A catalogue record for this book is available from the British library

Printed and bound in the UK by TJ International Limited
This book has been printed on paper that is sourced and harvested from sustainable forests and is FSC accredited

Pinter & Martin Ltd
6 Effra Parade
London SW2 1PS
pinterandmartin.com

Ṛtaṁ vadiṣyāmi
Satyaṁ vadiṣyāmi

[I will speak of what is right,
I will speak of what is true.]

Taittirīya Upaniṣad

Sarva maṅgala maṅgalye śive sarvārtha sādhike
Śaraṇye tryambake gauri nārāyaṇi namostute
Sṛṣṭi sthiti vināśānāṃ śakti bhūte sanātani
Guṇaśraye guṇamaye nārāyaṇi namostute

[You are the energy of Shiva all auspicious,
fulfilling all desires.
You are the refuge of all, you have three eyes,
salutations to You, shining radiant Narayani.
You are creation, preservation and destruction,
the eternal living energy.
You support the three qualities of nature,
which are your form, salutations to you, Narayani.]

from the Durgā Saptashatī [Devī Māhātmyam]

TABLE OF CONTENTS

CHAPTER THREE

CHAPTER FOUR

CHAPTER FIVE

CHAPTER SIX

CHAPTER TEN

CHAPTER ELEVEN

CHAPTER TWELVE

CHAPTER THIRTEEN

CHAPTER FOURTEEN

CHAPTER FIFTEEN

CHAPTER SIXTEEN

CHAPTER SEVENTEEN

PART THREE: FURTHER PRACTICES OF WOMB YOGA

CHAPTER EIGHTEEN

CHAPTER NINETEEN

CHAPTER TWENTY

CHAPTER TWENTY-FOUR

CHAPTER TWENTY-FIVE

CHAPTER TWENTY-SIX

PART FOUR: EXPANSIONS

CHAPTER TWENTY-SEVEN

CHAPTER TWENTY-EIGHT

CHAPTER TWENTY-NINE

AFTERWORD

APPENDIX

FOREWORD BY ALEXANDRA POPE

When Uma Dinsmore-Tuli first approached me to write the forward to *Yoni Śakti*, my instant reaction was 'yes' even though at that stage I had not read the book. In fact she had barely begun writing. But I knew Uma – her passion, her penetrating intelligence, and the deep tenderness and care in her teaching. I knew this book would be good, and even possibly one that could cause trouble – a trouble that is transformative. That I wanted to support!

My first taste of womb yoga outlined in this book was an hour's introduction as part of a menstrual health day at which I was also presenting. I raised myself off the floor after that first session to see the face of my colleague at *Women's Quest*, Sjanie Hugo Wurlitzer, grinning back at me. I knew instantly she was thinking the same thing as me: 'Wow, this is wonderful, we have to work with this woman.' And work we did and do, co-running Womb Wisdom Retreats.

What was it that Sjanie and I experienced that day that was so special? A yoga practice in which we felt our bodies and beings had been deeply engaged with rather than imposed on. Our bodies responded with an inner warmth and smile. We had been restored to a resting place of tender intimacy within ourselves, as well as feeling strengthened and balanced physically. And all in one hour. We wanted more.

There is an extraordinary movement, an awakening, occurring worldwide amongst women. It is both a yearning for, and a discovery and articulation of our own ways and practices to approach the sacred, to restore the power of the feminine. Uma Dinsmore-Tuli is one such woman stepping forward, nay compelled forward, by a deep intelligence to show us a yoga practice that is in service of women – physically, emotionally and spiritually. Practices must evolve with the times and with our evolving consciousness. Womb yoga is a fresh articulation of an ancient art that speaks deeply to and nourishes us as women.

For a long time I have argued that many spiritual practices, while worthy and great, can sometimes miss the mark for us as women. I would even dare to say that they were evolved by men to meet the needs and psychology of men, but not women. Women all along had a practice within their own bodies that was going unnoticed except by a few – it was the menstrual cycle. When approached with appropriate consciousness and time, the menstrual cycle can be an inner yoga that initiates a woman into a deep sense of intimacy with herself and the Divine. What is important about this female way is that it practises us. That is, we don't have to 'do' anything, rather, through a deeply felt engagement with the changing rhythms of our cycle, we can potentially enter a spiritual consciousness. Simple though this may sound, it is an inner discipline of a high order. When knowledge of the inner practice of women goes unnamed something immeasurable is lost to women and therefore to the world. It is rare for me to find other practices that understand this with any detail or discipline. However womb yoga explicitly embodies this. While working very thoroughly with all the structural aspects of our pelvis as a core part of our whole being it also engages with the energy dynamic of the cycle itself in both subtle and pragmatic ways that can give a woman a deeper sense of being 'in' herself. Uma also has a way of teaching that connects this deeply felt interior experience to a sense of belonging within mother earth. As one woman described it to me, 'I really love it when Uma gives each woman the opportunity to follow the phase of her menstrual cycle. We have a real sense of being taken care of and truly being ourselves. It's like opening a huge gate connecting my heart with my womb. And it makes me feel part of a great big womb, mother earth.'

Womb yoga speaks to women of all ages and in all stages of life – from menarche, through our budding sexuality, into the journey of pregnancy and birth, to the passage through menopause and beyond. It is for beginners as well as seasoned practitioners and teachers. It's both a revelation and a revolution; healing and nourishing; and restores a deep pleasure to our bodies.

Writing with authority and wisdom cultivated through many years of yoga practice, study and teaching as well as a very full life experience as partner, mother and woman dealing with all the vicissitudes of twenty-first century life, in *Yoni Śakti* Uma brings fresh 'sight' to the practice of yoga for women that will transform our experience of being women, and open doorways within that we didn't know existed.

This is vital work. Spread the word. Celebrate our wombs. Unlock the power of the feminine.

Alexandra Pope is author of The Wild Genie: the Healing Power of Menstruation, The Woman's Quest workbook, *and co–author of* The Pill: Are You Sure It's For You? *She teaches women about the power of the menstrual cycle.* **www.womensquest.org**

NOTE ON SHAKTI / ŚAKTI

The cover title *Yoni Shakti* is written with a 'sh' to ensure correct pronunciation for those who are unfamiliar with the more correct transliteration of this Sanskrit word as *Śakti* (and who may not perhaps get past the cover to reach this explanatory note). Throughout the rest of the book, however, the term is written *Śakti*, in keeping with the usual conventions of transliterating Sanskrit words into English, as outlined on pp.616–17.

AUTHOR'S PREFACE – OPENING PRACTICE: AN INVOCATION TO *YONI ŚAKTI*

Yoni Śakti is a celebration of women's power to heal and thrive. It describes how the practice of yoga and *tantra* can support the well-being of women everywhere, empowering us to reconnect to the wellspring of our vitality, our source power.

This opening practice of *yoga nidrā* includes a powerful diamond breathing pattern to raise consciousness of the key points of awareness in the cultivation of *yoni śakti,* the source power. It can be done seated, as a reading meditation, by allowing the awareness to follow the instructions described below (for 'close the eyes', simply read 'cast your eyes along the words on this page...') or it can be done lying down, as a listening practice, by playing the downloads available at **www.yonishakti.co**

TĀRĀ'S *YOGA NIDRĀ* OF ELEMENTAL INTEGRATION

Welcome home.
Lay flat like a star-web:
Hands and heels are celestial anchor points. The limbs, threads leading to the centre.
Close the eyes.
Exhale and allow the body to settle.
Feel the breath becoming spacious.
Observe the spacious, effortless breath settling the body deeper into stillness.
Be aware 'I am practising yoga nidrā, *I am practising* yoga nidrā, *I am practising* yoga nidrā.'
Let this be the form of awareness.
Be held by this state of consciousness.
Be safe within the vessel of the form of awareness which is yoga nidrā.
Exhale: drop the mind down into the heart.
Let the awareness be deep in the heart.
'I am my heart, I am my heart, I am my own true heart and my heart is open.'
Welcome the feelings or insights that arise in the heart.
Welcome the voice of the inner teacher.

Guide now the light of conscious awareness around the body.
The body remains still, but the awareness moves from point to point.
It is as if the body is a night sky,
and the light of mental attention shines at each point,
awakening the shining presence of a twinkling star –
so that the body becomes a constellation of shining stars in the night sky.

Inhale, and as the breath moves out
let a star shine bright at each point:
at the crown of the head,
between the eyebrows, and in the throat, between the collarbones.
Shine the bright stars of mental awareness down the right arm:
shoulder, elbow, wrist, thumb, index finger, middle finger, ring finger, little finger.
And back:
inside the right wrist, elbow, and shoulder.

Bring the awareness back to the throat, between the collarbones.

Shine the bright stars of mental awareness down the left arm:
shoulder, elbow, wrist, thumb, index finger, middle finger, ring finger, little finger.
And back:
inside the left wrist, elbow, and shoulder.
Bring the awareness back to the throat, between the collarbones.

Shine the awareness down into the heart space,
a bright star behind the middle of the breastbone.
A star shines in the left breast, and in the right breast.
Then bring the awareness back to the heart space,
so the star shines bright behind the middle of the breastbone.

Drop the awareness down into the navel. A star shines there.
Drop the awareness down into the yoni. *A star shines there.*

Shine the awareness over to the right hip, and feel stars shining down the right leg:
knee, ankle, big toe, second toe, third toe, fourth toe, little toe.
And back inside, stars shining in the right ankle, knee and hip.
Bring the awareness back to the light shining in the yoni.

Shine the awareness over the the left hip, and feel the stars shining down the left leg:
knee, ankle, big toe, second toe, third toe, fourth toe, little toe.
And back inside, stars shining in the left ankle, knee and hip.
Bring the awareness back to the light shining in the yoni.

And lift the awareness back to the star shining in the navel.

And raise the awareness back to the star shining in the heart space.
Be aware:
'I am practising yoga nidrā, *I am practising* yoga nidrā, *I am practising* yoga nidrā'.

Be aware of the whole constellation of the body shining in the night sky.
So many stars.
The whole body.

Inhale, and the space between the stars opens,
so the stars fill the full expanse of the night sky.
Exhale, the stars fall to earth, settling on the web of the body.
Inhale, stars rise and spread: spacious open dark between them.
Exhale, starlight like drops of rain descends,
landing on the star web body resting on the earth.
Light dawns.
Feel the star drops warmed on the body web as the sun shines.
Inhale, the earth is warmed,
the starlight drops drawn up from the body by the fire in the sky.
Exhale stars down to earth.
Inhale stars up to heaven;
exhale down to earth.

Pause between the breaths,
with awareness in the bright star in the centre of the heart space.
Awareness in the anchor points: heels, hands.
Awareness in the anchor threads, legs and arms.
Awareness in the spine and head.

Breathing on the web, anchored in the stars, breathing stars to earth.

Let the bright light of consciousness travel the triangles in the body web:
Exhale, breath moves down from yoni *to heels.*
Inhale, breath moves up from heels to yoni.
Upward-pointing triangle.

Pause to exhale, awareness at the yoni.
Inhale, breath moves up from yoni *to breasts.*
Exhale, breath moves down from breasts to yoni.
Inhale, breath returns to the breasts.
Pause to exhale, awareness at the breasts.
Downward-pointing triangle.

Inhale, breath moves up from breasts to eyebrow centre.
Exhale, breath moves down from eyebrow centre to breasts.
Inhale, breath moves up to eyebrow centre.
Upward-pointing triangle.

Let conscious awareness join the the upward-pointing triangle
to the downward-pointing triangle.
They meet at the breasts.
Let the breath move in the diamond of the body star web.

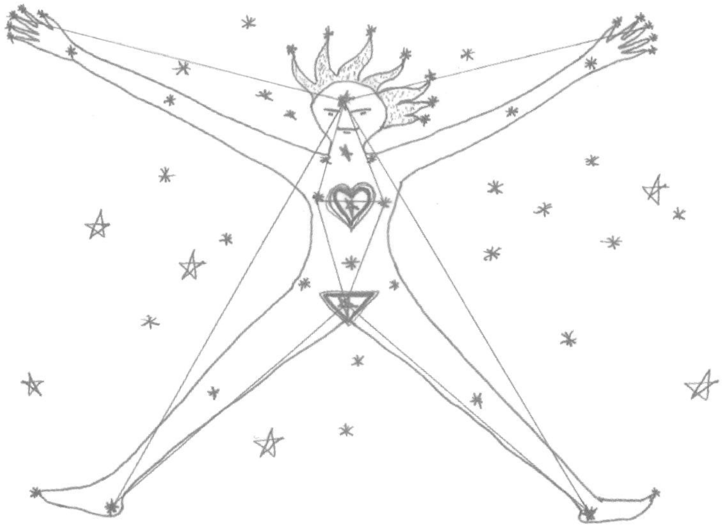

Shining diamond.
Exhale from eyebrow centre to breasts,
and pause to inhale.
Exhale from breasts to yoni.
Inhale from yoni *to breasts,*
and pause to exhale.
Inhale from breasts to eyebrow centre.
Exhale back to breasts.

Breath awakens consciousness in the diamond.
Diamond breath makes the shape vivid.
A shining diamond of awareness.
'I am practising yoga nidrā, *I am practising* yoga nidrā, *I am practising* yoga nidrā'.

Then
exhale all awareness from the edges of the diamond into the heart space
in the centre of the diamond.
Inhale awareness out to the edges of the diamond.
And back to the heart space.
Being in the heart space in the diamond in the web
feeling the stars shine.
'I am my heart, I am my heart, I am my own true heart and my heart is open.'
Breathe awareness in to the heart space.
Welcome the insights of the inner teacher, carried on the silent voice of the heart.
Welcome home to yourself.

Woman on the web of dreams.
Integrated.
Laying like a star-web.
Safe in the consciousness that is yoga nidrā.
Securely held by this state of awareness.
Safe within the vessel of the form of awareness which is yoga nidrā.

Know this practice of yoga nidrā *is coming to an end.*
Carry the blessings of the practice, the awareness of connection, out with you.
The practice of yoga nidrā *is complete.*
Stretch, yawn and open your eyes.
Let your breath be a bridge to a more everyday state of consciousness,
yet savour still the shining presence of awareness.
Hari Om Tat Sat.

introduction

WELCOME HOME

I invite you now to set aside everything you think you may know about yoga, its history, and its practice, and its present forms and lineages. Consider instead the possibility that this powerful spiritual practice, this technology for transformation and evolution, this global, grassroots phenomenon that brings peace and well-being to millions, this collection of practices we call yoga, is a naturally arising way of being in connection with elemental rhythms, and that it was perhaps, once upon a time, first inspired by reverence for the intense emotional, psychic and physical experiences of women's life cycles.

And recognise now with certainty that it is largely through women that the practices and benefits of yoga are caressing the globe, spreading a healing wave of positive energy. And now, allow your awareness to be open to the experience of yogic wisdom not simply living within you, but being inspired by the natural rhythms of your own physicality as a woman. Consciousness of yoga is in your body now. Welcome back.

Welcome home to your yoni śakti.
Welcome back to blood wisdom.
Welcome to womb yoga consciousness.

Welcome to a yoga of awareness, delight, and reconciliation with deep knowing. This is a book for women of all ages, and for the men who love them. It presents effective yogic means to live in freedom: to welcome joy, vitality, comfort and courage into daily lives that may seem to have no space left for peace. The practical guidance, stories and philosophical reflections in this book encourage you to reawaken, through an experience of womb-conscious yoga, your own inner guidance that leads you to a state of freedom. *Yoni Śakti* tracks routes for you to reconnect tenderly and respectfully with deep sources of wisdom and intuitive understanding. The practices of yoga and *śākta tantra* which are shared in this book all reveal, through the experience of our hearts and bodies, our wombs and our blood, a profound resonance with the patterns of elemental rhythms: that is the experience that points us to the source of our true wisdom and the state of freedom.

The very term *yoni śakti* locates the place of power [*śakti*] in our own bodies, in our *yoni*, a term that means both cunt or vulva, and womb or source. *Yoni* also means home, or place of rest. It is in and through the *yoni* that we encounter our connection to deeper knowledge, or *blood wisdom*. The term *blood wisdom* conveys a sense of the profound experience of 'knowing already', of recognising, sometimes not always so clearly, that this deep wisdom is present as a sense of spirituality in our lifeblood. The understanding of blood wisdom is that in our very cells, in our wombs, this knowing has never really been absent, and all that has been denied is access to the living consciousness of the true wealth that this wisdom brings, not just for women but for the whole planet. She is a deep and tender inner teacher. What she teaches is freedom.

Yoni Śakti is not just another book about adapting yoga for women's health. It is a contemporary *Tantra*: a handbook and compendium of practice and reflection, a treasure-house of resources, rituals and wild ideas, a powerful integration of philosophy and techniques for positive living. *Tantra* is often translated as a teaching that expands consciousness, but this understanding is also rooted in the literal meaning of the word *tantra* as a *loom*. So *Yoni Śakti* is a yogic weaving project: in and out through the warp of its structure are woven many different voices, experiences and strategies for living in freedom: there are fairy stories interwoven with instructions for nourishing, feminine practices of womb yoga, and there are radical and inspiring feminist perspectives on the origins and contemporary practice of yoga. *Yoni Śakti* is a rich fabric: it acknowledges the bloodroots of this powerful spiritual technology for awakening, and empowers you to reclaim your personal spiritual assurance in the urgent interests of the evolution of planetary consciousness and environmental healing.

So prepare to be refreshed, inspired and empowered. *Yoni Śakti* invites you to enter a newly embodied consciousness of the transformatory power of *tāntrik* yoga as a tool for global healing and freedom. The womb yoga that it describes moves beyond the biological and emotional aspects of yoga therapy for women's health to explore this deeper knowledge, a profound state of cosmic union, 'yoga', which enables us 'to restore a dignity and deeper meaning to a woman's cyclical nature' (Alexandra Pope 2001: 27). No longer do our yoga practices have to be 'adapted' or 'modified' to be appropriate for women, because they are, in the very essence of their genesis, the womb of yoga, and they lead us each back to our own blood wisdom: to the deep sense of knowing already exactly how to be free.

WHO NEEDS *YONI ŚAKTI*?

The philosophies and stories in *Yoni Śakti* explore the place of women in yoga past and present, and set out a theory of how women's lives now may be lived in freedom. The practices of womb yoga in *Yoni Śakti* are for any woman at any stage in her life who has an interest in yoga and consciousness, and a desire to support her own vitality, well-being, creativity, sexuality and spiritual consciousness. I have taught womb yoga practices to women of all ages in many different places, and have found that the techniques generally delight and astonish those who are new to yoga, those who are yoga teachers, as well as those who are thoroughly sceptical about yoga, and those who have been practising yoga all their lives. For many women the tender nurturing effect of this approach comes as a refreshing and rejuvenating relief in comparison to other more familiar (or imagined) ways of practising yoga.

Womb yoga is both accessible and esoteric: the techniques themselves are easy to follow, and positively supportive of women's health at every cycle of life. And though the instructions are clear enough for even a beginner to understand, the experiences that often result can open doors to profound levels of connection and peaceful awareness that are usually imagined to be accessible only after many years of advanced and sustained *tapas*, or yogic discipline. So the practices are open to all, but evoke different and individual responses in each practitioner, depending on their capacity and need. Once, after sharing the 'five dimensions of being' practice (pp.183–7) with a group of thirty experienced yoga teachers at a yoga festival, a *yoginī* in her seventies who had been teaching *haṭha* yoga for forty years approached me at the end of the session with tears of joy in her eyes to express her thanks for 'the most beautiful yoga practice I have ever done. My heart is melted.' In brief, the practices are enjoyable and powerful.

Yoni Śakti was born out of my own desire to understand more about the feminist potential of yoga as a radical force for deep change and freedom in women's lives. It is both a project of reclamation and a means to reconnection. Telling the histories of the women whose lives have been lived in freedom through the practice of yoga in the past reclaims their experiences for us all to learn from. This is the 'reclamation project': it is like picking over the leftovers and cooking up something tasty and sustaining. But reading other's stories will only bring us so far towards a state of freedom. Our lived experience of reconnection comes through our own practice. The 'reconnection project' of *Yoni Śakti* is in the practices it shares. All the instructions for the practices described in part three evolved at the request of women attending yoga retreats, my own students, clients, trainee teachers and colleagues who expressed a need for a comprehensive reference work that would present with detail and context all the practices they had encountered.

This book may be of especial practical use to yoga teachers, trainee teachers and yoga teacher trainers and yoga therapists. Because of the focus on women's health and women's experiences, *Yoni Śakti* may also be of interest to health care professionals and educators in the field of women's health, for example gynaecologists, psychotherapists, women's health physiotherapists, counsellors, midwives, childbirth educators, doulas and integrative health care providers such as acupuncturists, reflexologists, dance-movement and massage therapists.

WHAT IS WOMB YOGA AND DO I NEED A WOMB TO PRACTISE IT?

Womb yoga is part of *yoni śakti*. It is a means to realise freedom, a technology of transformation. To experience *yoni śakti* is to be empowered, and to practise womb yoga is a way to encounter this power.

It is not necessary to have a womb to practise womb yoga. The meaning and resonance of womb yoga is not tied or limited to the physical organ of the womb. Nor is it intended solely for women whose wombs experience menstrual cycles. It is a practice for all women of all ages, including women who no longer have a womb. In all phases of women's lives, it is the presence of the womb space energies, the energies of *yonisthāna cakra* (pp.141–2), which has a capacity to provide deep intuitive wisdom, and to reconnect us with the earthed and watery energies of creativity, fluidity, nurture and fertility that are characteristic of this energy centre. The *cakra* is not an anatomical feature. Historically, *cakras* have never been directly linked to particular aspects of biology: they are part of the energy body. For the purposes of mental focus during practice, however, it may be helpful to associate *yonisthāna cakra* with the physical organ of the womb, but even so, the qualities of experience it generates continue to be powerfully present in the absence of the womb herself.

As the locus of many women's significant life experiences, the womb and her energies can have a powerful presence in the female psyche. But whilst an awareness of womb life is, in the context of *yoni śakti*, the source of unfolding of cyclic wisdom and power, it is limiting to believe that women are simply 'womb carriers'. A central tenet of the women's liberation movement in the 1960s and '70s was to defy the oppression that occurred if a woman's biology was the only thing that determined her destiny. It is important for our sense of wholeness to see that our womb life is part of a whole world of experience that extends beyond our relationship with our womb, but it is not anti-feminist to admit that much of a woman's energy can be devoted to evolving her own understanding of womb life. Whether it be the practical challenges of menstruation, the emotional upheavals of menstrual cycles, concerns about conception or contraception, or anxieties about womb health in later life, including the presence of growths and fibroids, the effects of gravity and hormonal shifts, or issues about the value and function of her womb after menopause and beyond, the life of her womb often powerfully engages a woman's attention. That is why I have named this woman-centred yoga practice after the womb herself.

There are poetic, philosophical and political reasons for choosing to call this approach *womb* yoga. At a poetic level, the word *womb* has potently symbolic resonance as a place of nurture, safety and creativity. It is the place within the body where new life is nourished and protected. The womb is also a place within our embodied (or imagined) understanding of menstrual cycles that connects a woman's body to powerful cosmic rhythms and forces of elemental power. In the same way as the phases of the moon above exert gravitational forces strong enough to create tides in the great oceans, so too do the tides and flows of the body respond to the rhythmic cycles of the 'moon within'. With this understanding of the womb as an interface between individual and cosmic patterns, like the phases of the moon, then any yoga that seeks to support a growing awareness of our place in the order of the universe needs to attend to the rhythmic dances of the womb cycles. In the context of yoga and *tantra*, the word womb is pregnant with the metaphorical and spiritual meanings of the *hiraṇya garbha* – the golden cosmic egg or cosmic mother's womb, a metaphor for the endlessly fertile and creative cosmic mind that contains the whole universe. This Golden Womb is a manifestation of *śakti*, the feminine energy of creation in *tantra* and in yoga.

So for all these reasons, and at all these levels, *womb* yoga intends to heighten awareness and respect for this experience of the abundant creativity and fertility of *Śakti*, manifesting as the great Golden Womb, within whose nurturing boundaries all our needs are met, just like the child within the mother's womb. And for women, this has a double resonance, because even as we are all held within the Golden Cosmic Womb, so is the individual womb held within the woman herself.

OLD ROOTS

Ultimately, though, this approach to yoga is not really anything new. It is simply one amongst many means to reconnect to our innate wisdom, the knowledge that we hold within us and need only to attend to in order to realise that it has always been there. I have called this kind of knowing *blood wisdom* because of its resonance with the blood tides that flow at menstruation and in childbirth, and because it evokes a powerful primal and ancient sense of already having this wisdom embodied within us.

The spiritual and philosophical framework of *Yoni Śakti* is, appropriately enough for a work that is encouraging us to reconnect with our own ancient ways of knowing, many thousands of years old. The philosophy and practice of *śākta tantra* provides a detailed understanding of the living presence of the power of *Śakti*, the feminine energy of the creative life force, pulsing within each one of us. The full aim and intention of *śākta tantra* is the awakening of awareness to recognise and honour this living presence of the goddess as an everyday reality. Once this awareness is awakened, and with continued practice, the shift in consciousness which it makes possible is so powerful that it can literally change one's whole view of life, and can certainly support a newly confident and assured capacity to value the voice of the inner teacher and the blood wisdom within.

The practices of womb yoga are informed by this awareness, and to do these practices is to enter into consciousness that honours the power of *śakti* within us. In particular, womb yoga is nourished by the experiences of *śakti* consciousness expressed in the Sanskrit poem *Saundarya-Laharī*, which is discussed in chapters five and seven.

WOMB ECOLOGY AND THE SPIRITUAL DIMENSIONS OF FEMININITY

The experience of freedom through *yoni śakti* is rooted in an acknowledgement that those specifically female experiences that centre on or around the womb, such as menstruation, orgasm, childbirth and menopause, can be encountered consciously as potential doorways to spiritual power and heightened intuitive awareness.

This book provides both the philosophical context (in parts one and two) and specific practical yoga guidance (in part three) to enhance the spiritual experience of the great female *siddhis* (yogic powers) of menstruation, feminine sexuality, fertility, birth, postnatal recovery and menopause. The yoga practice is inclusive, holistic and comprehensive. It includes *āsana* (postures), *prāṇāyāma* (breathwork), *mudrā* (gesture), *bandha* (energy locks and seals), *yantra* (visual embodiment of energetic fields), *mantra* (sound), *pratyāhāra* (sense withdrawal), *dhāraṇā* (concentration), *dhyāna* (meditation) and *samādhi* (ecstatic trance). Womb yoga brings together all these forms of yoga in a creative and delicious synthesis of sound, breath, flowing movement and stillness that respects *śakti* (energy) as she flows within each of us, every day, whatever we are doing and wherever we find ourselves. It also includes simple rituals to reawaken consciousness to the deeper significance of life stages and female *siddhis*.

When we practise yoga that fully expresses our consciousness as women, and gives us freedom to feel the powerful forces of our feminine energy, or *yoni śakti*, then the whole world changes for the good. From the personal experience of physical and emotional benefits which lead to enhanced energy and creative thinking, comes an immensely positive influence on all areas of human life, from work to family, from intimate relationships to frameworks of national organisations and government. The healing effect of womb yoga leads from a personal rediscovery of a woman's blood wisdom to an evolved consciousness of union, to a healing global yoga experience that transforms the consciousness of all humans on the planet. It is the thread of reconnection that leads to freedom.

The practice of womb yoga guides us to rediscover a respectful connection with the inner wisdom of our womb cycles. It is an inner ecology of the womb, explored more fully in chapter twenty-seven. When this blood wisdom informs our life and work then we can honour the cyclical nature not only of a woman's life, but also of all life on earth. From the wisdom born of womb ecology follows a naturally arising global green consciousness rooted in a sustainable and respectful honouring of the natural cycles and energies of the earth, the womb that nurtures all life in our world. So it is through blood wisdom, this spiritual awareness that is literally encoded in the cycles of the female body, that we can access the deep healing that our planet, our earthly womb, urgently calls for now. We are in deep need of such yoga.

YOGINĪS AS AGENTS FOR GLOBAL JUSTICE

The free flowing *śakti* and woman-positive attitudes of *yoginīs* are potent antidotes to the poisonous misogyny of patriarchy. Eco-feminist understandings of ecological disaster and global inequality offer holistic perspectives that are entirely congruent with the teachings of yoga and *śākta tantra*. We can see from this viewpoint that the exploitation of women is part and parcel of unsustainable abuse of the earth's resources. Thousands of years of denigration, oppression and confinement of women's power has created a range of exploitative methods of control and disempowerment that are global, varied and effective. A key casualty of the patriarchal project has been female spiritual power and women's spiritual freedom; for the continued economic and political inequalities of power manifest also as an almost total eradication of any respectful honouring of women's access to our own spiritual authority.

Sadly, the yoga world is not exempt from oppressive misogyny. Many approaches to yoga teaching do not respectfully honour women's spiritual autonomy. In fact, the global yoga community is rife with inequalities of power that compromise women's freedom. This, I believe, is a deep structural problem. For many of the institutions that preserve and promote yoga teachings are modelled on patriarchal lines. They are hierarchical, commercial and often very secretive and controlling of power. These schools and centres are rarely good examples of how yoga can function as a positive force for social justice. Within such structures, women are often manipulated, disempowered and abused by those who wield authority. The nature of these structures encourages the abuse of power, and it is often women, especially (but not exclusively) younger women, who suffer this abuse most consistently and acutely in the form of sexual harassment by manipulative and exploitative male teachers. How can *yoginīs* fulfil our potential as agents for social justice when we, and the teachings we may share, 'belong' (or are seen to belong) to such organisations?

The good news is that these stories of manipulative abuse are now coming out into the open. Even better, as more *yoginīs* become aware of the anti-feminist and ultimately anti-spiritual activities of those in power within these organisations, then we can choose to leave these structures. We can choose not to give them further financial support. They will crumble, and the essential nature of yoga practice will be free to flourish, one woman at a time. This is a powerful route to profound change.

Because yoga lays such emphasis upon personal experience, it values shifts in individual consciousness as the starting points for global and cosmic change. This means that individual women's yoga practice can be an immensely effective way to rekindle global interest in the wisdom of a feminine experience of spirituality. Individual encounters with this wisdom through the practice of yoga point a way for everyone to live in freedom. Womb yoga and womb ecology are very effective tools for raising consciousness of the value of intuitive female wisdom and the earth-honouring spirituality which follows as a result. They offer positive practical responses both to the current ecological crisis and to the continuing disrespect and exploitation of women worldwide. Projects that are manifesting this work all over the world today are discussed in chapter twenty-seven. The lived, embodied experience of practices that awaken our trust in the inner guide and reawaken our sense of connectedness with the universe which we inhabit is pure yoga, and it has the potential to heal the world, one womb at a time, one menstrual cycle at a time, one birth at a time, one menopause at a time, one woman at a time. Each act of healing increases the collective *yoni śakti*, until we are all free.

HOW TO USE THIS BOOK

Yoni Śakti offers an integrated and holistic picture of the philosophy and practice of womb yoga and *śākta tantra* as a spiritual path that empowers women to live in freedom. Some of the practices are developments and combinations of yoga techniques that you may not have encountered before, and some are more familiar, and widely taught.

Yoni Śakti presents history and philosophy alongside practice and case studies, and is punctuated with fairy stories that communicate at another level of understanding. By intertwining a number of different 'voices', the book leads towards a synthesis of the many different ways of knowing; the intention of calling on all these different types of knowledge is to invite a complete encounter with many aspects of *yoni śakti*. The freedom which it describes affects all dimensions of our being: the intellect and the emotions, as much as the spiritual imagination and the body.

The first part, 'Foundations', includes the historical, philosophical and practical roots of *yoni śakti* and womb yoga. Chapter one opens with an overview of women doing yoga now, and tells the stories of how western women came to be initiated into lineages and schools of *haṭha* yoga from which they had once been excluded, and what benefits and limitations surround the experiences of women practising yoga in the contemporary yoga world. Chapter two covers the early historical development of yoga, including the presence of women teachers as *tāntrik gurus* and devotional mystics in the time before and during the growth of *haṭha* yoga. This is followed by a radical proposal to consider the female *siddhis* as an intuited and inspirational motivation for the genesis of *haṭha* yoga.

Chapters four to seven combine philosophy and yoga practice. They set out the most unusual and specifically womb-focusing yoga techniques, which are described in detail. These practices are gathered into three groups: 'Awakening to the feminine energy of the life force' (chapter four); 'Greeting the womb with love' (chapter five); and 'Honouring the feminine energy of the life force' (chapter six). These 'womb greetings' and 'honourings' combine movement, breath, sound and stillness with meditative gestures and attitudes, and they are the foundations of womb yoga. They promote a form of awareness that most directly enables you to connect with the presence of the womb or womb energies as an inner guide. These practices are especially useful to do at the start of any yoga session, since they use all means at your disposal to direct the focus of your mental attention to the womb: engaging the physical body, the state of mind and heart, the rhythm of breath, the direction of gaze and the voice. After the instructions for the 'greetings' and 'honourings' (chapters three to six), chapter seven ('Embodied spirit') shares two sequences that give an embodied experience of the philosophical structure of the whole *Yoni Śakti* project. The intention with these sequences is to use the totality of the yoga experience as a way to encounter, at deep levels, the elemental connections and metaphysical understandings of *śākta tantra* as manifesting in your own blood wisdom.

The second part, 'Life Cycles and the Wisdom Goddesses', presents a sustained examination of *yoni śakti* as she unfolds in a woman's life, and the practical use of womb yoga at every stage of a woman's life cycles, beginning in chapter eight with an investigation of how all these cycles overlap and interconnect. Each chapter in this part of the book, from chapter eight through to chapter seventeen, links female life stages and experiences to particular aspects of the Goddess in the forms of the ten great wisdom goddesses.

The third part, 'Further practices of Womb Yoga', includes a complete set of *yoga nidrā* practices specially developed to link to each stage of a woman's life (chapter eighteen). Chapters nineteen to twenty-six are practical instructions for yoga breaths, awareness, locks and energy seals, individual postures and flowing series of linked movements. Each of these chapters groups together a family of practices and the last chapter in this part presents suggested sequences for programmes and classes.

The final part, 'Expansions', offers explorations of womb ecology and the wider application of *yoni śakti* consciousness as an element of global and grassroots transition (chapter twenty-seven), and as the energising force that is generated and sustained by groups of women meeting together in *śakti* circles (chapter twenty-eight). These chapters are followed by a gathering of inspirational resources that support the manifesting consciousness of your own blood wisdom to live everyday life in a state of freedom.

If you prefer, you may use the book as a reference, to learn more about the particular practices or philosophical ideas which most appeal to you. Part two will be the most valuable resource if you wish to direct your attention to a particular time of life, or to discover those yoga practices which may be most appropriate during that time, since it is in these chapters that the cycles of women's lives are set out with most attention, from menarche to post-menopause, along with recommended practices for many experiences. These chapters offer a clear-sighted glimpse of the cycles of a woman's life from the perspective of a *yoginī*. It is not within the scope of this book to provide complete detailed anatomical or medical information, nor to outline in all their complexity the political and cultural influences that shape women's experience, and for this reason each of the chapters concludes with a set of recommended readings and pointers for further research.

Detailed instructions for all the practices not already described in chapters three to seven are set out in part two. The instructions pay particular attention to the internal awareness with each technique, in order to enable you to more fully understand how these, and countless other yoga practices not included within the scope of this book, may be used to create your own womb-conscious yoga practice.

The index of therapeutic applications at the end of the book (pp.657–61) also makes it possible for you to identify which practices may be of benefit as you encounter health challenges or life experiences that lead you to feel in need of yogic support. The second index, which lists individual practices, can guide you to the instructions for a particular technique (pp.662–4).

The colour *yantras* (geometric embodiments) of the wisdom goddesses (*Mahāvidyās*) in the appendix are for visual meditation (*tratak*); details of how to use them are on p.644.

However you decide to make use of this book, it is my hope that the material I present will be of service to each *yoginī* and *yogi* who encounters it. I trust that the experience of deep connection with the blood wisdom which this book endeavours to awaken will enable you to nurture with confident assurance the unique flowering of your own *yoni śakti*, the seed of which lies now within your consciousness.

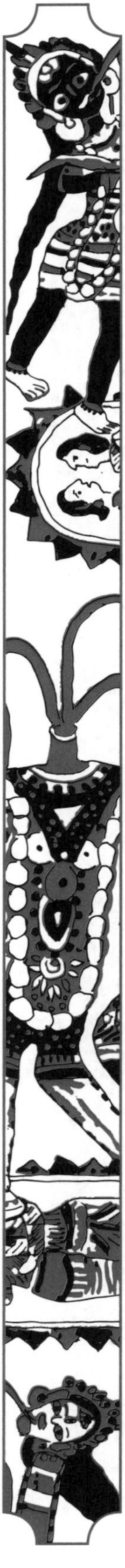

WHAT IS A *YOGINĪ*?

NOTES ON TERMINOLOGY

In contemporary yoga studios across the world, the Sanskrit term *yogin* is mostly used to mean women who are practising yoga. This is, at one level, what the word literally means, since it is the feminine form of th term *yogi*: a man who practices yoga.

But although technically speaking *yoginī* can literally refer to huma females who do yoga, the word *yoginī* carries quite a powerful charge of other meanings. In South Asian Hindu and Buddhist contexts, *yogin* are also ferocious and terrifying goddesses with astonishing and alarmi supernatural powers. In this sense, a *yoginī* is a demonic entity who ma steal babies, demand blood sacrifices, suck a man dry of his semen in t night, and then fly through the air to consort with her sisters and condu magical rituals on dark nights in secret temples. A sub-set of *yoginīs* is also associated with the spread of diseases such as smallpox and typhu and held responsible for miscarriages and stillbirths. As a group, these *yoginīs* inspire a combination of awed devotion and terror: they may bestow great powers upon those who worship them, but such worship may be performed out of fear that the unappeased *yoginīs* might use th powers to cause suffering or death.

In this context, human *yoginīs* are not simply female yoga practitio ers. They are seen to be women who, by virtue of their closeness to the *yoginī* goddesses and demonesses, may command superhuman powers *siddhis*. Because these powers are greatly feared, the human *yoginīs* ar both revered and reviled: they are women who may be in a position to use the supernatural powers gifted to them by the divine *yoginīs*, to pr vide assistance or protection, but they are also likely to be the scapego for inexplicable sufferings and diseases. A *yoginī*, human or divine, ca be a powerful protectress, but it is also wise to protect oneself from her

These dimensions of meaning to the word *yoginī* may not be immediately apparent to the millions of women doing yoga now, but it is important to be aware of their resonance. There are still *yoginī* temples standing in India, including two in Madhya Pradesh and two in Orissa. In these temples the *yoginī* images are placed in the walls of the templ forming a circle of power. These circular formations are also used in th practice of *tāntrik* rituals to invoke and embody the power of the *yogin* The *yoginīs*, like the groups of mother goddesses who are mostly worshipped as a collective, command even more power when they are assembled together than they had alone. The gathering of the *yoginīs* enhances their yogic *siddhis*.

The circular *yoginī* temples that were built in the tenth and eleventh centuries are noble ruins, testimony to a previously vibrant practice of worship. But even in their ruinous state, the circles of *yoginīs* in these medieval Indian temples remain the focus of great devotion, and there are certainly many other sites in India and Nepal where the powers of the *yoginīs* are celebrated and worshipped. In this sense the word *yoginī* still carries immense power that extends far beyond its literal meaning of a female yoga practitioner.

In *Yoni Śakti* I have chosen to use the word *yoginī* to describe all women who do yoga now. My choice is informed both by awareness of the fearsome powers attributed to the ancient *yoginīs*, human and divine, and by a desire to acknowledge that contemporary women are greatly empowered by the practice of yoga. It is a term we can use with pride, for it carries a powerful history that testifies to the immensely transformative power of yoga. When we call ourselves *yoginīs* we acknowledge that our practice of yoga brings us into direct connection with the capacity to heal and transform ourselves in ways that are every bit as magical as the supernatural night flights of the ancient *yoginīs*. The power of that magic rests in our own personal engagement with the practice of yoga, but it is amplified and extended by the collective presence of the other *yoginīs*: like the ancient *yoginīs*, contemporary women yoga practitioners find power in numbers: the circles of *yoginīs* are gathering today in yoga studios everywhere. The resurgence of *yoginī* power is a global phenomenon.

Yoginī śaktiki jai!

STRONG LANGUAGE: A CAUTIONARY NOTE ON TONE AND TERMINOLOGY

Yoni Śakti = Cunt Power.

The worst name anyone can be called is cunt. (Greer 1970: 39)

"Cunt" is related to words from India, China, Ireland, Rome and Egypt. Such words were either titles of respect for women, priestesses and witches, or derivatives of the names of various goddesses... Negative reactions to "cunt" resonate from a learned fear of ancient yet contemporary, inherent yet lost, reviled yet redemptive cuntpower. (Muscio 2002: 5–7)

I, personally, have a cunt... Cunt is a proper, old, historic, strong word. I like that my fire escape also doubles up as the most potent swearword in the English language. Yeah. That's how powerful it is, guys. If I tell you what

I've got down there, old ladies and clerics might faint. I like how shocked people are when you say "cunt". It's like I have a nuclear bomb in my pants, or a mad tiger, or a gun. (Moran 2011: 62)

The practice of yoga is a commitment to becoming fully established in the state of freedom. This is a book about women's spiritual freedom and empowerment in relation to the practice of yoga and *tantra*. It is both practical and philosophical. It contains technical instructions as well as fairy stories and poetry, and it brings together a wide range of different sources, from scholarly studies to sex manuals, from Sanskrit poetry to radical feminist menstrual rituals. Its intention is to share effective yoga teachings and resources to support the expansion and liberation of cunt power.

The yoga practices in this book are all informed by a particular aspect of *tantra*. *Tantra* is, to cut a very long story short, a set of practical and philosophical teachings that lead to the liberation of power (if you're interested to know more, there's a more detailed history in chapter six). *Śākta tantra* is, in brief, a Goddess-focused approach to *tantra*. It is this aspect of *tantra* that is presented together with the yoga throughout *Yoni Śakti*. Yoga and *tantra* are intimately linked, and all of the yoga presented in this book is rooted in, and expressive of *śākta tantra* philosophy.

I wrote *Yoni Śakti* because I knew the transformative power of yoga and *tantra* and sensed that the liberating potential of this powerful combination for women was truly radical. As a thinking woman who has been practising and teaching *tāntrik* yoga nearly all my life, I wanted to read about yoga and *tantra* and women, freedom and power, about yoga and sex and health and female spirituality. I was looking for a book that brought living yoga, *śākta tantra* and vibrant feminism together. I wanted to read about the sexual politics of yoga from the perspective that sees spiritual transformation as the most potent revolutionary force. I was searching for a book that considered how woman-centred yogic practice empowers women to encounter with remarkable awareness those experiences that define us as women: for example our expressions of creativity, sexuality and nurture, or our encounters with the powers of menstruation, birth, and motherhood. I was hunting for a book that explored yoga *tantra* in its absolutely broadest sense: historically and spiritually, and in terms that carried meaning into my everyday life as a mother, as a woman, as a wife, as a writer, and as a *yoginī*.

I began searching for this book in 1985, as a young woman encountering powerful transformative experiences through yoga and meditation. But however long I looked, I could find nothing substantial about the profoundly feminist potential of yoga as a transformational force to liberate women today, and I speak here of liberation in the deep sense of absolute freedom from suffering. I couldn't find the book I needed, so in the end I had to write it myself.

Motivated by the experiences of my own encounters of *yoni śakti* as a mother, as a wife, as a writer, and as a facilitator whose professional life brings me daily in contact with circles of women whose lives have been transformed and uplifted by the practice of yoga, I started reading around to find books that helped me make sense of what I knew. I found myself at sea on a great ocean of writings, and not one single text encompassed all that I wanted to see connected up in one place. None of the books about cunt power were included in the bibliographies of the women's yoga manuals. I thought it would be such a great resource to have the cunt power manifestos and the *yoginī śakti* stuff all in once place, so I felt certain that someone somewhere must have already written *Yoni Śakti*. My search for this book that I needed to read drew me down into fascinating whirlpools of scholarly research on the history of *tantra*, and carried me out on tides of inspiring spiritual autobiographies by contemporary *tāntrikas*, or practitioners of *tantra*, all over the world. My search carried me up into the great wild waves of contemporary writing on female sexual experience, conscious conception and primal mothering. Whilst I was out there at sea, I read writers currently surfing on the rising waves of menstrual and menopausal consciousness, not to mention all the available mainstream books on yoga and yoga therapy for women.

And throughout all this, I was listening to the stories that women on yoga retreats and training courses were telling me; hearing the ecstatic hymns of the ancient *tāntrik gurus*; and having the privilege to practise yoga with teachers like Swamis Satyananda and Satyasangananda Saraswati, who embody the living lineage of *tāntrik* yoga that thrives still in India. I hung out with the Italian menstrual enlightenment mothers in a Tibetan Buddhist retreat above Lake Garda, sang the names of the Divine Mother in the moonlight on the hills around Glastonbury Tor, and over the years sat in literally hundreds of circles of *yoginīs*, watching as women from over twenty-five different countries encountered the healing and transformative powers of yoga *tantra* that celebrates *yoni śakti*. It's been quite a trip.

I finally got washed up on the shore of my own growing awareness that the book I wanted to read had not been written. When I realised that there was nothing out there that could explain how all of this joined up, then I knew what the problem was. I was never going to find the book I wanted to read, because none of the people whose work I had encountered were talking to each other. The problem was not that the information was not available, but that it was so scattered across such an enormous deep ocean that very few people would ever get to sail out there on the high seas and bring it all together. None of the menstrual enlightenment mothers I knew were interested in those whirlpools of *tāntrik* scholarship (and even if they were, they had no time to read four hundred pages of tiny type). Even though the radical feminist cunt-lovers might be totally fascinated to discover a medieval Tamil *tāntrika*'s poetic guide to spiritual dimensions of cunnilingus (it comes in four parts, if you're interested: White 2003 (2006): 74–5), they would probably have no desire to plough through sixty pages of footnotes to locate the translation. I saw quite clearly that many women were practising yoga just because it made them feel good. They might love to read a little more about the history of the ancient *yoginīs*, but very few of them would see the point of sieving through a thirty-page bibliography to pick out what was truly relevant. It was with a sinking heart that I realised this was my job: the book that I had been searching for didn't exist. I would have to write it myself.

And so I came home, dried out, and started to write *Yoni Śakti* as a set of traveller's tales, a sharing from the treasure trove of resources and information that I have encountered in theory and practice over the past twenty years. During this process, I made some helpful discoveries. The most significant discovery was that if I wanted to read about *yoni śakti* from every possible dimension, and in relation to all stages of my life as a woman, then I would need to integrate my own experiences and the experiences of students, teachers and friends, with some of the astonishing histories and theories around women and yoga. It was my task to join up all the dots. Then I realised what a huge challenge it would be to find the right language to express all of these connections clearly and in relation to women's unfolding life cycles. So much of what we experience as women is never spoken of openly. To write a book about all the dimensions of yoga for women demands absolute clarity of expression. I discovered that I needed to think very hard about the language of such a book, in particular the words we use to describe women's bodies in light of all the different dimensions of being that these many different perspectives would create.

And so I've used four languages to write *Yoni Śakti*: there are several forms of English, which are so different in register that they can be thought of as separate languages. The first form of English you can read in this book may be described as 'coarse'. It is helpful when we need to be earthy and grounded, and to distinguish our cunts from our clits. The second form of English is a formal academic register (including simplified footnotes and references): this is useful in tracking arguments and histories. The last form of English is the poetic voice of the fairy stories and the practice instructions that use elemental metaphors from the natural world and a broadly *tāntrik* framework to describe bodily experiences as a microcosm.

The fourth language of the book is Sanskrit, of which there is minimal but sustained usage. For instance, some of the practice instructions use Sanskrit terms such as *prāṇa* (life force) and *cakra* (wheel/circle, and/or energy centre in the pranic body) because these technical terms have become quite widely understood, feel good on the tongue and are cumbersome to translate. *Yoni Śakti* has a Sanskrit title partly because the original language of yoga and *tantra* is Sanskrit, and partly because the English translation gets mixed reactions. When I was writing this book and people enquired what the Sanskrit title meant, I told them that *Yoni Śakti* meant 'Cunt Power'. This usually made people choke. If people didn't choke on 'Cunt Power' then the words would sometimes raise laughter, or eyebrows, or both.

And if 'Cunt Power' didn't raise eyebrows and laughs, it certainly raised hackles. Some of the women who laughed were laughing because they were so pleased and amazed to hear the word 'cunt' right next door to the word 'power': an unusual proximity. Feminists find it refreshing but others may find it alarming. Even Germaine Greer admits that 'cunt' is the only word in the English language that still has the power to shock. Sometimes the laughter was more of a horrified giggle that signalled deep embarrassment, like the friend with whom I watched a performance of the *Vagina Monologues*. When we were invited to shout 'CUNT' out loud along with four hundred other supportive and delighted women in the theatre, my companion squirmed in her seat whispering desperately, 'Oh no. Oh no. Oh no. There is absolutely no way she is going to get me to say that word in public.' She was mortified and resolutely speechless. Her lips remained closed as everyone else yelled out in glee at the top of their voices 'CUUUUUUNT!'

But to speak freely from a feminist perspective about the spiritual empowerment of women through the practice of yoga, we need to be able to be clear. And the language we use to describe our bodies and ourselves and what we do with them is really not very clear for women. 'Cunt power' is about as clear as it gets. And this is what *Yoni Śakti* means. Women are powerful. Yoga practice raises our awareness of the nature of that power: it reconnects us, and that reconnection enables us to live in freedom, confident of our own potency.

I have been intrigued by the fact that *Yoni Śakti* made people nod and smile but 'Cunt Power' made them choke. And so I feel obliged to offer this prefatory warning to readers who may not feel inclined to read any further. I do sometimes use the word 'cunt' in this book, along with many other words to describe female bodies and what they do, such as vulva, vagina, breasts, clitoris, blood and juice. This is a book about yoga, and not about anatomy, but since what we do in yoga can involve our physical bodies, and since the physical bodies about which I am writing are female, then there are only so many words to choose from. Many of these words are medical terms, and most of the others are not very complimentary. When mothers tell their little daughters what to call their genitalia, there are so few positive and acceptable terms available that some girls grow up believing they have a 'front bottom'. Really. This happens. Even now. At best, the term merely confuses the child, but at worst it is a shockingly denigrating disempowerment. A girl with a 'front bottom' either has a vulva that shits, or else, perhaps, in her body consciousness, she simply has no vulva, or no word for it, which amounts to the same thing. Instead, she has two arseholes, front and back. But then, what else would a nice girl call her cunt?

And this is the point. Language gives us power. To have no language to use about our bodies is to lose touch with ourselves. To be out of touch with ourselves is to be disempowered. For however passionately I may wish to convince you that the word 'cunt' is a fine term with an illustrious history and fascinating etymology, the fact that you have probably only ever heard it used as the nastiest kind of insult does make it hard to be enthusiastically cunt-positive. The fact that a term that so many people hold to be the most offensive word in the English language describes the most precious, beautiful, pleasure- and life-giving part of a woman's anatomy tells us a lot about the esteem in which women's bodies are held. And if our bodies are held in such contempt then there is not much hope for our spiritual empowerment.

Certainly there have been feminist defences of the c-word, and Inga Muscio, through her book *Cunt: a Declaration of Independence*, has relaunched a contagiously high-spirited movement to reclaim the word as a positive term. But right now, at least in the world of yoga, we are not really quite there yet. Let's be honest, yoga teachers mostly prefer pseudo-medical euphemisms. They call an arse 'your buttocks'. They talk about the 'anal sphincter region' instead of an arsehole. And when was the last time you even heard the word 'womb' in a yoga class, let alone 'vulva'? So to call *Yoni Śakti* 'Cunt Power' is probably several steps too far, at least on the cover. Which is why I've slipped the whole 'cunt power' discussion in here as an early warning to those who might just choke on it.

And what has all this cunt-talk to do with the spiritual empowerment of women through yoga? It's at the very heart of it. Yoga has an immensely healing and transformative potential to enable women of all ages to live in a state of freedom. *Haṭha* yoga works at many levels, and to do it we use the movement of body, breath and mind to shift energy and awareness. Initially at least, the mind needs the guidance of words. So the language we use to talk about who we are and how we experience yoga is important. Because if we don't have words that we are happy to use to describe our bodies, then we can't consciously bring energy to those places in ourselves, and if we can't do that then we cannot practise yoga with any awareness.

'Consciousness is made of language and we have no language for this: cock and balls have a thousand names, but uterus and ovaries have only their medical labels.' (Greer 1999: 48). We do have a few options to describe our *yonis*, as I have described, but even in yoga practices where we need to be clear about their effects on our womb, for example perineal locks or inversions during menstruation, then these organs are rarely named. It is as if they don't exist. Clear and precise verbal instruction is a prerequisite for the transmission of yoga teachings at most levels.

This is why I am making such a big deal at the start about the words I use in this book. Because I wanted to read / write a book that affirmed and empowered women's experience of yoga as a route to real freedom, I researched the historical texts of *haṭha* yoga to find positive and authentically yogic ways to describe *yoginī*s' experiences. When I discovered just how few women there are in the history of classical *haṭha* yoga, I widened my search to include earlier yogic ancestors such as the *Vedas* [earliest Indian sacred texts] and the *Tantras* [teachings on liberation], and practices contemporary with, but marginal to *haṭha* yoga, such as *śākta tantra* [goddess worship] and *bhakti* yoga [the yoga of devotion], both of which hold the spirituality and freedom of women in higher regard than the texts of the *haṭha yogīs* do. Whilst it was in the texts of *haṭha* yoga that I first encountered the term *siddhi* [magical power] which I use in this book to describe the liberatory potential of the female *siddhis*, for example of menstruation and birth, it was in the other sources that I found most of the language for *Yoni Śakti*.

Śākta tantra offered reverent terms for the vulva and the womb as cosmic gateways: the '*yoni*' or '*yonisthāna*' [place of the womb]; it also included vivid honourings of menstruation as '*yoni puṣpam*' [cunt flowers] and sexual secretions as '*yoni nāḍī*' [cunt juices]. In *śākta tantra,* I found the appreciative (sometimes overawed) descriptions of the fabulous powers of the circles [*cakras*] of *yoginīs* and *ḍākinīs,* embodiments of the potent *yoni śakti* that I have taken as the title for the book. The tradition of *śākta tantra* also offered the set of ten goddesses known as the *Mahāvidyās* [great cosmic wisdom goddesses], whose presence shapes part two.

The very term *tantra* itself can be literally translated as a 'loom', and is understood metaphorically as a set of teachings that liberates and extends the limits of consciousness. This meaning comes from the the Sanskrit words that form *tan-tra*: *tanoti* means s/he or it 'stretches' or 'extends', and *tra* is an instrumental suffix that indicates 'that which enables something to occur'. So in combination, these two words define *tantra* as 'that which enables expansion'. It is this state of *expanded awareness* that makes it possible to live life with authentic freedom and openness.

To write clearly about women's experience in yoga, I needed to create a women's yoga language that describes our bodies in a way that is alive with meaning.

By using Sanskrit terms from *yoga tantra* (e.g. *yoni*, *siddhi*, *yonisthāna*, *yoni puṣpam*, *yoginī cakra*) and by coining a few others in the same reverent spirit (e.g. *yoni-namaskāram* [womb-greeting], and *hṛdaya-yoni nādi* [the heart-womb river]), I developed a range of terms that could be used alongside clear (aka 'coarse') English words that are often avoided or ignored by yoga teachers (like cunt, arse, vulva, arsehole and juice). By weaving together these two languages with the third thread of metaphors from the *tāntrik* vision of the human body as an elemental microcosm, I have created a yogic language that is not just reverent and poetic, it is also precise and clear. Such clarity is empowering. It is helpful.

Haṭha yoga practice requires and promotes an open-minded curiosity and interest in the physical body as the vehicle for spiritual empowerment. It encourages plain-speaking and self-awareness. No daughter whose mother practises *haṭha* yoga and uses this kind of language is going to grow up thinking she has a 'front bottom', because her mother will know the difference between her *aśvinī mudrā*, her *mūla bandha* and her *sahajolī mudrā* and so will be able to explain to her daughter the different functions and relative locations of her bum-hole, her vagina and her pee-hole (if you don't know your *aśvinī* from your *mūla bandha*, see chapter twenty). Having clarified such crucial issues, the mother who has encountered her own physical experience through the spiritual language and practice of yoga may be able to offer her daughter, as she grows, terms of honour and respect for her menstrual blood. Such clarity of language empowers our daughters to live free from the confusion, shame or embarrassment that limited their mothers and grandmothers. This is a practical and inspiring example of yoga practice as a path to freedom for women.

Much of *Yoni Śakti* describes the practical application of yoga for women's health and well-being. In the middle of writing it, I shared some chapters with a group of thirty women on a training course for 'Well Woman' yoga as part of a yoga therapy diploma. These women were powerful *yoginīs* with such a commitment to the use of yoga to promote women's healing that they had signed up, paid up, and turned up for four days of intensive training on the subject.

By the third day we had enjoyed many passionate discussions about the root causes of women's suffering and the power of language to determine how we think about the world, and how that affects our practice and teaching of yoga. The mothers in the room had wept about how the *sādhana* [spiritual endeavour] of mothering was not truly acknowledged because there were simply no words to describe 'what mothers do', and the grandmothers in the room had regretted that for much of their lives, their intuitive wisdom and autonomy had been disregarded and disrespected, and the young women in the room had voiced their confusion and distress that there was no really respectful way to describe what it was to be a spiritually awake, sexy young *yoginī*. We even talked about how the word 'cunt' used to be a positive term related to the name of a goddess or a priestess, or any woman of spiritual power like a whore or a hag or a witch or any of the other terms that have now become insults. It was all pretty heavy stuff. But sharing these burdens had lightened everybody's load, and by the time we came to Saturday evening, these women were beginning to feel that they had some sense of sisterly solidarity and pride cultivated by the listening presence of the *yoginīs* around the room. This is the story of what happened next...

SATURDAY NIGHT ON THE TOWN

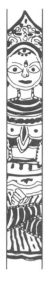

In December in England it gets dark very early, and as dusk began to fall in the afternoon we could hear revellers on the streets of London. I had taught in this studio before and had a number of bad Saturday night experiences, where young men had thrown insults and balls of spittle through the windows of the lower ground floor studio. As the thirty *yoginīs* settled into a powerful and meditative sequence of elemental womb yoga, I sensed that something very odd was about to happen. In my heart I echoed the teaching that had been shared with us the previous day when Mother Maya had come to address us on the subject of natural menstrual rhythms and the global crisis in women's health. Acknowledging that we lived in challenging times, and that many women were facing grave physical and emotional difficulties, Mother Maya had described a yogic tool for transforming of any challenge into a gift.

'When a difficulty arises' she had said, 'simply pause. In your heart hear the words of this *saṁkalpa* [yogic intention]: "This is my greatest gift". That awareness will change everything.'

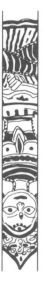

As I heard the drunken voices of the teenage boys who were gathering right outside the window of the studio, I perceived a grave difficulty arising. I was holding the space for thirty women to practise a deep, quiet meditation that resonated tangible female energy and power. And the drunken lads outside were kicking off big style. Just by being there, in the beautiful yoga studio, all women together practising yoga, we were offending these young men. The women in meditation seemed oblivious to the approaching challenge. Because I had no wish to leap up and disturb the group's deepening meditative experience, there was absolutely nothing I could do to prevent what was about to happen. And so I resolved to welcome whatever disturbance was about to occur as our greatest gift.

Just as the women settled deeper into the final phase of the meditation, the group of young men outside the window began to laugh and shove each other up against the glass. Their faces lined up at the open window and the bravest of them stuck his head through the gap and yelled in a very loud voice, 'You CUNTS!' Then he gobbed a fat blob of spit through the window onto the floor. There was a pause. I silently repeated the

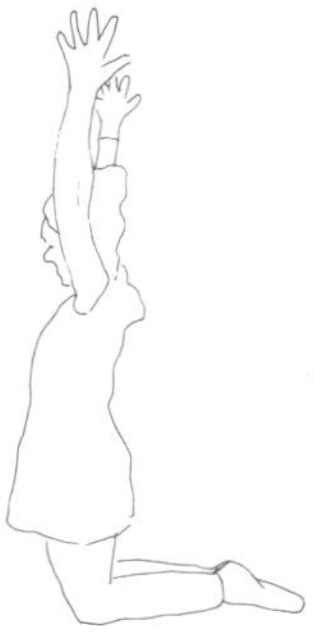

saṁkalpa,
and waited to see
the challenge transform into our
greatest gift.

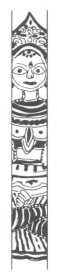

First I spotted a twinkle in the eyes of the woman opposite me in the circle. I watched as she spread out the fingers of her left hand. Then she curled her fingers, clenched her fist and slowly raised it above her head. Everybody else's eyes were shut, but, as if the movement had been choreographed and rehearsed for months, thirty-one fists, including mine, simultaneously clenched. Thirty-one women's arms raised straight up to the sky. As the fists punched the air, with one powerful voice, every woman in the room shouted an affirmative response:

'YESSSSS!'

Thirty-one *yoginīs* with powerful lungs and voice projection shouting together in a low-ceilinged room are very loud indeed. The noise was astounding. The boys at the windows disappeared and we heard them running down the street. They left behind them a palpable aftershock of deep surprise and utter bewilderment.

As swiftly as they had been raised, the *yoginīs'* fists were lowered. The meditation continued peacefully and we ended the session. There were a few smiles as we left, but it was not until the next morning that any of us thought to observe: 'What happened last night, that was a truly remarkable thing'. Having encountered similar disturbances in the same place previously, I had a context for the 'You CUNTS!' 'YESSS!' dialogue that we had experienced. I knew it could only have happened on that evening because our consciousness of the power of the word 'cunt' had been raised by our discussions about language and spiritual empowerment the day before. When similar disturbances had occurred in the past, most of the women had been upset by drunken louts calling us 'cunts' whilst we tried to practise yoga: in the past it had seemed that we had nowhere to put their intrusive words and intentions, and so they hit us where it hurt most and we felt vulnerable, afraid and disrespected. But this time it was different.

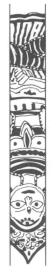

Two things had changed: in the first place this group of *yoginīs* had helped each other to reach a conscious understanding of the uses and abuses of the word 'cunt' itself.

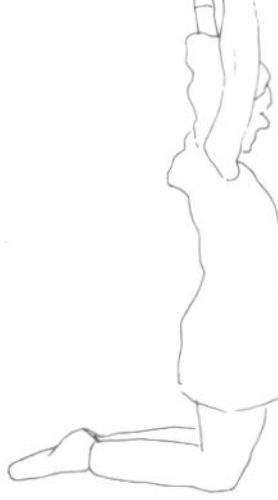

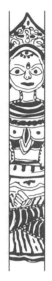

And in the second
place we had been gifted a
powerful teaching that showed us how
to turn something negative into something
positive: 'This is our greatest gift' was the spirit in
which we received what had been intended as an insult.

And so it became a compliment, an honorific title that we accepted with vociferous pride and triumphant air punching, as if we were footballers in a World Cup final celebrating a winning goal. Our collective consciousness had the power to turn the 'insult' into an enquiry as to our status which we were happy to answer: the drunken lad had yelled 'You CUNTS!' but we heard 'You 'CUNTS?' and by answering 'YESSSS!' we confounded our abusers and they ran scared into the night. What happened that evening in the yoga studio was a beautiful and spontaneous manifestation of the possibilities of groups of women literally changing our reality through yogic means. Conscious use of language is a yogic practice of awareness. This is how Inga Muscio, author of *Cunt: A Declaration of Independence*, describes it:

> *Based on the criteria [sic] that "cunt" can be neither co-opted nor spin-doctored into having a negative meaning, venerable history or not,* it's ours to do with what we want. *And thanks to the versatility and user-friendliness of the English language, "cunt" can be used as an all new woman-centred, cuntlovin' noun, adjective or verb. I, personally, am in love with the idea. (Muscio 2002:11)*

What we did that evening was to use conscious awareness to turn an insult into a 'positive force in the language of women'. When the *yoginīs* said 'YESSS!' together, punched the air, and continued with the meditation, then the negative power of 'cunt' simply '...fell in upon itself, and we [were] suddenly equipped with a word that describes all women...' (Muscio 2002: xxvi).

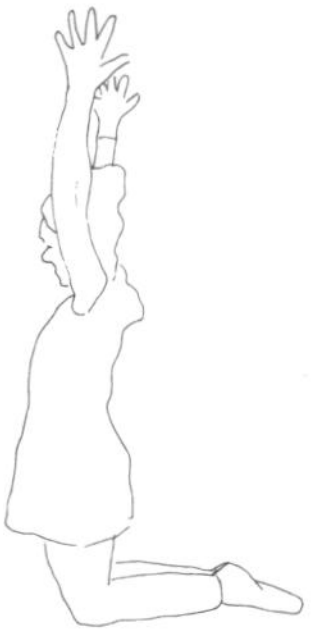

This is not to say that we need always and everywhere to use the
word 'cunt'. That would be silly, and probably inappropriate
in most places. But it is helpful to identify that, when
speaking of ourselves and our genitalia, 'cunt'
can be one viable option. I take this
option sometimes in this book.
Just so you know.

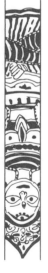

QUESTIONS AND REFLECTIONS

I invite you now to explore your own experience of the effects of the language we use to describe ourselves and our bodies by asking yourself some of the following questions:

1. What feelings do you experience when you hear (or read) the word ‘cunt’?
2. Re-read the ‘Opening practice: invocation to *yoni śakti*’ (pp.17–20), this time, replace the word *yoni* with the word cunt. How does the practice sit with you now? What changes when *yoni* is cunt?
3. Listen to the pair of audio downloads at www.yonishakti.co, ‘Opening practice: invocation to *yoni śakti*’: one uses the word *yoni*, and one uses the word cunt. Which do you prefer? Why?
4. What word/s do you usually use to describe your cunt? Do you use different words in different situations, when talking to different people? Where do those words come from?
5. What words do other people in your life use to describe female genitalia? What words have you ever heard in a yoga session that acknowledge the presence of these parts of ourselves?
6. What word/s would you love to use to describe your cunt? What words would you love to give to your daughters, nieces, goddaughters, granddaughters, or other little girls in your life to describe themselves?

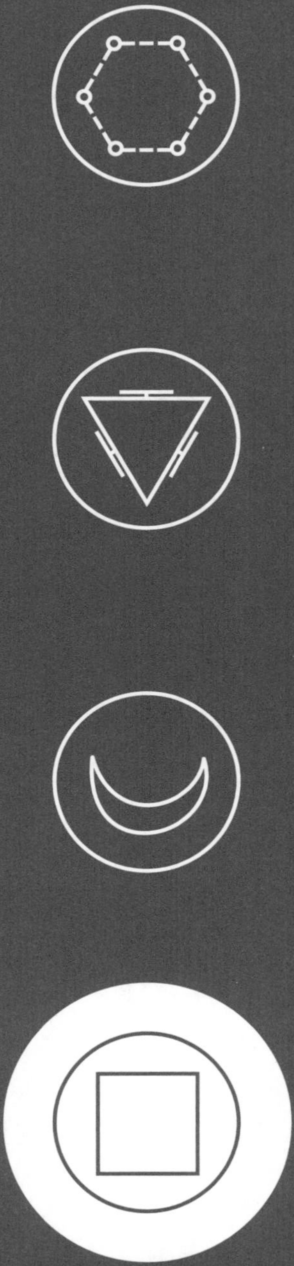

PART ONE
FOUNDATIONS

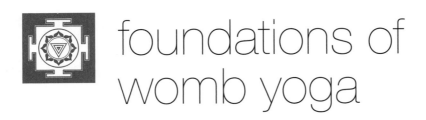

foundations of womb yoga

THIRTEEN GATES

Haṭha yoga is a collection of practices that all work to achieve spiritual connection through the physical body, breath and mind.

All foundational *haṭha* yoga texts were written by men, and until very recently most yogic lineages were preserved and perpetuated only by men (information about women teachers within the *tāntrik* traditions are explored in chapter two).

All the *haṭha* yoga practices in these written texts and preserved through male lineages of transmission were originally designed for a male body with 'nine gates' or orifices: two each of eyes, ears and nostrils, plus one mouth, an anus and penis.

Female bodies have twelve gates: the first eight are the same as in the male body, the ninth is the urethral opening, and the tenth gate is the cunt: a 'cosmic gateway' or *yoni* through which blood, mucus, female ejaculate, the rhythmic release of energy through orgasm, and babies can all move from the womb into the world. Additionally, there are two further gates in the form of a woman's nipples that can open to allow milk flow.

Although the *yoni* as the tenth 'cosmic gateway' is mentioned in a number of yogic and *tāntrik* texts (see chapters two and three for further details and explanation), it is never usually integrated as one of the nine 'gates' of the *haṭha* yoga tradition.

Womb yoga honours with inclusion the cosmic gateway of the cunt as the tenth gate in the 'human city' and the female nipples as the eleventh and twelfth gates. These gates have their own place in the practices of womb yoga.

Womb yoga offers practices that attend to the spiritual significance and potential of the whole of a woman's body and experience at all stages of her life. In particular, these practices honour and amplify the powerful energies of the womb, the entrance to whom is through the tenth gate of the cunt.

In both male and female bodies the final gate through which the soul leaves at death is in the top of the head: in men this is referred to as the tenth gate.

In women the gate at the top of the head is the thirteenth gate.

All the original practices of *haṭha* yoga are intended to bring about altered states of consciousness and heightened awareness of the cosmic powers of those *yogīs* who envisioned their microcosm as a nine-gated city: these heightened and altered states give the *yogi* access to special powers which are described as *siddhis*.

Womb yoga recognises that the twelve-gated nature of a woman's body and the powerful rhythms of her body open up feminine routes to these heightened states of consciousness and awareness, and womb yoga honours these experiences as female *siddhis*: naturally arising feminine experiences such as menstruation, female orgasm, pregnancy, birth, lactation and menopause.

Womb yoga proposes a radical revisioning of the roots of *haṭha* yoga to recognise that the naturally arising altered states of consciousness which women can experience during menstruation, birth and menopause, for example (there are other examples), were possibly both the inspiration and the goal of all *haṭha* yoga practices.

Womb yoga does all this because this is the time that we need to respect and honour feminine consciousness in yoga, in order to reconnect with *yoni śakti* and live life in freedom.

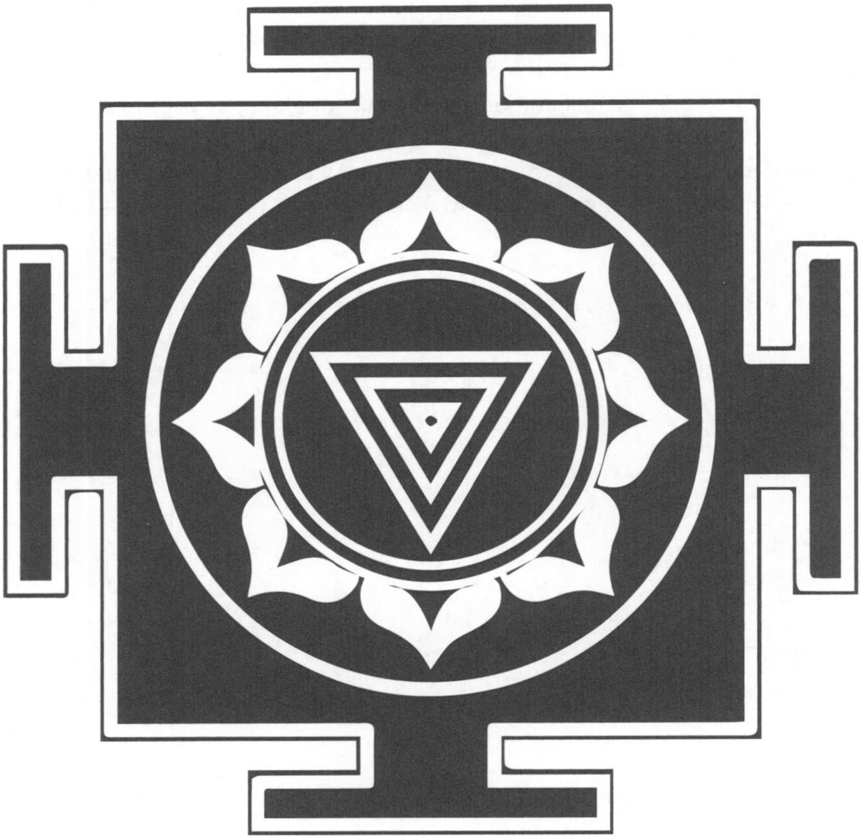

CHAPTER ONE

from exclusion to initiation: men teaching women, women teaching the world

> *. . . [there is] an eternal light, and right out in front, shining ahead of a woman, like a presence which goes a little bit before her and reports back to her what it has found ahead. It is her perpetual reconnaissance. . . . Yet, when one sees and senses thusly, then one has work to do something about what one sees. To possess good intuition, goodly power, causes work. It causes work firstly in the watching and comprehending of negative forces and imbalances both inward and outward. Secondly, it causes striving in the gathering up of will in order to do something about what one sees. (Estés 1993: 108)*

SO MANY WOMEN

Haṭha yoga started out as an activity strictly bounded by the walls of the 'nine-gated' city of the male body. It was developed by men for men, and passed from teacher to pupil as a closely guarded secret. But now yoga is an open secret shared by a huge global community. This community is largely female. The practice and teaching of yoga in the UK, the US and Europe is predominantly a women's activity. Most of the yoga teachers and teacher trainers in this country are women and most of their students are female. An estimated fifteen million people in the US practise yoga, and seventy-two percent of them are women. In the UK the total number of yoga practitioners has been estimated at 2.5 million (Hunt 2010, Singleton 2008) which includes between 300,000 and 450,000 regular students, of whom seventy to seventy-five percent are women (Statistic Brain 2011, Fox 2005).

Approximately twenty to thirty thousand yoga classes are taught each week in the UK (calculations based on combined figures from the British Wheel of Yoga and Fox) many of them in gyms and health clubs, but a sizeable number are held in dedicated yoga spaces. I estimate that there are currently over three hundred such yoga studios in the UK of varying scale, and the majority are run and staffed by women. New yoga studios are opening every month. There is a proliferation of urban and rural 'micro-studios' where a single teacher creates a yoga teaching space in his or her home, workspace or garden to teach small groups and individuals.

There are certainly men involved in some of these studios and the training courses they host, and there are male studio-owners and teachers and teacher trainers too, but they are in a small minority. There are around ten thousand active yoga instructors in the UK, involved in teaching yoga either full-time or part-time, and over three quarters of them are women. From my observations as a trainer of yoga teachers and yoga therapists, I see that for every thirty trainees on any given training course, approximately twenty-eight of them will be female. In certain areas of yoga training, the norm is for courses to be one hundred percent women. For example, over the past eight years across six different European countries I have trained over five hundred yoga teachers and yoga therapists in specialist approaches to yoga for women's health. Only eight of these teachers are men, half of whom are married to pregnancy yoga teachers and the other half of whom are devotees of a female swami (or, more properly, '*svāmī*', which means 'renunciate') who leads an international yoga training organisation based in India. Clearly, training sessions to share yoga for women's health work are bound to attract more women then men, but even so, the gender proportions are striking.

The ratio of six hundred women to eight men in my training courses is extreme, but the situation at this far end of the spectrum reflects the pattern across the whole of yoga now. All forms of access to yoga, from weekly classes in village halls and gyms to international training intensives in huge London yoga studios are largely offered by and for women. The largest yoga organisation in the UK is currently the British Wheel of Yoga, with over eight thousand members, four thousand of whom are teachers. Most of these members are women. At the BWY South West regional yoga festival in 2011, 171 out of 175 attendees were women: this is a typical gender split at BWY events across the country. At the 2010 event, the gender split was similar, except that of the four men present at a gathering of over 150 people, one was a volunteer officer on the BWY organising committee and the other three were male tutors running sessions at the festival, of whom one was offering workshops based on a text of *Vijñāna Bhairava Tantra* translated by Swami Satyasangananda Saraswati, the top female swami in the Satyananda yoga tradition. The male-female ratio within the BWY is possibly more extreme than those of other organisations, but it clearly demonstrates a powerful female presence in UK yoga.

Why are women practising yoga in such numbers? There are so many good reasons that it is hard to know where to start. But, in brief, the simplest answer is because yoga makes you feel good. It is a system of self-care and spiritual development that does just about everything you can think of to optimise physical and mental health: it increases flexibility, strength, balance and immunity; it improves heart function, strengthens bones, and improves co-ordination; it reduces stress, lowers blood pressure, and helps people to lose weight; it also promotes a positive outlook, a happy sex life, a sense of well-being and equanimity. In relation to women's health in particular, yoga has a balancing effect on hormones, which helps to effectively manage menstrual and menopausal difficulties, boosts fertility and supports healthy pregnancy, birth and postnatal recovery. Very many of the health problems that women experience have their roots in stressful living patterns that deeply disconnect women from our natural life cycles, leaving us exhausted, irritated and often ill. The practice of yoga, which can be translated as 'union', literally reconnects women to the source of health and vitality, offering the possibility to enjoy positive physical and emotional health.

This experience is, of course, open to men too, but it is of especial value to women. For the original source of the disconnection which causes so much of women's ill-health in the first place is deeply rooted in our cultural expectations of what it is to be a woman, or even to look like a woman; it is almost as if, in a world where we live by men's values and according to men's expectations, the very fact of being a woman at all is a source of struggle and disease. Female bodies are subject to so many cultural, sartorial and medical controls and 'improvements' that it is almost impossible to open a catalogue, travel on public transport, or watch the TV without being overloaded with images of what women need to do in order to be 'real women'. From adverts for crash diets and make-up, to the phenomenal rise in the numbers of cosmetic surgeries to change the shapes of our vulvas and our breasts, the experience of being female is hedged about on all sides with pressures to change or fix or alter ourselves in some way that our culture teaches us will make us more desirable. To be just plain happy in our own woman's skin is sadly a rather rare experience. Many women spend their whole lives looking for a way to feel 'at one' with who they really are. And then we find ourselves in a yoga class where we are taught to accept where we are, how we are, right now, just as we are, and just to be at one with that. No wonder women like yoga so much.

The fact that yoga improves women's well-being at a truly profound level is the clear and simple explanation for why so many women are doing it; but this explanation does not really get to the bottom of why there are so many *more* women than men in the yoga world. The ratios do vary across different forms of practice, and there are certainly some schools of yoga where there's a more even gender spilt, but as a whole women outnumber men to a very high degree. Many yoga classes are entirely female, not because they are 'women-only' sessions, but just because no men show up. And this state of affairs is remarkable, especially when we consider that all the usual histories of *haṭha* yoga show it to be a male-only practice in origin. This is explored in more detail in the next chapter, but for now it is enough to know that virtually no women at all appear in the original texts of *haṭha* yoga on which contemporary practice rests. They were written by men, and for men.

As I explore in the next chapter, although there are certainly women in the early history and pre-history of yoga, you have to hunt very hard indeed to discover them, or to find any practices designed for female bodies. So how did it happen that this male-only activity is now almost entirely taught and practised by females? There are a few different ways to answer this question. We can look to recent history, and we can explore much further back. As I demonstrate in chapter two, there are some fascinating hidden stories to be revealed about the pre-history of yoga, the part that women may have played in its embryonic development, and the likelihood that there were female teachers in the early growth of yoga and *tantra* before the classical texts were written. But nowhere do we ever find conclusive proof of any of this. This is not to say that these histories did not happen, because maybe they did. But since the stories we hear today were written by and for men, it is more difficult to hear the stories of these early female teachers.

Although some precedents for women as teachers may be found within the *tāntrik* tradition, especially within *śākta tantra* and its precursors, we need to admit that these women were certainly exceptions to the rules that forbade women from practising yoga prior to the modern period. Prohibitions and restrictions on women's involvement with yoga, and upon their access to and knowledge of Sanskrit in which the texts were written, ensured that there was generally very little access for most women to the usual lineages of *haṭha* yoga teaching even up until the very end of the nineteenth century. Although, as I describe in chapter two, there were certainly some remarkably free-spirited *bhakti yoginīs* in the early history of yoga who clearly were practising forms of *haṭha* yoga, these women were extremely unusual in their flouting of orthodox Hindu roles for women. It is only after the beginning of the twentieth century that women in any significant numbers, especially western women, have had access to these teachings. Read on to discover how this access was gained.

WESTERN WOMEN LEARNING YOGA 1890–1960

There were two basic routes through which the teachings of yoga came to be shared with western women. One route was the 'export' route, through which yoga philosophy and practice was brought out of India by Indian teachers and delivered to the West. The other was the 'collection' route, through which women came to India to receive teachings, and then brought them back home with them.

All the Indian teachers involved in both the 'delivery' and 'collection' modes of the transmission of yoga teachings since the late nineteenth century have been men. Swami Vivekananda, a key disciple of Ramakrishna, attended the World's Parliament of Religions in Chicago in 1893, lecturing on *vedānta* (philosophy) and later teaching *prāṇāyāma* (breathing practices), whilst a fellow disciple, Swami Abhedananda, taught *āsana* (yoga postures). Vivekananda's US lecture tours were supported and managed by a largely female network of followers, including Josephine Mcleod [Jaya], and Sarah Bull and Sara Farmer who sponsored Vivekananda in Boston. After meeting Vivekananda in London in 1895, Irish-born Margaret Elizabeth Noble accompanied him on his return to India in 1898, where she became the first western woman to be initiated into the vows of *brahmacārya*, taking the name Bhaginī [Sister] Nivedita [dedicated to god] as part of her identity as a renunciate within the Ramakrishna order of monks. Sister Nivedita travelled with Vivekananda in India, accepted from him the mission of working for women's education in Bengal, and later was an active campaigner in the struggle for Indian independence from the British. Nivedita was a proponent of '*karma* yoga', the yoga of selfless service, and although she did not teach *haṭha* yoga, she studied Indian philosophy, and her *Cradle Tales of Hinduism* and other writings demonstrate her knowledge and love of the myths and stories of ancient India, and the yogic philosophies that developed from them. Her understanding of yogic philosophy was the inspiration for her radical desire to serve the needs of Indian woman both by providing education and health-care, and by working towards Indian independence. Nivedita clearly understood that these philosophical, social and political projects were intimately connected, and she felt that improving the health, status and education of Indian women was crucial to India's independence. The energy and commitment that Sister Nivedita poured into this form of *karma* yoga was so prodigious and so well-received that the epitaph on her tombstone reads: 'She gave her all for India.' The integration of yoga philosophy with social and political activism that guided Nivedita's life and work thrives today in the many women-led yogic projects for education, social support and global healing through environmental responsibility around the world. These projects are explored in chapter twenty-seven.

Sixteen years before Sister Nivedita arrived in India with Vivekananda, the Russian Theosophist Helena Blavatsky established the international headquarters of the Theosophical Society near Madras. Blavatsky had first travelled to India as a spiritual seeker in 1852. She lived there for two years, returning in 1856, and living for several years in Tibet, where she is reputed to have studied Tibetan Buddhism with a variety of teachers. Although she disdained *haṭha* yoga, Blavatsky did much to popularise yogic thought and philosophy in the Victorian era through her books, which sold out in multiple printings, and even more significantly through the founding of the Theosophical Society in 1875. Through its publications, the Society revived nearly moribund interest in Patanjali's *Yoga Sūtra* in India, and certain scholars of yoga history, for example Anne O'Brien and David White, are of the opinion that the Theosophical Society's works may well have influenced even such figures as Vivekananda and Krishnamacharya. As a result of the wider impact of the society which she founded, Helena Blavatsky '...despite her rather well earned reputation as a charlatan, can be regarded as an important pioneer in terms of popularising the idea of yogic wisdom, and fuelling a growing interest in the West for all things Eastern' (O'Brien 2012). Blavatsky's influence on the popularity of yoga in the west is the focus of more detailed analysis in an unpublished master's thesis on the history of western women's influence on the popularity of yoga (O'Brien 2012).

US yoga scholar and *yoginī* Anne O'Brien shared some of her research on the history of women in yoga in the recent documentary, *Yoga Woman* (2011). Additional research commissioned by the film's producers from yoga teacher Eric Shaw offers an interesting perspective on what he identifies as a particularly feminine aspect of yoga practice. In his review of western women in yoga since 1890, Shaw identifies philosophical and political integration as one of the key contributions that women yoga practitioners have made to the development of contemporary yoga as a way of life. He also refers to other early female promoters of yogic philosophy including Annie Besant, who was groomed by Helena Blavatsky for the task of finding and supporting the young Jiddu Krishnamurti as the 'World Teacher', and Theosophist Katherine Tingley, who led the Theosophy movement in America and established the Rājā Yoga School in Point Loma, California. These women, although not directly involved in the teaching of *haṭha* yoga, were influential in raising awareness of yoga philosophy in the west. More directly involved in the early spread of *haṭha* yoga in the US was Blanche DeVries, the first woman to open a yoga studio in New York in 1938. DeVries had learnt yoga from her husband Pierre Bernard, who had first encountered the discipline during a visit from a *tāntrik* master to Nebraska in 1888 (Shaw, E. 2011).

Around the same time as deVries' husband was learning yoga in Nebraska, Queen Victoria took yoga lessons in London. She met Shivapuri Baba, a visiting south Indian mystic who was one of the first Indian spiritual teachers to gain wide publicity in the west (he also met US President Theodore Roosevelt and some European heads of state). Shivapuri's spiritual awakening at the age of fifty led him to travel widely, and his teachings focused on the search for spiritual wisdom as a source of peace and happiness. Since he is reputed to have lived to be 137 years old, he had the time to share his teachings with many people. Although he did not identify what he taught as 'yoga', his message was clearly informed by yoga philosophy, and this is what he shared with Queen Victoria. She was receptive and positive enough about Shivapuri's teaching to have eighteen private meetings with him during his visits to London during the 1890s.

DeVries, Sister Nivedita and Queen Victoria were all fortunate enough to have their first encounter with yoga on home ground. But most of the women involved in the beginnings of the popularisation of *haṭha* yoga in the west needed to travel to India to find their teachers. Because of the original exclusion of women from the practice of *haṭha* yoga, the teachers that these travelling western women found were all men. Fortunately, the men they found had the prescience to welcome the western visitors, and Indian women, as their students. It is through these male teachers that the practices and philosophies of yoga have been protected, preserved and passed on, often in recent years, as we will see, through women. Amongst the Indian *yogīs* who have had most direct influence on the forms of yoga practice in the west today, there are two general groupings: the householders (married men with families), and the swamis (monastic renunciates).

The householder side has as its key lineage holder Tirumalai Krishnamacharya (1888–1989), a great scholar of the *Vedas* and Indian philosophy, whose *haṭha* yoga teacher for seven and a half years was Yogeshwara Ramamohan Brahmachari. There are several versions of the story of how and when Krishnamacharya found Brahmachari, but most concur that at the time Krishnamacharya studied yoga with him, Brahmachari was living in a cave in the mountains of Tibet with his wife and three children. His two daughters were his students, and legend has it that one of the treasured gifts that Krishnamacharya took with him after his studies with Brahmachari was a parchment book of drawings of yoga *āsanas* done by one of the daughters. In this text, most unusually in the context of other sources for *haṭha* yoga, half of the poses were demonstrated by female figures. In exchange for sharing yogic practices with Krishnamacharya, Brahmachari is said to have instructed Krishnamacharya to get married, raise children and lead a householder life. In this way, the daily presence of women would form part of the context for his yoga practice.

The four key teachers who learnt from Krishnamacharya have had an immense impact on the spread of yoga to the west, and between them are responsible for some of the most popular forms of yoga practised today. In chronological order, they are

Indra Devi (1899–2002), K. Pattabhi Jois (1915–2009), Krishnamacharya's brother-in-law B.K.S. Iyengar (b.1918), and his son T.K.V. Desikachar (b.1938).

It is significant that the first and most effective promoter of the yoga learnt from Krishnamacharya was a western woman. Indra Devi (Latvian born Eugenie Labunskaia) not only began to spread her teacher's teachings earlier than Kirshnamacharya's other prominent students, but she extended the reach of these teachings more rapidly and into farther corners of the world than any of the three key male Indian students. Her legacy of teachers is vast. In 1948, Devi pioneered the idea of writing books to popularise yoga, long before Iyengar published *Light on Yoga*. O'Brien identifies Indra Devi as the foremost of Krishnamacharya's key students in terms of the global reach of her influence (O'Brien 2012). She has observed that Devi's decision to direct her 1953 US publication *Forever Young, Forever Healthy* to a female readership was crucial to its immense popularity. Additionally Indra Devi's '…high profile celebrity students added much to her visibility and launched her fame. She cultivated her own high profile through lectures and appearances and then ultimately through her books… Winning endorsements from Gloria Swanson, Linda Christian, and other celebs of the day helped sales as did Devi's personal appearances at women's clubs, health conferences and Theosophical lodges, sometimes including asana demonstrations, to promote the book; by 1960 her book was in its 18th printing.' (O'Brien 2012).

Devi's remarkably successful global popularisation of yoga was rooted in the appeal her approach had for women. *Forever Young, Forever Healthy* 'is primarily about many aspects of health. Discussion and demonstration of *āsana* appear only in the last several pages of the book. Devi modeled many of the poses herself in modest shorts, a sleeveless top and a simple hairstyle. At fifty-four years of age, she embodied what she taught; she appeared toned, healthy, and younger than her age.' (O'Brien 2012).

The teachings of Indra Devi, as well as those of Jois, Iyengar and Desikachar, were all shared, as indeed Krishnamacharya had shared his teachings, within the rhythms of family life: yoga sessions and classes were part of everyday life, and institutes and schools were set up to enable students to take yoga classes and have one-to-one yoga teachings during the day. Even today, schools and *śālās* inspired by these four pioneers are generally non-residential, often urban institutions attended by students and staffed by paid teachers who all return home at the end of the working day to their family life.

Interestingly, it is partly through the presence of the women in these families that the preservation and promulgation of yoga techniques to female students became a possibility. B.K.S. Iyengar's daughter Geeta Iyengar, author of *Yoga: A Gem for Women*, is perhaps the most famous example of this transference of power to the domestically proximate. However, Krishnamacharya himself also taught Vedic chanting and yoga to his female family members, most significantly to his daughter-in-law Menaka Desikachar, whose remarkable contribution to the worldwide spread of this previously male-only spiritual discipline will be considered later.

In contrast to this familial sharing of yoga teachings with daughters and daughter-in-laws, the teachings of Swami Sivananda (1887–1963), who is the key lineage holder for the renunciate stream of influential yoga teachers, were offered in the context of *aśram* life. This meant that his students were *aśram* visitors and residents, many of whom had renounced their families and the world. Those visitors to the *aśram* who displayed appropriate commitment and devotion were initiated into the monastic order, and many remarkable disciples of Swami Sivananda transplanted this model of *aśram* life, renunciation and volunteer work (or '*karma* yoga') to the various centres and yoga schools that they set up all over the world.

The householder lineages stemming from Krishnamacharya, and the renunciate lineages of Sivananda have both taught yoga to Indian and western women. It is without doubt the vision of these two men, who overturned centuries of prohibitions against women practising yoga, that facilitated the huge expansion of yoga worldwide. Their insight into the future global power of women in the field of yoga gave them the courage to break rules in the face of immense opposition and opprobrium.

It was in 1930 that Krishnamacharya first overcame his initial profound scepticism about teaching yoga *āsana* and *prāṇāyāma* to a western woman, and accepted as his student one of the first European women to study yoga in India, Indra Devi. At the outset, he rejected her request to study with him, and it was only after considerable persistence on her behalf that she succeeded in persuading him to teach her. Such was her facility, passion and love for yoga, that Indra Devi went on to become, as described earlier, the foremost amongst Krishnamacharya's key pupils. She had an immensely powerful influence on the teaching of yoga in the US, China, South America and Europe, both through her books (translated into ten languages and sold in twenty-nine different countries) and through her teacher training programmes and international tours. Amongst the numerous US teachers whom Indra Devi inspired was Hollywood dancer Magaña Baptiste, who opened her own yoga centre in San Francisco in 1956, and whose son and daughter, Baron and Sherri Baptiste, have also become influential as yoga teachers themselves (Shaw, E. 2011).

When T. Krishnamacharya began to teach Vedic chants to his daughter-in-law Menaka Desikachar in the 1970s, he was well aware that the teachers and students at every single Vedic chanting school in India were male, and that access to traditional teaching for accurate chanting of the *Vedas* was absolutely forbidden to women. But Krishnamacharya believed the future survival of Vedic culture lay in the hands of women, so he broke all the prohibitions of the tradition of which he himself was a product. His beliefs have been thoroughly vindicated. Today not only is Menaka Desikachar one of the leading world teachers of Vedic chant, but most of the chant teachers, senior trainers and students in the Krishnamacharya Yoga Mandiram (KYM) tradition of Vedic chant worldwide are also women: the 20:1 female-to-male ratio of students on the most recent UK Vedic Chant Teacher Training Course is typical. However, as I observed in the introduction, the majority presence of women, even in positions of authority, is no guarantee that female students within such yoga organisations are safe from exploitation and sexual abuse by male teachers.

The example set by Krishnamacharya as a teacher who welcomed female students inspired his own students to share yoga with western women. The Italian Vanda Scaravelli (1908–1999) first studied with Iyengar in her late forties, and later also with Desikachar. Developing her own unique response to what she had been taught,

Scaravelli was most interested in finding waves of energy in the body, teaching students how to work with gravity in their poses, and exploring the power and subtlety of breath in yoga. A powerful yogic luminary in her own right, Scaravelli's evolution of the practices she learned developed into a very feminine and responsive approach to yoga practice that has been deeply influential to many internationally respected teachers, including Donna Farhi, Angela Farmer, Dona Holleman, Esther Myers and Diane Long. Scaravelli's approach has also been significant in the field of yoga for pregnancy, through teachers such as Sandra Sabatini, whose work has inspired the approach to yoga taught in the Active Birth movement.

Swami Sivananda also demonstrated remarkable openness to sharing yoga with western women. In 1956 he initiated Swami Sivananda Radha (the German-born Sylvia Demitz, 1911–1995) into 'sannyas' (or more properly, '*saṃnyāsa*': renunciate vows), and at his request she went to Canada to establish the Yashodhara *aśram*, an international network of Radha House yoga centres, and *Ascent* yoga magazine. By initiating Swami Radha, Sivananda set an important precedent for his own disciples to initiate women into various kinds of *sannyas*. The most influential of Sivananda's many powerful disciples in this respect were Swami Satyananda, whose Satyananda Yoga is largely promulgated by a network of female swamis and *karma saṃnyāsins* in Europe, Swami Vishnudevananda, whose Sivananda Yoga Vedanta Centres worldwide are staffed by predominantly female teams of *brahmacāris* (celibate renunciates), swamis and volunteer *karma yogīs*, and Swami Satchidananda, whose Integral yoga system has been spread by a combination of mostly female renunciates and volunteers including, between 1972 and 1991, Nischala Joy Devi, whose recent translation of the *Yoga Sūtra*s of Patañjali brings an explicitly feminine perspective on this traditional text.

Like Nischala Joy Devi, who worked closely with Swami Satchidananda for twenty years before leaving the *aśram* to have the freedom to explore her own more feminine approach to sharing yoga, most of the early female seekers after yoga in India initially remained closely associated with the teachers from whom they had learnt. But not all of the women who came to 'collect' yoga directly from Indian teachers remained closely aligned with the teacher's structures and systems of practice. For example, Dublin-born Mollie Bagot-Stack has been identified by yoga scholar Mark Singleton as an influential teacher of what were effectively yoga *āsanas* under another name in the UK during the 1920s and 1930s (Singleton 2010). Stack went to India in 1912 and learned what were described as 'imagesanas' from a teacher called Gopal. She later incorporated these yoga-based practices into the gymnastics programmes taught in London in the 1920s through the organisation she founded, the Women's League of Health and Beauty. Mollie Stack clearly felt free to adapt what she had learnt in India to render it more suitable and appealing to the ladies of the Women's League of Health and Beauty under the title: the 'Bagot-Stack Stretch and Swing System'. Singleton claims Stack's creative incorporation of the yoga she learned into her own system of teaching is a pre-echo of some of the more feminine approaches to yoga taken by other pioneering women teachers more closely aligned with the traditions of yoga and the teachers from whom they learnt.

ADAPTING THE TEACHINGS: WESTERN WOMEN SHARING YOGA INSIDE AND OUTSIDE TRADITIONS, 1960–2010

> *A yoga lineage provides a human link to the tradition and its various branches. To become part of a yoga tradition is not just an outer formality of joining one group or another, but the ability to connect to great teachers and teachings at a heart level. Great gurus have created roads that we can drive on. There is an 'inner tradition' that we can access within ourselves if we gain the right receptivity.*
> *(Frawley 2008: 230)*

Many inspirational and powerful women teachers of yoga have taken a creatively adaptive approach to yoga practice. Janice Gates, in her charming and informative survey of women in yoga past and present (*Yoginī: the power of women in yoga,* 2006), identifies this tendency to adapt as a feminine characteristic. Through her interviews with fourteen of the world's most influential female yoga teachers, she reveals a keenly experienced sense of femininity informing all of their work. Coming as they do from a variety of different yoga traditions and schools, it is apparent that, within the diversity of their work and lives, the shared feature of their engagement with yoga has been a responsiveness, a readiness to adapt and adjust the traditional forms of yoga to the needs of women.

For example, Angela Farmer studied for ten years with B.K.S. Iyengar, striving to perfect his system of alignment and 'correct poses' in her own practice, before going on to develop a more fluid and feminine approach to *āsana*. She and her fellow Iyengar yoga teacher and husband Victor Van Kooten began to offer what they described as 'Un-trainings' to encourage teachers and practitioners to experience a more easeful yoga practice 'from the inside out'. Angela Farmer's work has influenced Donna Farhi, whose practical integration of structure and responsive spontaneity, and reflective writings on the subject invite practitioners to encounter yoga as an opportunity for spiritual discovery and exploration beyond form.

But the 'feminisation' of yoga that Gates describes has not just been about bringing softness and fluidity to *āsana* form. For Angela Farmer, and eventually also for other women teachers who were rooted in a particular tradition, like Nischala Joy Devi, the growth and expression of their own experience of yoga entailed leaving their yoga 'homes'. Such departures are not always easy. When Farmer and Van Kooten began to offer teachings that were different from what Iyengar had taught them, they were cut off from their teacher and the structures that had supported them: 'It was like being excommunicated,' says Farmer. When Nischala Joy left Satchidananda's *aśram* she described it as 'a difficult time'. Even Mother Maya, an influential teacher and writer on yoga and *āyurveda*, recently renounced her monastic title (Swami Mayatitananda) and the formal, traditional structures within which it held her in order to 'walk a simpler life'. Although she maintains a positive relationship with the *guru* who initiated her into the monastic order, she has chosen less orthodox means to share her practices of yogic meditations, ceremony, *prāṇāyāma* and *āyurvedic* self-care with a worldwide community.

What the stories of all these teachers tell us is that, at a certain point, the traditional lineages and structures that have grown female teachers within them may no longer serve to nurture those teachers' developing gifts and understandings. For Angela Farmer as well as for Donna Farhi and Nischala Joy Devi, the shift in focus that prompted their departure from their original lineages came about because they began to see yoga practice from a feminine perspective. This same feminine perspective also underpins Mother Maya's understanding of the profound connection between women's health and the ecology of our planet, and shapes her work in presenting *āyurvedic* and yogic breath, food and sound *sādhanas* (practices) as a form of environmental awareness.

But the sense of needing to change the usual perspectives of a traditional lineage of teachers is not an exclusively female experience. There are certainly many male teachers who have negotiated such shifts and transitions, notably Natanaga Zhander (known as Zhander Remete) and John Friend, both of whom began their teaching lives within the Iyengar yoga school, and subsequently 'left home' to formulate their own approaches: Shadow yoga and Anusara yoga respectively. Remete and Friend's departures from their yogic 'home towns' were motivated partly by discoveries that called for a new approach to practice, partly by philosophical and practical questioning of the principles operating in their original trainings, and partly by their own personal histories. Ultimately these combined influences led them to a shift in the focus of their yogic attentions, a profound alteration of outward forms and methods of practice, and the creation of two new 'yoga traditions'. The process can be seen as a form of 'career development' motivated at a deeper level by the specific personal and emotional circumstances of the teachers involved. This process is not gender specific. Elements of the same process are evident in the trajectories of many female yogic adventurers who depart from their original modes of practice.

Although there are clearly some shared experiences that link such enquiring and creative *yogīs* and *yoginīs*, there is a very specifically feminine aspect to the pressing need some women practitioners feel to leave the formal structures of yoga traditions. For many *yoginīs*, the urgency to leave structured and rigid yoga practice is completely rooted in their experiences as women. The necessity to 'move on' for these *yoginīs* has a primal, physical and emotional urgency that comes very directly from the experiences of womb cycles, from life-changing experiences such as pregnancy, birth or miscarriage, or from personal experiences of physical vulnerability that are fundamentally to do with being female. For example, Donna Farhi and Angela Farmer identify traumatic early experiences of sexual abuse and/or deep physical and emotional suffering as the most profound motivating factors in their keenly felt desires to develop more responsive and sensitive approaches to yoga practice for women. Their experiences as vulnerable girls and young women opened up a heightened perception about their own needs and the needs of other women in the yoga world, and this led both of them away from teachings which emphasised rigid ideals of alignment and correct practice within the context of a strictly enforced hierarchy of power and control. Both Farhi and Farmer have worked instead to create safe environments and approaches to yoga that empower women to let go and be nourished by a practice that naturally arises from within.

Like John Friend or Natanaga Zhander, Angela Farmer's departure from Iyengar yoga may well also have been motivated by some general concerns about structure and freedom, or methods of teaching. But unlike Friend and Zhander, Farmer's commitment to the evolution of a yoga practice that ultimately caused her to leave Iyengar was motivated by being female. She experienced a deep sadness that everything she had been trained to do had never actually met her needs for a practice of yoga that acknowledged her femininity. Above all she left, neither because it was a good career move, nor because she needed the creative space to develop her own 'tradition', but because of a gnawing sense that everything she had been taught had never answered her desire for a practice that met her as a woman. Moreover, as a woman who was teaching other women, Angela knew that she was perpetuating collective female disempowerment every time she stood in front of a class of female yoga students and taught them what she had learned from Iyengar.

So now, even thirty years later, when Angela Farmer speaks about her reasons for parting company with Iyengar yoga, she still touches her heart, and reflects on her own personal need for emotional and spiritual growth and her responsibility to other women: 'I just couldn't do it anymore', she says, 'I knew that this practice could not respond to where I was, and so I simply could not continue to share it with other women. So one day, I had to come clean, and I had to share the practice that I had allowed to move through me. It was a practice that was nourishing me as a woman, and that's what I knew I had to share with the other women.' (Farmer 2012) The name she gives to the work is 'The Feminine Unfolding': and this name speaks of the deep sensitivity and gentleness that illuminates her approach to yoga: 'I find my focus is more and more about reclaiming one's power, one's body and one's personal space. By this I mean that many, if not most women, due perhaps to historical suppression, early trauma, sexual and other abuse or physical and emotional injuries, have only a partial sense of their "beingness"... My approach is to create a space/setting where there is a feeling of safety and support to take the journey inwards to where these old traumas hide within our bodies, Instead of forcing or avoiding these places, we begin by giving them space and loving concern, as a mother might do to a frightened or injured child.' (Farmer 2012)

Other feminine vulnerabilities: developing maternal adaptations to yoga practice

In addition to the encounters with vulnerability, such as those that led Farmer and Farhi to discover more feminine approaches to yoga, for women who choose to bear children there are other experiences that can lead in the same direction. Pregnancies, the effects of births or miscarriages, and the experiences of postnatal recovery can all change a woman's relation to her yoga practice and lineage. Sometimes also the desire to move out of a rigidly defined structure of practice or a framework of teaching and learning that is rooted in the control of power may be motivated simply by a perception that these approaches to yoga do not provide sufficient opportunity to honour the cycles of her womb or cycles of life experiences that come with age.

For example, my own encounter with the experiences of being pregnant and practising yoga within the structure of the traditionally maintained Satyananda yoga lineage was largely positive, but led me to question, from the point of view of my own physical and emotional needs, the traditional guidelines which I was being encouraged to follow, particularly in relation to *prāṇāyāma*. I experienced that the standard approach to most *prāṇāyāma* taught in Satyananda classes was fundamentally unsuited to the needs of myself as an expectant mother, and I was concerned for the effects that this would have on my unborn child. It was hard to put my finger on it, but it just didn't feel right. There were no good answers within the tradition to the questions I asked. In fact, there was a general distaste for asking any questions at all. My unanswered questions generated a profound experience of dissatisfaction with what that lineage could offer, and it was that experience that eventually prompted me to look elsewhere for answers, a search which culminated in writing *Mother's Breath*, which was the book I felt I needed during my second pregnancy.

Similarly, when I returned to yoga as a postnatal woman after the birth of my eldest son, I perceived discrepancies between my physical and emotional needs as a lactating woman recovering from birth, and the standard yoga programmes that Satyananda yoga had to offer. I sensed that there were many valuable practices that would promote healing, but knew instinctively that what was usually being suggested in these classes would often be more harmful than beneficial. There was also a discrepancy between my desire to practise with my baby son close by, and the usual expectations for a reverent silence to be maintained during class. Whilst there was an initially very warm welcome for the presence of the infant, as a kind of delightful novelty, that welcome soon cooled when it became apparent that I hoped his presence could become a regular part of the yoga class experience. For months I struggled to fit my changed perspective as a new mother back into the old Satyananda yoga box I had so loved to inhabit. But it simply didn't fit. I needed to acknowledge both the current physical unsuitability of the teachings I had previously so enjoyed, and the slowly dawning sense of exclusion I experienced as a 'disruptive' new mother in relation to the lineage holders' desires to maintain power and control over their classes and retreats. This was a painful experience. But in comparison with the experiences of other postnatal women wishing to practise yoga within traditional hierarchies, my difficulties were minimal (for details of the challenges faced by postnatal women within yoga communities, see chapter fourteen).

In the end, such discrepancies between the shifts in my life as a woman and the lineage's restrictive expectations about behaviour and forms of practice created a profoundly creative tension. This tension pushed me into finding and developing new approaches to yoga practice, to the yoga teaching environment and to the relations between yoga teachers and students, in which new mothers and their babies could be welcomed and nurtured. I was relieved at this time to discover the inspirational approach to yoga practice for mothers pioneered by Françoise Freedman and her teachers at Birthlight. Attending Freedman's classes with my first son opened up for me the realisation that some key elements of this more informal and welcoming approach could helpfully be combined with those beneficial practices that I had experienced within the formal confines of Satyananda yoga. It was the polarised experiences of these two very contrasting approaches to yoga that prompted me to develop for my own practice and teaching a very feminine hybrid that met my own needs for nourishing postnatal yoga practice, and later formed the basis for the wider application of womb yoga for menstrual health. Reflections on these practices and this approach to yoga are explored in the postnatal recovery section of chapter fourteen.

The quest that started from a place of resentful exclusion ended with the happy discovery of a whole community of displaced female yoga practitioners who positively embraced the new ways of sharing and teaching yoga. Some of these teachers had found their home within the Birthlight organisation, or within the Yogabirth network of teachers, and some were connected to the yoga for pregnancy approach developed by Janet Balaskas and her colleagues at the Active Birth Centre; but many others were simply out on their own, unable to return to their usual yoga classes after the births of their babies. For, of course, my experiences were not unique. There were, as I slowly began to realise, many women practising yoga who appreciated the need for more responsive and nurturing classes. Initially the focus of the classes I began to teach at this time was purely on meeting the needs of pregnant and postnatal women, but as I began to discover, yoga that is so specifically designed to support the life of the womb during periods of immense challenge such as pregnancy, also appeals greatly to women at all stages in their lives. Having experienced the quality of self-nurture and delight that arises during the very feminine practices of yoga for pregnancy, women became reluctant to return to other forms of practice. So all sorts of women who were not pregnant started to come to the 'pregnancy yoga' classes. I decided then that a more appropriate name for what I was offering would be 'womb yoga', for its practices were well suited to many other stages of a woman's life. Women recovering from miscarriage, and those seeking to conceive, all find the approach helpful and healing. Women with menstrual difficulties discover the practices of womb yoga to be supportive. Perimenopausal women appreciate the nourishing and rhythmic aspects of womb yoga, and post-menopausal women delight in the spacious and sensual experiences of the practice. My colleague Sofya Ansari, after attending a particularly nourishing womb yoga practice in Bristol recently described it as 'pure yin [feminine, nurturing energy]; you can feel the nourishment feeding you, physically, emotionally, even at the levels of the organs themselves. It's abundance of yin. It pours into you.'

The inner teacher and the outer structures: womb yoga, women and yoga lineages

Womb yoga is rooted in an environmentally aware, responsive and adaptive approach to yoga to support women's lifelong health. It uses yoga as a technique to encounter a profound understanding that resides in the very blood of the menses, the walls of the womb and the rhythms of a woman's life, to give a completely clear and true source of guidance and teaching for that woman. The intention of womb yoga is to facilitate a lived experience of communion with an inner wisdom that is primal, profound and powerful. From this experience flows a quiet but truly secure confidence, a total trust that an inner, embodied understanding, a deep knowing, is founded on and expressed through the blood wisdom of a woman's body. No outer teacher can come close to the deep sense of right wisdom and understanding that flows through a woman who is absolutely and profoundly connected with her own intuitive understanding. So womb yoga, like many of the other approaches to yoga practice that have been developed by women over the pasty fifty years, is not about following the teachings of particular tradition, text or lineage. It promotes direct access to the presence of the inner teacher.

This is not to say that there is no value or goodness in traditions and lineages. On the contrary, it is right to give thanks and praise to those robustly maintained traditions and lineages that have protected and preserved the teachings of *haṭha* yoga for so long and so well. We need to be very glad that they exist at all, for without these traditions and lineages we would have no yoga. They have functioned very effectively as protective vessels for the export and distribution of yoga worldwide.

To learn and practise yoga within the boundaries of any particular tradition or lineage may bring many benefits, but it also imposes very strict limitations. From my own experiences and those of colleagues who have chosen to depart from or remain within the lineage hierarchies, I can see that the role of the student in most traditional yoga lineages is quite clearly defined. To study within a lineage, students are required simply to accept the teachings, as obediently as we are able; diligently to listen to the teachers within our chosen tradition, and to do what has been taught in the honest belief that the chosen tradition is offering the right answers, and that those answers should not and need not be questioned. A clarity and depth of trust and understanding may come from this kind of faithful engagement and subscription to any particular tradition. This can be a deeply comforting and valuable experience that creates a powerful sense of belonging. It may also place a student in a position of great vulnerability. Students who put their entire trust in their lineage's power-holders may find that they exert powerful pressures to conform to the values of the lineage, and to protect it from any outside criticism. For certainly, engagement with any particular tradition or initiation into a specific lineage entails a responsibility on the part of the initiate to uphold the traditions of that lineage. As the stories I have already told demonstrate, and as recent revelations show, there can evidently be deep challenges associated with this. The challenges can be particularly difficult if the tradition is a male lineage and the initiate is a woman, especially if the exploitation of women is accepted as part of the power structure of the organisations that have grown to protect the teachings, and not the students.

The organisations which have grown up around the desire to preserve and disseminate (I use the word advisedly, since the teachings have usually been offered by male teachers) precious teachings usually involve strictly enforced protocols, titles, hierarchies and other demonstrations of respectful humility to the senior teachers, as well as intense trainings and commitment on behalf of the students who wish to have access to their teachings. For example, the hierarchical structures of different levels of initiations and experience, which are the organising principles of the global families of Satyananda yoga or Kundalini yoga organisations, create a sense of belonging and a trust in the wisdom of the *guru* which is often very pleasing and nourishing to those who are happy for their yoga experience to be held within the boundaries of the tradition or school. In organisations that have clear hierarchies of initiation that derive from a monastic structure of *saṃṇyāsa*, then these structures are overt, and offer a clear route for accessing power and influence within that particular organisation, and well trodden pathways for deepening one's own personal engagement with the teachings. So some traditions offer clear outer signs of one's progress along the path of that particular tradition. But in other traditions where there are no different-coloured robes or beads to wear, and no 'inner circle' of higher initiates, then these hierarchies are less overt, but equally powerfully maintained. Such invisible hierarchies are not signalled by the colour of a person's robes, but through very strict enforcement of different levels of teacher training and experience. Examples of this can be found within the Iyengar tradition and within the community of practitioners and teachers of *aṣṭaṅga vinyāsa* yoga, or surrounding the circles of teachers associated with the Krishnamacharya Healing and Yoga Foundation. This is why a teacher like Angela Farmer, certified as an advanced Iyengar teacher, could experience the sense of being 'excommunicated' when she could no longer align herself with those teachings which she had been authorised to share. Students were cautioned not to attend her classes, and colleagues shunned her. This experience is not unusual, for it is what happens to any yoga teacher who starts inside any kind of tradition and then begins to question it, or to step outside of it. To exclude those who question the tradition is a necessary function of the tradition: it ensures its survival.

For whether overt or covert, these various hierarchies and structures all exist to guard and share the teachings of a particular tradition by creating a community of people who 'belong' to that tradition. Students are expected to demonstrate respect and honour for the teachers within that tradition. This is intended both to deepen their own experience of the teachings of that approach to yoga, whilst also reinforcing the power structures of the organisation that has grown up to preserve and protect those teachings from being diluted or contaminated. This experience of 'belonging' to a group of people committed to a particular lineage can be an important aspect of building confidence and an experience of authenticity for a teacher, because that teacher understands that they are merely passing on the authentic practices with which the tradition or the teacher has entrusted them, and that this level of authenticity and adherence to tradition provides an integrity to their practices which they are able to share.

All of this can be good, and can offer a sense of nourishment and protection to those who belong to the lineage. However, there can come a point (and the stories I have already told in this chapter show how many women in yoga today have already reached beyond this point) where the boundaries of tradition and lineage can be not just a confining limitation, but a cloaking device for the sexual exploitation and disempowerment of women. For just as the strict enforcement of hierarchy protects and preserves precious teachings, so also can that same structure of power permit the continuance of exploitative and manipulative behaviours by lineage holders. It is this kind of power-holding that makes it possible for traditions to continue to function commercially even in the face of accusations of immorality and abuses of power at the highest levels. The power can become so centralised that leaders simply dispense with any critical senior teachers, retain or promote those teachers who are too blind, scared or bedazzled to dissent, and together welcome in the next batch of unsuspecting new (largely young, female) students upon whom they continue to prey.

Paradoxically, even as yoga in its broadest sense offers women empowerment by the reconnection or 'yoga' with our inner teacher, so the practice of yoga in its most limited sense, as the unquestioning replication of specific practices promoted by a single tradition – even if they are no longer appropriate for the student, and even if they abuse and exploit the trust of students – can utterly disempower us as women.

When this happens, then the incredible potential of yoga to liberate women from suffering and sadness is lost. Instead of offering us the keys to freedom and self-acceptance, this kind of disempowering yoga becomes a kind of prison. This is a tragic paradox. The very practice that offers the most complete empowerment and freedom to be ourselves can end up as a disempowering burden which confines us by disconnecting us from the inner teachings of our own awareness. This disconnection depletes and disempowers women.

There is no simple equation between traditional lineage-based yoga and disempowerment. There is no simple equation between non-traditional or out-of-lineage based yoga and freedom. For some women, the freedom to practise the yoga that nourishes their own awareness best is experienced within the safe boundaries of a traditional hierarchy. For other women this is simply not possible and they feel their own consciousness stifled by the structures, or unsuited to the practices, or else they find themselves exploited, abused or expelled by those who hold the power within the lineage hierarchy. It depends on the lineage and upon the teachers. For some women, the freedom to experience the yoga which truly feeds her deepest sense of well-being and acute awareness is experienced in the practice of 'eclectic' styles of yoga which are currently proliferating. For others, these out-of-lineage hybrids create confusion and unease that hinder the development of our own conscious awareness. Again, it depends on the appropriateness of the practice to the student, and upon the responsiveness of the teacher sharing the practice.

The key concern for any woman doing yoga now is to discover an approach to yoga practice that empowers her to listen to the wisdom of her body, especially the cyclical rhythms of her womb life. This empowerment gives a woman confidence to engage in a responsive yoga practice that can fully nurture and nourish her in respect of the different cycles of her womb or the stages of her life. This kind of empowering practice can be found both within and without traditional structures of yoga teaching. Equally, yoga practice that disempowers women can be experienced as much within eclectic, 'free style' contemporary approaches to yoga as within the confines of more traditional lineage-based yoga hierarchies, as I explore in the stories which follow.

STORIES FROM TODAY'S STUDIOS: DISEMPOWERMENT OF WOMEN IN YOGA THROUGH DISCOURAGEMENT, DISRESPECT, DISREGARD AND DISCONNECTION

The paradox of yoga that actually disempowers a student is that it clouds the very light of awareness that yoga practice is intended to clear. For women, the light of awareness shines most brightly when we attend to the rhythmic cycles of our wombs and to the changing needs of our physical and emotional bodies at different stages in our lives. To disempower women yoga students is to teach them yoga in such a way that they become unable (or unwilling) to discern and respond to their own needs. This disempowerment is especially relevant to women practising yoga now, and it happens through four basic means: discouragement, disrespect, disregard and disconnection.

In the first place disempowerment occurs through the discouragement of questioning. This form of disempowerment relates mostly to the experiences of students within a particular tradition. It can result from a belief, which can be promoted through certain lineage structures, that we need to look outside ourselves for the answers we need. Sometimes a reliance on the external focus of the outer teacher in a particular tradition can distract us from the true presence of our inner teacher. Ideally, of course, devotion and respect for the teachings of the *guru* or the tradition leads directly to a rediscovery of our own inner teacher, because in the end the outer *guru* and the inner *guru* are one and the same: we are yoga, and it is already in us, as much as we are within the tradition. But even within traditions that preach the discovery of the inner teacher, there can remain powerful discouragements to question, or to delve deep into the sort of investigations that lead us back home to the inner teacher. Sometimes the sort of questions that help us find the light of the inner teacher are not very well supported within the structures of Indian yoga traditions. This is understandable. Those who ask these questions pose a threat to the tradition simply by the act of asking: traditions are not maintained by people who ask questions about them, they are maintained by people who accept the tradition and feel no need to ask questions about it because they believe that the traditional answer is always right. We have seen what happens to those members of a tradition who insist on asking questions: eventually they have to look outside of the tradition to find answers. For women asking questions about yoga practice, the best answers tend to come from inside.

Discouragement

'Don't ask us, we don't know... but we need you to believe that we do'.

No single lineage has access to all of the wisdom of the whole of yoga. It may often be simpler at the start of a yoga journey to narrow one's focus to a particular yoga tradition. But when it comes to finding effective and complete yoga therapies for a particular individual, then to remain bounded by the limitations of one lineage alone can at best be a disadvantage, and at worse, be a disrespectful disservice to those who are seeking help to find a yoga practice to heal and empower them.

For example, if yoga teachers are not respectful of the range of research and information that may exist outside of their own tradition, it can be easy to provide unhelpful answers to students' questions. This is exactly what happened at a yoga retreat that I attended, which was organised by one of the world's leading foundations for yoga therapy. The subject of the retreat was yoga for women, and the leaders of the retreat were two very senior female teachers within this tradition. Many inspirational and empowering practices were shared at this retreat. However, such was the deeply respectful honour in which the two senior teachers were held, and such was their conviction that their tradition offered absolutely all the answers, that there was no possibility for students to get full and complete responses to the many complex questions about women's health and well-being that were raised during the formal question and answer sessions held each evening of the retreat. The intention of these question and answer sessions was to give retreatants the opportunity to access the wisdom of their senior teachers' long experience. Often this is what happened, but equally often the senior women teachers were in fact able to offer only incomplete and inaccurate information that disregarded recent relevant research. This happened more out of ignorance that anything else, but such answers created experiences of disempowerment for the women who had asked the questions.

For example, an elegant *yoginī* in her early fifties, named Susie, raised a question about the practice of headstand (*śirṣāsana*) after menopause. Susie made it clear that she was seeking clarity and guidance for her own practice; 'I love *śirṣāsana*,' she explained, 'but someone told me it was not wise to continue this practice after menopause.' She presented the hearsay to her senior teachers in an honest and humble search for good information on the subject. What she received from these women in response was a very funny, but utterly disrespectful answer that equated her desire to continue her own private practice of *śirṣāsana* with the desire to show off: 'So you want to be on TV and show everyone what you can do?' quipped the teachers. The elegant *yoginī*'s protests that she had no plans to do this were drowned in gales of laughter. This was the first disempowerment, to ridicule the *yoginī*'s desire for guidance on appropriate practice by taking her enquiry out of context. Having done this, the senior teachers then proceeded to liken this *yoginī*'s pleasure in practising *śirṣāsana* in private to the desire of an ageing former pole-climbing champion to continue shimmying up greasy poles at village fairs. They offered the explanation that greasy pole climbing was a popular Indian festival activity that involves climbing up an oiled pole to retrieve a bag of money at the top. 'Listen,' said the most senior teacher very seriously, 'in our yoga centre we knew a man who had been the champion greasy pole climber of the whole of India.' Susie stared at her, utterly baffled. What did this greasy pole champion have to do with her question? 'He didn't want to stop either,' explained the senior teacher, 'He was continuing to climb greasy poles when he reached the age of sixty.' A hilarious anecdote ensued, about the sad injuries that had followed such a foolish choice. 'He fell and broke his neck.' The senior teacher looked sternly at Susie as she spoke about the unfortunate end of the ageing greasy pole-climbing champion: 'He is bedridden now. It is not wise. I think I have answered your question?' And so, thoroughly ridiculed and disrespected, the *yoginī* was advised to plan on abandoning any 'difficult' postures after menopause for fear of falling and breaking her bones.

Seeking some sort of clarification on this question, and knowing the most recent research on the importance of weight-bearing exercise as a way to build bone in osteopoenic women (Fishman and Saltonstall 2000), I followed up the greasy pole story with an enquiry about which weight-bearing *āsanas* were recommended for the purpose of building bone strength in post-menopausal women. In response I received the same ridicule and bad information: weight bearing was absolutely bad for bones, and the tradition did not advise *āsana* practice post-menopause. It was dangerous. I am pleased to report that, according to all reputable authorities, this is absolutely not the case. For information and guidance on yoga and bone density please see chapter sixteen.

The ridicule of Susie's question effectively discouraged other women on the retreat from asking further questions on this topic. The disrespectful response to the perspectives and research from outside of the tradition effectively denied all of the women in the room access to information that would have helped them to make informed choices about their own health and the health of their students simply because the teachers representing this tradition had no knowledge or understanding about the other schools of yoga that had conducted the research into bone building yoga practice for menopausal women. Even when this very useful information was brought to their attention by my contribution to the discussion, it was dismissed and disrespected as irrelevant because it did not originate from within the tradition that was hosting the retreat. The senior lineage holders' disrespect for other traditions utterly disempowered Susie, and left her not only humiliated but also ignorant of yoga practices that could be beneficial to her own well-being in future years.

Sometimes, strict adherents to a single tradition, especially if it is a tradition that does not admit that any valuable offerings can be found outside of itself, will simply deny that any other approaches are really yoga at all. This attitude promotes a kind of inter-tradition rivalry that is never helpful. It is particularly inimical to the positive practice of yoga for women, whose cyclical experiences may well be better served by engaging in a range of complementary practices to suit different times in the menstrual cycle, for example. Having practised a number of different yogic disciplines, sometimes in parallel, during different times of my life, I have observed that this kind of inter-tradition disrespect can create absurd situations that benefit no one and can often cause suffering and harm.

For example, Nell was a yoga teacher who was motivated to train as a pregnancy yoga teacher herself after her yoga experiences in her first pregnancy. She was dismissed sobbing from an Iyengar yoga class that she had been attending regularly for over six years: 'My teacher refused me access on the basis that she wasn't insured to have a pregnant woman in the class. Even though I'd been her student for six years, she felt I didn't know well enough how to practise safely in my new state of health. It wasn't so much the eviction that made me upset,' recalled Nell, 'I completely understood the insurance position. But what really got me sobbing was the fact that she was so deeply rude about any other kind of yoga, and that she utterly discouraged me from going elsewhere – she made it seem to me as if I had been cast into the outer darkness, and that there was simply nothing else for me to do but sit at home and watch the telly: "There's no point bothering with that pregnancy yoga rubbish" she said as she pushed me out the door, "It's a total waste of space. It isn't even yoga."'

At the other end of the perinatal spectrum, Sarah was warmly welcomed back into her *aṣṭaṅga vinyāsa* class six weeks after the birth of her first baby. 'No need to bother with that poncy postnatal and baby yoga nonsense,' smiled the teacher as he began to offer full intensity adjustments through a led primary series class.

After thirty minutes, Sarah was a trembling wreck, and collapsed on her mat in tears. The teacher's arrogant discouragement of the therapeutic practice of healing postnatal yoga revealed his own unhelpfully judgmental stance on the relative status of different forms of yoga. His readiness to disrespect yoga forms other than his own chosen practice masked a complete ignorance of the physiological and emotional needs of a woman who had only recently given birth. His discouragement of more appropriate practices not only persuaded Sarah that her recovery would be better served by his own approach to yoga, but also caused her profound damage both physically and emotionally.

Disrespect

'Yoga? That's not yoga. Only what we do is yoga.'

The second method of disempowerment is disrespect. This can take the form of disrespect for those individuals who have chosen to step outside of a tradition to which they once belonged, or it can be a general disrespect for any approaches to yoga that differ from our own. This form of inter-tradition disrespect arises when adherence to a particular way of doing yoga (not necessarily, but often, a traditional form) can condone disrespect towards the valuable contributions made by other traditions and approaches. Frequently this form of disrespect is rooted in ignorance, or a fear that other ways of doing yoga may somehow dilute or pollute the preferred choice or tradition.

In the South London yoga world in the 1990s, two lineage-specific yoga schools were located relatively close to each other. There were a few dedicated *yoginīs*, including myself, who could see the relative benefits of both Satyananda and Iyengar approaches to yoga practice, and who would cycle between south-east and south-west London to attend classes at both the Iyengar School of South East London and the Satyananda Centre. By doing this, we gained the advantages both of an attentive approach to alignment-based *āsana* in a fully-equipped Iyengar studio, and exposure to the broad range of *mudrā*, *prāṇāyāma*, *svara* yoga and teachings in *kuṇḍalinī tantra*, *yoga nidrā*, meditation and *bhakti* yoga that were taught in the Satyananda school. We felt at the time that this was an especially positive combination of approaches to yoga practice that supported both the needs of the physical body and engaged with more esoteric realms of spiritual practice. Teachers in both establishments offered excellence in the teachings of their own traditions.

As an open-hearted young *yoginī* and yoga teacher I thought the arrangement of learning from both sets of teachers was a great gift. But because of the profound disrespect which senior teachers openly displayed to each other's traditions, it was unpleasant and unwise for students who practised in both centres to let anyone know about this. We had to pretend that we never went to 'the other place'. Whoever so much as named the other approach to yoga would be subject to ridicule, and jokes would be made about some aspect of the other way of practising. The best way to avoid this awkward experience was to pretend that the only yoga was that taught by the tradition in whose centre you found yourself at that moment. It was as if these two approaches to yoga practice were two separate worlds, each determined to maintain the belief that the other did not exist. Were inhabitants of one world to be reminded of the existence of the other world, then disparaging comments would be made about the invalidity of the other tradition's approach to yoga. This was a pity, because many of those women practising the more esoteric meditations would have benefited from some of the strength building and restorative *āsanas* practised so assiduously in the Iyengar school. Equally, some of the more body-focused practitioners in the Iyengar school would have gained enormously from the subtle breathwork and nourishing *bhakti* and *yoga nidrā* techniques taught so well by the Satyananda teachers. Additionally, from a menstruating woman's perspective, it made sense to me to attend the class that best matched my cyclical rhythms at the time: for example, when energy was high at ovulation it made perfect sense to do an Iyengar back-bending workshop, but when a more mystical frame of mind was present, for example at menstruation, then chanting *mantras* at the Satyananda centre was more appropriate. As a discerning *yoginī* becoming attuned to the inner world, I could sense there was a deeper rhythm at work. Having access to very different forms of yoga (albeit surreptitiously) supported my attempts to honour my inner rhythm.

More prosaically, having practised in both places I could see that there were also some students who had clearly and unfortunately just ended up in the wrong place, and that an alternative approach to yoga would suit them much better, but this possibility was never raised by the teachers. These 'out of place' students often just left, thinking that yoga was not for them, never considering that they simply might be practising a form of yoga that was simply unsuited to their needs at the time. The senior teachers' mutual disrespect effectively disenfranchised their students, because even if techniques or approaches offered by a different tradition may well have been more appropriate for a certain student, this option could absolutely never be mentioned. This disenfranchisement extended also to opportunities for further training and development across different traditions, because the teachers within certain traditions routinely refused to provide any supporting documentation that might be needed to enable their students and teachers to access further or specialised training in other schools of yoga. For example, yoga students from one lineage who chose to pursue their yoga teacher training with another, perhaps more eclectic training organisation, would discover that their teachers would not provide them with references. This was troublesome for all students, not just women, but it caused especial difficulty for women interested in pursuing studies in yoga for women's health, because the organisations offering pregnancy yoga trainings were not recognised by their usual teachers' lineages.

This form of disempowerment is rooted in a belief that one's own tradition offers all the answers. It is rooted in a disrespect for wisdom from other sources, and is not especially helpful for women practising yoga now. There are other forms of disempowerment that can in fact be injurious to women. Disrespect for other sources of wisdom may be limiting, but disregard for the voice of the inner teacher in the form of our body's own wisdom can be harmful, as the following story shows.

Disregard

'Don't mention the wombs. Let's pretend nobody has one.'

Lou was in tears outside the hall. She was weeping with sadness, pain and rage, because the specific needs of her womb-life had been disregarded: she had been encouraged to practise yoga techniques unsuited to her, and to a large number of other women yoga students in the class she was attending. Inside the enormous hall, eighty-two women and seven men were taking a break from a yoga workshop. Over the past three days, a popular North American yoga teacher trainer had been skilfully laying out some of the *tāntrik* technologies for spiritual development in relation to yoga practice. He was visiting London as part of his international yoga-teaching schedule, and many of those present were devoted yoga practitioners and long-time students. The teacher was knowledgeable, experienced, generous in the sharing of his knowledge, and charming and engaging in his relaxed modes of communication.

He was covering a lot of profound and complex materials with efficiency and lightness, sharing teachings from the *tantras* that he himself had learned from his own teachers, all of whom had been men. The practical techniques which he shared involved a number of powerful pelvic lifts, abdominal contractions and yogic manipulations of the breath and pelvic and abdominal muscles, all of which practices impacted very powerfully upon the pelvic organs, in particular the womb, the vagina and the ovaries. Some the practices involved held exhalations, pumping breaths and inverted held contractions and lifts of the abdominal wall. The teacher had been sharing these practices for three days. At no point had he issued any precautions relating to how the techniques might be unsuitable for women at certain points in their menstrual cycles or life stages.

For Lou, who had flown specially into London to take her yoga practice to a deeper and more responsive place through this workshop, some of these practices were not only unsuitable but deeply uncomfortable. Lou had been practising yoga for twelve years and teaching for nine. But she wasn't just a *yoginī*. She was a mother, and she was still lactating, having arranged for her child (who usually had a feed of breastmilk only at night) to be cared for by family members. At the time of the workshop, Lou was nearing the onset of her menstrual bleed. Her periods had recently returned after a long period of lactational amenorrhoea (for more guidance on yoga suited to breastfeeding mothers please see chapter fourteen). At this time of the month, her joints were still soft, and her breasts and womb were both very full. She felt as if there was no space in the teaching style and content for her needs to be respected, or for other more suitable practices to be suggested. Some of Lou's discomfort was also experienced by a number of other women who were menstruating or close to menstruation, but none of them felt able to voice their difficulties with the practices, until I brought the issue into the open by publicly asking the teacher to give some guidelines for women's practice of these techniques. I waited until the third day of the event before doing this because initially I had trusted that such a well-regarded teacher would naturally include sensible precautions and alternative practices for menstruating women. No such precautions had been voiced on the first day, and so halfway through the second day I had politely and privately requested that he share these precautions, suggesting that it would be good practice to demonstrate awareness of how to meet women's needs since there were so many yoga teachers in the group who may well model their teaching on his approach. But after the private suggestion was not followed through, I began to worry that in fact the teacher saw no need to identify any of the practices as unsuitable for women at certain times in our lives.

I had initially been mildly irritated by the fact that the visiting teacher continually referred to us all as '*yogīs*' instead of '*yoginīs*', even though there were only seven *yogīs* in the room, including him, and so women outnumbered men by eleven to one. But it began to dawn on me that this grammatical slip was actually evidence of a kind of gender blindness based on an inability to understand that women may experience things differently from men. This is not equality, it is ignorance, and it can be harmful. After a particularly intense practice of *uḍḍīyāna bandha* and *agnisāra kriyā*, one of the women students reported in the group Q&A with the teacher that she had felt discomfort in her pelvis as she did this technique. In his response to her, the teacher made no mention of the impact of such pumping abdominal lifts on the womb. He wondered instead how she was holding her lower spine, and expressed a belief that the practice should cause no pain if it was done with the spine in the right position. At this point, his disregard for the presence of the eighty-two wombs in the room was so clearly inimical to women's health that I felt the need to voice my concerns in public. 'During menstruation,' I offered, 'this practice is not comfortable.' The teacher nodded. 'I usually suggest women practitioners avoid it at this time. Would you say this is a wise precaution?' He said that it was. The twenty-five percent of the women in the room who were menstruating began to wonder why he had not issued this precaution in the previous two days, but he smiled a gorgeous smile, and they forgave him.

Sensing that something useful might come out of this I followed up with the observation that during ovulation these practices could also cause discomfort, 'Ovulation?' he said incredulously, 'Really? How would you know?' I assured him that it was entirely possible for a woman to know when she was ovulating, and that tenderness in the belly at this time could make these practices uncomfortable. He was ready to admit that perhaps during menstruation or pregnancy there were precautions to be observed, but seemed surprised to learn that there were other aspects of womb life that might also be observable, and that these parts of the cycle might also demand respect. Chancing my arm, I offered the final observation that women seeking to conceive would do well to avoid all these pumping breaths and strong *bandhas*. The teacher was so evidently astonished about the suggestion that ovulation might be a noticeable disincentive to the practice of *agnisāra kriyā* that he seemed keen to disregard this last observation about the adverse effects on the energies of conception. He continued to teach these practices for the next two days to eighty-two women with no further mention of the need for anyone to amend or adapt any of the practices.

I heard later from Lou that after I had left the training (a prior obligation meant I could not stay for the final two days), the issue of menstrual cycle awareness had come up again. I was not surprised. Out of the eighty-two women in the group, it was likely, at a conservative estimate, that about eighteen of them could have been menstruating. Lou explained that the visiting teacher had moved on to speak about *svara*, and the need for respect for the cycles of breath: 'He addressed the different qualities of awareness within those cycles. It seemed like a great opportunity to get his perspective on the *mahā svara* – the great cycles of womb life, and so I asked about the different qualities of consciousness at times in the menstrual cycle and what yoga practices he would suggest to support these experiences.' Like many of the people attending this workshop, Lou was a yoga teacher herself, and she was looking for guidance to share practices safely with her students. She had been teaching for nine years, and for six of those years she had focused her attentions on yoga for women's health. Lou had been hoping that the master teacher would have some understanding of what she was talking about, and that his yoga experience would enable him to offer practices that would both assist her professional development as a teacher, and deepen her encounter with the spiritual dimensions of the changes in awareness she experienced as part of her cycles of menstruation.

But he simply denied that there could be any shifts of consciousness associated with the cycle. 'He looked a bit perturbed about the question. First he asked where Uma was,' laughed Lou 'he said she was the "womb expert round here". Then he mentioned a couple of books on the subject. But in the end he just squashed the question. He said that shifts in consciousness were not part of the menstrual cycle.' Shocked by his denial, Lou pointed out to the teacher that she had herself experienced visionary psychic awareness during menstruation, and other forms of consciousness at other points in her cycle, and that the awareness she had developed through her yoga practice helped her to perceive these shifts. 'He didn't want to hear it. He said it didn't happen. He said the menstrual cycle was just a physical thing.' What astonished Lou was not so much that the teacher had no good answer to her question, but that he used his position of authority to deny the reality of her own experience. 'It would have been fine for him just to say that he did not know, that it was out of his experience. But he didn't say that. He said that he did know, and he told me what I had experienced in my own cycle awareness was simply not possible.' She decided not to go back to this particular teacher. 'But what about the other women there?' I asked, 'Did anyone else respond?' Lou told me that the women on either side of her had commented that the answers the teacher had given were ' "Not very satisfactory". They weren't very pleased either.' But he had smiled and everyone stayed on for the rest of the workshop. No one mentioned menstruation again.

It is one thing to be ignorant of the effects on a woman's consciousness of the menstrual cycle, but it is quite another thing to speak with authority on the subject, thus presenting ignorance as knowledge. When international teachers arrive in town, they carry with them a reputation for knowledge and wisdom. Unfortunately, sometimes that knowledge can be patchy, and one of the gaps in many teachers' knowledge relates to the experiences of women in yoga. Because the training he was offering had been identified as *tantra*, and because the teacher identified himself as a 'master teacher', I had arrived with the impression that he would have some knowledge of the *tāntrik* tradition of reverence for female teachers, which I discuss in the next chapter. But when he was asked to speak about these lineages of female *tāntrik gurus*, he professed that he knew of no such people. Perhaps this was out of respect to female teachers of his acquaintance whose identity he may have had an obligation to protect by secrecy, and perhaps it was because he was genuinely ignorant of these lineages of female teachers. Either way, his ignorance of the place of women within the tradition of which he claimed to be so knowledgeable seemed directly linked to his denial of the spiritual relevance of changes in consciousness through the menstrual cycle. At the level of physical practice, his utter disregard for the presence of eighty wombs in the room was rooted in his own ignorance of what difference it might make to a yoga practitioner to have a womb or a menstrual cycle at all. His responses to our queries seemed not to be motivated by any deliberate desire to cause harm or discomfort, but rather simply revealed the fact that he had just never thought about what it might be like to practise *agnisāra kriyā* with a womb whose lining was full of blood, or how a woman's state of consciousness might truly expand at menstruation. Any person who has thought this through would at least acknowledge the massive shifts in awareness that can accompany the menstrual cycle and would certainly offer menstruating women options for alternative practices or rest times. And this is what some teachers in the Iyengar and *aṣṭaṅga vinyāsa* traditions of yoga practice often do.

In Iyengar yoga schools, menstruating women are often offered the opportunity to practise more restorative poses within their usual class under the guidance of their teacher, and in the practice of *aṣṭaṅga vinyāsa* yoga, especially as it is practised in Mysore, the home of the late Pattabhi Jois's yoga *śālā*, the preferred approach is to encourage menstruating women to take a 'ladies' holiday'. These holidays are in addition to the observation of 'moon days', where practice at full and new moons is cancelled. So for women who bleed at either of these times, then the observation of the moon days in itself constitutes an opportunity to avoid practice at menstruation, and the 'ladies' holidays' additionally provide this option for women whose cycles are not in synch with lunar phases. So built into the rhythms of this practice, and within the structure of the usual Iyengar yoga teacher trainings, is the opportunity for women to respond to the rhythms of their own cycles and either to skip practice or to work in a more restorative manner during menstruation. But women do not always choose to do either of these things. From the numerous reports I've received from female practitioners of *aṣṭaṅga vinyāsa*, many women students and teachers pay little attention to the changing needs of the female body during menstrual cycles, and sometimes also during pregnancy and postnatal recovery. The long-term effects of a continued and uninterrupted daily practice of vigorous yoga *āsana* that disregards the cycles of women's lives can result, judging from a plethora of anecdotal evidence, in subfertility, constipation, prolonged second stage labour and cessation of menstruation altogether (often for years at a time). Whilst the traditional manner of sharing these teachings of *haṭha* yoga offers opportunities to honour women's cycles, these opportunities are not always taken.

Disconnection

'If you don't tell me, how will I know you're bleeding?'

Over a period of about ten years I had the good fortune to attend workshops with a leading senior teacher from the Iyengar tradition who travelled and taught internationally. His approach to yoga as a form of self-discovery and empowerment was rooted in the Iyengar approach to *āsana*, and suffused with a clarity of thought and expression that flowed from his own experience, including early encounters with Integral yoga as taught by Swami Satchidananda. His classes were full of philosophical gems of understanding and awareness, expressed with wit, humour and humility. His annual visits to London provided me with opportunities for great learning that I valued immensely. At a certain point he recommended that the best way to go deeper with this approach to yoga would be to attend a teachers' retreat.

When I arrived at the beautiful Italian retreat space, a number of the participants had already been in residence for a previous week of yoga. There were nine women and four men. A feature of the place where we were staying was that some of the women shared a communal bathroom with a metal bin for the disposal of sanitary towels and tampons. This bathroom was used by all the women during the day, so that we were inevitably aware of each other's sanitary disposal activities. When I began menstruating on the fourth day of the retreat I knew that I was not bleeding alone. Judging from the contents of the bin in the women's bathroom, I estimated that through the week about four other women had also been bleeding, and my estimate was confirmed by the massage therapist working at the retreat, who had massaged all of the women on retreat, and who expressed her concern that women were 'pushing themselves too hard' in the twice daily classes, especially when they were menstruating. And this is also what I saw for myself.

Despite the fact that at least four of us were bleeding during the time of the retreat, it was only me who shared this experience with our teacher. As a well-trained and highly experienced senior Iyengar teacher, he was familiar with a whole sequence of supported restorative seated and lying poses that are perfectly suited to encourage a positive experience of menstruation as a cleansing, quiet and rejuvenative experience. I was glad to engage with these practices over the heavier flow days of my period, and to return to the general programme after a couple of days. I felt nourished and refreshed by the experience, and had enjoyed the opportunity that our teacher gave me to encounter this approach to practice.

I was also astonished that none of the other women who had their period during the retreat told our teacher that they were menstruating. If they had, they knew that his duty of care to them would have obliged him to encourage alternative practice. His obligation to do this was rooted in the fact that his training and experience led him to view menstruation as a time to avoid most standing poses or any vigorous forms of yoga practice. From a professional point of view, if he knew a woman was menstruating, it would be irresponsible for him to allow her to continue with the demanding level of practice that he was offering in the class. His skills and understanding as a teacher obliged him to respect the experience of menstruating students by offering a type of practice that supported and nourished their flow. But his capacity to respond appropriately to menstruating students depended upon him being informed about whether or not a woman had her period. By not telling the teacher that they were menstruating, the women on the retreat disempowered themselves and their teacher: they denied the reality of their own experience and refused the opportunity for rest, regeneration and nurture which the alternative practice offered. Rather than accept the nature of the cyclical wisdom which menstruation can teach, they preferred to carry on as usual. By this practice of denial they created a relationship with themselves and their teacher that was based on deception. Being thus deceived, the teacher was denied the opportunity to encourage more suitable practices that would empower the women to honour their cycle. Having thus deceived themselves, the women were free to practise the general yoga programme during menstruation. As a result of this, they were sustaining physical and emotional injuries. To deny the presence of the menstrual cycle is a form of self-harm. The self-harm affects every level of being, and there was a lot of suffering as a result of this on the retreat. The massage therapist, who was privy to these experiences, expressed her concerns about what was occurring, and placed the blame squarely on the teacher: 'He is really pushing everyone very hard'.

From her perspective, it was the practices that the teacher was offering which were causing the injuries and emotional disturbances; they were 'too demanding', the schedule was 'too intense', and the energy in the class was a powerful incentive to 'overdo it'. The injuries his students sustained were his fault. Certainly this was the reputation that this teacher carried. However, from another perspective, this was only half the story. The perspective which I had, as a menstruating woman whose physical and emotional experiences had been caringly and expertly supported by this teacher, revealed that the injuries and harm sustained by female students in these classes were largely caused by their own refusal or inability to respect themselves: because they did not honour their menstruation by informing the teacher, they actually had placed him in a position where he was unable to offer the support and nurture which he clearly, willingly and ably offered to me.

The paradox is very clear; in this situation, the offer to receive skilful support and respect for the experience of menstruation is refused, and the capacity for yoga practice to nurture and nourish women's embodied experience of their own wisdom is turned against itself. For all sorts of profound and complex reasons, many women in yoga now seem to find it very hard to accept the invitation to honour their own cyclical nature, even when that invitation is offered with love and respect. It is as if, when women in yoga are offered the keys to freedom and self-knowledge, we may use those keys to lock ourselves inside an ersatz-yoga prison of our own making. The yogic keys to self-acceptance become tools for self-denial and confinement. This paradox lies at the heart of my deep concerns about how yoga can end up harming women, and contribute to our failure to own any self responsibility and spiritual authority, instead of helping us to grow in freedom, confidence and strength.

The paradox of disempowerment through yoga is that we may embrace its practice in such a way as to deny ourselves access to the results of that practice. If we allow ourselves or others to be discouraged from asking important questions of our lineage holders; if we collude with inter-lineage disrespect; if we permit our teachers to disregard the presence of our wombs; if we disconnect our own consciousness from the wisdom of our bodies, then we will always need to be looking outside for the source of the light that shines from within, and we will experience a profound disconnection from our own inner teacher. It is this disconnection that disempowers us.

There is a vicious circle here: for it is because of the profound disconnection from our own inner sense of what is right for us that we choose to practise the forms of yoga which further disempower us. In particular, when we adhere rigorously, and without regard for our own life cycles, to those versions of yoga practice that focus on maintaining power over the body, rather than experiencing power moving through the body, then we imprison ourselves. Practising these forms of yoga in this way is not really yoga at all: it has become instead a response to the cultural pressures of our society that leads us to feel that we need to practise yoga in the first place. Donna Farhi has described how certain approaches to yoga practice are now 'being used to create a very strong, explicit identification with the body… It has become part of the pathology of the culture and it's feeding into that pathology' (Farhi in Gates: 45).

It is as if the disconnection that is a feature of our own culture has become a characteristic of the forms of yoga that we seek to practise. Yoga was traditionally taught within sacred, philosophical frameworks and in the context of the temple or the forest hermitage. Contemporary yoga, on the other hand, is most often located in a health club, or a gym. There are many stories to be told about how and where the yoga transformed into a variety of physical culture. Whether or not this happened before or after yoga got out of India and headed west, it is undeniable now that contemporary yoga is largely about the practice of *āsana* for health and beauty. These side effects of yoga have become the central focus of many contemporary *yogīs*' attention. Many yoga centres feel more like a health club than a temple or a forest *aṣram*. The governing body for yoga in England (the British Wheel of Yoga) was selected and endorsed by Sport England. This relocation of yoga from the temple to the gym, and its identification as part of the 'body beautiful culture' of health clubs has not only altered the environment in which yoga is transmitted, but has soaked deep into the fabric of the practice of yoga. Mother Maya puts it like this: 'Yoga came to the west to change the west. But the west has changed yoga.' We have created forms of yoga in the image of our own disconnection. Practising in this way simply mirrors our own disregard for our inner guide.

EMPOWERMENT OF WOMEN'S YOGA PRACTICE THROUGH EXPLORATION, WELCOMING, OPEN SHARING, HONOURING AND RECONNECTION

As the previous quartet of stories from today's studios show, there are many aspects of contemporary yoga practice that can disconnect female practitioners from the light of their own inner truth. It is disheartening to know that such disempowerment is widespread. But once we identify the forms and causes of these disempowerments, then we are in a position to replace them with their opposites. This is a practice of *rājā yoga* called *pratipakṣa bhāvana*, and is described by Pātañjali in the *Yoga Sūtra* (2:33). Once we learn to recognise the adverse impact of the discouragement of questioning, or of disrespect for other traditions, or of the negative energies of secrecy, of disregard for womb cycles and disconnection from the inner teacher, then we can find an antidote for their ill effects. These four negative aspects find their positive opposites in the key qualities of a more feminine approach to yoga.

The antidotes to these constraints empower women: by encouraging exploration and questions, welcoming and sharing openly relevant wisdom from all traditions and lineages, honouring womb cycles and life cycles, and reconnecting to the inner teacher. This approach leads to an empowered and intelligent, responsive practice of yoga. It is of relevance to everyone who practises yoga, but it is of special significance to women practising now, when there is a staggeringly wide range of traditions, lineages and organisations offering trainings and classes. These four qualities of exploration, welcoming, honouring and reconnecting can be hard to find in many of the most popular forms of yoga taught in huge classes in commercial studios. But if you search diligently, then it is possible to uncover these positive qualities both within traditional lineage-specific approaches to yoga, and in the contemporary hybrid and eclectic approaches to yoga. It depends more upon the responsiveness and sensitivity of the teacher than upon the label they give to the yoga they teach.

These four qualities are clearly evident in the work of many women teachers who have contributed to the development of yoga practice since 1890, and whose stories were told at the start of this chapter. This empowering approach to the teaching and practice of yoga can be found in the work of male and female teachers: it thrives wherever awareness is acute enough for teachers to perceive that to serve yoga students well is to empower them to heed the wisdom of their inner teacher.

There is a global proliferation now of yoga teacher training courses. Many of the better courses have embraced the challenge of offering an eclectic range of teachings that compare traditional lineages, whilst empowering graduates of the trainings to ask questions, explore their own experiences and respect and honour their own inner guide. Teachers trained well in such a way can be more inclined to empower their own students because the model of their own formation as a teacher is rooted in exploration: a process of discovery rather then reception. Teaching yoga with an attitude of openness to questioning, and a welcoming and open sharing of the wisdom of other traditions can lead students to respect their own needs and reconnect with the source of insight and wisdom that eventually renders their good teachers redundant. The students walk free.

When these four qualities are all present, then yoga ceases to be a prison that constrains women by discouragement, disrespect, disregard and disconnection, and it can become an experience of real freedom and spaciousness. Instead of discouraging questions, this approach to yoga encourages exploration. Instead of disrespecting traditions other than our own, we welcome all relevant wisdom, and share what we know with others. Instead of disregarding the presence of the womb, we honour and respect her cycles. Instead of creating situations that disconnect students from the wisdom of their own bodies, we promote a rediscovery of embodied insight. This experience of rediscovery and reconnection empowers students to find and follow the guidance of their heart. Such an approach to yoga empowers us to love and respect the inner teacher. This experience is at the heart of womb yoga.

Extract from a Burren yoga retreat diary – Womb yoga

I am writing this by the light of a samhain (hallowe'een) full moon in the west of Ireland – just before dawn on 23 October 2010. The full moon is shining above in the sky, which is still dark, and a cock is crowing. Asleep but now stirring in the retreat house are fifteen women who have travelled here from all over Ireland and England, and from the Czech Republic to do yoga that gives soulful experience and succour at this time of struggle and change.

The work that I have come to share with these women is part of a kaleidoscope of unfolding beauty and creative engagement with haṭha *yoga and related disciplines of self care, ritual and spiritual insight. Women are ready to hear what is being said, and to engage with what is being shared. I have a clear sense now that all those teachers who have been shining the light of yoga into the dark and difficult corners of women's lies and lives, have been bringing the consciousness of yoga to illuminate the challenges of mothering, menstruating and birthing, or menopause and menarche. Through the practice of empowered yoga, consciousness and heightened awareness has been brought to these experiences in order to enable women to sense for themselves that these challenges are special gifts and special times, special abilities,* siddhis *in fact. Once that awareness is gained then change can happen – once there is a change in the consciousness of the women about the remarkable capacities of their own bodies and an acknowledgment of their own spiritual authority through the possession of these siddhis.*

It is a deep blessing to have the opportunity to lead retreats and yoga holidays here at the yoga and meditation centre in the Burren, a place of great wild beauty in the west of Ireland. The first three times that I came to work at this magical place it was to run training course and retreat weeks that were exclusively aimed at women only. But this time the retreat director decided to open the work up to men, and so the retreat was advertised simply as a yoga weekend open to men and women. It is a full moon weekend, at Samhain, the turning of the year, a time traditionally believed to be full of magical openings and opportunities, and this year it is fortuitously blessed by Irish governmental bureaucracy with an official national holiday (whose specific placement, on the last Monday in October, means that this particular bank holiday chimes very beautifully in with the Samhain full moon, even though as a national holiday it is not primarily intended to honour lunar cycles). The bank holiday has made it a very attractive time to get away, since the whole country has the Monday off. The retreat has sold out.

As I was travelling towards County Galway all I knew was that all fifteen places on the retreat were taken, and the last three places had only been booked in the final week. When I arrived and began to meet the retreatants I discovered all fifteen were women. Had we planned for this women only group, the women asked? No. But the message is clear. Women need yoga. Each one of the women has been moved to join the retreat because of issues and challenges in their lives that are specifically feminine, and one after another on this first evening of individual interviews before the group class, the women spoke of their experiences: two have had hysterectomies in the past year, some are recovering from relationship break-ups or are grieving for the loss of their partners, there are two sisters together, come to support and encourage each other, one who has come because her sister herself was a yoga teacher and had encouraged her, another has been guided by a woman friend who had worked with me previously. There are young women at turning points in their lives, realising that the working environment in which they have been struggling was not nourishing them, and there are older women who are looking for something deeply soulful to nourish and heal the special sort of suffering that comes to women of spirit who find no place in their lives to express and honour their femininity. There are mothers whose bodies and minds are exhausted from decades of giving and serving their families. There are teachers and nurses, mothers and maidens, women who work outside in the country, and women whose bodies are stiff and painful from years of being sat inside at computers. Above all, they are tired. They come to yoga to get back into their bodies, for all their physical limitations, they come to yoga for healing, comfort, guidance, direction, pain relief, insight, and deep rest.

These women on this retreat are a microcosm of the whole universe of women in yoga. It is my privilege and honour to serve these women through the teaching and sharing of yoga. In response to their very specific, but universally representative needs, I share with them an approach to yoga that is adaptive and responsive. I share womb greetings and teach techniques that encourage each women to foster her own connection between heart and womb, between love and power. I teach fluid sequences and deep resting poses, and hand gestures of elegance and strength. Each woman is part of the group, sharing the core of the practices, but working in respectful response to her own needs.

Together in this practice of womb yoga we are evolving an approach to yoga that cultivates joy and freedom in women's lives and different life stages. We encourage questions, and openly draw from the wisdom of many different traditions and lineages. We honour the cycles of the women's wombs, the place of no-wombs, and the points in their life cycles. We share practices that help these women to reconnect to their own inner teacher, so that they may bring home with them the joy and freedom of practising yoga together in this place, and take this experience into their daily lives.

All that we do here can helpfully be understood as a process of 'un-doing' what has been done to the inspirational source of yoga: the great power of female siddhis.

WATCHING THE TIDE TURN: GUIDELINES FOR A PRACTICAL FEMININE YOGA CONSCIOUSNESS

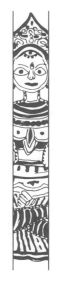

Think of the body of yoga knowledge and practice as a great ocean. It has waves and tides. I've been practising yoga since 1969, and have been involved in the training of hundreds of yoga teachers and yoga therapists. Over that time I have observed that the tidal patterns in the ocean of yoga have been changing.

I believe that the plethora of women doing yoga now is in fact a return to the source of yoga's initial inspiration. If we can see, as I propose in the next chapter, that the source motivation for all yoga practices may be a desire to develop technologies to catch the elemental connections that can be experienced as a naturally arising and powerful force within the vessel of a woman's body at certain times in her life, then the vast numbers of women 'doing yoga' is a sign that the ocean tide is turning. It is coming back in.

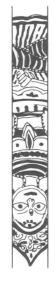

The ocean I imagine when I consider the vast sea of yoga is the part of the Atlantic off the south-west coast of Ireland in County Clare, where the ocean comes up against the most westerly edge of Europe. Here, at the south end of the semicircular bay of Kilkee Beach, is Duggerna Reef. On the inner edge of this reef, all along the shoreline, is a set of extraordinary pools called the Pollock Holes. The Pollock Holes are remarkable wells in the reef that fill with seawater so that during low tide, they remain full and deep (and quite chilly). They are beautiful, fascinating and perfect swimming holes. But when the Atlantic tides turn, the ocean comes back in and they disappear.

This is the way I understand what has happened with all the different schools and lineages of yoga: the great ocean tide of the original inspiration for all the yogic practices has gone out, and left us with a set of Pollock Holes, each one a perfect little ocean in itself, salty like the ocean and deep like the ocean and full of all the same fish and sea life that exist out in the deep ocean, but contained in a more accessible size, close to the shore, safe for us all to swim in. Indeed when the tide has gone out, then the Pollock Holes are the only place left to swim. They are magical places and much visited. The scale, depth and numbers of Pollock Holes are awe-inspiring. Calling Pollock Holes 'rock

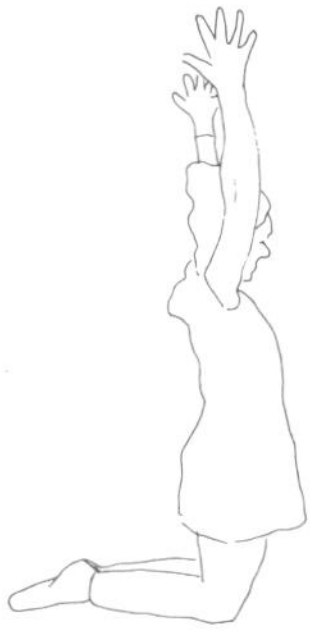

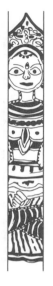

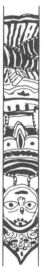

pools' is like calling the ocean a puddle. The Kilkee Pollock holes are to ordinary rock pools what Swami Sivananda or Sri T. Krishnamacharya are to the average yoga teacher in your local gym. There is simply no comparison.

But marvellous though they be, if we swim only in the Pollock Holes, then we miss the great force and abundance of the Atlantic that continally re-fills and renews them.

The inspirational source of the yoga project, the experience of women's mysteries, the female *siddhis* (presented in the next chapter) – that is the ocean. The marvellous range of Pollock Holes – that is the myriad of yoga lineages and schools that the ocean has filled. Although each different Pollock Hole may have its own unique micromarine ecosystem, they all share a common oceanic origin. The tide is turning, and the power of women's mysteries are returning, and when it does, the Pollock Holes will all overflow and become one with the ocean. Right now, at low tide, we can argue amongst ourselves about which lineage we're attached to, or which teachers are more authentic, or what place women have in any of this, as if we were debating which Pollock Hole we enjoy to swim in. But in the end, we were only swimming in the Pollock Holes in the first place because the tide had gone out; and the point of swimming in these magical rock pools was to prepare ourselves for the open sea. In the end, it doesn't really matter which Pollock Hole or lineage we're in, because the great flood tide of the ocean will inundate every hole until they all become one. And when that happens we will see that the Pollock Holes, and the yogic lineages they represent, are a set of separate containers for a superabundant force that is ultimately bigger and more powerful than all the lineages put together. The containers were very useful to preserve and maintain aspects of sea life at low tide, but when the waters of the ocean return, then the containers become redundant.

In terms of practical guidance for women doing yoga now, this is very good news. So much of the disempowerment of women in yoga has grown out of the disconnection from our inner teacher due to the limitations of lineage-specific teachings. And so much of the disregard for individual student needs that is especially inimical to women's well-being has been rooted in the disrespectful relations between different lineages. As the great ocean of yogic wisdom floods back in and reconnects all these separate rock pools, then practitioners are in a better position to connect with those forms of yoga practice that are most appropriate to them.

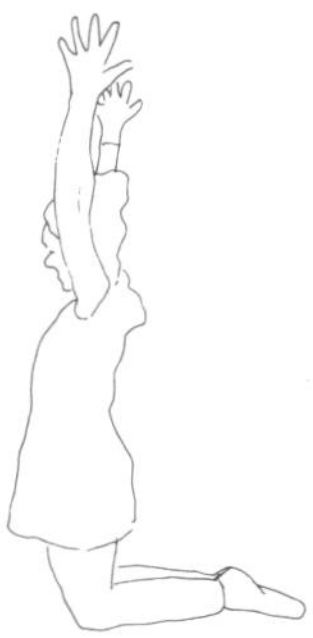

for women doing yoga now

I suggest that a respectful responsiveness to cyclical changes in our bodies is the most important aspect of our yogic awareness. It is our 'inner yoga'. To develop awareness of this kind it is crucial to hold women's bodies in respect. And to do this it is necessary in the first instance to withdraw our financial and energetic support from any organisation that exploits or abuses women under the guise of teaching yoga, for to support such structures is to dishonour ourselves and our sisters. Once we have reclaimed our energies from these structures, it is then possible to focus our attention on the cultivation of the kind of awareness that nourishes and respects our cyclical lives. To do this, it is helpful to include the following elements in all our yoga practice sessions, classes and trainings:

1. A warm and respectful welcome for each woman in the class: an opportunity to inform the facilitator of the group of our current place in the seasonal menstrual cycle, or in the cycles of our life experience. This can be offered briefly and poetically through a shorthand that refers to the 'inner seasons' of our menstrual cycles, for example 'I'm in high summer today,' or 'Last night I entered the first day of winter.' (For details on the seasonal metaphors for understanding the menstrual cycle, see chapter ten).
2. Good information about the effects of yoga practice on women, to enable informed decisions to be taken about whether to practise, for example, pumping breaths, *bandhas,* etc.
3. Accessible alternatives and modifications for women seeking to conceive, as well as for those who are pregnant, menstruating, lactating, and peri-, post-, and menopausal women, including those with osteoporosis and osteopaenia.
4. Respectful referrals to other forms of yoga practice that may be more suited to students than the form currently being shared.
5. A willingness for teachers to admit their/our ignorance when it comes to an understanding of the effects of a woman's monthly/life cycle experience on her yoga practice: a deference to the superior wisdom of each woman's inner teacher, the awareness that comes to her through her own recognition of her cyclical wisdom: she knows best what practices suit her.

(There are more complete guidelines and practical suggestions for 'womb-friendly' yoga practice on pp.582–8).

By expanding our yogic awareness to encompass these widely experienced aspects of women's health, then the practice of yoga becomes a way to connect to inner wisdom and guidance, respecting the body and her cycles, and honouring the cycles of the moon without and within. In the context of the great ocean of yogic wisdom, as the tide flows in with the cumulative knowledge and power of the whole history of yoga practice, then it is possible to respond appropriately to our life cycles as women by choosing wisely those practices that most support our health and well-being in the service of our spirit. In this environment, sharing and openness are the touchstones for a feminine practice of yoga. When we practise with full awareness of our femininity then yoga is an immensely powerful tool for the empowerment and uplift of women's spirit. Yoga then becomes a way of being at ease with oneself, a means to live consciously in a state of freedom. The practice of womb yoga can help this to happen.

The four chapters at the end of this first part of the book outline the practices of a yoga that awakens us to the feminine energy of the life force (chapter four), greets the womb with love (chapter five), honours the awakened energy of the life force (chapter six), and sets the whole experience of blood wisdom and womb yoga in a wider philosophical framework that has very ancient roots (chapter seven).

All of these practices trace their origins back to the earliest developments of the traditions of yoga and *śākta tantra* in the first few centuries of the common era and before. We are fortunate to have access to such an ancient system of guidance and empowerment. As with any ancient technology, it can be helpful to know the early history of its origins and development. And so, in the next chapter the pre-history of yoga as a path to freedom is explored from the perspective of contemporary *yoginīs*.

QUESTIONS AND REFLECTIONS

I invite you to explore your own experience of practising yoga by asking yourself some of the following questions:

1. How many of my own teachers, or authors of favourite yoga books, have been women, and how many of them have been men?
2. Are there differences and/or similarities between the yoga teachings that I have received/am receiving from male and female teachers, especially in relation to my experiences of menstruation / pregnancy / menopause?
3. How can I describe those differences and/or similarities, and how did/do they affect me?
4. How do my female teachers handle the fact of their own menstruation / pregnancy / postnatal recovery and/or menopause in relation to yoga? For example, are they open about their place in their own menstrual cycle, and do they make any changes to their manner of teaching or

demonstrating during menstruation/pregnancy? What impact does this have upon their ability to empower me to live in freedom with who I am and how my body is when I attend their classes or do the practices I have learnt from them?

5 What has been the relationship between my experiences of menstruation / pregnancy / postnatal recovery and/or menopause and my desire to practise yoga?

FURTHER READING AND RESEARCH

The most comprehensive and detailed history of female yoga teachers in the west is **Anne O'Brien**'s unpublished thesis (2010), which is the basis of her forthcoming book on the subject.

The surveys of women in yoga produced by **Janice Gates** (2006) and **Eric Shaw** (2011) are both accessible starting points to find out more about the contribution of women teachers to the development of contemporary yoga.

The perspectives of **Elizabeth de Michelis** (2004) and **Mark Singleton** (2010) on the evolution of Modern Postural yoga both provide detailed historical evidence that is fascinating to read if you are happy with footnotes and scholarly arguments.

For practical guidance on inspirational feminine approaches to yoga practice, the writings and teachings of **Judith Lasater** (1995, 2000) and **Donna Farhi** (2003) provide excellent guidance.

The resources produced by **Angela Farmer** (2000), and at **www.angela-victor.com** and by **Mother Maya Tiwari** (2000, 2010) both offer precious and profound insights from the perspective of *yoginīs* whose life and practice have been shaped by their experiences of vulnerability and deep challenge as young women.

The explorations of *cakras* by **Caroline Shola Arewa** (1998) provides a valuable feminine approach to esoteric anatomy and yoga practice that is uniquely informed by African perspectives.

More traditional guidance on yoga practice for women from within the established Indian yoga lineages of Iyengar and Satyananda respectively are to be found in the work of **Geeta Iyengar** ([1983] 2002) and **Swamis Satyananda** and **Muktananda Saraswati** ([1977] 1992).

CHAPTER TWO

women in the pre-history and early development of yoga

> *...Yoga is not a myth, buried in oblivion. It is the most valuable inheritance of the present. It is the essential need of today and the culture of tomorrow. (Saraswati, S 2007)*

> *As a category for thinking about yoga, 'authenticity' falls short and says far more about our 21st-century insecurities than it does about the practice of yoga... Beyond mere history for history's sake, learning about yoga's recent past gives us a necessary and powerful lens for seeing our relationship with tradition, ancient and modern. At its best, modern yoga scholarship is an expression of today's most urgently needed yogic virtue,* viveka *("discernment" or "right judgment"). (Singleton 2010a)*

> *...any authority that women assume today will not be a dramatic new development made possible by Western feminism, but a reclamation of the precise dynamics that gave rise to this [*tāntrik*] tradition. (Shaw, M 1996: 5)*

HOW DID WE GET HERE? CONSIDERING THE ROOTS OF YOGA, EXPLORING THE ROUTES OF YOGA

The longer something has been around, the more stories there are to tell about it. Yoga has been around a good long while. The simple story is that it is certainly very old. Some stories tell us that people have been practising yoga for six thousand years. The written accounts of *haṭha* yoga are medieval, but the philosophies upon which *haṭha* yoga rests are at least three thousand years old. There is no doubt that the practice of yoga preceded any written documentation. This is why some inspired practitioners, eager to claim truly ancient Indian roots, trace yoga back over six thousand years, and some scholars settle for three thousand years.

Most of the traditional lineages that train yoga teachers have an investment in maintaining the 'mythic' or pre-historic origins of yoga, and discouraging too many difficult questions about exact dates and historical evidence. These kinds of stories seek to create a sense of unbroken tradition that reaches back into the 'mists of time' in order to imbue the current *guru*s of any given lineage with a quasi-mythic authority to speak on behalf of the ancient seers. From these perspectives, it can seem as if the ancient practices of yoga were handed directly down through the tradition, perfectly preserved, like a fossil.

In contrast, more recent researchers have revealed that many yogic lineages' claims to have preserved the 'mythical origins' of yoga practice are questionable. Contemporary yoga scholars have observed, for example, how complex political and social influences have prompted many different transformations of yoga, all of which have their own perspectives on the origins of the practice. Alternative, feminist perspectives on the history of yoga have offered arguments for global matriarchal, Palaeolithic origins of yoga practice in ecstatic dance and shamanism.

If you are looking for explanations of the origins of yoga, then there are many versions from which to choose, each one taking a different angle. Indeed there are many different perspectives on what yoga itself can be, and many possible explanations for the 'origins' of each 'yoga'. This creates a kaleidoscope of overlapping, sometimes contrasting accounts of all of these different 'origins'. Some have more scholarly credentials than others. There are academic studies, hagiographies, philosophical explorations, radical feminist rewritings, neo-pagan poesy and much controversy and confusion raging around the claims to have found the authentic origins of yoga.

When things are this old, so many stories have been told that it is hard to be completely certain about how they started and who started them. The proliferation of stories means that to endeavour to pin down one particular origin as the pure source of 'authenticity' of a single yoga tradition is neither truly possible nor especially valuable. It is far more fruitful to engage in careful historical and textual explorations of the many ways in which yoga has been practised, developed and changed over time, as Mark Singleton has very helpfully pointed out in relation to his own investigations of 'Modern Postural yoga' (Singleton 2010).

What we know about the origins of the yoga we practise can have an effect on our experience of yoga. To a degree our understanding becomes part of what we think we are doing when we practise yoga. The stories are powerful. And if there are so many stories to be told, then it does matter which ones we hear, because what we hear is part of what we experience as yoga. So it is helpful to encounter this tangle of tales as a manifestation of yoga's profound significance to very many different types of people, and to recognise that there are quite a number of perspectives to be taken on the evidently ancient origins of yoga. If each of these views together creates a fuller picture of the whole yogic project, then we can better place ourselves and our practice in a reverent and informed relation to that impressive and now sprawling range of technologies for transformation that we call yoga. It is worth listening to at least some of the stories with attentive ears, especially if they are not so widely told. The intention of this chapter is to open our ears to some of the stories that help us to understand a little more clearly the place of women in the history of yoga.

For example, in recent years, alternative histories of India, yoga and matrifocal spirituality have helped us to see that although women have been at the periphery of major lineages and traditions of *haṭha* yoga, the female presence 'outside' the orthodoxy has certainly shaped and informed the growth of yoga (Gates 2006, Noble 2011). Equally, stories being told now about the study and living practice of *śākta tantra*, in particular encounters with devotional structures related to *Durgā*, the sixty-four *Yoginīs* and the Great Wisdom Goddesses (Amazzone 2010, Chopra 2006, Frawley [1994] 1996, Johnsen 1999), show how some of those traditions on the fringes of what most people understand to be yoga may hold the key to an holistic living yoga practice that is especially resonant for female practitioners. These alternative perspectives help us to recognise that what may be seen to be absent from the usual histories of yoga, in particular the bloody nature of women's mysteries, may well resonate profoundly with the original inspirations and aim of the broader *tāntrik* yoga project: to harness the energy of our awareness to help us realise a vivid encounter with the power of pure consciousness.

Opening our ears to hear all these stories helps us to know what yoga can be for us now. This chapter shares a selection of yoga origin stories. I bring together the orthodox and unorthodox, the his-stories and her-stories of yoga's development, so as to invite awareness of how the simultaneous presence of all these different tales opens space to welcome some of the mysteries in yoga: in the form of the possibilities of woman-centred, intuited mysteries of womb yoga in the next chapter.

HISTORIES OF YOGA: THE DEVELOPMENT OF *HAṬHA* YOGA

Most orthodox histories of *haṭha* yoga, especially those delivered on yoga teacher training courses, are usually told through a limited survey of those written sources readily available in English translations, starting with the *Ṛg Veda* and winding towards Patañjali's *Yoga Sūtra* and Svātmārāma's *Haṭha Yoga Pradīpikā*, leaving unaccounted the centuries of development that lies between these three texts. They usually stop at that point, leaping over a six-hundred-year gap until the arrival of contemporary yoga schools. The notion that the *Yoga Sūtra*, the *Haṭha Yoga Pradīpikā* and other medival manuals such as the *Śiva Saṁhitā* and the *Gheraṇḍa Saṁhitā* in fact comprise a 'canon' of *haṭha* yoga manuals is a modern idea, the result of a revived textual tradition. There may well be a huge gap between this newly created, 'textual history' of yoga and the reality of how the medieval *haṭha yogīs* actually lived and practised.

Recent yoga scholarship, for example by Singleton and De Michelis, and new translation projects by Mallinson, are all helping to bridge that gap, and the first chapter of this book has also endeavoured to reveal the important place of women in the historical growth of modern yoga practice. To understand all these histories of yoga, it is helpful to see links between the practical foundations of *haṭha* yoga (in texts from the third to the seventeenth centuries), and the philosophical soil in which these practices grew.

The earth that nourishes the roots of the philosophies from which yoga developed is very rich. It comprises many different types of soils, all mixed together, including the Vedic and shamanic traditions, early *tantra*, and a complex network of Indian philosophies that includes Buddhism. The oldest elements of this loam are Vedic: by broad definition this includes all the collections of rituals, incantations and philosophical reflections from ancient India, starting with the four collections which form the *Vedas* proper, up to and including the *Upaniṣads*. The oldest Vedic scripture is the *Ṛg Veda Saṁhitā* that was composed (or received, depending on your perspective) by nomads in the Punjab nearly four thousand years ago, between 1700 and 1500 BCE. It wasn't actually written down until the turn of the common era. Just like the later yogic texts, which codified systems of practice that had been well-established long before they were ever recorded in writing, the written text of the *Ṛg Veda* is widely understood to have been preceded by an older, purely oral tradition, in which the hymns it contains were sung and chanted, and preserved and passed on through memory. The other three *Vedas*, *Yajur*, *Sāma* and *Atharva*, were composed (or received) around three thousand years ago (1200–900 BCE). Scholarly debates about the origins of the *Vedas* are endless and, depending on your taste for this kind of discussion, varyingly fascinating or pointless. Each of the *Vedas* has within it a number of different parts. The earliest parts of the *Vedas* explaining rituals and sacrificial ceremonies are referred to as the *Brāhmaṇa*, whilst the portions that are believed to have been composed by later forest dwellers are referred to as the *Āraṇyaka*.

The *Upaniṣads* (literally, to 'sit close by and listen') are the most recent, more philosophically reflective parts of the Vedic literature. There are only about twelve to fourteen of these *Upaniṣads* that are considered to be truly 'Vedic'. These earliest *Upaniṣads* were composed c.700–600 BCE and the later ones, of which there are hundreds, were composed between 400 BCE and the turn of the common era. It is the *Upaniṣads* that offer the most reflective examination of the philosophical truths that grew out of, and in response to, the Vedic world-view. It is only in these later *Upaniṣads* like the *Kaṭha* and *Śvetāsvatara Upaniṣads* (c.300 BCE) that we find any direct mention of yoga or any practical instructions for the practice of yoga. Yoga, in so far as it is both a means and an end (the process of cultivating heightened awareness and the awareness itself), is in the *Upaniṣads*. But texts specifically about yoga techniques to attain such awareness generally (with the exception of the *Kaṭha Upaniṣad*) come after the *Upaniṣads*, and were influenced by the post-*Saṁhitā* Vedic philosophies such as *Sāṁkhya* (see chapter seven). This means that, in addition to being steeped in the *Vedas*, the later codifiers of yogic practice and philosophy would also have been familiar with philosophies such those in *Sāṁkhya* and the *Upaniṣads*. In particular, the development of the practice of yoga as a tool for self-discovery can be seen partly as a reaction against the emphasis on ritual for ritual's sake that is characteristic of the earlier parts of the *Vedas*. The later yogic codifiers would also have been familiar with the philosophical developments of Buddhist thought. From this rich soil, in which were combined both Vedic and non-Vedic philosophical and spiritual influences, grew the fertile tree of *haṭha* yoga, which has borne, and continues to bear, many remarkable fruits.

The oldest extant written reference specifically and exclusively for yoga practice is the *Yoga Sūtra* of Patañjali, which is usually dated somewhere between the first and second century CE, but is generally accepted to codify a system of practice that existed for many years prior to being written down. The *Yoga Sūtra* is a set of aphorisms that tersely condense a profoundly rich approach to meditation, ethics and spirituality. There is no description of complex physical postures or *āsana* in the *Yoga Sūtra*, save for the guidance that the *yogi* should be able to sit steadily and comfortably.

It is in later works such as the *Haṭha Yoga Pradīpikā* (c. sixteenth century), the *Gheraṇḍa Saṁhitā* (c. eighteenth century) and the *Śiva Saṁhitā* (c. sixteenth century) that the more complex technologies of breath and body control and cleansing are set out. These are some of the texts upon which rest all the *haṭha* yoga lineages which now present yoga to contemporary practitioners, even though, as yoga scholars and practitioners such as Mark Singleton (2010) and Georg Feuerstein (1998) have pointed out, many (but not all) of the forms of yoga now taught in the west sometimes bear little outward resemblance to the practices laid out in these early yogic texts. Certainly historical, cultural and economic pressures have come to bear on the development of yoga, and these medieval practices have taken many complex routes before arriving at the contemporary forms of yoga that are currently so popular. That is another story, well told in other places (Singleton 2010). But ultimately, when modern yoga practitioners and teachers look for roots, many claim to find at least most of them in the philosophy and practices set out in the *Yoga Sūtra*, the *Haṭha Yoga Pradīpikā*, the *Gheraṇḍa Saṁhitā* and the *Śiva Saṁhitā*.

'NO WOMEN PLEASE, WE'RE YOGIS.' WAS CLASSICAL *HAṬHA* YOGA FOR BOYS ONLY?

It is important to understand that, in the context of the medieval yoga world, the emphasis upon asceticism, concerns about 'pollution' (especially from menstrual blood) and a range of other strictures related to caste and gender indicate that all of these texts are written entirely from the male perspective, and that they clearly describe practices intended for male bodies, taught by men to men. From reading these texts it is clear that hardly any women were invited to the *haṭha* yoga party. With the exception of three verses in the *Haṭha Yoga Pradīpikā* that describe how both male and female practitioners of *haṭha* yoga are able to practise the perineal lift known as *vajrolī* (3:85) and how women are able to use this technique to raise subtle energies through their bodies (3:99, 100), women are barely mentioned in any of the *haṭha* yoga texts, other than to observe that their presence can be distracting or polluting.

There are definitely quite a few women's voices to be heard in the earlier Vedic texts that precede the *haṭha* yoga manuals, and certainly there is a powerful female presence in the *tantras* that were composed both prior to them and around the same time (we'll hear their stories shortly). But so far as the texts of *haṭha* yoga instruction let on, *haṭha* and *rājā* yoga are almost exclusively women-free zones.

Those rare places in the *haṭha* yoga manuals where women are described are mostly concerned with ritual practices focused around sexual intercourse. For example the *Haṭha Yoga Pradīpikā* includes an account of post-coital ash-smearing as a shared ritual for males and females (3:92, 93), and the seventeenth-century *Haṭharatnāvalī* recommends the technique of *vajrolī* for women, and equates menstrual blood with semen in terms of its life-giving magical properties: '*Rajas* [vital energy] is permanent … in the reproductive organ of a woman. The *rajas* should be saved during menstruation like *bindu* [semen] is to be saved. The woman should practise *vajrolī*, after that she should draw up the *rajas* if possible.' (2:101, 102 quoted in Muktibodhananda Sarasawati 1999: 362).

The *yoginīs* in the *Haṭharatnāvali*, like their sisters in the *Haṭha Yoga Pradīpikā*, only make an appearance when the actions of their cunts and juices are being described in relation to the success of certain techniques, usually variants of *vajrolī*. This is not to say that the *yoginīs* were simply being exploited for their cunt juices. The techniques described clearly have equal status and benefits for both men and women: both are engaged in the drawing up of *rajas*. There is equal access to these practices. But there is not an equal presence of *yogīs* and *yoginīs* in these texts. It is striking to me as a female reader that the only *haṭha* techniques in these manuals that mention women seem to be practices that involve their cunts. I have been hunting fairly hard to find solitary medieval *haṭha yoginīs* in these manuals, and I have observed that whenever the women do appear, they are not alone, but are mostly engaged in sexual yogas with the men. This does not of course completely exclude the possibility that women ever practised other aspects of *haṭha* yoga for themselves alone outside of the techniques of *vajrolī*, but these experiences are not described in any detail in these texts. Whilst this does not necessarily mean that no women ever practised *haṭha* yoga independently of men at that time, there is certainly very little evidence for it in the surviving texts, which in themselves, as I described above, are not necessarily a clear indication of the true nature of the lived practice of medieval *haṭha* yoga.

There is an alternative, grammatical explanation for the general absence of references to women in these *haṭha* yoga texts. It could simply be that the female practitioners are only mentioned when it is necessary to specify that there are anatomical differences in the form of practice. For example, with techniques that involve the muscular contraction of cunts and/or penises, there are clearly gender-specific variations, whereas most of the other practices described could equally well be done by male or female bodies. Following through this grammatical line of thinking, it is possible to see that the fact that the texts say *sā yogī* (masc.) instead of *sā yoginī* (fem.) is not proof that women did not practise *haṭha* yoga, it's just proof that the language which was used to describe it was gender biased. In the same way as it was standard English usage until very recently always to use the masculine pronoun 'he' to mean 'he or she', perhaps the word *sā yogī* (masc.) actually refers to yoga practitioners of either gender, unless anatomical differences need to be clarified. It's certainly encouraging to imagine that the female practitioners may well have been a presence in the living world of *haṭha* yoga, and that their textual rarity is just a linguistic effect, but this does not in itself give us any more reason to believe that they were.

Some recent enthusiastic claims have been made by US yoga practitioners and writers that women have always been involved in *haṭha* yoga practice (Shaw, E

2010, Gates 2006), and although these claims are very attractive and appealing, especially to contemporary *yoginīs*, there is minimal textual evidence of women doing the kind of yoga practices described in the standard handbooks of medieval *haṭha* yoga. Of course, as I pointed out above, even the 'canon' of *haṭha* yoga texts is itself a fairly recent creation, and so there may well be other texts, as yet undiscovered or untranslated, that present quite different perspectives on the lived experiences of medieval *haṭha yogīs* and *yoginīs*.

The *haṭha* yoga texts were written in Sanskrit and, generally speaking, women had far less access to this language than men. In Sanskrit plays, women usually speak dialect, whilst the men speak Sanskrit. 'Women were forbidden to study the most ancient [Sanskrit] sacred text, the *Veda*, but the wives, whose presence was required at Vedic rituals, both heard and spoke Vedic verses' (Doniger: 36). Even though many women probably did comprehend, speak and possibly even write Sanskrit, and there are some women characters in Sanskrit plays who also speak Sanskrit, this does not mean that these women were ever part of the *haṭha* yogic project in any way that we can discern from the *haṭha* yoga texts. Whilst the women may have been able to understand the Sanskrit used in religious rituals, they were certainly not active in writing *haṭha* yoga manuals. Women are almost totally absent from these texts, partly by simple virtue of the fact that they could not inhabit the foundational structure of the 'nine-gated city' – the male body with only nine orifices – for which the practices are intended. It is evident that some of the practices were considered to be equally accessible to women (for example 'bringing *nāda* into *bindu*' in the *Haṭha Yoga Pradīpikā* 3:99, 100), but in the context of medieval *haṭha* manuals, yogic co-education is a rarity.

Although in the handful of previously cited verses in the *Haṭha Yoga Pradīpikā* Svātmārāma does observe that the practices can be done 'by men or women' (*vajrolī* 3:84 and *sahajolī* 3:91), the only other mention of women in relation to the practice of yoga in the *Haṭha Yoga Pradīpikā* is in verse eighty-three of the third chapter (on *mudrās*) when the *yogi* is informed that he needs to find a woman to practise certain variants of *vajrolī mudrā*, in particular the collection and retention of a woman's cunt juices within the penis. As in the instructions for *vajrolī* in *Haṭharatnāvalī*, the women's juices are described with the same word, and accorded the same status as semen: (*rajas*), but other than this, women are generally absent from these texts.

The *Śiva Saṁhitā* does mention the presence of the 'beautiful *yoni*' (2:22) and even includes in chapter four a rhapsodic *tāntrik* paean to the *yoni* as 'brilliant as tens of millions of suns and cool as tens of millions of flames … [and] above [this] a very small and subtle flame, whose form is intelligence' (4:2). But in this ascetic context, the practitioner is instructed to 'imagine' the union between himself and that flame whilst performing a perineal squeeze, so that the practice involves no real live nude girls. The muscular contraction aspect of '*yoni mudrā*', minus the solar visualisation described in the *Śiva Saṁhitā*, is similar to those techniques described as *mahā bandha* in the *Gheraṇḍa Saṁhitā* (3:18–9). Both these *yoni mudrā* practices involve contraction of the male perineum, and not worship of the vulva. Indeed, in the third chapter of the *Śiva Saṁhitā*, the 'companionship of women' is clearly listed as one of those aspects of life that a *yogī* should renounce, along with twenty-two other obstacles to spiritual advancement, including theft, pride, duplicity, untruth and 'too much eating'. Clearly, girls are not held in high regard, and certainly are not usually envisioned as yogic practitioners in these texts.

The only ostensibly early *haṭha* yoga text in which we can find any extended consideration of the practice of yoga for women is the *Yoga Rahasya*. And this text is not usually included amongst the set of classic foundational texts of the modern renaissance of *haṭha* yoga described above. Although the *Yoga Rahasya* is said to have been written in the ninth century by the *Vaiṣṇavite* saint and *yogī* Nāthamuni, it was apparently lost for many centuries. It is claimed that the text was mysteriously rediscovered by the modern teacher T. Krishnamacharya, and translated into English in 1964 at his request by his son T.K.V. Desikachar. However, Krishnamacharya's long-time student Srivatsa Ramaswami has reflected that in fact the text may well be 'the masterpiece of my own *guru*, inspired by tradition and devotion' (Ramaswami 2000: 18). Whatever the provenance of the *Yoga Rahasya*, it certainly addresses in some detail the application of yoga as a therapeutic tool for women's health, including specific *āsanas* for contraception, pregnancy and preparation for labour. It is now one of the central texts in the training of yoga teachers and therapists associated worldwide with the Krishnamacharya Healing Yoga Mandiram in Chennai, but remains relatively little known outside of this particular school.

In contrast to the almost total absence of women from all the other texts of *haṭha* yoga, the past thirty years have produced a plethora of books specifically on *haṭha* yoga for women. This wave of women's *haṭha* yoga books is a very recent phenomenon indeed. For six hundred years women barely get a mention, and then there is a tidal wave of writings especially for women. The wave was a very long time coming, so by the time it hit the shore in the 1970s it was huge. Jeannine Parvati Baker's visionary book *Prenatal Yoga and Natural Birth* was published in the US in 1974, and was followed three years later by the Indian publication of the first general guide to address all aspects of yoga specifically for women, *Nawa Yoginī Tantra*, written by the Australian woman Swami Muktananda, under the direct guidance of Swami Satyananda Saraswati, founder of the Bihar School of Yoga. Both these texts blended a broadly *tāntrik* approach to women's spiritual power with practical techniques adapted from *haṭha* yoga. In 1983, a more *āsana*-focused guide to *haṭha* yoga for women was presented in Geeta Iyengar's *Yoga, a Gem for Women*.

These three influential books were the first wave of an incoming tide of yoga titles by and for women. Women had written books on yoga before this, such as Indra Devi's influential *Yoga for Americans* (1953), and still other books came after, for example Sivananda Radha's *Kuṇḍalinī Yoga for the West* (1978), and Vanda Scaravelli's *Awakening the Spine* (1991). But this first wave of women's yoga teachings was different, because the books were specifically aimed at women yoga practitioners and addressed their needs as women. Rather than offering yoga as something in which women may have a general interest, they present yoga in the service of women's well-being: they are specifically about a feminine approach to yoga. These writings and those that follow them reflect the interest of a powerful majority presence of female teachers and students in the yoga world. The first wave of 'how to' manuals created a wide general awareness of the possibility of feminine yoga practices specifically to support women's health. Once this awareness was established, it in turn gave rise to a later series of increasingly philosophical explorations about yoga as a way of life. This second wave included books that were not specifically about 'yoga for women,' but were clearly grounded in feminine, and sometimes motherly responses to the application of yoga principles to daily living, for example Sandra Sabatini's *Breath: the Essence of Yoga* (2000), Judith Lasater's *Living Your Yoga* (2000), and Donna Farhi's *Bringing Yoga to Life* (2003), which includes a very womanly translation and interpretation of yogic ethics and moral precepts.

But even these successive tidal waves of yoga books by women, for women, or inspired by women's experience of life and yoga, are such recent phenomena that they have had, in some ways, very little impact on the yogic ocean as a whole. Bear in mind that the since the late nineteenth century, the growth of modern *haṭha* yoga as a global practice has been traced through lineages that have been until now almost exclusively headed by men, and that the old texts that form the basis of this practice have not changed: the nine-gated city is still the basic model for *haṭha* yoga practice, even for women. So it is not surprising that female practitioners have felt the need to feminise and expand the range of yoga manuals available. What is quite astounding is the vast proliferation of work on this topic, and the absence (until very recently) of any sustained examination of how it is that so many women came to be doing *haṭha* yoga in the first place.

The contribution that women teachers and practitioners have made to the development of yoga in the west, and their acquisition of power and leadership roles in the contemporary yoga world has been described in detail in chapter one. In a bid to find some historical precedence for those remarkable stories of women's initiation into once exclusive yogic hierarchies, some yoga practitioners and feminist scholars have searched beyond the usual textual histories of *haṭha* yoga. Their searches have unearthed some fascinating stories and characters, which are outlined below.

HERSTORIES OF YOGA: 'ARE THERE ANY GIRLS IN HERE?' LOOKING FOR WOMEN IN THE PRE-HISTORY OF YOGA; GODDESS WORSHIP AND THE GLOBAL MATRIARCHAL NETWORK OF NURTURE

Even though many readable scripts describing *haṭha* yoga have survived and been ably translated, we still have only fragments of the whole *haṭha* yoga project. These written texts were only a small part of the whole living culture of yoga, and the texts can only tell us so much. Current yoga scholarship, in particular projects such as Mark Singleton and Jim Mallinson's plans to translate many more of the previously untranslated texts in the yoga tradition, may yet reveal more fragments of the whole picture, but right now there is only partial understanding. If we are seeking to uncover any of the older layers of the pre-histories of yoga, then we have even less to go on, because this kind of pre-history cannot be done through textual histories: there are no written records that we can read. We need to dig deeper. And so scholars have turned to archaeology, and to the explorations of archaeo-mythology, through which the material culture of what is literally found in the mud is examined in the light of mythology, the histories of religion and the ethnographic study of folklore and living practices of worship and devotion, such as ritual, trance, ecstasies and shamanism. This is the rich mix of different disciplines that have come to be used to explore the pre-history of yoga and the possibilities of its female origins. Just as the stories that we can hear through the usual histories of the yoga texts are necessarily partly conjecture, so too these alternative muddy stories are partly improvisations on basic themes.

The objects that many argue provide evidence for the earliest beginnings of yoga were made over six thousand years ago in the pre-Vedic culture of the areas now known as the Punjab and Sind in Pakistan. The urban centres of the Indus Valley Civilisation (IVC) began to develop along the banks of the river Indus and its tributaries in north-west India c.2500 BCE and did not decline until 2000–1500 BCE. The area covers 750,000 square miles and included two major cities, Harappa and Mohenjo-Dāro, over four hundred miles apart. At the height of this civilisation, during the period 2200–2000 BCE, over forty thousand people lived in the city of Mohenjo-Dāro. The remains of the material culture of this city and thousands of other sites in this part of north-west India include many terracotta figurines and stone seals that have provided the basis for scholars to offer all sorts of explanations for what life was like then (Doniger 2010, Kinsley 1987).

A particular soapstone seal less than an inch tall, for example, is often referred to as the 'Indus Valley Proto-Śiva (Seal 420)'. It was found amongst several thousand other seals in Mohenjo-Dāro, and is believed to date from c.1500 BCE. The image is frequently presented as the earliest material evidence of *haṭha* yoga practice and is most widely interpreted as a depiction of a male meditating figure, or sometimes as the god of the *yogīs*, Śiva. But this is conjecture, and it is wise to be aware that scholars have come up with at least ten different interpretations of the meaning of the image on this seal, including that it is not a god at all, but a goddess. For, with only a slight shift of perceptual awareness, as suggested by Janice Gates, in *Yoginī:*

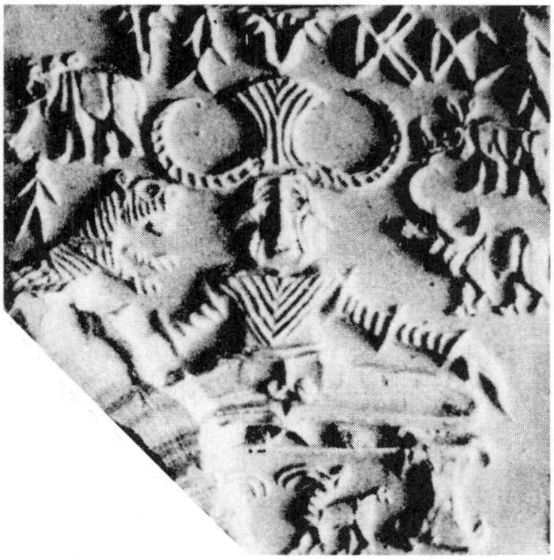

Indus Valley Proto-Śiva

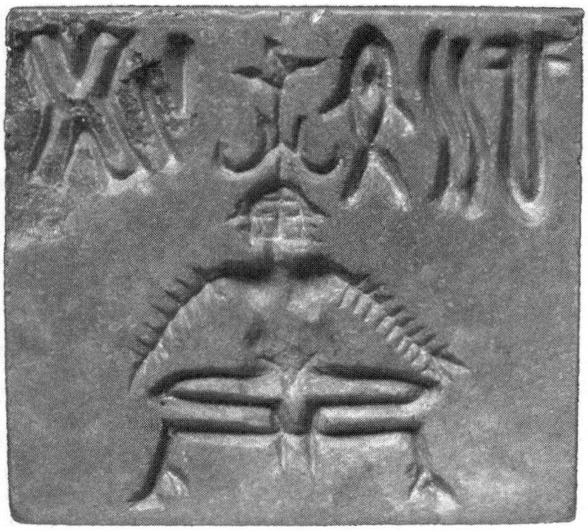

Indus Valley meditating figure

the Power of Women in Yoga, it is perfectly possibly to see these kinds of supposedly male meditating figures as feminine – a woman with outstretched arms wearing bracelets.

And it is also quite possible to see the Indus Valley meditating figure on the previous page, which was made in the same place at the same time, to be a pregnant woman wearing a lot of bangles on her arms and doing a posture which could be a birth preparation practice. Gates goes further and argues that 'Considering the number of women practising this posture in prenatal yoga classes today… it isn't difficult to imagine that some yoga postures were created by women, possibly in preparation for childbirth.' (Gates 2006: 11).

Yoginīs who are hungry to find proof of women in the pre-history of yoga may readily accept such images and items as the remains of evidence for the practice of yogic techniques by women during these times. And to be honest, their conjectures and interpretations seem just as valid as any of the many other previous interpretations that have been prompted by a desire to understand the culture that created these artefacts: colonialist scholarship has created colonialist interpretations, and feminist perspectives create feminist interpretations.

Feminist shaman, *yoginī* and women's studies author Vicki Noble was inspired by her own yogic practice to study women's role in the development of spirituality and yoga. In her article entitled 'The Life Cycle and Yoginī Roots' she asks directly 'Did Women Invent the Ancient Art of Yoga?' and explores the pre-history of yoga in relation to the late Neolithic frescoes and sculptures found in the Cucuteni culture in Western Ukraine, and in the Vinca culture in Bosnia in the fifth century BCE. Her research into these images and figurines leads her to suggest that '…women had invented yoga by the 7th millenium BCE, and that the varied poses shown in these early sculptures, as well as frescoes, murals, and rock art through the ages, are expressions of an ancient and widespread female-centred communal practice of yoga which was eventually codified into the formal schools that we recognize today'.

The cultural life of the civilisations that created the images to which Noble refers was matrifocal, egalitarian and centred around the peaceful worship of the earth's rhythms and the fertility of women. The existence of such cultures in 'Old Europe' during the late Stone Age was first highlighted by the Lithuanian archaeo-mythologist Marija Gimbutas, author of *The Civilization of the Goddess* and numerous other books that combine archaeological spadework with ethnographic and mythological interpretations of the pre-history of religion. Gimbutas' original contribution to the understanding of pre-history was that she provided evidence to support the existence of goddess worship in peaceful Neolithic agricultural civilisations, where weaving and pottery were practised. The rhythms of this mother-focused, egalitarian way of life honoured the cosmic order, in so far as it manifested as the cycles of the moon and sun, and as the turning of the seasons of the year, the growing and ripening of crops, and the birth and growth of all forms of life.

The publication of Gimbutas' work fortuitously coincided with the rise of the second wave of feminism in the United States, and with the growth of eco-feminism and neo-paganism. Her ideas were warmly embraced by a wide range of feminists, including long-time *yoginīs* such as Noble, for whom the vision of an ancient culture

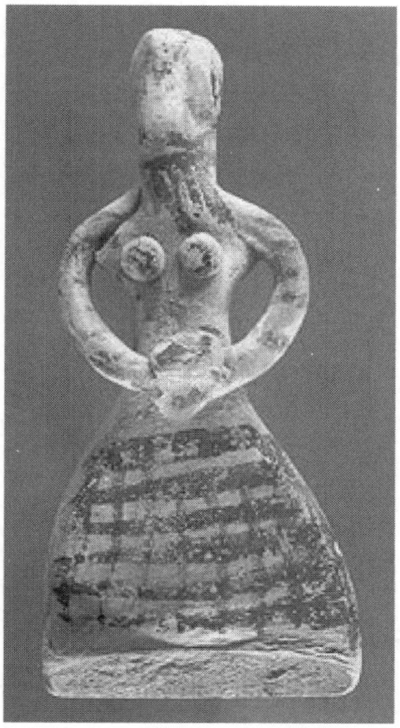

Indus Valley terracotta female figurine with infant

of goddess worship connected straight into a powerful story of yoga's origins in which women played a significant role. The fact that most of the figurines unearthed in the Indus Valley were female is the Indian link from the matriarchal Palaeolithic civilisations to the pre-history of yoga: 'The widespread depiction of women in the IVC [Indus Valley Civilisation] artefacts suggests that they were highly valued. In contrast with the predilection for macho animals (including men) on the seals, the many terracotta figurines are mostly women, and there were so many thousands of them that there was probably one in every household in the IVC. Some of the figures seem to be pregnant, or to hold on their breasts or hips small lumps that appear to be infants...' (Doniger: 76–7).

Taking these figurines as her starting point, Janice Gates's history of women in yoga identifies the Indus Valley Civilisation as female-oriented (citing the number of female figurines unearthed and the total absence of weapons). She describes how the desire to honour and reverence the rhythms of the earth's seasons was manifested in rituals where 'women's inclusion was...considered auspicious, even necessary, for the presence of the divine, and women were positively associated with fertility, growth, abundance and prosperity' (Gates 2006: 12). Gates traces a direct line from this early peaceful mother-focused culture, through certain forms of sacred dance and movement, to the development of a practice of yoga that included women.

Others have also told a similar story. For example, the influential Belgian yoga practitioner and author André van Lysebeth, who was a student of Swami Sivananda and K. Pattabhi Jois, sees '[the] cult of the feminine' at the origins of yoga and *tantra*. His perspective is that yoga's beginnings are rooted in early *tāntrik* practices whose seeds lay in the Harappa civilisation, and that these rituals revered divine powers that were vested in women, so that the focus of worship, practice and philosophy was entirely feminine: 'All women are goddess' (Lysebeth 1988).

Lysebeth's story, and the stories told by Vicki Noble and Janice Gates, all connect the spiritual project of yoga into the ecstatic dance and meditation practices of female-centred spiritual traditions of mother worship and earth reverence, which are understood by feminist historians to have been a global phenomenon. Yoga practitioner and scholar Mikel Burley has offered an interesting variant of this story, contending that the spread of the early roots of the practice of *haṭha* yoga was so extensive that there could certainly have been *yogīs* in ancient Europe. His perspective views the European fascination with yoga as less of an orientalist delight in the exotic and more of a homecoming to ancient roots and feelings that stem from an earlier European practice of yoga (Burley 2000). On the same theme, in a conference address to an international gathering of Satyananda yoga practitioners at

Aix les Bains in 1997, Swamis Niranjananda and Janakananda Saraswati both cited archaeological evidence in the form of figurines and rock carvings from Colombia, Mexico and the Mediterranean that had led them to believe yoga was an ancient global phenomenon, practised by women and men. Swami Satyananda also held this view, and linked these pre-historic feminine roots of yoga to the greater facility that women currently have for yoga practice. Recent scholarship tracks the roots of *tantra* into the pan-Indian presence of many mother-goddess cults (Joshi 2009: 40), and identifies numerous sculptural and architectural forms that carry images of groups of mother-goddesses. These images date back as far as 1300 BCE, and are understood by some scholars to form a network of local goddesses whose worship pre-dates Vedic religion, and whose presences were subsumed within the Vedic pantheon. They then resurface in the forms of ferocious mother-goddess groups and *yoginīs* in texts describing ritual practice and in temple sculptures, especially during the ninth and tenth centuries.

FEMALE VOICE AND PRESENCE IN THE *VEDAS*

These conjectured histories of yoga's possibly feminine pre-history link *haṭha* yoga into a broad and ancient context of ritual practices to propitiate and connect with goddesses whose powers were experienced as elemental forces. Worship of deified elemental forces is present in the *Vedas*, mostly in relation to male deities. A significant exception is the goddess Vāc, who was revered as a deified form of the creative energy of sound. The Vedic goddesses are certainly in a small minority, but there may be, as recent scholarship on the roots of *tantra* has indicated (Harper and Brown 2002), some thematic and symbolic continuity between the possible early mother-reverence of the Indus Valley Civilisation and Aditi, the mother of the gods praised in the *Vedas*. In the *Ṛg Veda*, Aditi is praised as the goddess of creation in whose cosmic womb the whole universe was held, and who gives birth to all the gods: 'In the earliest age of the gods, existence was born from non-existence. After this the quarters of the sky, and the earth, were born from her who crouched with legs spread' (v 4 in Doniger 1981: 38–9). Aditi's position with her knees up and her legs spread wide [*uttāna-pad*] is both a posture for giving birth, and an *āsana* in *haṭha* yoga. Even Wendy Doniger, scrupulously resistant to hindsight, comments that 'this position is later associated with yoga and might have yogic overtones even in this period' (Doniger 2010: 127).

Aditi is not the only powerful female figure in the pre-history of yoga. The clearly articulated female voices in the *Vedas* testify to the high standing in which some women were held during the Vedic period. For example in the *Bṛhad-āraṇyaka Upaniṣad*, Maitreyī, the insightful wife of sage Yajñavalkya, discusses the nature of the absolute self with her husband. In the same *Upaniṣad*, Gārgī, 'the virgin philosopher', engages in a public debate on the nature of the eternal soul with Yajñavalkya, and proves herself to be the most sensible of the eight Brahmin inquisitors. In the *Ṛg Veda*, the erudite princess Lopāmudrā is able to convince her husband, the sage Agasthya, of the value of a holistic approach to spiritual life that encompasses domestic responsibility, marital duties and spiritual purpose (Das 2011;

Radhakrishnan 1953). The voices of these women are strong and clear, and their involvement in the pre-history of yoga's philosophical and spiritual life is complete. In his lucid commentary on the principal *Upaniṣads*, Radhakrishnan observes tersely of the conversation between *Yajñavalkya* and *Maitreyī* on the Absolute Self that 'This section indicates that the later subjection of women and their exclusion from Vedic studies do not have the support of the *Upaniṣads*' (Radhakrishnan 1953 [1996]: 201).

But the relatively high status, spiritual involvement and sexual freedom of some women that is evident in the *Vedas* does not last. After this period women's ritual roles and social status begin to be downgraded through a series of increasingly restrictive Brahminical laws. The Laws of Manu were characterised by a deeply phobic attitude to the possibility of pollution by women's menstrual blood, sexual desire and other uncontrollable expressions of femininity. These were composed c.100 CE and by the second century powerfully influenced all attitudes towards women (Doniger 1991). The laws sought control over women through early betrothal and marriage, and effectively barred women from many aspects of life. Part of what closed down for women at this time was the option for involvement in the early development of the spiritual technologies that led to medieval *haṭha* yoga. In the intervening years, as we shall see when we explore women's involvement in the worlds of *tantra* and *bhakti* yoga, the spiritual experiences of some women were highly revered. But there were no such opportunities in relation to the growth of *haṭha* yoga, and so women are almost totally absent from the classical *haṭha* yoga texts. It is only through an investigation of the *tāntrik* influence upon *haṭha* yoga that we can discover any female presence in relation to this spiritual technology.

TĀNTRIK YOGINĪS: WERE THE WOMEN TEACHING MEN?

Practically everybody who writes anything about *tantra* usually begins by explaining that nobody can really define what it is. The term has a long and complex history that is not confined to a specific single sect or religion. In the simplest understanding, it refers to texts called '*Tantras*' written by Hindus and Buddhists all over India. 'The word "*Tantra*" is a reference to ancient texts that deal with yogic practices, magical rites, metaphysics and philosophy, and which straddle the world of Hindu Vaiṣṇavites and Shaivites, and cross over not only into Jainism and Mahayana Buddhism, but even Chinese Daosim and some forms of Sufi Islam' (Dalrymple 2012: 213). Most scholars of *tāntrik* history observe that the wide range of Indian religious practices and philosophies we describe as *tāntrik* can be traced to texts written between 650–800 CE (Flood 2006, Harper and Brown 2002). However, some see this period as a revival of an earlier *tāntrik* period around the turn of the first millennium (White 2003: 258). Others date the roots of *tantra* even earlier, regarding the existence of sculptural forms of proto-*tāntrik* goddesses such as Chinnamastā (cf chapter fourteen) as evidence that certain elements of *tāntrik* ritual worship date back as far as 1300 BCE (Joshi 2002: 40). What we can conclude from all this scholarly debate is that the roots of *tantra* go back so far that no one quite knows where it starts. It was certainly a pan-Indian phenomenon: some see that it had shamanistic origins and others believe it to have been an elite practice of worship that trickled down from royal patronage (White 2003: 261).

Some perspectives see that *tantra* developed partly in response to the misogynist shut-down of access to Vedic spiritual knowledge and practices that had begun during the first and second century CE, and continued to impact on lower castes as well as women (Flood 2006: 41). Whatever historical roots are claimed for *tantra*, and wherever its practitioners gathered, one of the key features of its rituals was an emphasis on the power of female deities and practitioners. In contrast to the exclusivity of Brahminical Vedic practice, *tantra* offered a more inclusive and often transgressive approach to spirituality, characterised by an openness towards physical experience (including female experience) as a means to access spiritual power, through rituals which enabled devotees to embody the powers of deities, especially ferocious goddesses. However the later developments of what David White has described as 'high Hindu *Tantra*' between the tenth and the twelfth centuries '... especially involved the subordination of the feminine – of the multiple *yoginīs*, Mothers and *Śaktis* (and their human counterparts) of Kaula traditions – to the person of the male practitioner, the male *guru* in particular.' (White 2006: 219–20)

There are over sixty-four different schools of *tantra*, each with its own specific approach, so it is hard to generalise, but at its heart *tantra* is concerned with the transmutation of energy, liberation of the mind, and attainment of power. On the one hand this power may be experienced as a spiritual connection to deities, and on the other it may be used to gain worldly powers, as in the case of the politicians and businessmen who still today worship the *tāntrik* holy women and goddesses at the *Tārā* shrines in Bengal by offering blood sacrifice in the form of goats. Feeding the goddess is a means to ensure that financial and political ventures are protected and supported by the power of *śakti*, the feminine force. *Śakti* is a central aspect of all *tantra*, but is especially revered in *śākta tantra*. It is in the texts and practices of *śākta tantra* that the ten great wisdom goddesses described in part two originate.

Like the early *Vedas* and the later *haṭha* yoga texts whose philosophies and practices were established long before they were written down, *tāntrik* rituals and stories were in circulation for many years before they made it into the written texts called *Tantras*. And like the *haṭha* yoga texts, there is debate about how far back the origins of these practices can be traced. Scholars give the seventh century as the earliest start date, but very many contemporary yoga and *tāntrik* practitioners claim that the living practice of *tantra* preceded this period by very many centuries, and in fact can be seen as the origin and root of yoga: 'Yoga is the son. *Tantra* is the mother' announced Swami Satyasangananda Saraswati in her keynote address to an international conference on *tantra* and daily life in 2009. Certainly at a philosophical level, there are resonances and overlaps between yoga and *tantra*: 'Yoga in the deeper sense is also inherently *tantra*, an integration of the forces that weave the fabric of our lives. Similarly, *tantra* is inherently yoga or inner integration. *Tantra* provides a form and a vehicle for these powers of yoga, making them out of the dry field of mere techniques and personal strivings, into tools of worship, adoration and exaltation beyond the mind and ego' (David Frawley in the foreword to Chopra 2006: v).

When we open our ears to hear the different stories of the origins of yoga, what resonates most clearly from the histories of *tantra* is the place of women in philosophy and practice. For in direct and deliberate opposition to the pollution-conscious exclusion of women, especially menstruating women, from the practice of later Vedic rituals '…in the *tāntrik* practices of India, it was the "menstruating *Śakti*" who was held as a *guru* capable of initiating the (male) adept into the sacred sexual rites that she performed during her "red" period' (Noble 2009). Judging from the presence of the menstrual *vajrolī* instructions in the *Haṭharatnāvalī*, traces of *tāntrik* reverence for menstrual blood were clearly evident in some medieval *haṭha* practices. In *tāntrik* texts the feminine is worshipped, and women can also be teachers. The tenth century open air circular *yoginī* temples such as those in Madhya Pradesh and Orissa (Dupuis 2008) are reputed to have been the gathering places where *tāntrik* practitioners conducted sexualised rituals to worship the powerful *yoginīs* depicted in the temple sculptures. These rituals involved the veneration of the vulva and her fluids, especially menstrual blood. Carvings at these temples illustrate such rituals, and recent scholarship testifies to the significance of the collection and consumption of sexual fluids, including menstrual blood, as a means of worshipping the *yoginīs*, to access their power and protection (White 2003: 68). *Yoginīs* in such rituals held power and were spiritual initiators of the male practitioners.

So from the point of view of contemporary women yoga practitioners searching for the presence of women in the history of yoga, and keen to discover evidence for some women teachers somewhere amongst all the men, it certainly seems as if *tantra* is a promising place to look. And, judging from what can be known about *tāntrik* ritual, women were not simply admitted, but could be accorded unique and valuable status. Gates writes that 'In the *tāntrik* texts, women are revered as representations of *Śakti* and accepted not only as practitioners but also as teachers.' (Gates 2006: 21). But whilst we may be glad to welcome into our women-focused stories of the history of yoga the marvellous discovery that *tāntrik* sects had, and still have, women teachers, it is wise also to understand, that even within the *tāntrik kulas* ('families'), where ritual worship of women was at the heart of philosophy and practice, we cannot really be sure of the exact status of women and their roles as teachers. Because these practices are so old and the interrelationship between the different schools is so complex, it is impossible to know exactly what was taught, by whom, to whom and in what context.

When scholars endeavour to get good answers to these questions they usually end up admitting this. In the first place, it's hard to hear the women's perspective because most of the existing texts (with the exception of some of the Buddhist *tantras* described in the next section) so far as we know, were written by men (Flood 2006:167). In the second place, many of the rituals described in the *Tantras* were intended primarily to gain power for the male *yogīs* through association with the female *yoginīs*, so that the worship of female goddesses and practitioners can be seen to be less a liberation for women than a means for men to acquire access to and control over feminine power, both human and divine. (The acquisition of magical powers by *yogīs* and *yoginīs* as a result of their spiritual practice is explored in the next chapter). So although *tāntrik* rituals clearly offered the potential for women's participation and empowerment, we cannot really be sure whether this potential was actually realised: '... the evidence we have suggests Buddhist *tāntrik* cults, and doubtless also the *Saivite Kaula* and *tāntrik* cults, were male-directed and male controlled.' (Samuel 2008: 302–3). Wendy Doniger concludes her discussion of *tāntrik kula* ritual by reflecting that the answer to 'what was in it for the women?' is 'not much'. She also concludes that the *tāntrik* rituals involving worship of women were designed largely to give pleasure to 'those who had *lingas* and not those who had *yonis*'.

This is the general consensus amongst the scholars of Hindu *tantra*. But, on the contrary, in relation to women in *tāntrik* Buddhism, Miranda Shaw's recent studies have uncovered historical and textual evidence that women were indeed *tāntrik* teachers of considerable power and acknowledged authority. Not all scholars of this period are convinced by her evidence (Samuel 2008: 302), but Shaw certainly offers a range of writings by female *tāntrikas* that support her understanding that women were active participants in the spiritual practices of Buddhist *tantra*. David Kinsley, who has written and researched extensively on the topic of goddess worship in Hindu *tantra*, has welcomed Shaw's arguments that 'male spirituality in general, might be understood to reflect female experience' (Kinsley 1998: 250), and he considers it only a matter of time before similar discoveries are made in studies of Hindu *tantra* rituals and texts. Amongst other *tāntrik* texts translated and examined by Shaw is an influential eighth-century Sanskrit treatise on liberation through ecstasy called 'Realization of Reality through its Bodily Expressions'. This treatise is written by a female teacher, *Sahajayoginīcintā* (her name means the Spontaneous Jewel-like *Yoginī*), and it is directed to a female audience of *yoginīs*. The treatise articulates the relationship between bodily pleasure, bliss and enlightenment. The teachings of the Spontaneous Jewel-like *Yoginī* show clearly that the practice of *tāntrik* Buddhism was co-created from the outset by women in the role of *guru*s, and that their disciples were often men. 'Some of the men who today are acknowledged by the tradition as authoritative formulators of the practices received the teachings from women,' asserts Shaw: 'The male transmission of the teachings does not preclude their female origins' (Shaw: 1994).

Although there were some conflicts and disagreements between Buddhist and Hindu *tāntrikas* during the early development of these practices, there is a close relationship between Buddhist and Hindu *tantra*, and there are striking similarities between the teachings and the goddesses in both pantheons. The research and analysis conducted by Miranda Shaw is powerfully indicative of the fact that women in *tāntrik* Buddhism played an important role in the development of these teachings from the start: 'Since women were among the early teachers of this genre of practice, it is reasonable to maintain that women did not create or view this practice as one in which they would be manipulated and exploited. It was conducive to women's enlightenment because women helped to design it.' (Shaw, M: 1994). If this is the case with Buddhist *tantra*, it is also reasonable to understand that it may be true also of Hindu *tantra*, even if the usual histories dispute this. The scholarly debates are complex and contradictory, but the textual evidence uncovered by Shaw is powerful testimony to the presence of women *tāntrik guru*s during the early period of *tantra*'s development within Buddhism.

Scholars are not the only people telling stories about this period. There is a considerable and growing body of work from practitioners and visionaries in India and elsewhere who clearly believe that the tradition of women teaching men was usual, and still continues in the practice of *tantra*. In these practitioners' experience, the sacred and ritual role of women within *tantra* offers powerful models for contemporary *yoginīs* to embrace their spiritual awareness. The power of women as spiritual teachers, and the divine manifestation of that power in the form of goddesses, informs the mystical writings of Shambhavi Lorain Chopra in her spiritual autobiography *Yoginī: Unfolding the Goddess Within*, and also resonates with a growing literature of goddess-focused *tāntrik yoginīs* and writers in the US, including Laura Amazzone, Vicki Noble and Linda Johnsen. For all these women, it is their personal encounter with the presence of the goddess in their lives that ignites their desire to explore the female presence at the heart of yoga and *tāntrik* experiences. Amazzone's passionate diaries of her embodied connection with goddess Durgā in Nepal is interwoven with feminist history and anthropological studies of *tāntrik* ritual practice in *Goddess Durgā and Sacred Female Power* (2010); Linda Johnsen's *The Living Goddess* (1999) roots an exploration of Śaktism, 'the heart of *tantra*', in her own engagement with practitioners, rituals and temples in order to 'reclaim the tradition of the Mother of the Universe'; Vicki Noble, in *Shakti Woman* (1991), spins together her own spiritual autobiography of awakening as a woman, a mother and as a shaman, linking these stories to her analysis of feminist *tāntrik* spirituality as the roots of contemporary female shamanism.

But it is not only female commentators who acknowledge the power of women as spiritual teachers and honour their capacity to give *tāntrik* initiation. Amarananda Bhairavan writes of his childhood spiritual initiation in a Kālī-worshipping village matriarchy in South India. In *Kālī's Odiyya* (2000), Bhairavan tells the story of life in a matriarchal culture whose principal spiritual directors and power-holders were all women, and he describes with vivid detail the respectful (sometimes fearful) awe in which the female elders and spiritual guides were held. Bhairavan's autobiography includes first-hand accounts of *tāntrik* shamanic rituals and his experience of the living power of the goddess Kālī as accessed through female *tāntrikas*. His motivation for sharing these stories is that he wishes to preserve knowledge of the powers of the female *tāntrik* teachers because he fears that they may be forgotten or misunderstood. The experiences Bhairavan describes occurred during the 1950s and 60s, but elements of *śakta tāntrik* practice continue today. William Dalrymple's vivid contemporary account of female *tāntrik gurus* still living and teaching in Bengal includes perceptive interviews with Manisha Mā Bhairava and her fellow Tārā devotees, and includes observations of *śakti tāntrik* ritual and daily life at the Tarapīth cremation grounds. Politicians and businessmen come to Manisha Mā and her partner Tapan Sadhu in their home in the burning ghats to honour the power of the goddess Tārā (see chapter ten), whose power they see embodied in Manisha Mā.

The contemporary respect for women's spiritual authority that Bhairavan and Dalrymple both describe finds parallels in the interpretations of ancient *tāntrik* ritual offered by some historians of *tantra*. For example, one of the most influential early western apologists for *śākta tantra*, Sir John Woodroffe (aka Arthur Avalon,

1855–1936), quotes from the *Kubjika Tantra* (c. 900 CE) in his *Hymns to the Goddess* (1913): 'Whosoever has seen the feet of woman, let him worship them as those of his *guru*' (Woodroffe 1913: 15). Woodroffe also writes with admiration in *Śakti and Śakta* about the place of women as spiritual teachers in Shaktism: 'A glorious feature of the *Śakta* faith is the *honour which it pays to women*. And this is natural for those who worship the Great Mother, whose representatives all earthly women are… the *Śakta Tantras* enjoin the honour and worship of women and girls, and forbid all harm to them' (Woodroffe 1918: 109. Italics in original). After referencing the *Mahānirvāṇa Tantra*'s (c.1600) strictures against husbands who speak rudely to their wives (they should fast for a whole day), and applauding the same text's encouragement of the education of girls, Woodroffe concludes 'The *Śakta Tantras allow of women being a Guru*, or a spiritual Director.' (Woodroffe 1918: 109).

Woodroffe also sadly observes that, at the time he is writing, in 1917, the honouring of women as *guru*s was a 'reverence the West has not (with rare exceptions) yet given them'. He praises the spirit of *śākta tantra* as bringing a spiritual dimension to the honouring, cherishing, education and advancement of women (Woodroffe 1918: 109). Woodroffe's respect for what he saw as the egalitarian philosophies of *Śakti*sm led him to take issue with more sexist contemporary commentators who used the language of the early nineteenth century to complain about *tantra* as a '*Religious feminism run mad*… a doctrine for *suffragette* Monists'. Woodroffe dismisses these 'ignorant notions', pointing out that 'the Śakta Sadhaka does not believe that there is a Woman Suffragette or otherwise, in the sky, surrounded by members of some celestial feminist association…' (Woodroffe 1918: 110). Instead, he correctly identifies the unity of Śiva (male principle of consciousness) and Śakti (female principle of energy) in *tāntrik* philosophy: '…both are one and the same. Śakti is symbolically "female" because it is the productive principle. Śiva in so far as He represents the *cit* or consciousness aspect, is actionless, though the two are inseparably associated, even in creation' (Woodroffe 1918: 111).

It is important to recognise that Woodroffe's understanding of *tantra* was based on interpretations which distanced him from the possibility of a more literal, or indeed accurate, interpretation of the *tāntrik Kaula* rituals he describes (Wood 2006: xii; Flood: 166). Recent *tāntrik* scholarship has effectively cleared colonialist and other westernised misperceptions on the subject of *tantra*. In particular, David White's impressively vast and detailed study of '*tāntrik* sex' in its South Asian contexts: *Kiss of the Yoginī* (2003), the product of over thirty years of scholarly exploration of the subject, argues that *tantra* is '…a perennial and pervasive form of religiosity that has persisted on the Indian subcontinent since well before the emergence of the *Kaula* sects [c.1000 CE], down to the present day' (White 2003: 258). By re-situating *tāntrik* texts and practices in their original contexts, White restores the dignity and power of the people who invented them, highlights the powerful intentions and actions of the Indian *tāntrikas* (past and present), and reveals many of the opinions of Woodroffe (whom he calls 'Father of Western *tāntrik* scholarship', White 2003: xii), and other western 'tantrists' who have built upon some of his interpretations, to be misunderstandings.

Nonetheless, Woodroffe's genuine admiration for the honouring of women's spirituality that he saw in Śaktism is palpably heartfelt. He was evidently moved by the respect paid to feminine power in *tantra* in so far as he was able to understand it. This element of his work still carries a powerful charge, above and beyond the misperceptions or misunderstandings upon which his interpretations were based. For example, Woodroffe's championing of the *śākta tantra* respect for the place of women as spiritual teachers has been recently echoed by Mike Magee, whose translations in the *Worldwide Tantra* project have made many *tāntrik* texts available online in English. Magee affirms in the introduction to his translation of the *Yoni Tantra* that: 'The Kaulas regarded female *guru*s very highly and there were many examples of *yoginīs* or female *tāntrik*s. In *Yoni Tantra* Patala 7 we find: "Women are divinity, women are life, women are truly jewels." This sentiment is echoed in many other *tantras* such as *Śakti Saṅgama Tantra*, *Devīrahasya* and elsewhere. A woman is the goddess: 'Worship carefully a woman or a maiden as she is *Śakti*, sheltered by the *Kulas*. One should never speak harshly to maidens or women' (*Kaulajñānanirṇaya*: Patala 23).

The spiritual power of a female *guru* has been explored more recently from a male perspective by Daniel Odier in his autobiographical book *Tantric Quest: an Encounter with Absolute Love* which, he claims, documents his initiation into higher states of consciousness by the *yoginī* Lalita Devī. He also explores the same ideas in his book *Desire: the Tantric path to Awakening*. The teachings of Lalita Devī have many interesting parallels with the stories of the female *tāntrik* teacher Aghori Narayani in Bhairavan's autobiography. Whilst it is not possible to determine to what degree Odier and Bhairavan's experiences are in fact entirely autobiographical, it is absolutely evident from the focus and nature of their subsequent writings and teachings on *tantra* that everything they have to share on the subject is gratefully attributed by both men to the teachings of their female *tāntrik gurus*.

The late Swami Satyananda Saraswati, founder of one of the most respected and influential schools of *haṭha* yoga (Satyananda yoga, previously known as the Bihar School of Yoga) also received spiritual teachings from a female *tāntrika*. He describes in his early works, and in his encyclopaedic *Systematic Course in the Ancient Tāntrik Techniques of Yoga and Kriyā*, his initiation as a young man by a *śākta tāntrik* female *guru* or *bhairavi*. Her name was Sukhman Giri, and Satyananda was her disciple from 1940–3, between the ages of seventeen and twenty. What the young Satyananda learnt from this *yoginī*, prior to his monastic ordination by Swami Sivananda of Rishikesh in 1947, was a profound formative influence on his spiritual empowerment. Many of the most significant of his publications focus on the *tāntrik* aspects of yoga, for example, *Kuṇḍalini Tantra*, *Yoga Nidra* and *Meditations from the Tantras*, all of which present in accessible form many of the teachings of *śākta tantra*.

Swami Satyananda's willingness to share these teachings contrasted with the attitudes of his *gurubhai* (spiritual brothers) at the Sivananda *aśram* in Rishikesh, who regarded *tantra* with disdain. 'The truth is, he was for many years *persona non grata* among his fellow Rishikesh swamis because he had the audacity to teach about *tantra* – which they considered to be left-handed, debased. He was the "rebel" among them' (Bhavananda 2010). Disdain for *tāntrik* teachings among the more orthodox *haṭha yogīs* of Sivananda's lineage manifested in a desire to exclude these teachings and those who shared them from yoga teaching environments. For example, on a visit to Los Angeles in 1983, when Satyananda had established an international reputation for publishing *tāntrik* teachings through the Bihar School of Yoga, he was denied access to the Sivananda Yoga Commuity space in West Hollywood. Apparently the refusal was rooted in dismissive attitudes towards *tantra*, and Swami Satyananda ended up delivering his lecture in a garage in Santa Monica instead (Bhavananda 2010).

After leaving the Bihar School of Yoga in 1988 and living for some time as a wandering monk, Swami Satyananda was guided by a vision to settle at Rikhiapīth, a remote rural area of Jharkhand (previously Bihar). He explained later that he was drawn to this place precisely because of its significance in *śākta tantra* as the *smaśan*, or cremation ground of the heart of the great goddess Satī, Śiva's first wife. Satī's dismembered body is believed to have fallen to earth at various places in India known as *śakti pīṭhas*, which were especially popular places for pilgrimage during the eighth and ninth centuries, and are still held in reverence in this regard by many modern Hindus. In relation to his decision to base himself at this site of *tāntrik śakti* worship, Swami Satyananda said that '...the cremation ground of Satī will also be the place where Śakti will resurrect herself in the Kālī *yuga* [present age]. Deoghar is the seat of Devi's [the goddess's] heart. It is also the birthplace of the new Devi.' (Satyananda Saraswati 2007: 74) It is significant that Swami Satsangi, senior female disciple of Satyananda, who continues to reside at Rikhia since her *guru*'s death, has devoted her considerable energies to a highly effective programme of girls' education amongst the previously illiterate and disrespected young women of the local tribal peoples, in particular teaching the girls Sanskrit in order that they may be able to lead community recitations of the key *śākta tāntrik* text *Saundarya-Laharī*. Over the past ten years, Swami Satsangi has established Rikhiapīth as an internationally renowned centre for the teaching of *tāntrik* yoga meditation practices such as *tattva śuddhi* (elemental purification), *ajapa japa* (*mantra* repetition), *yoga nidrā* (the meditative heart of yoga) and *antar mouna* (inner silence). Most of the teachers, and the majority of seekers attending these courses, are women.

BHAKTI YOGINĪS: DEVOTION AS A DIRECT LINE TO SPIRITUAL AUTHORITY

Whilst Satyananda's Rikhiapīth has become a centre for the living practice of *tāntrik mantra* and meditation, it has also incorporated other elements of yoga into its daily activities. Significantly, *bhakti* yoga (the yoga of devotion) in the form of daily *kirtan* (devotional song) and chanting of devotional scriptures, is part of the programme of holistic yoga on offer to those who come to study meditation, *āsana* and *prāṇāyāma*. The inclusion of *bhakti* yoga is now also widespread and popular, often as a weekly or monthly event, in many UK, US and European yoga studios, even if the emphasis of the classes offered in these studios is usually upon the more physical practice of yoga. In some approaches to contemporary yoga, such as Jivamukti and Sivananda yoga, the *bhakti* elements of *kirtan* and chant are integrated into daily *āsana* and *prāṇāyāma* classes.

Historically, the path of *bhakti* yoga was a development arising initially in medieval Tamil Nadu through the popularity of devotional poets and saints. From around 1300–1600 CE the *bhakti* movement thrived all over India, partly as a response to ruling Muslim pressure to convert to Islam. It was a hugely influential, popular and egalitarian form of Hindu spirituality in which the value of an authentic, personal, and often passionate devotion to the chosen deity overshadowed or eradicated boundaries of caste and class. Most of the famous *bhaktas* were men, but in this open-hearted religious context, women devotees were warmly accepted and revered.

Female *bhakti yoginīs* often lived as ascetics, and were held in high esteem as spiritual teachers. Like the female *gurus* in *tāntrik* Buddhism, these women were honoured as highly evolved *yoginīs*, and their songs, prayers and poems were written down and accorded serious study and respect. Their intense spiritual experiences led them to leave the traditional confines of women's lives as wives and mothers, and they often lived free from social constraints, empowered to speak their spiritual truth in courageous and often defiant voices that expressed a boldness that was very unusual in Hindu women of the time (Gupta 1991:195). For example, the most famous and prolific of all *bhakti yoginīs* was Mirābai (c.1498–1573), whose poems not only express her experience of deep union with the spirit of *Kṛṣṇa* but also convey her frustrations and conflicts with her in-laws' expectations of obedient female behaviour. Mirābai created around four hundred devotional poems, and nearly a thousand more are attributed to her. Her feminine voice was held in high regard by the whole *bhakti* yoga community, men and women alike. Similarly, the devotional poems written by Karaikkal Ammaiyar, the earliest example of a female *bhakti yoginī*, were highly revered many hundreds of years after her death. Karaikkal was a forest-dwelling *Śaivite* poetess saint who lived in the sixth century, devoted herself to the worship of *Śiva*, and identified herself as a 'spirit companion' of *Kālī*, one of the ghosts who sing to accompany the dance of *Śiva*. Her powerful voice expressed a female spiritual experience, and what she said was highly respected by her brother ascetics.

Other influential female devotees whose songs and poems were revered by the male *bhakta* world include Akka ['Older sister'] Mahādevī, a twelfth century *Śaivite* renunciate from Karnataka and Lalla [Granny] Ded who lived in Kashmir during the fourteenth century. Mahādevī wandered naked, praising *Śiva* and defying people who challenged her 'unsuitable' or disruptive behaviour by composing poems: 'To the shameless girl / wearing the White Jasmine Lord's / light of morning / you fool, / where's the need for cover and jewel?' (Gupta 1991: 194). Lalla followed the life of a *tāntrik* renunciate and *yoginī* whose devotional and philosophical sayings were deeply respected and carefully preserved by her fellow Kashmir *Śaivites* as well as by Sufis. She was recognised as 'a *tāntrik* master (*siddha*) who has realized the true nature of Reality and who has thus reached salvation … [and] is indifferent to social and religious laws and norms' (Gupta 1991: 201):

I made pilgrimages, looking for God
Then I gave up, turned around, here God was inside me!
... In the form of a love that fills your heart. (Lalla Dad)

The devotional compositions of both Lalla and Mahādevī, like Karaikkal before them, were much admired by their co-religionists who accorded them the status of great spiritual teachings. Such admiration and respect was possible in the context of the Śaivite sects of Hinduism (which includes *Śakti* worship), and it was this which 'enabled people to understand these women and to accept them. For women *guru*s are familiar and even preferred in *tantra*' (Gupta 1991: 208).

The tradition of *bhakti yoginīs* as powerful spiritual teachers is alive and well in contemporary India. The Bengali mystic Anandamayi Ma, the ('bliss permeated mother') who left her body in 1982, was widely recognised in her lifetime as one of India's greatest sages, admired as much by scholars and politicians as by the village people who first recognised her sanctity. Her teaching was simply to be, rather than to praise, but the deep love at the heart of her presence inspired profound devotion in those who came into contact with her. Her profound spiritual authority was honoured throughout the world. The most widely known contemporary female *bhakti yoginī* is probably Ammaci, the 'hugging saint'. The foundation of her spiritual practice and those of her devotees is *bhakti* yoga, devotional worship of the goddess. The fruits of this devotion manifest in the environmental initiatives and other charitable projects described in chapter twenty-seven. Ammaci is honoured by her devotees as a living embodiment of the goddess and is a Hindu member of the advisory committee to the World Parliament of Religions.

Other contemporary *bhakti yoginīs* whose spiritual authority has been recognised in recent times include those female devotees of spiritual leaders who now hold responsibility for the direction of *aśram*s following the death of their male *guru*s. For example, Gurumayi Chidvilasananda became the spiritual head of the international *Siddha* yoga organisation following the death of Swami Muktananda in 1982, and Swami Satyasangananda ('Satsangi') was appointed the Pīṭhadhiśvari (guardian and teacher of the place) of Rikhiapīth (home of Sivananda Aśram and Sivananda Math, the charitable foundation associated with Satyananda yoga) by Swami Satyananda in 2007, and she continues to control the running of these institutions since Swami Satyananda's death in 2009. The *bhakti*, or devotion, of these women to the living memory of their *guru* grants them a tangible spiritual power. Whilst Gurumayi and Satsangi have found themselves travelling worldwide in the service of their *guru*s' massive international organisations, Narvada Puri, the widow of her husband and *guru* Srī Santosh Puri Baba, remains on the island *aśram* established in Haridwar by her husband, and receives international visitors. All three women demonstrate such powerful *bhakti* that they are felt by many devotees to manifest the living spirit of their *guru*'s teachings.

The power invested in these past and present *bhakti yoginīs* is reminiscent of the spiritual authority that was so respected in the female *guru*s of Buddhist *tantra*. Clearly, Mirābai, Karaikkal, Mahādevī, Lalla Ded and the Buddhist *yoginīs* were remarkable women whose yogic paths of self-realisation and intense *bhakti* will always be a rarity rather than the norm. Their examples may not be easy to follow, but when viewed in a broader perspective, the intensity of these medieval *yoginīs*' spiritual quest, and the courageous, intuitive and specifically feminine nature of their expression in the form of their devotional poetry, can be heard to echo in the contemporary growth of *bhakti* yoga as a spiritual path. The fact that some of these devotional *yoginīs* (for example, Lalla) were singing about their experiences of *kuṇḍalinī śakti* yoga, brings the practices of *bhakti* and *haṭha* yoga into a closely embodied relationship, as if their practice of *haṭha* yoga gave them access to the devotional states that are expressed in the practice of *bhakti* yoga.

From this perspective, the *yoginīs* who sing *kirtan* and chants in today's yoga studios can be seen as the inheritors of the fruits of these medieval women's practice of *bhakti* yoga. This creative path of devotional spiritual practice is certainly an aspect of yoga for which contemporary *yoginīs* can find ample inspirational female role models, both in the medieval past and in the present day, through the voices of western *bhakti yoginīs* such as Wah!, Deva Premal, Narayani, Hari Pyari and Snatam Kaur Khalsa, and the powerful guidance of Indian female *gurus* such as Ammaci, Anadamayi Ma, Swami Satsangi and Narvada Puri.

For those seeking evidence of the missing female presence in the origins of yoga, the tracing of a *tāntrik* line of female *gurus* and a tradition of female *bhakti yoginīs*, including those who sing about *kuṇḍalinī śakti*, connects to a vivid living heritage. The spiritual teachings of these women can nurture the global unfolding of feminine approaches to yoga practice which are being shared by the contemporary female yoga teachers outlined in chapter one. The existence of many female *gurus*, mystics and teachers in the wider spiritual history of yoga and *tantra*, who both pre-date and surround the development of *haṭha* yoga, can be a powerful source of inspiration to contemporary female practitioners whose exposure to yoga teachings may hitherto have been confined within the male worlds of *haṭha* yoga lineages. The medieval *yoginīs* and *tāntrikas* were revered not only for their *tapas* and deep meditative revelations, but also for the distinctively womanly qualities of cyclical, psychic and emotional wisdom that they brought to their yoga quest. The *bhakti yoginīs* of medieval and modern times demonstrate huge spiritual power and deep love in the feminine forms of goddess worship and devotional and humanitarian service. By widening our perspective to include such women teachers in the broader history of the development of *haṭha* yoga, present day *yoginīs* have the opportunity to connect with the free spirit and abundant creativity of early *tāntrik* and *bhakti yoginīs*, and to embrace their awareness of ritual, poetry, intuitive insight and devotion as the heart of yogic experience. Consciousness of the heritage of our female yogic ancestors may help us to find a place for female spiritual empowerment in the contemporary practice of yoga. The possibilities for this are explored in the following chapter.

QUESTIONS AND REFLECTIONS

I invite you to consider now your own 'pre-history of yoga' by asking yourself some (or any, or all) of the following questions:

1. When I first practised yoga, did it ever feel like a 'homecoming' to me? What things may I have done or felt before anyone 'taught' me yoga that could have made the practices seem already familiar? (Consider the spontaneous arising of prayers, dreams, dances, deep resting, *kriyās*).
2. Before I read this chapter, what did I know or imagine about the presence of women in the pre-history of yoga and/or *tantra* and/or *bhakti* yoga?
3. Now I have read this chapter, how do I understand women's place in the development of yoga and their relationship to yoga and/or *tantra*?
4. What difference does any of the new information I have encountered in this chapter make to my own practice of yoga and/or *tantra*?

FURTHER READING AND RESEARCH

On the subject of Vedic literature, and for some helpful practitioner-focused explorations of the links between Vedic and *tāntrik* thought, **Swami Satyadharma Saraswati**'s 2003 translation of and commentary on the *Yoga Cūḍāmanii Upaniṣad* is a useful reference. **Wendy Doniger** (2010) presents a fascinating alternative history of the Hindus, including everything from the place of women in the Indus Valley Civilisation to the treatment of dogs in contemporary Hinduism. There is a useful appendix on goddesses in the Indus Valley Civilisation in **David Kinsley**'s *Hindu Goddesses* and some detailed scholarly accounts of the origins of mother-goddess worship in **Katherine Harper** and **Robert Brown**'s edited collection of essays, *The Roots of Tantra* (2002).

Absolutely the most authoritative and comprehensive scholarly study of the place of the *yoginīs* in the original rituals around *tāntrik* sex is **David White**'s *Kiss of the Yoginī*. **Katherine Harper** and **Robert Brown**'s *The Roots of Tantra,* and **Gavin Flood**'s *The Tāntrik Body* (2006) are also helpful if you want scholarly detail and historical perspective. On the other hand, for goddess-feminist visions inspired by yoga practice, read anything by **Vicki Noble**, and for a classic feminist exposition of goddess worship as a global phenomenon from Palaeolithic times to the Greeks and the eventual suppression of women's rites, **Merlin Stone**'s *When God was a Woman* (1977) is the place to start. **Laura Amazzone**'s and **Linda Johnsen**'s contemporary goddess-feminist work is also rooted in *śākta tantra*. The spiritual autobiographies of **Odier** (1997), **Chopra** (2006) and **Bhairavan** (2000), as well as the interviews of **Dalrymple** (2010), present first hand accounts of *tāntrik* initiations and rituals.

Richard Lannoy's photographic essays on Anandamayi Ma (1996) are evocative depictions of this powerful female mystic, and **Linda Johnsen**'s writings (2004) convey the living tradition of *bhakti* yoga as practised by the women saints of India. **Narvada Puri**'s spiritual autobiography (2009) and **Swami Satsangi**'s *Light on the Guru and Disciple Relationship* (1984) are both vivid accounts of *bhakti* yoga in the form of devotion to the *guru*.

CHAPTER THREE

female *siddhis*: intuited origins for a new perspective on yoga

ANGELA FARMER'S 'LEGEND': ANOTHER WAY OF SEEING IT

Angela Farmer told me this story during an interview. It shone brightly in my heart for days afterwards, making me smile. Whenever I shared it with other *yoginīs*, they smiled too, because the basic idea at the heart of the story resonates beautifully with many women's experiences of yoga. It also offers a sweet inversion of the usual arrangement in most *tāntrik* sources, where it is Pārvatī who asks her husband to answer her questions about yoga. In Angela's charming vision, it is Pārvatī who teaches Śiva: in this imaginary explication of the origins of yoga, the teacher's wisdom, as is more common in *śākta tantra*, is rooted in her femininity.

Before sharing the story, Angela reflected:

> *It's always been my belief that yoga evolved through women. I believe that because I see how many women love yoga but how often they get really hard and tight with sticking to and following a system. Then when you give them the opportunity to become more free to feel and go inside and make those connections with places inside that want to be heard and express themselves instead of putting the pose on top of them, they start to shine. They become beautiful and their movements are beautiful. It makes me so happy seeing this and I love nothing more than when the whole room is all doing something different but it's actually all coming from the same essence and the same feeling of divine connection. It was in one of my women's retreats that I created a little skit on Śiva and Śakti. Well it was Śiva and Pārvatī (one of Śakti's incarnations), and I just told this story because it just came up in my mind at that moment and so I had fun telling it sometimes to help people feel the difference.*

And the story goes like this…

PĀRVATĪ AND ŚIVA

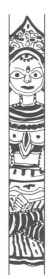

Pārvatī was Śiva's wife and she was very beautiful. She just enjoyed her life and she had a lovely home to live in. She had a bath made from a shell in which she would bathe herself and rub sandalwood paste on her body and she would stretch out in the morning in the sunshine, and she would feel her body. It was so delicious that she would twist this way, and twist a little back that way, and then maybe she would lean back over a rock or a sofa and breathe. She just felt good doing this.

Sometimes Śiva, who was madly in love with her, would creep up behind a pillar and watch her. He would peek secretly, because this was her private time. He loved to see her enjoying herself so much. Then suddenly his mind started ticking, and he said to himself 'Well, maybe I could do this too?' So he watched her very carefully and then went out in the jungle and he tried to try to do some of the things he had seen her doing so beautifully in the early morning light.

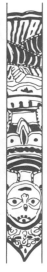

Being Śiva, and being male of course, he began to *perfect* these movements and these positions. He organised them and he codified them and he practised very hard to get them all right. When some of his devotees heard about this, they said 'Lord, please will you teach us?' So Śiva thought about this, and then he spoke. (At this point in the story, Angela Farmer clears her throat and adopts a brusque sergeant major voice, loud and very bossy.) 'Very well, all of you, line up. One, two, three, four! And now you've got to JUMP! Three feet apart, left foot in, right foot out! STRETCH your arms! More, more, more!' Bang crash! And he *trained* them.

After some time he said 'Mmm. OK, I'm going to give some of you certificates.' He handed out the certificates and then he sent them off out into the world to open up *aśrams* and yoga centres, and yes, we know the rest of the story!

But what about Pārvatī? Oh, she's still at home, enjoying the beautiful sunshine, taking her bath, rubbing herself with sandalwood paste, doing a twist here and a backbend there and just feeling so delicious! One morning she might wake up and say to herself, 'Well I don't know what's going on in the yoga world out there, maybe I should come out and show them where it all comes from?'

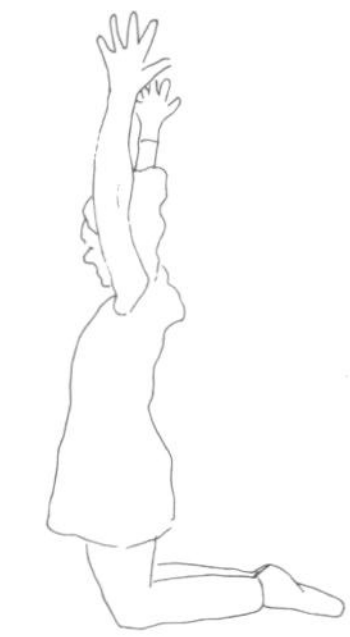

AN INVITATION TO A RADICAL NEW PERSPECTIVE

The intuitive 'rightness' of Angela Farmer's charming tale links the legendary histories of the beginnings of yoga with a feminine perspective on why so many women love to practise yoga. It's the perfect opener to a radical new perspective. In the previous two chapters I have told the inspirational stories of women in the global growth of yoga as a grassroots revolution in consciousness, and the stories of women's presence and absences in the early development of yoga. I share here in this chapter a radical and 'intuited' history that connects the central intention of yoga directly with the experience of women's blood mysteries and the potential for planetary change through shifts in personal awareness. This is *radical* because it returns afresh to the sources of both the orthodox and the unorthodox histories, showing a way to envisage the yogic future. It is *intuited* because it arises from insights gained through lived experiences: of myself, my students and the teachers I have trained to share yoga especially for women.

The practice of yoga for pregnancy, or for heightening menstrual cycle awareness, or for coping with menopause has created a range of opportunities which are unprecedented in all the past written histories of yoga. It has made possible a heartfelt and intuitive welcoming of yoga practice into women's most profound and initiatory life experiences, for example menstruation and orgasm, labour, birth and lactation, and through the intensities of the perimenopausal challenge. Because women have now brought yoga awareness with them into these transitional moments of deep challenge, we can now tell other yoga stories, different from those told before. We can hear, through the voices of these 'women's mysteries', that the very experiences which were originally excluded from the *haṭha* yoga project are now feeding the roots for the future growth of yoga. It is these stories that tell us how the potential for intuitive states of heightened consciousness can reside right here in the bloody cycles of women's lives. It is these stories that are both the origins and outcome of womb yoga.

The insights I have gained as a yoga practitioner and yoga therapist, as a teacher and as a teacher trainer in the field of yoga specifically designed to support women's health throughout the whole of the female life cycle, have given me an unusually vivid context for my perspectives on the new stories and future purpose of yoga. The context is red. It is the context created by honouring the rhythms of women's experiences of menstruation, conception, pregnancy, miscarriage, postnatal recovery, lactation and (peri) menopause as female *siddhis*. Rather than regarding these experiences to be peripheral or incidental (or indeed, as many find them to be, inimical) to yoga practice, my particular personal and professional perspective has enabled me to put these initiatory experiences at the very centre of an evolving yoga practice: womb yoga. I invite you to take a radical shift of perspective, and to hear yoga's past and future histories as they echo in women's experiences of blood mysteries: to bring these barely heard whispers from the edges of the yoga histories right into the centre, and to attend to the resonances that arise from this different way of listening.

MAGICAL MYSTERIES IN YOGA: *SIDDHIS*, THE SUPERNATURAL POWERS IN *HAṬHA* AND *RĀJĀ* YOGA

The previous chapter laid out a selection of different stories about the absence and presence of women in the early development of *haṭha* yoga. Whether or not these histories 'prove' the existence of women teachers in the pre-history of yoga, we end up in the same place: a twenty-first century world of yoga almost entirely populated by women. From whatever roots they have come, and by whatever routes they have travelled, the *haṭha* yogic practices from which females were once excluded have at last come into (or returned to) the hands of contemporary women. Knowing the end of the story now, it is helpful for us to revisit those first histories that were explored at the start of the previous chapter: the classical texts of *haṭha* and *rājā* yoga.

With the echoes of these 'women-invented yoga' stories in our ears, I now invite us to reconsider some of the least explored aspects of these yoga texts. Having heard about the possible feminine origins of the early, male-only *haṭha* yoga, and knowing that this practice has ended up today in the hands of women, it becomes possible now to re-engage with the original texts of this tradition from an entirely new perspective. This new perspective sheds light on some of the least celebrated aspects of the *haṭha* yoga texts, the stories they tell about magical superhuman powers.

For all of the classic texts – the *Yoga Sūtra*, the *Haṭha Yoga Pradīpikā*, the *Gheraṇḍa Saṁhitā* and the *Śiva Saṁhitā* – contain fabulous accounts of magical powers and supernatural capacities. Across the often falsely made distinctions between *haṭha* yoga, and *rājā* yoga, and in the overlaps between these traditions and the philosophies and practices of the *tantras*, there exist the most incredible stories of *yogīs*' superhuman feats. These amazing tales sit cheek-by-jowl with more sober philosophical considerations of the nature of suffering and what we may do to avoid it. In the *Yoga Sūtra*, for example, after the tersely elegant guidelines for making wise choices about life, after the teachings about honesty and non-violence and equanimity come these tales of the *siddhis*, stories of how a particular yogic practice can confer invisibility, clairvoyance or the ability to fly.

These are the parts of the old texts that contemporary *yogīs* do not really broadcast too widely. If you are in the business of convincing ordinary folk that yoga is a perfectly relevant and positive way of life that promotes well-being and clarity of mind, or that yoga therapy is an effective remedy for stress-related disorders, then it's a bit awkward to deal with all these fantastical claims about magical powers lurking in the texts. And so when male and female contemporary *yogīs* call on these texts (the *Haṭha Yoga Pradīpikā*, the *Yoga Sūtra* and others) to bear witness to the value of practising yoga now, they focus on the benefits of yoga to mental health and physical well-being, or yoga's value as a philosophy to promote non-competitiveness and harmonious community. The stories about flying *yogīs* tend to get left out, dismissed as overstatement or nonsense, or at the very least are seen to be 'no longer relevant'. It is as if they are the 'forgotten *sūtras*' that contain all the weird and embarrassing stuff none of the popular promoters of yoga ever talk about. Personally, I find these parts of the classic yoga texts to be the most fascinating and deeply relevant, but that may be because I bring an unusual perspective to them.

Having had the experience over the years of sharing the contents of the *Haṭha Yoga Pradīpikā* and other yoga texts with groups of yoga teachers, trainees and keen practitioners, I can testify to the fact that in any given group of dedicated contemporary yoga practitioners, most of them are going to regard these portions of the texts as entirely irrelevant to their own practice. One or two of them may embrace the whole text with deep love, and quite a few of them will get very angry that they have been asked to read such pieces of 'arrant and offensive nonsense' in the first place. If they are offended, it is usually by the nitty gritty of practices such as *amarolī*, *vajrolī* and *sahajolī* (see chapter twenty). If they see these parts of the texts as nonsense, it is because they have taken at face value all the outrageous claims that yoga can empower you to raise the dead, or make you fly, or live forever, or become as large as a giant, or other magic tricks. 'What relevance at all do any of these stories have for twenty-first century *yogīs*?' they ask. And I reply that if we listen carefully, then these fantastical stories are a precious gift, for they give us a powerful new way to understand the deep relation between yoga and the rhythms of human lives, in particular the often intense cyclical experiences of female bodies.

These magical powers are called *siddhis*. They are supernatural abilities that come to dedicated *yogīs* either as side effects, or as the intended goal of their yoga practice. *Siddhi* is a Sanskrit noun that can be translated as 'attainment' or 'accomplishment', in the sense of successfully perfecting a skill or power. The *Yoga Sūtra* states that such powers may be attained through the use of herbs, or by the diligent application of sustained effort (*tapas*). *Siddhis* are also said to manifest in those practitioners who attain *samādhi* (non-dual experience of cosmic consciousness) and some people are simply born with these powers (chapter 4, verse 1). The *siddhis* are also described in the key texts of *haṭha* yoga, including the *Haṭha Yoga Pradīpikā* (c.15th century), and the *Śiva Saṁhitā* (c.14th–16th century). The number of *siddhis* varies according to the text, but in *haṭha* yoga eight primary ones are generally presented (*aṣṭa siddhis*). The first one, *aṇimā*, gives 'minuteness of the soul' (Rele 1927 (2007): 70), by which means the *yogī*'s energy, condensed to the size of an atom, can penetrate all beings and even, in higher levels of accomplishment, bring the dead back to life. The second, *mahimā,* enables the *yogī* to expand to fill the universe, thereby experiencing the whole of creation within himself. These two *siddhis* offer power over scale and physical boundaries. The third and fourth *siddhis* relate to power over the forces of gravity. *Laghimā* is the power to become weightless. *Garimā* is the power to become very heavy.

The fifth *siddhi* is *prāpti*, which gives unrestricted access to every place in the universe, or to all desired objects. It also gives clairvoyance, clairaudience and the capacity to predict the future and to understand all languages. The sixth *siddhi* is *prakāmya*, the power of realising apparently impossible desires including eternal youth. In some texts, the benefits of *prakāmya* are classified as belonging to *prāpti*. The seventh *siddhi* is *vaśitva*, or the capacity to bring the elements and all living creatures, including humans, under one's control. The eighth and final *siddhi* is *īśatvam*, or dominion at a universal level, which gives the ability to control cosmic powers in this world and others.

In addition to these primary *siddhis*, there are also ten secondary and related *siddhis*, such as being able to see, hear and smell far away things, teleportation, and choosing the time of one's death. There are also a host of minor *siddhis* that relate to mastery over the energies in particular *cakras*. For example in the *Śiva Saṁhitā*, the *Yoga Sūtra* and the *Yoga Cūḍāmaṇi Upaniṣad*, specific gifts and powers are associated with the mastery of techniques pertaining to individual energy centres. In the *Śiva Saṁhitā*'s section on the knowledge of the *cakras*, each of the *siddhis* relates particularly to powers rooted in knowledge of that energy centre and its related element. For example meditation on the heart centre, *anāhata*, gives dominion over all who move in the air, and 'When the *Yogī* contemplates the *Maṇipura* lotus, he gets the power called the *pātala-siddhi* – the giver of constant happiness. He becomes lord of desires, destroys sorrows and diseases, cheats death, and can enter the body of another. He can make gold, etc, see the adepts (clairvoyantly), discover medicines for diseases, and see hidden treasures' (*Śiva Saṁhitā* 5:81–2). Other minor *siddhis* associated with mastery over particular yogic techniques include becoming 'eagerly desired by celestial maidens', 'walking in the air, whenever he likes' (*Śiva Saṁhitā* 5:85–6), destroying all past *karmas* and all present fears (*Śiva Saṁhitā* 5:111 & 114), and total freedom from disease, death, hunger and thirst (*Yoga Cūḍāmaṇi Upaniṣad* 5:53–5).

In essence, the secondary *siddhis*, like the eight primary and other minor *siddhis,* all offer the diligent yogic practitioner *power over* aspects of life which are usually experienced as uncontrollable. As a result of unification with the energies of the universe, the *yogī* is able to transcend all usual human limits. *Siddhis* are '... acquired by the particular mode in which the *Yogī* concentrates and merges himself in the divine Spirit (the Cosmic Power) or contemplates it within his own self.' (Rele 1927 (2007): 68).

Most of the yogic techniques described in the medieval *haṭha* yoga texts offer the possibility that diligent practice of them will lead at some point to the acquisition of a *siddhi*. Such is the tenor of delight with which they are described that it can sometimes seem that the whole point, or 'benefit', of any given practice is in fact to acquire the related *siddhi*. But the *siddhis* that are described as evidence of accomplishment in *haṭha* and *rājā* yoga can also be identified as distractions from the ultimate aim of practice, for example the *Yoga Sūtra* (3:37) defines the *siddhis* as being in contradistinction to the highest spiritual vision.

A *yogī* who attains *siddhis* is referred to as a *siddha* – one who possesses *siddhis*. Above all, the *siddhis* are seen as evidence of an altered state of consciousness that confers supernatural powers. The establishment of this altered state of consciousness is proven both by the presence of the *siddhi* and by the *yogī*'s response to it. Having acquired by diligent yogic practice the capacity to be everywhere at once, for example, the truly accomplished *yogī* would not utilise this ability to steal, to play foolish tricks, or to attain political power. Rather, his sanguine response to the presence of such a supernatural ability would demonstrate the *siddha*'s higher state of consciousness every bit as much as his possession of the *siddhi* itself.

So the acquisition of the *siddhi* is a sign of accomplishment, but yet it is also a test: for if the *yogī* delights in the *siddhi*, then his progression to the next level of establishment in yoga is halted, and the authenticity of his continuing bliss (*samādhi*, or other yogic state) is in doubt. The way the *yogī* chooses to respond to the acquisition of the *siddhi* is in itself an initiatory trial. The yoga he practises brings him to the threshold of the initiation: the *siddhi* gives the sign that the threshold has been crossed, but his further response to the powers bestowed upon him by the acquisition of the *siddhi* is the deeper initiation. For, if he fails to respond appropriately to this initiatory trial then all his previous efforts will have been in vain, and his quest to become fully and permanently established in the ultimate state of yoga – *samādhi* – will ultimately have been futile. The initial acquisition of a *siddhi* simply signifies that the *yogī* has secured sufficient mastery (or good birth, or enough herbs) to encounter supernatural powers without fear, but the subsequent testing of the *siddha* is in order to discover whether he is sufficiently evolved to allow this power to flow through him. For if he desires to maintain his power over the force and to abuse it, then his yogic accomplishment becomes a burden and not a gift. Maintaining power *over* the *siddhi* is a less refined spiritual attainment than respecting and honouring the power that flows *through* in the form of the *siddhi*.

A key characteristic of the astonishing powers of the *siddhis* in the *Śiva Saṁhitā* and elsewhere is the importance of keeping them secret in order to maintain their power: 'there is no greater secret than this throughout the three worlds. This should be kept secret with great care. It ought never to be revealed' (*Śiva Saṁhitā* V:140). *Siddhis* are to be kept secret because they are precious. They are rare, hard-won opportunities to reach the edge of worldly awareness before making the leap into transcendental consciousness. Secrecy is advocated because *siddhis* are uncovered in the intimate privacy of the *yogī*'s own spiritual practice, often at the point where this practice has led to the very limits of human endurance. To acquire a *siddhi*, a *yogī* needs to go to the edge. So the experience of *siddhis* is often associated with liminality: with particular junctions or transitions, turning points.

These junctions are seen as portals to liberation and to certain *siddhis*. Sometimes the junctions are real places, for example the confluence of the holy rivers: 'The sacred Triveni (Prayaag). Between the Ganges and the Jamuna, follows this Saraswati: by bathing at their junction, the fortunate one obtains salvation' (*Śiva Saṁhitā* V:132). Sometimes the junctions are in the esoteric anatomy of the *yogī*, and the process of 'bathing' is a meditative form of absorption in the inner world that can open a portal to cosmic consciousness: 'He who performs mental bathing at the junction of the White (*Ida*) and the Black (*Pingala*) becomes free from all sins, and reaches eternal *Brahma*… At the time of death let him bathe himself in the water of this Triveni (trinity of rivers): he who dies thinking on this reaches salvation then and there' (*Śiva Saṁhitā* V:134 and V:139). In both cases, whether the junction be geographic or somatic, the experience of a *siddhi* is seen to mark a key turning point, to signal a transition between one way of being and the new wisdom which the *siddhi* brings. Even if the *siddhi* manifests as a form of magical control over worldly powers, the yogic practice through which it was acquired is intended to prepare the *yogī* to encounter the power of the *siddhi* as a form of surrender. Acquiring a *siddhi* is a threshold between worldly and transcendental awareness. The *siddhi* occurs at the junction between the two and passing through it is a kind of initiation. This aspect of a yogic *siddhi* is also a defining characteristic of the potential for specifically female *siddhis* that I discuss in the next section.

FEMALE *SIDDHIS*

The yogic *siddhis* are described by men, and at this point in the history of *haṭha* yoga, the practitioners who may have been seeking to acquire them would have been almost exclusively male. But within the earlier literature of Hindu and Buddhist *tantra*, there are many *yoginīs* who displayed the *siddhis* described later in the classic yoga texts. For example Miranda Shaw's impressive catalogue of magical powers possessed by *tāntrik* Buddhist *yoginīs* includes the *yoginī guru* Dinakara who possessed the power of flight; Kaṅkana *yoginī* who could render herself invisible; the *yoginīs* Dombiyoginī and Menaka who were both able to walk on water; and the princess *guru* Gangadhara who could change shape at will, and once turned herself into a wolf. Yogic *siddhis* are accomplishments open to men and women equally. In fact, in the oldest of the Buddhist *tantras*, the *Guhyasamāja Tantra* (c.350 CE [*Secret Assembly*]) clearly and repeatedly identifies sexual union with women and ceremonial worship of women and girls as a key part of ritual practice for accomplishment of all *siddhis*: 'To achieve ultimate *siddhi* he should offer to all the Buddhas a girl like a mine of jewels, adorned with many jewels' (8:18)... With various forms he should love all the women who dwell in the three worlds, born of the three *vajras*. This is the most wonderful sacred law (chapter 17:17. All from *Guhyasamāja Tantra* trans. Freemantle).

The association of women with the acquisition of *siddhis* is a characteristic of the early *tantras*, which were composed approximately nine hundred years prior to the key texts of *haṭha* yoga. Perhaps the clearest expositions of the close relation between women and the acquisition of *siddhis* occurs in the *Yoginī Tantra* (c.1350) which predates the *Haṭha Yoga Pradīpikā* by about one hundred and fifty years, and the *Yoni Tantra* (c.1650), which was composed around the same time as the *Gheraṇḍa Saṁhitā* (c.1700). Both these *śākta tantras* set out complex ritual and sexual worship of women as goddesses, and both clearly state that any human or divine being desirous of access to the great powers of the *siddhis* should focus their devotions upon the power of *śakti* embodied in women.

For example, in the sixth section of the *Yoginī Tantra*, Śiva describes the *siddhi* conferring worship of the 'three *bindus*' (or spots of brightness) in the form of a young woman: 'The first is as bright as 10,000,000 dawn suns, extending from the head to the breasts. The second extends from the breasts to the hips and the third from the *yoni* to the feet. This is the Kamakala form, the very essence of Brahma, Viṣṇu and Śiva' (*Yoginī Tantra* 6). In the first section of the *Yoni Tantra*, it is stated that: 'If a person worships with menstrual flowers [a symbol for menstrual blood], he also has power over fate. Doing much *pūjā* in this way, he may become liberated.' (*Yoni Tantra* 1). In the next section of the same *tantra*, the acquisition of the highest *siddhis* of immortality and liberation are said to accrue to the practitioner who '... sees the *yoni* full of menses' and offers the '*yoni* flowers' [menstrual blood] as part of his *pūjā* [worship] (trans. Magee 1995:11). In these *tantras*, menstrual blood is a crucial component of worship and is seen to contain immense spiritual power and to confer *siddhis*.

Whether they are associated with women, as in the texts of *śākta tantra*, or reserved mostly for men, as in the classic manuals of *haṭha* yoga, fundamentally, what all these accounts of yogic and *tāntrik siddhis* affirm is that human consciousness holds the potential for superhuman capacities. This potential can manifest as *siddhis* when focused awareness invites unified alignment with cosmic powers. These magical encounters with power have a particularly direct relevance to female experience. In the yogic texts the *siddhis* are the result of intense ascetic yoga practice and in the *tantras* they are the result of ritual ceremony and *mantra* recitation. In relation to women, though, there are certain times in our lives when we encounter naturally arising, intense physical experiences that invite us to embrace the power of specifically *female siddhis*.

Awareness of these female *siddhis* dawned on me when I began to realise intuitively what the fabulous stories about flying *yogīs* and their magical powers could really be about. When we recognise that the yogic *siddhis* are about acquiring a *connective* power to cosmic forces, it is also possible to see that these are the same cosmic forces that can set the rhythms of women's cyclical life experiences. The wild tales of the *siddha*s tell of experiences of connection with transcendent power. The mysteries of women's life cycles reveal that this very same transcendent power is fully tangible, and immanent: the birthing or menstruating woman, or the menopausal woman drenched with sweat as she burns in the heat of a raging hot flush, are all experiencing the powers of elemental forces flowing unbidden through their female human frame. These experiences are evidence of connection with transcendent power. They are potential power, or *proto-siddhis*.

I identify the eight female *siddhis* as those apparently purely biological functions of the human body that are exclusively female. I say 'apparently purely biological', because a crucial feature of all these functions is that they are hormonally driven, and thus powerfully under the influence of a woman's emotional life, her familial, cultural and social milieu, her environment, nutrition, general health, occupation and the nature of her spiritual awareness. This means that conscious experience of the eight female *proto-siddhis* can be suppressed, overlooked, refused or otherwise altered for many reasons and by many factors, which are explored later in this chapter, and examined in detail in chapter eight. It is when they are consciously recognised and encountered that these *proto-siddhis* become female *siddhis* proper.

In the order in which they are encountered in a woman's life, these eight female *siddhis* are:

1. The onset of menstruation at menarche
2. Menstrual cycles
3. Female orgasm
4. Pregnancy

5 Miscarriage

6 Labour and birth

7 Lactation

8 Menopause

Because four or five of these eight female *siddhis* are experienced by nearly all females, the numbers of women who can encounter these potential *siddhis* is huge. In contrast, the level of commitment required to maintain the sustained quality of practice or devotions needed to manifest any given yogic or *tāntrik siddhi* means that the number of men who would have the correct circumstances to begin to attempt to achieve such *siddhis* is very few.

Because the female *siddhis* are naturally arising physical experiences, it is important to notice the difference between experiencing their physiological aspects as bodily functions, and recognising these experiences as potential *siddhis*. It is conscious recognition that transforms the physical experience into a *siddhi*. What is crucial here is the level of awareness required to perceive that the hormonal, emotional and physical experiences of the female *siddhis* have the capacity to be experienced as spiritual initiations into power. Christiane Northrup expresses this with great clarity when she writes: 'Unconscious biological instinct and biological instinct that is honed and refined by consciousness and choice are two different things.' (Northrup 2005: 22). If women are to identify these physical and emotional experiences as *siddhis*, or as sources of wisdom, insight and spiritual growth, then it is necessary to encounter them with conscious awareness. Yoga helps us to do this.

There are interesting parallels and contrasts between the yogic and *tāntrik siddhis*, and the female *siddhis*. All *siddhis* have initiatory and signal functions: they are at once an initiation and a sign of having been initiated. Yogic, *tāntrik* and female *siddhis* can also be understood to be particular talents, special gifts or capacities. The difference is that the yogic *siddhis* can only be accomplished by protracted and disciplined practice, and the *tāntrik siddhis* can be obtained through ritual, whereas female *siddhis* naturally unfold in the life cycles of a female body. This means all women have the potential to experience female *siddhis* just because they are women.

There are very rare occurrences in which a male body may experience (even vicariously) one of the female *siddhis*, but these anomalies are so unusual as to be considered miraculous. For example, the story of the 'lactation' of Saint Bernard of Clairvaux describes how the saint's deep meditative absorption in the maternal qualities of the Virgin Mary were rewarded by a stream of her heavenly milk touching his eyes and lips to bless his vision and speech. St Bernard's vicarious lactation is depicted in many paintings (most famously those by Bartolomé Esteban Murillo, 1666 and by Alonso Caro, 1650), as a form of spiritual nourishment. In these images, Mary's capacity to lactate is tranferred to her saintly devotee, who is then described as having experienced 'miraculous lactation'. Mary's lactation is presented as a divine gift or *siddhi* with the essential quality of compassionate spiritual nurture. Divine status is also accorded to the capacity to breastfeed in Saint Ephrem the

Syrian's *Hymns on the Nativity* (c. fourth century), in which Jesus Christ is described as the 'Living Breast of living breath'. In the fourth of this series of hymns, Mary's ability to nourish by lactation is metaphorically transferred to her son: 'He sucked Mary's milk / and from His blessings all Creation sucks. / He is the Living Breast of living breath; by his life the dead were suckled, and they revived… as indeed He sucked Mary's milk, / He has given suck – life to the universe.' (Hymn 4:149–53, trans. McVey).

With the miraculous exceptions of Jesus Christ and Saint Bernard of Clairvaux, lactation, and all other female *siddhis* are usually experienced only by women, and only in specific sequence. In the same way as the yogic *siddhis* usually manifest in a particular order in relation to the *yogī*'s spiritual development, the female *siddhis* also tend to unfold in a certain order. For example the opportunity to give birth comes after pregnancy, and lactation usually follows after birth but not after menopause, although these 'norms' are not absolute. For example, I have heard of instances where young girls who have never been pregnant have begun to lactate as a manifestation of their deep love for the babies for whom they cared (Ina May Gaskin, at Birthlight conference 2005), and it is certainly possible for women of any age (whether or not they have ever been pregnant) to lactate in order to breastfeed grandchildren or adopted children.

The special gifts and capacities of the female *siddhis* are encoded in the female body, and naturally arise in response to cyclical tides and waves of hormones as they circulate through the female body in a delicate and complex dance. These tides work through women in the same way that the seasons of the year are played out in the earth. A fuller exploration of the significance of these inner 'seasons' is given in chapter ten in the section on menstruation. A sustained examination of the significance of the womb / world metaphor is worked out in chapter twenty-seven. Each of the female *siddhis* in relation to life cycles are laid out in full in chapter eight.

As the female *siddhis* unfold in a woman's life, they offer a series of initiatory challenges and experiences that potentially bring an embodied understanding of the great powers of cyclical change and growth that echo the phases of the moon in the sky, or the tides in the sea. The female *siddhis* are opportunities for learning this wisdom as it is encoded in the body. Some of the *siddhis* may recur frequently, like menstruation or orgasm, others are less frequent, such as birth/s, or miscarriage/s, whilst others occur infrequently but perhaps over a more protracted period, such as pregnancy, lactation or the experiences of the perimenopause. But, in the same spirit as the yogic *siddhis* confer supernatural powers and deep clarity of vision, the female *siddhis* all offer the potential for initiation into wisdom, power and insight that can transform our understanding of ourselves and the world we inhabit. For example, the moments before menstruation, if observed with attentive awareness, can transform a woman's vision of the world:

> *One of my most beautiful memories of college is of a day when my period was due but hadn't yet arrived. I was sitting in my living room, studying, and I felt an unaccountable surge of joy. I looked up from my book and was dazzled by the air. It was so clear, so purely*

> *transparent, that the objects in the room were sharply etched and proud against it, and yet it was as though I could see the air for the first time. It had become visible to me, molecule for molecule. My mind was focused and free of anxiety, I felt for a moment as though I had taken the perfect drug, the one that has yet to be invented… (Angier 2000: 98)*

And the *siddhi* of birth can bring a woman into such a vivid encounter with the power of life itself that her perspective on the world is utterly transformed:

> *I see you dart into the world*
> *Pearly pink like the inside of a shell*
> *Streaked with silver.*
>
> *Look! Look!*
> *I am shouting with joy, rising up*
> *Like a phoenix from my pain*
> *With my eyes I behold you*
> *In the flesh I behold you*
>
> *So a holy man waking into death*
> *from a life of devotion or*
> *martyrdom in flames*
>
> *Might look into the shining face of god*
> *and see at once*
> *he had never believed.*
>
> *I see you with my eyes*
> *I see you in glory.*
>
> – *Transformation*, by Jeni Couzyn (in *Palmira* 1990: 92)

The pre-menstrual woman is 'calling in the vision' with mystical clarity, and the birthing woman and the visionary *yogī* both have the opportunity to 'look into the shining face of god'. In both the yogic *siddhis* and the female *siddhis*, the person encountering these special powers has to face this 'glory' not only in order to experience its force, but also to acknowledge it. For women, part of the process of acknowledging the wisdom gained through the experiences of the female *siddhis* comes through sharing. In direct contrast to the necessity for isolation and total secrecy in order to acquire or maintain yogic *siddhis*, for women it is the sharing of experiences that raises consciousness of them as potential *siddhis*. The power of circles of women to honour and celebrate the wisdom gained from our conscious encounter with female *siddhis* is fully explored in chapter twelve.

Yogic *siddhis* are powers that give *yogīs* dominion over the usual restrictions of human life on earth, conferring immortality or the capacity to defy the usual limitations of time and space. Female *siddhis*, in contrast, align the physical body of a woman with the elemental forces and cycles of the earth herself. The gift of the female *siddhis* is neither to control nor transcend natural forces and cycles, but the ability to embody their powers. The embodied experience of powerful natural cycles enables a conscious surrender to their force. It is this conscious surrender that can enable a woman to come more completely into harmony with the earth herself. The female *siddhis* are not evidence of dominion over nature's power, but a direct and embodied experience of that power at work. The female *siddhis* demonstrate a living connection with the cyclical powers of creation, nurture, sustenance and death. To embrace the power of the female *siddhis* is to encounter the deep rhythms of these cycles through the experiences of the female body.

One of the most recent and vivid descriptions of this elemental aspect of the yogic *siddhis* is described by Yoga Manmoyanand in his spiritual autobiography, *Sivananda Buried Yoga* (2008). He describes how his master *tāntrik* teacher actually manifests the elements of earth and water, fire and air in his own body: his consciousness is so aligned with the powers of the universe that he is able to create fire and hold it in his hand without burning his skin. This *siddhi* was attained as a result of many lifetimes of intense spiritual practice. At an embodied level, such experiences are naturally encoded in the cycles of the female body: a woman can be thoroughly 'earthed' by the experiences of late pregnancy and birth, she can be reconnected to the presence of watery flow in her body by her menstrual tides, and literally feel that she is 'burned alive' by the sheet-drenching hot sweats of *kuṇḍalinī* rising in a menopausal hot flush. The elements are encountered directly through these experiences, as we simply live through the cycles of our lives, our female *siddhis*. To achieve this merging with the cosmic forces by means of yogic *siddhis* requires years and lifetimes of *tapas*. All that is required for the female *siddhis* to confer their power is to pay attention: to notice that these *siddhis* arise naturally, to bring consciousness to these experiences. Paying close attention to these experiences feeds the power of the wild *yoginī* within, and nourishes the global empowerment of women.

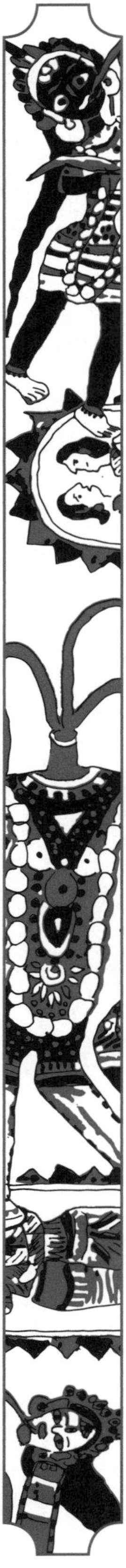

FEMALE *SIDDHIS*

THE ORIGINAL INSPIRATION FOR YOGA?

The practice of yoga helps women to bring awareness to our encounters with the elemental forces that are made very tangible in women's bodies through the female *siddhis*. The greatest '*mahā*' *siddhi*, or at least the *siddhi* that is most openly honoured in women, is the *siddhi* of giving birth. 'Birth is the most obvious expression of "what is" that we can experience...' explains Parvati Baker, author of the first western book on prenatal yoga (1974). 'For a conscious woman, childbirth is self-evidently holy.' (Baker 2001: xii).

Women who have the opportunity to encounter the *siddhi* of birth with fully conscious awareness, either through their own births or through attendance at other women's labours, frequently voice this understanding of birth as a great *siddhi*. Community midwife Ali Woozley, who has practised yoga for over twenty years, is able to perceive from a yogic perspective that the *siddhi* of birth is the ultimate manifestation of union with power, and as such she regards it as an inspiration for all yogic practice: 'The whole of yoga seems to me to be motivated by men's desire to create for themselves the powerful feelings that naturally arise in the body of a woman giving birth'. I believe Ali is right. And what she says about birth is also true of our experience of other intensities arising during the female life cycle, for example, menstruation and menopause.

I invite you now to feel the possibility that the inspiration for the earliest genesis of yoga may be rooted in a quest to emulate the experiences of female *siddhis* such as birth and menstruation. Consider that the development of *haṭha* yoga as a form of spiritual alchemy and transformation could have been motivated by a desire to elicit in men the kind of transcendental experiences that can come to women through conscious encounters with the naturally arising female *siddhis*.

This is not to say that women 'invented' the practice of yoga, but rather to hold that a reverent response to women's evident physical and emotional connection with the rhythms of cosmic order may have inspired men's search for yogic *siddhis* that would link them, through disciplined practice, to the kind of connection with pure power and being that comes to women through the female *siddhis*. From this perspective, yoga practice, and the whole technology of yogic techniques and disciplines, can be seen as a means to elicit the direct experience of elemental powers that work unbidden through women's bodies. Whilst the *haṭha yogīs* created a system of practice that is consciously imposed with force from without, the *yoginīs' siddhis* arise from within, and their power is experienced by consciously acknowledging what occurs quite naturally without any force.

If the inspiration or original model for the states of transcendental consciousness and superpowers of the yogic *siddhis* can be seen to lie in the female *siddhis*, then that changes how we understand the relationship between women and yoga now. It means that the predominantly female bias of contemporary yoga practice can be seen not as a colonisation of a previously male space, but instead as a kind of homecoming. It is not that women just have the power to 'feminise' *haṭha* yoga, but rather that we are now able to reclaim our connection to the female origins of the practice's inspiration. And this has a powerful impact, not just for how we relate to the past histories of yoga, but for how women practice now. For we live in a time when conscious encounters with the female *siddhis* are the exception rather than the norm.

We inhabit a world where many women have been disconnected from the experience of menstruation, or actively seek to avoid any conscious encounters with any of the other physical experiences that signal the female *siddhis*. For example, many millions of women worldwide experience the menstrual cycle as a source of physical pain, discomfort or inconvenience, and do their best to manage the monthly cycle in such as way as to minimise its impact upon their lives. There is a multi-billion pound global industry marketing hormonal contraception and disposable menstrual products to women. The intention of these forms of contraception and 'sanitary protection' is to obliterate the effects of the menstrual cycle upon women's lives, partly to render menstruation invisible, to avoid the shameful or inconvenient experience of having other people know a woman is menstruating, and partly because it is believed that naturally occurring menstrual cycles somehow limit a woman's sexual and physical freedoms, or at least are simply annoying.

If the menstrual cycle is approached with shame and annoyance, then it cannot be experienced as a *siddhi*. And as it is the 'mother cycle' around which all the other female *siddhis* circle, our cultural attitudes to menstruation have had a profoundly damaging effect upon women's capacity to encounter consciously any of the other female *siddhis*. But if the physiological and emotional changes of the menstrual cycle are recognised with full awareness, then the experience of shifts in consciousness around menstruation can be experienced as powerful meditative states that lead directly to deep insights, an experience of yoga, or union with cosmic rhythms. To menstruate with this awareness is a *siddhi*. It is not just the process of menstruation that offers the woman the *siddhi*, it is rather the attentive awareness to the subtle shifts of energy and consciousness that turn this capacity of the female body into a potential *siddhi*. Evidently, the more a culture and society honours, respects and acknowledges the significance of women's 'moon times', the more likely it is that the powerful experience of menstruation is understood by women themselves to be a *siddhi*. The culture of shame, disrespect, denigration and control that currently surrounds menstruation has cut women off from the possibility that they could experience menstruation as a spiritual initiation into higher realms of consciousness and awareness. The nature of the menstrual *siddhi* is discussed at much greater length in the section on menstruation in chapter ten. But the same process of denigration and control can be seen in patterns of response to all the other female *siddhis* too.

Almost every aspect of every one of these female *siddhis* has been systematically eradicated and/or brought under the control of the protocols and practices of a dominant orthodoxy of western medicine that regards most of the female *siddhis* as a set of medical problems to be fixed. Birth has been medicalised and controlled to the degree that many women lack any confidence that they are able to birth their babies. The *siddhi* of conscious menstruation has been rendered inaccessible to the hundreds of millions of women whose cycles are synthetic 'false cycles' created by contraceptive pills, injections and other strategies. These hormonal contraceptives have a profound effect upon the experience of the *siddhi* of female sexuality, lowering libido and altering female sexual response and the emotional context in which it unfolds. The *siddhi* of breastfeeding was almost entirely lost during the 1960s and 1970s in Europe and the USA, where women's natural rhythms of lactation and feeding were doubly controlled by medical misconceptions and the marketing power of companies selling artificial milk. This combination effectively stopped women lactating, or made them believe that they had insufficient milk, which had the same effect (see Palmer 2009). Access to the *siddhi* of menopause is widely denied by the use of hormone replacement therapy, whilst the experience of menarche is so hidden and ignored, or made the focus of such shame and disgust, that its status as the primary initiation into the conscious experience of the rest of the female *siddhis* is lost.

For many women, all of these *siddhis* have effectively been reduced to the status of medical problems, inconveniences or difficulties which need to be fixed or eradicated by a model of medical care that prizes intellectual order, controlled restraint and linear progression above emotional sensitivity, experiences of surrender, and the cyclical unfolding of wisdom. This systematic eradication of women's access to the sources of feminine spiritual wisdom can be reversed. The reversal is made possible by conscious acknowledgement and awareness of the powers of the female *siddhis*.

It is through the experiences we have gained by the practice of yoga that women can now bring consciousness to the female *siddhis* in their own lives. For example, the practice of pregnancy yoga encourages conscious awareness of birth as an initiatory encounter with cosmic power, and the practice of womb yoga encourages reverent honour and respect for the experiences of perimenopause and for the subtle shifts in consciousness through the menstrual cycle – especially the capacity for visionary insight in the time preceding and surrounding menstruation itself. Evidently, respect for these experiences can arise without practising yoga, but it is more common these days for these experiences to be encountered with zero conscious awareness of their spiritual significance.

So what yoga offers women is a very precious gift indeed: it is an attitude and an awareness, created by practice, that helps us to recognise these female experiences as potential *siddhis*, so that we can respectfully encounter them as initiations into power. Through such conscious initiation, we can become more open to the spiritual insights and deep understandings that are the inner power of the female *siddhis*. Yoga is helping us to reclaim our blood wisdom.

The insights I share are voiced by other women yoga practitioners and feminist scholars, and I hear similar discoveries expressed every day by the women with whom I work in the field of yoga for women's health. I am privileged to have heard these many voices, so what I am able to share now is an authentic appreciation of the phenomenal opportunity which yoga offers women and the men who love them to effect a planetary shift of awareness. The shift of awareness which yoga makes possible is to welcome the significance of the cyclical experience of time and consciousness as it plays out through the cycles of women's lives in the female *siddhis*. Yoga practice, especially womb-friendly yoga practice, encourages us to embrace the initiatory states of liminality and pure being of the female *siddhis*.

The following four chapters set out the foundations of womb yoga. In part two, we explore ten *tāntrik* goddesses known as the *Mahāvidyās* ('great wisdoms') who are representations of female power and cosmic wisdom. Understanding these goddesses can help us honour our own encounters with the female *siddhis* through each stage of a woman's life.

QUESTIONS AND REFLECTIONS

I invite you to consider now your own female *siddhis* by asking yourself some (or any, or all) of the following questions:

1. What experience do I have of altered and/or heightened states of consciousness and awareness arising through (or during) the practice of *haṭha* yoga and meditation?
2. What experience do I have of altered and/or heightened states of consciousness arising through the female *siddhis*, eg at menstruation, orgasm, lactation or childbirth?
3. What is the relationship between the female *siddhis* in my life and my practice of yoga? E.g. do I stop practising yoga when I menstruate, or do I stop menstruating when I practise yoga?

FURTHER READING AND RESEARCH

Fundamentally, further research into the experiences of the female *siddhis* can only be conducted in the laboratory of your own body, and by sharing your experiences with your female friends. In so far as I have been able to discover, there is no previous mention of the existence of potential female *siddhis* in the literature of *haṭha* yoga. But for an inspirational Goddess-feminist vision of women's experience that is rooted in a practice of yoga, I recommend **Vicki Noble**'s spiritual autobiography *Shakti Woman: Feeling our Fire, Healing our world: The new female shamanism* (1991), and her 2011 article 'Women and Yoga: Did Women Invent the Ancient Art of Yoga?

For accessible translations and commentaries on key *haṭha* yoga texts, **Swami Muktibodhananda Saraswati**'s (1999) translation and commentary of *Haṭha Yoga Pradīpikā* is a good place to start. The poetic rendering by **Mukunda Stiles** (2001) of the *Yoga Sūtras* is inspiring as a means to bring the teachings alive in everyday experience.

CHAPTER FOUR

awakening to the feminine energy of the life force: *prāṇa śakti* and the foundations of womb yoga

WELCOMING THE POWER OF LIFE

To breathe with reverence is to honour *prāṇa śakti*: the power of life itself. Our breath is a vehicle for the life force. There are other vehicles, for example food, and light and other beings, but the breath is of especial significance as a means to access vital energy. In yoga philosophy this energy is understood to be a feminine force, a form of the goddess known as *prāṇa śakti*, which literally means the power of the life force (*prāṇa* = life force; *śakti* = power). When we breathe we allow for this *prāṇa śakti* to enter our bodies. Most human breathing is an entirely unconscious business, and most people most of the time have little awareness that they are even breathing at all. And so, by neglect, the power of the life force within us can atrophy. We grow tired, and become ill, listless or unhappy for lack of vital energy. When we neglect to notice the rhythms of the flow of the breath that carries into us the very power which sustains us, we risk losing access to it entirely. Consciousness of the breath, and a positive attitude of welcome to the *prāṇa* which it brings us is key to our well-being.

Thankfully, yoga offers us a complete technology for heightening consciousness of our breath: *prāṇāyāma*. The range of yogic *prāṇāyāma* practices and the literature accompanying these practices is huge and complex. Generally speaking these techniques seek to heighten awareness and control over the natural flow of the breath in order to maximise the life force that can be 'extracted' from each breath, like pressing olives to extract the oil.

In the history and development of yogic lineages and schools, the practice of *prāṇāyāma* is hedged with cautions and characterised by controlled systems of measurement and restraint that can become very rigid. In *Mother's Breath* (2006),

I explored a more feminine and fluid approach to *prāṇāyāma* that is rooted in consciousness of naturally arising spontaneous breath patterns, for example observation and awareness of moments of transition in the breath as 'thresholds', or using the voice on the breath as a bridge between will and surrender. Such fluid and responsive approaches to *prāṇāyāma* not only provide therapeutic applications for use during pregnancy, birth, postnatal recovery and mothering, but also refine and feminise the more rigid types of breath control *prāṇāyāma*.

But whichever approach to *prāṇāyāma* is taken, whether rigidly measured and controlled, or fluid and feminine, the ultimate and simple intention of all *prāṇāyāma* is to heighten consciousness of the ebb and flow of *prāṇa śakti*. In *śakta tantra*, this awareness has a reverential or devotional attitude or *bhava* at its heart. For to bring awareness to the passage of our breath is to give a conscious invitation to *prāṇa śakti* to enter us. By issuing a conscious invitation to her to be our guest, we are more able to prepare for her arrival, and thus we are empowered to honour her. When we welcome *prāṇa śakti* fully through conscious breath, she is able to give of herself more completely, and so each conscious breath can access the vital energy of the life force more effectively. It is as if, when we know a guest is arriving at our home, we endeavour to make things pleasing to receive that guest so that she will be more comfortable when she arrives, and more likely to stay longer with us, sharing her wisdom and gifts. The wisdom which *prāṇa śakti* shares is that the life energy is precious and to be revered; the gift she gives is vitality. The foundations of womb yoga practice enable us to cultivate a reverent awareness of the movements of *prāṇa śakti* through conscious breath.

The practices described below embody this key understanding. The practices move from the simple to the complex, starting with observation of the natural flow of breath and ending with a rich combination of directed breath and hand *mudrās* (gestures) with visualisations. The practices can be done individually or joined all together into one longer sequence. Each practice is described from two perspectives: how to do it and why to do it. The 'how' section gives instruction on the physical form and energetic flow of the technique; the 'why' section offers guidance on the nature of the inner feeling or *bhava* to evoke in order to encounter the effects of the practice at the level of emotional connection and spiritual insight.

CIRCLE OF FLOWING BREATH: WELCOMING THE RHYTHMIC BREATH CYCLE

The circle of breath brings clarity of awareness to the rhythm of the natural breath cycle. All practices in this book rest upon this practice. It provides a vital foundation for everything that follows, and so even though it appears to be so very simple, its stages are described in detail. To begin, it works well to follow the breath as you read the instructions. That way, you are not struggling to remember the points at each breath. To read and breathe with awareness is in itself a meditation that can cultivate the attitude of reverence to the breath that makes this practice so special.

STAGE ONE

How to do it: form and flow

Choose a comfortable seated or resting position.
Let yourself yawn a few times. Close your eyes. Then settle deeper into your chosen position and just let the breath come and go, in and out through the nose.
Notice when the breath comes in.
Notice when the breath goes out. Just observe this coming and going.
Allow for the breath to move at an easy and natural pace – if there are quick breaths, notice them. If there are slow, deep breaths notice them.
Be aware of the rhythm of two parts: inhalation – exhalation.
A coming in, and then a going out. Understand the two parts as being part of a circle of breath – one half going out, and one half coming in.

Why to do it: bhava or inner feeling

The intention with this practice is to heighten and deepen awareness of the presence of the precious life force in every breath. Evoke an attitude of welcoming each breath: know that *prāṇa śakti*, the life force, is riding in on each inhalation and riding out on each exhalation. Honour her arrivals and departures. Feel each breath welcoming her into the body, and then bid her farewell as she leaves.

STAGE TWO

How to do it: form and flow

Begin to notice the rhythm of shifts from in-breath to out-breath.
Then notice the place where the inhalation turns into the exhalation.
Then begin to notice the place where the exhalation turns into the inhalation.
Watch these places, and acknowledge the turning of the breath at these places.
As your sense of the rhythm of the breath becomes more acute, begin to notice how these pauses are not really pauses, but little places all of their own.
The rhythm of the breath, as you observe the inhale and the exhale – to a rhythm based on the relationship between four – the inhale, and the place between inhale and exhale; the exhale, and the place between it and the next inhale.
The circle of the breath expands into this awareness: inhale, and the place between in and out; exhale, and the place between out and in.

Why to do it: *bhava* or inner feeling

Observation leads to insight. The point of observing the breath so intently is to learn what *prāṇa śakti* has to teach. Each rhythmic cycle of the breath is unique, and part of a pattern. Know that within this continuous rhythmic cycle of circles, everything is the same, and everything is changing. The breath keeps coming, and the breath keeps changing. Every breath is a complete rhythmic cycle: in, and the pause that follows it, out, and the pause that follows it.

Every rhythmic breath cycle contains within its circle all that we need to know. Things always change: the inhalation turns into the pause; and the pause turns into the out breath; and the out breath turns into the pause.

Know that the truth of the breath circle is just this: right now, vitality is coming in on the breath; right now I am watching the breath turn to leave; right now I am breathing out; right now I am waiting for the breath to turn back in. The cycle is complete but the rhythm continues. Watching the rhythmic breath cycle, we see the patterns of change, pause, and release. Over, and over and over again – each rhythmic breath cycle is unique, and each one part of a pattern. A rhythmic pattern of change, pause and release.

Within our recognition of the patterns of the breath cycles comes clear attention to the spaces between the component parts of each breath: especially of the spaces between inhalation and exhalation. Awareness of these spaces between the breaths brings us a great gift. The gift is an intimate encounter with the very ground of being. For the relationship between Śakti and breath is like the relationship between Śiva and conscious awareness. We encounter Śakti when we notice her riding into the body on the vehicle of the breath, as *prāṇa śakti*. We encounter Śiva, the consciousness of pure being, when we notice him riding into our awareness on the vehicle of conscious attention.

In the same way as we feel the enlivening effects of *prāṇa* in and around us when energy comes into the body on the breath, so too can we drop into a state of pure being when we focus mental attention on conscious awareness.

If the most vivid object of focus can be the feeling of breath, especially at its turning points, then the awareness of Śakti on the breath and the experience of pure being through conscious awareness become simultaneous: simply by becoming aware of the turning points of the breath, there is a connection to both *prāṇa* (Śakti) and the stillness of pure being (Śiva) – thus arises an experience of the unity of Śiva / Śakti: pure energy and pure consciousness as one.

Integration

When you are ready take the awareness gently away from the breath, and back to the position in which you are lying or sitting. Take a big breath in, yawn and stretch. Open your eyes. Even when you stop this conscious practice, the attitude or *bhava* of reverence continues. Every breath in the circle is an opportunity to honour the life force as she rides in on the breath. Every pause in the breath circle is an opportunity to experience the stillness of pure consciousness. Each circle of breath can lead our awareness to an intimate encounter with the powers of pure energy and pure being.

If you become comfortable with the pause places at the end of the exhale and at the end of the inhale, then allow yourself to rest there momentarily. Don't let this resting disrupt the naturally occurring rhythmic flow of the breath cycle. There should be no holding or forcing – just resting with the pause and waiting for the rhythm of the breath to take you over into the next change. Noticing the turning moments between inhalation and exhalation can impart a sense of spaciousness, as if the circle of breath expands to accommodate our heightened awareness of its rhythmic pauses.

These pauses offer the potential for profound insights and deep calm, as Sandra Sabatini recognises:

the pause at the end of the exhalation
and the pause at the end of the inhalation
is a special place
where nothing happens or nothing seems to happen
yet the old air is travelling away from us
and the new breath is ready to move in

in that space in between
there is silence
more than anything else
silence... and space
(Sabatini: 79)

The foundation of this understanding is clearly communicated in the following dharanas or meditative concentration practices given in the *Vijñāna Bhairava Tantra*, a ninth-century Kashmiri philosophical and practical treatise on the state of *bhairava*, or that form of consciousness experienced at the realisation of the individual soul's desire to be united with universal consciousness. From the feminine perspective of womb yoga practice, it is the tender observations of the natural pauses and releases in the breath that lead to the encounter with the nature of pure consciousness itself:

> *By fixing the mind at the two points of generation (of upward moving and downward moving energies), the state of fullness results' (Dhāraṇa 24). 'When the ingoing pranic air and the outgoing pranic air are both restrained in their space from the (respective points of) return, the essence of Bhairava manifests' (Dhāraṇa 25). 'When Śakti in the form of* vāyu *or pranic air is still and does not move swiftly in a specific direction, there develops in the middle, through the state of* nirvikalpa, *the form of Bhairava. (Dhāraṇa 26).*

FULL YOGIC BREATH: WIDENING THE CIRCLE, INVITING THE GUESTS TO LINGER

If the honoured 'guests' whom we welcome in the circle of breath practice described above are the very essence of yoga – pure energy and pure being united in consciousness – then it is natural for us to wish to make our guests as comfortable as possible in order that they may wish to linger. The intention of the full yogic breath is to encourage our breath circle to be as full and wide as possible, by making space in the body.

How to do it: form and flow

In this practice, the breath becomes like a wave flowing up the body on the inhalation and down the body on the exhalation. Inhaling, the breath flows up from the pubic bone to the base of the throat. Experience the rising up of the abdomen and the full sideways expansion of the ribcage.

Feel the shoulder blades moving down the back and pressing the spine forward, sense that the sideways lifting upwards movement of the ribcage allows for a full inhalation. Allow for the lungs to expand completely, and take the breath right the way up to the collarbones. As the breath leaves the body the movement of 'deflation' flows down from the base of the throat to the pubic bone. Feel the ribs coming back closer together, the whole ribcage settling back down into its starting position, and the belly moving back towards the spine a little.

Why to do it: *bhava* or inner feeling

The intention with full yogic breathing is to create a more powerful and spacious vehicle on which *prāṇa śakti* can enter the body. If watching the natural breath is like inviting *prāṇa śakti* to enter and leave seated on a little pony, then watching the full yogic breath is like providing her with a sleek thoroughbred. The heightening and deepening of awareness cultivated through the circle of breath practice is rendered more powerful by applying the observations to the full yogic breath. Never compromise your own ease: you should be comfortable and relaxed enough with the rhythm of the breath to allow the full yogic breath to flow in a gentle pattern that enables you to breathe completely, but at an easy pace. Watch as the rhythm settles in – there may be some shorter breaths, followed by longer ones – take an interest in the rhythm and cultivate awareness as you watch for the comfortable rhythm to arise. After a while it should feel effortless, as if the breath and the body have become great friends, so that the breath simply lets itself into and out of the body without effort. Because breathing in this way creates more space and time for each circle of breath, the experience of the pauses between the inhalations and exhalations is intensified, and a more intimate understanding of the relationship between energy and consciousness arises: the breath is bigger, so the pauses can be longer, and with longer pauses there is more time to honour the guests and their gifts.

VICTORY AND SURRENDER: THE OCEAN–GOLDEN THREAD COMBINATION

This combination of two naturally arising breath patterns creates a powerful physical incentive for all parts of the breath circle to become spacious. Victorious breath (*ujjāyī*) is used on the inhalation and the Golden thread breath on the exhalation. Both promote a gradual lengthening of the flow of breath. By lengthening the inhalation and exhalation, the mind has space and time to rest in the conscious honouring of *prāṇa śakti* and to witness the arising of pure conscious being in the open spaces created by this technique. At an emotional and spiritual level, each cycle of breath alternates between the experiences of victory and surrender.

How to do it: form and flow

First observe the naturally arising circle of the breath. Then establish a complete yogic breath with an easy rhythm.

GOLDEN THREAD

Now invite the Golden thread breath to arise on the exhalation. Take several yawns, releasing the jaw and throat. Circle the jaw, and move it from side to side. Let there be a big breathy sigh: 'AAAH' next time you exhale. Open your mouth very wide to allow the loud sigh to escape. Repeat three times, or more if you feel the need to stretch and release the jaw and throat. Yawn again if you feel any tension in the jaw and throat. Soften your lips, either by stretching and releasing through movement or flipping the lips with your fingertips, whichever feels softest. Take a few more loud sighs, but with more power to the exhaling breath so that the soft, relaxed lips flap open and close as the breath moves through, making a BHRRRR, BHRRR sound like a horse blowing breath away.

Now reduce the volume of the sighing sound and let the lips be still but open, so that you can feel the breeze of the breath moving through them. Let the sound of the sighs gradually reduce to silence. Have the teeth and the soft lips open at whatever distance apart feels comfortable as the breath exits through the mouth.

If it feels comfortable, but only if it feels comfortable, gradually reduce the distance between the lips so that they remain soft but only very slightly apart – just enough of a gap so that you might imagine a piece of tissue paper held between the lips. Watch the easy natural rhythm of the breath as it exits through the lips. The heart of this exhale is softness. You are not pursing the lips, or making them tight as if to whistle. The lips are perfectly soft, and the breath that passes out between them is perfectly gentle.

If the reduction in the space between the lips is effortless, but only if it is effortless, then gradually allow there to be only a very small gap between the top teeth and the bottom teeth, between the top lip and the bottom lip. It's such a small gap that it's practically invisible.

Breathe in through the nose. Breathe out between the slightly parted lips.

Feel a fine cool breeze passing out between the lips. Have the cheeks, lips and face utterly relaxed. There is no pursing or holding the lips. They are soft. Feel the breath now travelling in through the nose, and out through the mouth. Have the lips at whatever distance feels easiest and either simply focus on the sensation of the breeze of the breath leaving, or allow the breath to be so fine that it feels as if a golden thread is spinning out between the lips. It's a thin, golden thread, like embroidery yarn, smooth and silky, soft and supple, and it is spinning out and out and out and out with every exhalation. Feel the breeze of the exhalation travelling out between the lips, out into the air, in front of your closed eyes.

Allow the focus of the mental attention to travel out with each breath. Let the end of the golden thread carry the mental attention farther and farther away with each exhalation. It is as if the final point of the outgoing breath were carrying the mental focus completely out of the body.

Keep on with the easy rhythm of this Golden thread breath exiting through the lips, but now prepare to exhale through the nose instead of the mouth. Temporarily depart from the Golden thread exhalation as you invite the Victorious breath (*ujjāyī*) to arise.

UJJĀYĪ

Ujjāyī is a naturally occurring, slow and softly audible breath that happens every night when we are deeply asleep. The following instructions enable you to evoke this naturally arising breath consciously.

Exhale with the sound HAAAH and the mouth wide open. Repeat several times. Feel the sound creating movement in the bottom of the throat. Then after the next inhale, close the lips and exhale with HAAAH behind a closed mouth. You will be exhaling through the nose, whilst maintaining the same sound and feeling in the throat, but behind the closed lips. Now the power of the sound is retained inside the body, and you can direct it wherever you like. As your mind follows the sound of the breath, healing energy can be directed to wherever the mind visits: 'Where the mind flows, there energy flows.' (*Haṭha Yoga Pradīpikā* 2:2, p.134)

Continue to breathe through the nostrils, but feel now as though the sound of the breath is coming in through the throat. Feel the breath passing over the base of the throat, almost as if you had bypassed your nose, and were breathing directly through imaginary gills. Allow there now to be a gentle sound in the base of the throat, rather like the soft beginnings of a snore (but not so hard as to make a snoring sound), or the breath you make at night as you drift off to sleep.

Let this sound be very gentle, so that although the throat is slightly constricted, there is ease and softness. Be sure the breath is still actually coming in and out through the nose, even though it feels as if it is in the throat. This is *ujjāyī* breath

After the next *ujjāyī* breath inhalation, return to the feeling of the Golden thread exhalation by opening the lips to let the breath out. At the end of the exhalation close the lips softly but completely and use *ujjāyī* for the inhalation. Alternate now in an easy rhythm between *ujjāyī* breath inhaling and Golden thread breath exhaling.

Why to do it: *bhava* or inner feeling

The intention with this combination of two *prāṇāyāma*s is to evoke an experience of rhythmic alternation between restraint and release, an embodied understanding of the dance between victory and surrender. The lengthening of the exhalation with the Golden thread is achieved effortlessly and softly: it is a physical experience of slow and total surrender. Simply because the gap through which the breath passes is small, it takes a long time for all the breath to get out. There is no sense of force; you simply watch the breath lengthen, following it out into the limitless space and silence in front of you. The end of the exhalation marks the completion of the experience of letting go, a surrendering of effort: the silence of absolute release. The use of *ujjāyī* on the inhalation creates, by contrast, an audible sense of restraint and focus. The sound of *ujjāyī* breath signals that the inhalation is being guided and held by the sensation in the glottis. The sensation in the throat is enticing or drawing the breath in under circumstances of soft restraint, providing boundaries and form, a way to feel and hear the breath.

When both these *prāṇāyāmas* are partnered in this pattern, the breath moves in a metaphorical dance between the experiences of victory and surrender. It is as if the audible form and tangible sensation of the offers a victorious vehicle on which *prāṇa śakti* can enter the body: you can actually feel and hear her entering. Then as the

Golden thread releases the breath through the exhalation and beyond into the spaces that may follow, we discover the possibility of an open encounter with pure being: a soft release into consciousness. It is limitless and silent. Together the experiences offered by this pair of *prāṇāyāmas* invite the guests of power and being (Śakti and Śiva consciousness) to inhabit us: she rides in on the *ujjāyī*, and then as she leaves on the silent Golden thread breath it leads into a limitless space of stillness and quiet in which to encounter pure consciousness.

Refinements

Ujjāyī slows the breath, lengthening both the inhale and the exhale, by breathing through a slightly narrowed glottis. Adopting *ujjāyī* consciously plays a clever yogic trick on the body, sending it signals to enter a deep state of rest ('sounds like I'm asleep'). Continued and regular use of *ujjāyī* breath can reduce high blood pressure, probably due to the calming effects of the lengthened inhales and exhales. *Ujjāyī* can be done very quietly, so that only you can hear it. It can also be done more loudly, so that it is louder than your thoughts. Or it can be like the sound of the waves of a far distant ocean. It can be very helpful to imagine, as you listen to the sound of this far distant ocean in your throat, that the breath is lowering you deeper down to the source of all peace, to a place of profound quiet, where you can rest absolutely undisturbed.

The temptation when learning *ujjāyī* is to create the sound at the expense of the rhythmic cycle of the breath. The soft sound of *ujjāyī*, when done properly, should enhance and not compromise the easy pace of the rhythmic breath cycle.

A common problem when learning the Golden thread breath exhalation is that a struggle arises because the gap between the lips is too small for your rate and depth of breath. Never compromise the free release of the breath for the desire to reduce the gap between the lips. Always allow the gap to be a sufficient size for the breath to leave comfortably. The lips need to be soft and the exhalation free and easy if the pratice is to lead into any experience of quiet and stillness.

OPENING THE LOTUS TO *PRĀṆA ŚAKTI*: INTEGRATED SOUND, BREATH AND *HASTA MUDRĀ* (HAND GESTURE) MEDITATION

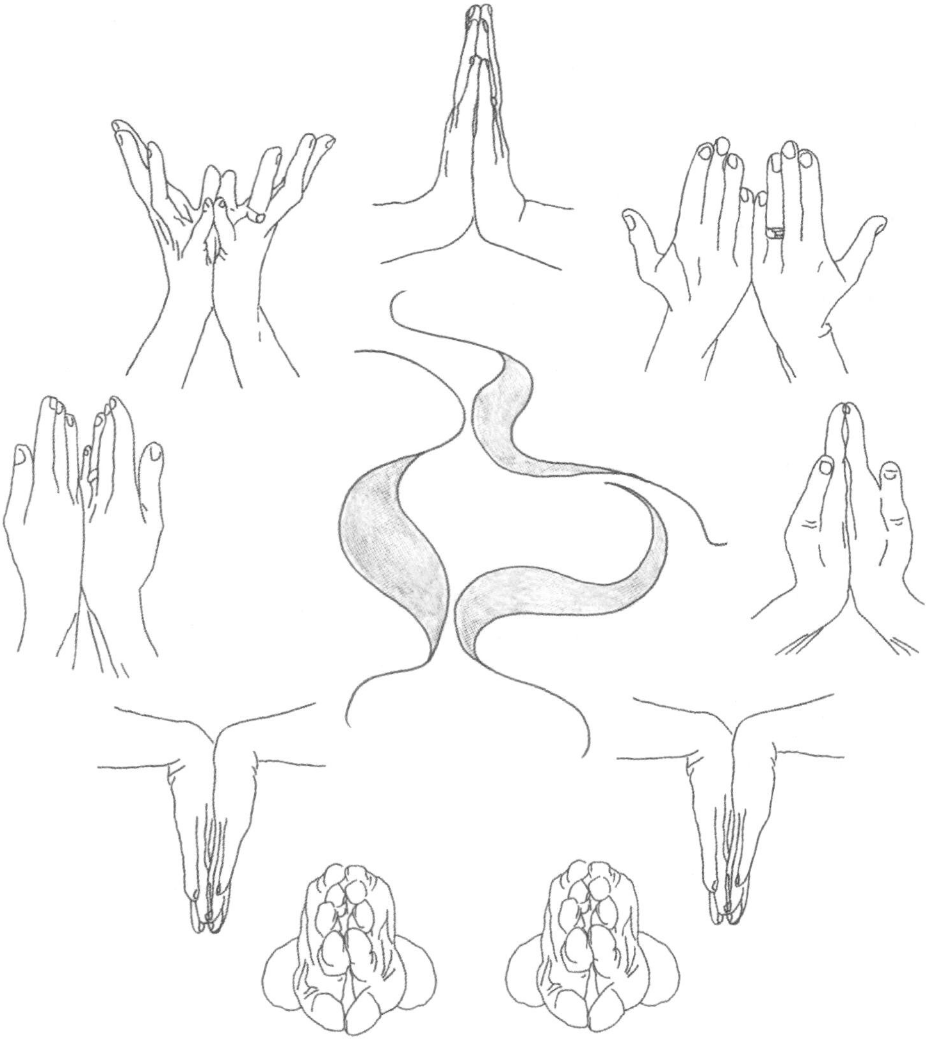

Opening the lotus to *prāṇa śakti*

This beautiful practice floats a fluid *hasta mudrā* (hand gesture) sequence on the ocean of the previous *prāṇāyāma* pattern. It can be accompanied with optional *bīja mantra* chanting. The integration of breath and hand movement with sound and awareness serves to deepen the encounter with surrender and release that arises in the previous practice.

How to do it: form and flow

Sit comfortably and establish a comfortable rhythm of easy full yogic breath. Now establish the dance between Golden thread exhalation and *ujjāyī* inhalation. Utilise this *prāṇāyāma* throughout the following practice. It creates a good foundation for the natural voicing of the *mantras*.

Place your hands in the closed lotus position – *namaste* – either with palms flat together, or with a tiny space between the palms and fingers like a little cave. Have the fingertips touching, and pointing upwards, with the thumbs resting on the breastbone. Inhale.

On Golden thread exhale, move the hands forward rolling open the palms as if you were opening the pages of a book (palms facing chest, with the sides of the little fingers touching). Look down into the pages of the 'book' of your hands.

Keep the outsides of the little fingers touching like the binding of the book, and continue to open out the palms, letting the wrists turn and pivot against each other until the backs of the hands are touching and the fingers point in towards you, touching the breastbone. The elbows will move up and out to the sides.

Keep pivoting the wrists against each other with the hands rotating inwards and down so that the fingertips are pointing downwards. The fingertips may stroke down the breastbone.

Then the *namaste* has been turned upside down and 'inside out'.

Let the hands keep turning, backs touching, so that the sides of the little fingers are uppermost.

Keeping the backs of the hands together, turn the wrists so that the fingertips point away from you, straightening the elbows and stretching the arms out straight at the height of the heart. The fingertips will now point forwards and out.

Now pause the hand movement and inhale *ujjāyī* breath into your 'inside out' *namaste*.

On a Golden thread exhale bend the elbows outwards, and draw the 'inside out' *namaste* closer in, turning the wrists to let the fingertips point straight down. Keep the backs of the wrists touching and continue the exhale as you roll the fingertips to point in towards the body. Let the fingertips touch the breastbone, stroking upwards as you turn the wrists until the fingertips point upwards.

Then open up the palms like the pages of the book again, and use the meeting point between the two little finger sides as the binding and bring the palms back towards each other.

At this point, bring the hands into the open lotus position – keeping the sides of the two thumbs touching, and maintaining contact between the outer sides of the two little fingers – but opening up the other fingers into as wide open a lotus bloom as you choose: anything from a barely open bud, where the tips of the fingers are quite close and the fingers are bent, to a fully open bloom, where the fingers are straight, widely spaced and the finger tips stretching away from each other.

These instructions take you through one whole cycle of the opening of the lotus to *prāṇa śakti* – inhale – exhale – inhale – exhale.

Practise the breath and hand gestures together until it feels as if the rhythm of breath and the pattern of the movement have synchronised.

Then prepare to voice the breath.

Inhale *ujjāyī* with your hands in the closed lotus position – *namaste* – with palms flat together, fingertips pointing upwards and thumbs resting on the breastbone.

On an exhale, sound YAṀ as you roll the palms open, turn the fingers down and out to the inside out *namaste* with straight arms out in front.

Now pause the hand movement and inhale *ujjāyī*.

On an exhale, sound YAṀ as you bend the elbows and draw the 'inside out' *namaste* closer in, turning the wrists and returning to the open lotus at the heart.

Refinements

The basic *hasta mudrā* sequence described above offers 'open' or closed lotus options at the start and/or finish. It can be placed at a single energy centre (*cakra*), or it can be placed at different heights in the body, to 'open' the lotus of each energy centre in a sequence, moving from the earth centre (*mūlādhāra*) up to the crown of the head (*sahasrāra*) with the open lotus gesture, and then from the crown of the head (*sahasrāra*) back down to the earth centre (*mūlādhāra*) with the closing lotus gesture. The instructions above are for the focus at the heart centre, where the sound is YAṀ. If you choose to transpose the gesture to other energy centres, you can match each location in the body with the appropriate *bīja mantras* as described below:

Earth *cakra* (*mūlādhāra*), *bīja mantra LAṀ*: start and end with the *namaste* / lotus resting at the pubic bones.

Water *cakra* (*svādhiṣṭhāna*), *bīja mantra VAṀ*: start and end with the *namaste* / lotus resting above the pubic bones and below the navel.

Fire *cakra* (*maṇipūra*), *bīja mantra RAṀ*: start and end with the *namaste* / lotus at the navel.

Air *cakra* (*anāhata*), *bīja mantra YAṀ*: start and end with the *namaste* / lotus at the breastbone as described above.

Space / ether *cakra* (*viśuddha*), *bīja mantra HAṀ*: start and end with the *namaste* / lotus at the throat.

Beyond the five elements:

Third eye *cakra* (*ājñā*), *bīja mantra AUM*: start and end with the *namaste* / lotus at the third eye.

Crown *cakra* (*sahasrāra*), *bīja mantra AUM*: start and end with the *namaste* / lotus on the crown of the head.

Take the practice up from earth to crown, opening all the lotuses and then down from crown back to earth, closing the petals.

Why to do it: *bhava* or inner feeling

The fluid hand gestures which accompany the victory / surrender breath patterns and sounds present a manual metaphor. The experience begins with the lotus as a closed bud (palms together), moves through a period of intense upheaval, in which the bud is turned upside down, and inside out, to come to a pause where the practitioner has a moment to nurture herself through the breath. After this moment of nurturing in the midst of upheaval (with the lotus upside down, inside out and stretched 'out there') the closed bud returns to the heart space as a fully blooming open lotus. It is through the challenges and upheavals of life, which turn our sense of ourselves upside down and inside out, that our hearts come to open fully, and bloom with love and acceptance. This metaphorical encounter with the transition from closed, to out of control, to happily open, can be helpfully applied to many of the experiences of growing into ourselves as women. For example, the initial letting go of the palms' first opening, can be like falling in love, when letting go of one's individual boundaries and closed heart is pure delight; but the second release, which comes from a place of challenge and confusion, is more like the process of choosing to sustain a relationship in the midst of difficulty, choosing to open again to the forces of love even in the face of fear or resentment. The practice can also helpfully be understood as a metaphor for labour and birth, where the first letting go, as labour begins, is welcomed with excitement, but the release into second stage labour, at a time of exhaustion or desperation, can sometimes be terrifying or painful.

However you choose to apply this 'second letting go' metaphor to your experiences, the attitudes of acceptance and open-hearted embracing of change make 'Opening the Lotus/es' a practice that we can helpfully invite to live in our hearts. The experience of the sound, breath and hand gestures in this practice can be interpreted in such a way as to sustain us through many challenges. To meet the demands of being a woman requires acceptance, courage and compassion. The metaphor of this practice can be a means to invite these qualities into our lives: the turning of the hands demonstrates the shifting upheavals (upside down and inside out) which we need to accept, reminds us that courage (whose root word is *cor* – Latin for heart) requires an open heart, and shows us that the opening of the heart can be a beautiful blooming into a maturity that allows for deep compassion and understanding.

From a spirited perspective, this practice provides an engaging synthesis of breath, hand movement and sound that invites us to encounter balance between the need for release and the need for nourishment, strength and protection. There is both poignant surrender and letting go (as the hands open up on the exhale), and an experience of returning home (as the inhale brings the hands back to the starting place). It can be as if the inhalation, when *prāṇa śakti* enters on the breath, gives us the strength and the energy to allow the total release of the exhalation. At the time when the first letting go has led to a place that is palpably out of control (with the *namaste* inside out, upside down, and fully extended away from us), then the arrival of *prāṇa śakti* on the inhalation is a welcoming renewal of strength. It is her nurturing presence on this second inhalation that provides the capacity to let go once again from that point of chaos; and it is only through the release of the second exhalation that we are able to fully allow the blooming of the lotus in the heart as we move into a place of expanded consciousness and spacious opening.

CHAPTER FIVE

greeting the womb with love: nine core practices of *yoni namaskāra*

...By the Yoni Mudrā the fingers form a triangle as a manifestation of the inner desire that the Devī should come and place Herself before the worshipper, for the Yoni is Her Pīṭha [place] or Yantra [geometric representation]. (Woodroffe: 351).

RECONNECTION

These practices reconnect your awareness to your womb or womb-space as the seat of a nourishing inner wisdom. They are simple but powerful greetings that use movement, breath and gesture to direct consciousness into the heart of the womb. The practices integrate awareness of the womb as a physical organ or literal space, and as a symbolic connection with mother consciousness. This consciousness exists energetically within every woman as the sacred potentials for love, nurture, generosity and creativity: the qualities of the womb herself. To experience these qualities as real powers in our lives is to embrace our ancient blood wisdom. This embrace is initiated by offering loving greetings to the womb or womb-space within us.

HEART-WOMB RIVER: THE CHANNEL OF ENERGY BETWEEN LOVE AND CREATIVITY

All of these greetings begin with consciousness in the heart and bring it to the womb. The channel through which the awareness flows is the heart-womb meridian, a pranic link between the the heart and the womb. This particular meridian is acknowledged both in Traditional Chinese Medicine (heart-uterus meridian) and in *āyurveda*, the ancient Indian medical system that shares the same philosophical framework of understanding (*sāṁkhya darśana*) that underpins the whole of yoga. I refer to this energetic connection between heart and womb as the *hṛdaya-yoni nadī*, which literally means the river (*nadī*) of energy that flows between the space of the spiritual heart (*hṛdaya*) and the source of creation or the womb (*yoni*).

In āyurvedic understanding of the energy body, and in particular the approach to *āyurveda* pioneered by Maya Tiwari in her Wise Earth School of Ayurveda, the womb is revered as a portal to universal consciousness: 'the cosmic gateway through which the universe's rhythm and memory exchange with human life'. The energies residing in the womb (or in the space that organ may once have inhabited) manifest the very powers of creation: 'In essence your *śakti* energy is the Mother Consciousness on planet earth' (Tiwari 2007: 5). By practising the greetings in this chapter with an inner feeling of love and respect for the womb within us we honour this part of ourselves as a microcosmic manifestation of the creative energies of the universe. These greetings are the foundation of an approach to yoga that honours the energies of the womb as the source of our creative vitality. By greeting the womb with love we not only reconnect to the *śakti* or life power in the womb or womb space, but also revive the loving energies of the heart by bringing them into conscious connection with the nourishing potential of the womb space energies.

YONISTHĀNA CAKRA: PLACING THE WOMB BETWEEN EARTH AND WATER

In yogic esoteric anatomy, the *cakra* system generally places the womb specifically in relation to the second *cakra*, *svādhiṣṭhāna*, which is associated with the water element. Relating the womb's qualities to water at an energetic level helps us to experience the energies of the womb as flowing tides. Certainly at a physical level, we experience the functions of the womb's cycles as a series of fluid flows: menstrual blood flow, cyclical changes in mucus, the sometimes gushing release of amniotic waters, and the juices which flow at sexual arousal and orgasm are all evidence of the fluidity which the womb and vagina create, harbour and release in response to our monthly rhythms. The shifts in these flows are our part of a cosmic dance whose rhythms can respond to lunar phases, and whose intricate pattern of 'inner seasons' responds to the cycles of our emotional and spiritual life (for a more sustained examination of these cycles in relation to menstruation and female sexuality, see chapter eleven).

It is helpful to understand that the rhythmic patterns of womb life flow in waves and tides like oceans and rivers. But the water element is not the only force at work in the womb. If we are fully to connect with her powers then we need also to experience that there is an earthed quality to the womb opening; for the vulva, the 'cosmic gateway' to the womb, is in fact directly associated with the earth herself. In terms of the usual pattern of understanding *cakras*, then the first energy centre, *mulādhāra,* is linked with the element of earth. And so, if we envision the vulva poised within this *cakra*, connecting with the earth, and the womb above filled with fluids and governed by the cyclical flow of lunar tides, we can begin to recognise that the womb's qualities are composed of both earth and water. The two mingle.

To heighten our consciousness of the co-mingling of earth and water in the energies of the womb, it is valuable to recognise that in fact she occupies her own special place in the anatomy of the energy body. This place is more than a simple 'junction' between *mulādhāra* (earth *cakra*) and *svādhiṣṭhāna* (water *cakra*). The womb's location in relation to the other *cakras* can be identified as *yonisthāna cakra*, which literally means the 'special land of the womb', or 'the place of the cosmic gateway'. *Yonisthāna* is an additional feminine refinement in our understanding of the *cakra* system, the womb's special place where water and earth meet in creative fusion. A fuller exploration of *yonisthāna* and the relationship between the elements of earth and water in relation to womb energy is given in the next chapter, where seated and standing sequences provide an embodied understanding of this relationship. For now, it is helpful to acknowledge this energetic placement of the womb between *svādhiṣṭhāna* and *mulādhāra cakras*, and to know that when we greet the womb with reverence in these practices, we embrace the qualities of earth and water as they mingle within in the microcosm of the female body, manifesting as our capacity to be rooted and stable, creative and nurturing.

HOW TO USE THESE PRACTICES

The series of techniques described in this chapter stand alone as a complete yoga meditative practice that is rewarding and delicious to encounter in full, just as it is presented below. However, the techniques also fit very well in the context of a more general yoga session involving other *āsana* (postures) and *prāṇāyāma* (breathing practices). For example, the semi-supine practices can be utilised at the start of *āsana* practice and the seated greetings make a very positive closure, or vice versa. The techniques can also be practised individually, or integrated a little at a time within other approaches to yoga in order to provide a softer or more feminine feel to the experience. Although the first three practices are here described as seated techniques, they can fruitfully be transposed to standing poses and incorporated within *vinyāsas* (sequences) of many other poses, as described in chapters seven and twenty-six.

A NOTE ON BREATH AND *MUDRĀ*

The breath patterns described can be used with a simple yogic breath, or overlayed with the *ujjāyī* / Golden thread combination *prāṇāyāma* described in the previous chapter, according to your preferences and intentions. The flat, open form of *yoni mudrā* (womb gesture) is used in the majority of the practices because it is the most simple and easily moveable version of the *mudrā* to incorporate into movement. A variety of more complex variations are presented in the sixth practice, 'womb power sacred gestures sequence' (pp.149–52).

HEART-WOMB RIVER SACRED GREETING GESTURE: RIVER-LOTUS FORM (INNER)

How to do it: form and flow

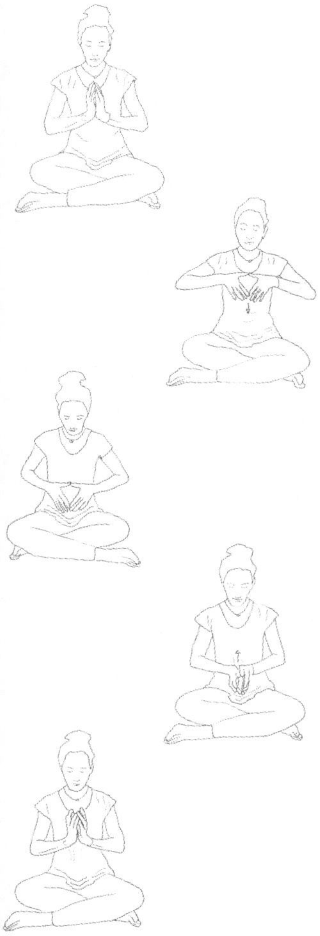

INHALE as you sit comfortably. Begin with the palms together and outer edges of the thumbs resting on the breastbone in *namaste*.

EXHALE as you keep the thumb tips touching and slide the palms of both hands outwards across the top of the breasts, until the hands rest flat and soft on the chest, with the index fingertips touching to create an open *yoni mudrā*, the downward-pointing triangle inside the space between the outstretched thumbs and index fingers.

Continue to **EXHALE** as you slide this *yoni mudrā* down the central line of the body until it comes to rest over the womb, with the thumbs beneath the navel and the tips of the index fingers on the pubic bones. Let the hands rest here until the exhalation is complete.

INHALE with the hands resting over the womb in simple *yoni mudrā*.

EXHALE keeping the thumb tips touching and sliding the palms of both hands inwards towards each other across the belly until the outside edges of the little fingers touch and the two hands form a lotus.

Continuing to **EXHALE**, point the fingers outwards and pivot the wrists until the lotus petals of your fingertips come to point upwards, and then the palms come back together as you roll the *namaste* gesture back into the starting position, resting on the heart.

INHALE with the hands in *namaste* at the heart, and repeat as many times as you enjoy, synchronising hand movements with breath.

HEART-WOMB RIVER SACRED GREETING GESTURE: RIVER-LOTUS FORM (OUTER)

How to do it: form and flow

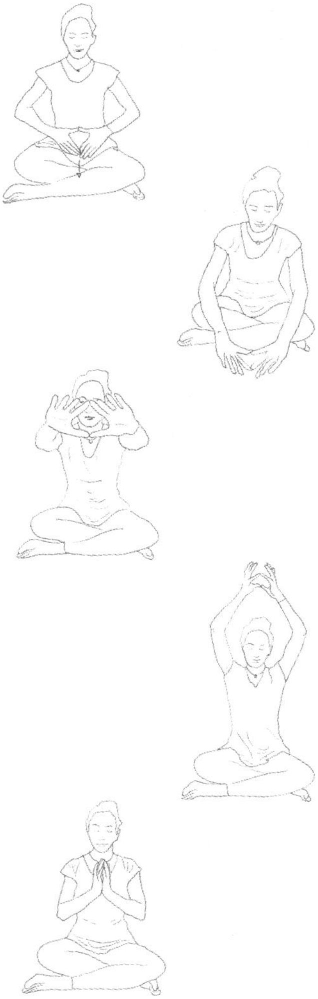

This simply extends the journey of the inner form described on the previous page, so that the flow of the river extends down into the earth and then up above the head before returning to the starting point; follow the first three instructions on the previous page, but then:

Continue to **EXHALE** sliding this *yoni mudrā* down the central line of the body, over the womb and on down towards the earth, stretching the arms and torso forwards from the hips so that the *yoni mudrā* triangle reaches down and out towards the earth, or touching the earth, whichever is most comfortable for you.

INHALE maintaining *yoni mudrā* as you reach the hands up above the head in a long arc, arms straight. Look up through the triangle into the sky.

EXHALE keeping the thumb tips touching as you bring the sides of the little fingers together so that the two hands form an open lotus above the head, and then draw this *mudrā* back down past the third eye and the nose, thumbs touching forehead, nose and chin as you draw the *mudrā* down through the central line of the body. When the hands reach the heart, press the palms back together into *namaste*.

INHALE with the palms together and the outer edges of the thumbs resting on the breastbone in *namaste*.

Repeat this exercise as many times as you enjoy, synchronising the hand and arms movements with the breath. You can also alternate between the short (inner) and longer (outer) flows of this river-lotus form of the womb greeting.

Why to do it: *bhava* or inner feeling

These gestures build connections between the heart and the womb by greeting the womb with love. They also offer the opportunity to let the inner river of energy between heart and womb flow down into the earth and up into the heavens. The lotus that blooms in the womb is offered back to the heart, and the river of energy flowing from the heart nourishes the womb. On the longer form, the lotus blooms in the heavens and its spiritual energy is drawn down into the heart. Both forms of these gestures bring the loving compassionate energy of the heart down to honour, heal and nourish the womb, and invite the creative and fertile energy of the womb to rise up and enliven the loving energies of the heart. The gestures also feed the flow of the river of energy that runs between heart and womb. This *nadī* is a magical river that flows in both directions, up to the heart on the inhalation and down to the womb on the exhalation. The experience of the practice can be deepened by resonating a hum (see *bhrāmarī prāṇāyāma*, pp.469–70) or an Aum on the exhalation.

These are beautiful and powerful gestures that make perfect opening and closing practices for any yoga session that a woman does with the intention of honouring and respecting her womb or womb space energies. Each can be practised alone, by repeating several times with different intensities and speeds, or they can punctuate other practices, for example in the variations described in chapter twenty-six or indeed as a pausing practice in between rounds of other flowing sequences such as sun and moon salutations (*sūrya* or *candra namaskār*, see chapter twenty-three). For use in this way it is pleasing to use the outer form of the river-lotus practice described above or the more expansive ocean form described below.

HEART-WOMB RIVER SACRED GREETING GESTURE: LOTUS-OCEAN FORM

How to do it: form and flow

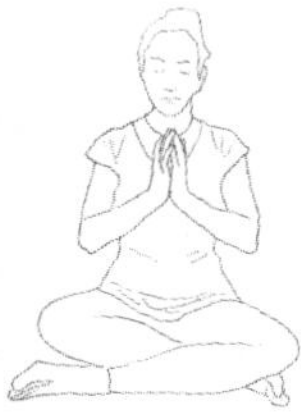

1

INHALE begin with the palms together and the outer edges of the thumbs resting on the breastbone in *namaste*.

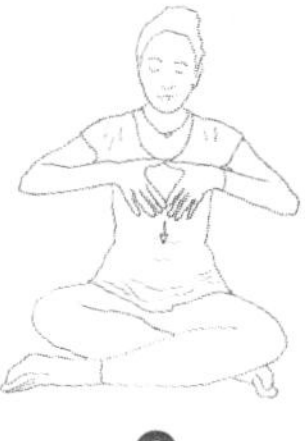

2

EXHALE keep the thumb tips touching and slide the palms of both hands outwards across the top of the breasts, until the hands rest flat and soft on the chest, with the index fingertips touching to create *yoni mudrā*, the downward-pointing triangle inside the space between the outstretched thumbs and index fingers .

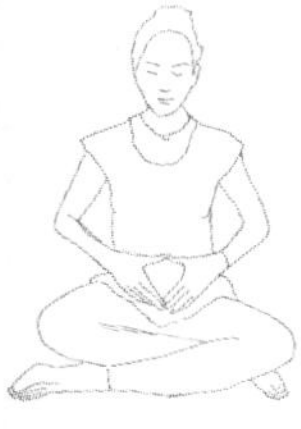

3

SAME EXHALE continue sliding this *yoni mudrā* down the central line of the body, over the womb and on down towards the earth, stretching the arms and torso forwards from the hips so that the *yoni mudrā* triangle reaches down and out towards the earth, or touching the earth, whichever is most comfortable for you.

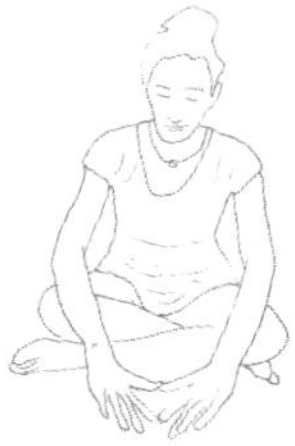
4

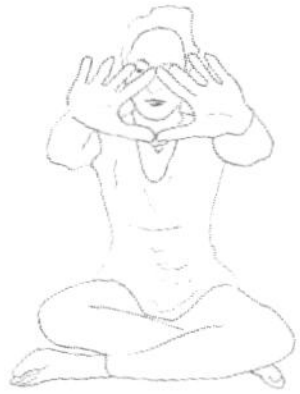
5

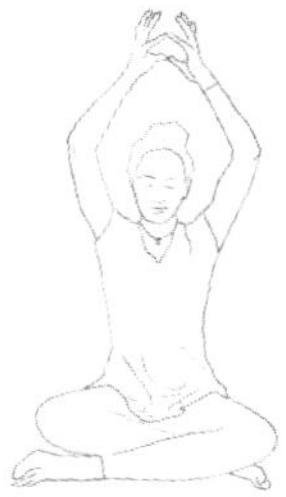
6

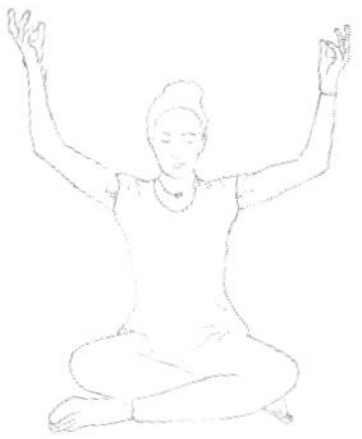
7

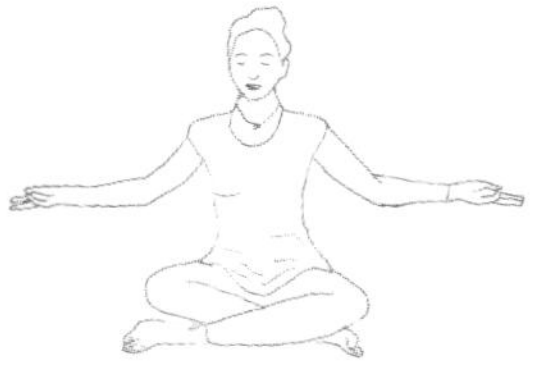
8

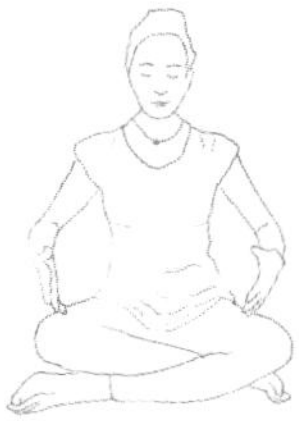
9

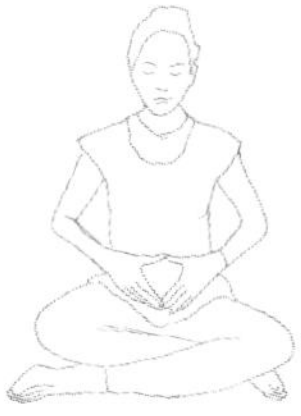
10

INHALE maintaining *yoni mudrā* as you reach the hands up above the head in a long arc, arms straight. Look up through the triangle into the sky (6).

EXHALE bend the elbows, drawing them back behind you and separating the two hands so that they travel down behind the head; then pivot the forearms outwards and scoop the cupped hands back in towards the womb, starting with the palms facing upwards and ending with the palms facing in towards the body in *yoni mudrā*, over the womb (7–10).

Repeat as many times as you enjoy, synchronising the hand and arms movements with the breath. Use a transitional INHALE to bring the *yoni mudrā* hands back up to *namaste* so as to return to the starting point at the heart.

Why to do it: *bhava* or inner feeling

This gesture feeds the flow of the river of energy between heart and womb until it grows to meet the ocean of *prāṇa* around the body. It offers a sense of profound connection with all the elements: with earth as the *yoni mudrā* travels down from the womb, and then up through water, fire and air until the energy and focus is lifted up into the heavens (6 and 7), which can be viewed through the shape of the *yoni mudrā* triangle. It literally embodies the experience of the *yoni* as a cosmic gateway: the heavens enter our vision through the *yoni mudrā*. On the exhalation, the space around the back of the head is 'combed' with the hands and the energy of all the elements is gathered up in the cupped palms and guided in towards the womb herself (9 and 10). The practice gives the option to close with the focus on the womb in *yoni mudrā* or to return to the heart with *namaste*, depending on where you prefer to direct your energies at the end of the practice. As with the river-lotus form, the experience of the practice can be deepened by resonating a hum (see *bhrāmarī prāṇāyāma* in chapter nineteen) or an Aum on the exhalation as the hands descend.

HEART-WOMB RIVER MEDITATION

Of all the yoga practices that can reconnect you to womb awareness, this one is probably the simplest, and the most beautiful and powerful. It centres your attention on your heart and your womb or womb space energies. It is best to do the practice sitting in any comfortable position, but you can also do it standing or lying too.

How to do it: form and flow

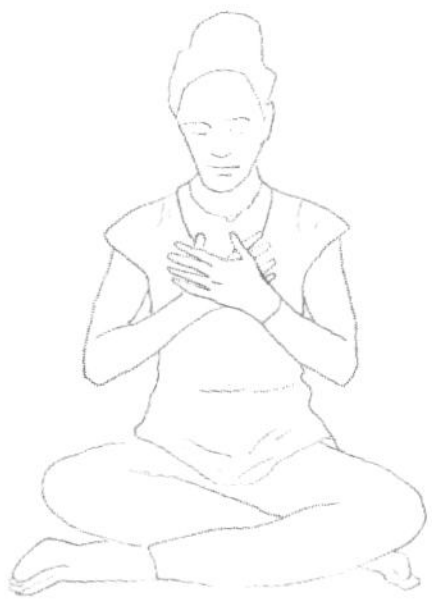

EXHALE as you settle into a comfortable position and close your eyes, bringing your attention to the movement of your breath.

INHALE placing the palm of the left hand flat over the heart, and cover it with the right hand. Feel the breath moving into the chest, as if the heart is breathing. Tip the chin slightly down and let the exhale travel out through the lips as if greeting the heart. Let the breath nourish the heart. Evoke a feeling of gratitude in the heart by calling to mind whoever has helped make it possible for you to be doing this practice right now.

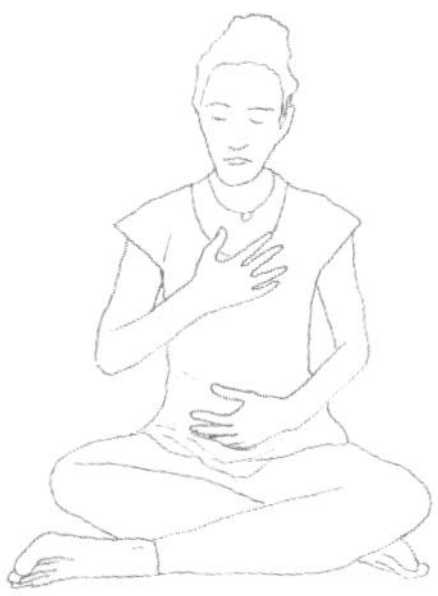

EXHALE when the heart feels fully nourished and full of gratitude, and let the right hand slide down the centre line of the body to come to cover the womb. The hand brings with it the loving gratitude from the heart and directs it into the womb or the womb-space. Let the hand rest wherever you feel you have the best connection with your womb. Imagine a golden thread connecting the heart and the womb or simply feel and hear a connection between womb and heart on the breath as the nourishing experience of gratitude flows between the two.

INHALE carry the mental attention up to the heart.

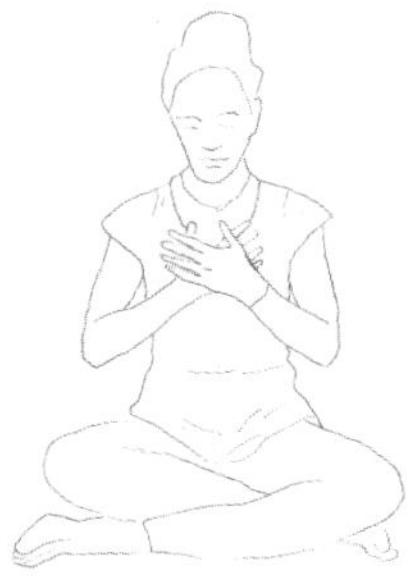

EXHALE carry the mental attention down to the womb. Let this awareness continue as you breathe: up to the heart and down to the womb. Stay with this breath and meditation for as long as you like, but for at least two minutes.

INHALE to close, sliding the right hand back up to cover the left hand, and if you like, repeat the affirmation (silently or voiced, as you prefer) 'With great respect and love, I honour my heart, my inner teacher.'

Why to do it: *bhava* or inner feeling

Simply and with great power this meditative act invites healing into the heart, into the womb and into the river of energy that flows between them. It integrates feeling, breath, body and mind into one unified focus that nourishes the central channel for the movement of *prāṇa* to increase our *śakti* or life force. There are a number of options for the position of the 'heart' hand: either directly over the organ of the heart, to the left of the breast bone, or on the centre of the sternum over the space of *anāhata cakra*, or slightly to the right to connect with the space of the spiritual heart *hṛdayākāśa*. Choose whichever one feels right to you.

HEAD-HEART SACRED GESTURE MEDITATION

I learnt this peaceable and profound gesture from Ayurvedic massage therapist and yoga teacher Sofya Ansari (**www.sofya.org.uk**), who learnt it from her Sufi sheik and spiritual guide. It integrates very well with the heart-womb sacred gesture meditation, and can be established before, after or during that meditation to carry the focus more profoundly into the heart energy.

How to do it: form and flow

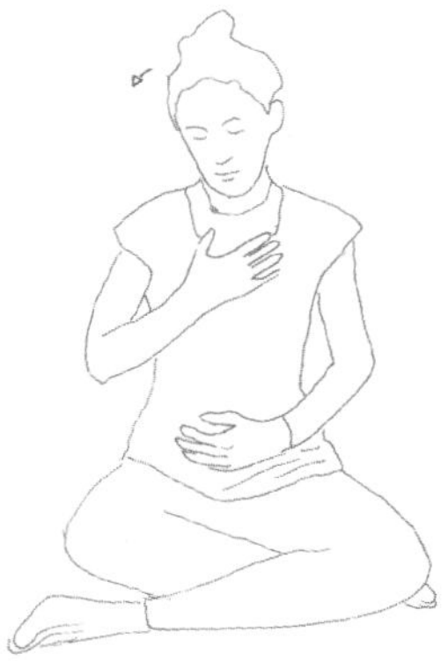

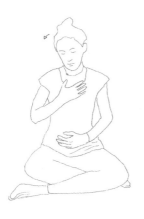

EXHALE settle into a comfortable seated position and establish an easy breath. Watch until it feels as if the rhythm of breath is completely effortless

INHALE and lengthen the spine and neck

EXHALE then gently drop the chin a little and tilt the head very slightly to the left, as if the left ear feels heavier than the right. Sense that the slight tilt of the head encourages the focus of the mental attention to shift completely from the world of thoughts into the world of feelings.

INHALE let the head remain where it is. Draw the mental attention up into the head.

EXHALE deepen the attention on the heart, by 'dropping' the thoughts from the head down into the heart. Lock the mind in the heart.

Sit breathing with this practice for as long as you feel comfortable. The focus is on the exhalations dropping the thoughts into the heart. At the end of the time you want to give the practice, return the head to an upright position and bring the palms together in *namaste*.

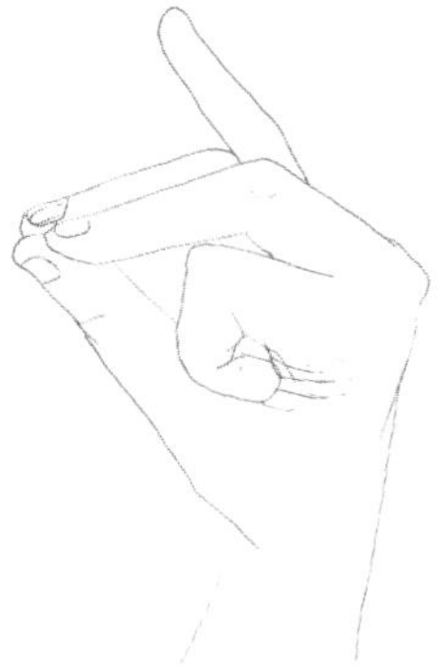

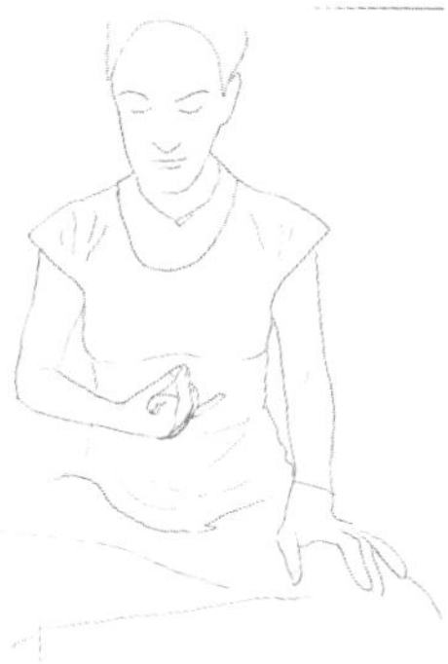

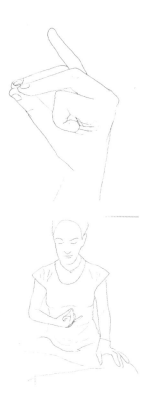

Breathe three more rounds and then open the eyes.

If your hands are not already in the position for the heart-womb meditation sacred gesture, then the heart-focusing effect of this meditation can be amplified by the use of the heart gesture *hṛdaya mudrā*:

With hands resting palms up, comfortably on the knees or thighs, lightly touch the tip of the index finger to the tip of the thumb. Then slide the tip of the index finger down along the length of the thumb, bending it until the tip of the index finger is tucked into the root of the thumb. Keep it in this position, whilst you touch the tip of the thumb to both tips of the middle and ring fingers together. The little finger remains relaxed, or outstretched, whichever feels most comfortable to you. Traditionally this *mudrā* is held with palms up, but if it feels easier to have the palms down, then turn the hands over. This hand gesture connects to the space of the heart, enhancing qualities of compassion, love and understanding.

Why to do it: *bhava* or inner feeling

The awareness with this practice settles very naturally into the heart. It is as if all the thoughts, concerns and anxieties that endlessly revolve in the mind can be poured into the ocean of the heart. The gesture of tilting the head indicates that the superior wisdom lies not in the mind but in the heart. The continued focus on 'breathing down' into the heart brings the proliferation of mental difficulties into the limitless ocean of the heart, where the exact and perfect solution to every difficulty naturally arises. It reminds us that the solution is always in the heart. It also teaches us that the heart is a powerful healer, and that the boundless ocean of love in the heart is available to fill the womb.

WOMB POWER SACRED GESTURES SEQUENCE

There are many variations on the basic open *yoni mudrā* described in the first two practices. All are intended to provide a refined and powerful connection to the energies of the womb or womb space energies so that *prāṇa śakti* can flow into the womb to nourish and heal.

The following sequence combines three *yoni mudrā* variations with a sacral *mudrā* and *śakti mudrā* to nourish the power of the womb.

How to do it: form and flow

Each of these sacred hand gestures (*hasta mudrās*) can be practised individually, and held for longer periods during meditation and for their specific healing energies. In the following sequence they flow together to optimise all the powers of the *śakti prāṇa* in the womb and to support the earth element in the body.

Downward-pointing triangle / Open *yoni mudrā* (simple)

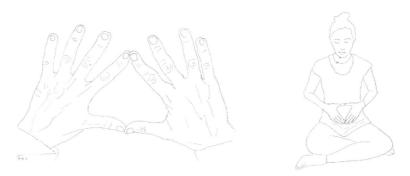

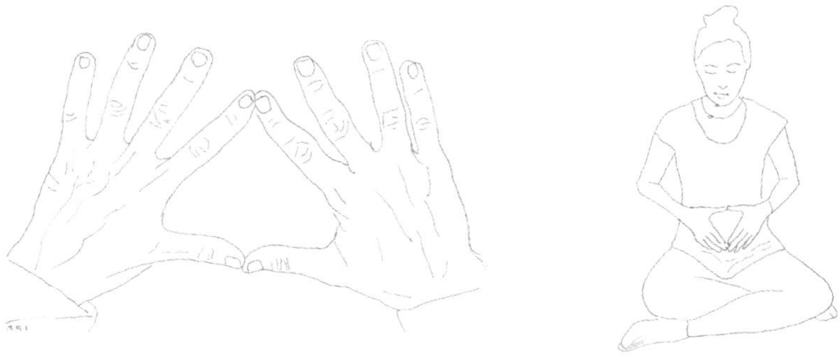

Thumb tips touch, index fingers touch, and the palms and wrists rest flat against the belly. The remaining fingertips rest on the pubic bones or the curve of the belly. Breath into the *mudrā* for nine breaths.

Angled downward-pointing triangle diamond / Interlaced open *yoni mudrā*

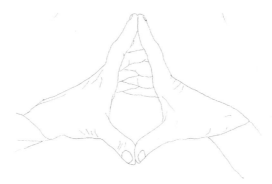

Thumb tips touch, still resting on the belly, and index fingers touch and point downards, strongly extending to create a downward-pointing triangle or extended diamond. The remaining fingertips interlace lightly and are slightly curved so that the outer edges of the little fingers rest on the pubic bones or the curve of the belly, and a little 'cave' appears as the palms of the hands curve upwards. The wrists rest on the belly. Breath into the *mudrā* for nine breaths.

Directional *vesica pisces* / Interlaced extended *yoni mudrā*

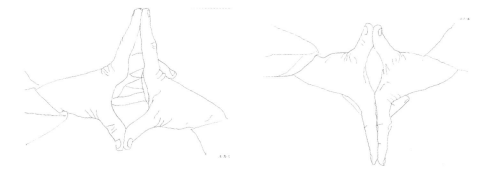

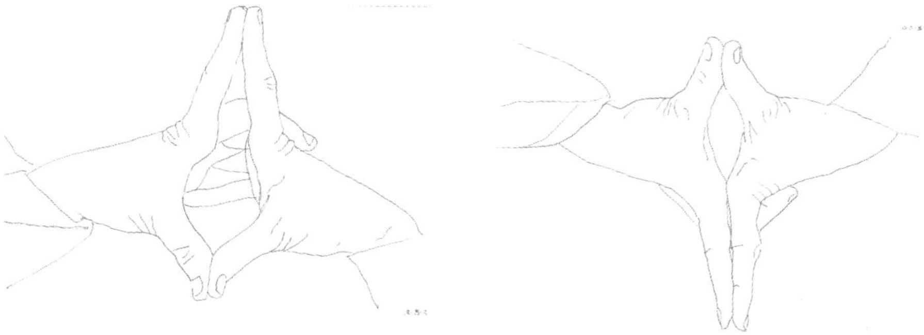

This follows from the previous practice, but now the pads of the thumbs touch, and point up, drawing the base of both index fingers together to touch, and lining up the whole length of the two index fingers together. An ovoid shape reminiscent of the opening to the vagina (*vesica pisces*) appears in the space between the two hands where the skin is stretched between the base of the index fingers and the base of the thumbs. The remaining fingertips interlace more closely to hide the inner 'cave' of the previous practice. The wrists can still rest on the belly. Breath into the *mudrā* for nine breaths. In her classic reference text on *hasta mudrā*, *Yoga in Your Hands*, Gerturde Hirschi describes this same *mudrā* as *uttarabodhi mudrā* or 'the gesture of the highest enlightenment', and she recommends its use for times when we need 'a flash of inspiration'.

Power gesture / *Śakti mudrā*

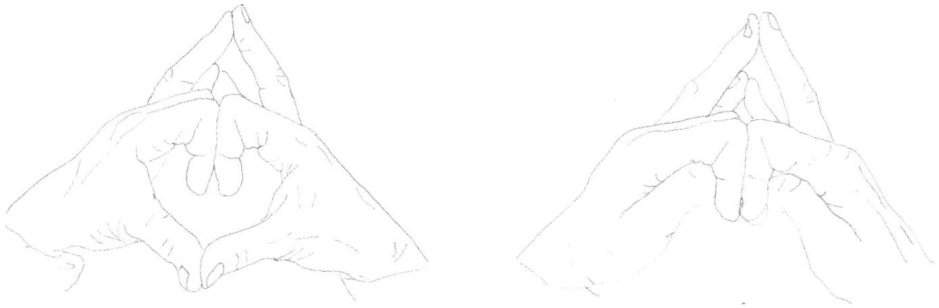

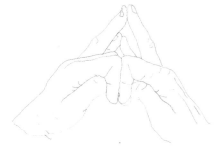

This follows from the previous practice, but now the tips of the index fingers turn in and downwards, until the backs of the top two finger joints and the fingernails are touching and pointing straight down. The pads of the thumbs tuck into the palm. Then the middle fingers follow the example of the index fingers tucking down the tips until the fingernails are touching. The tips of the two ring fingers rise up to touch each other and so do the tips of the two little fingers. Breath into this *mudrā* for nine breaths.

Great sacral gesture / *Mahā mulādhāra mudrā* in two parts

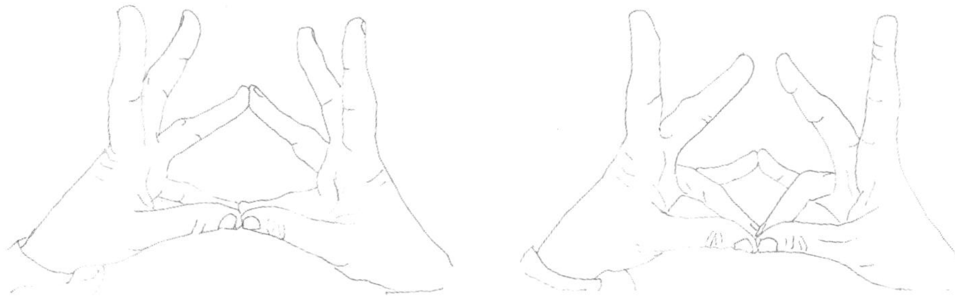

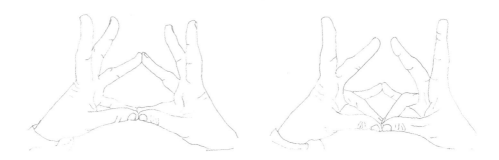

This can follow from the previous *mudrā* or flow from a simple open *yoni mudrā*. With the hands at chest level, touch the tip of each thumb to the tip of the little fingers and bring them all together. The tips of the ring fingers touch and lift up, creating a diamond shape between the little fingers and ring fingers. The index and middle fingers on both hands stretch up and open. Hold this *mudrā* for nine breaths before swapping the positions of the ring fingertips and little fingertips so that the ring fingertips point down to join the thumb tips and the joined little fingertips point upwards. The other fingers remain in the same position as for the first part of the *mudrā*.

Why to do it: *bhava* or inner feeling

When the exhalation focuses on the contact points and energy circuits created by these sacred hand gestures, then *prāṇa* is directed very powerfully into the womb and the ovaries (or the space in the pelvis that these organs once inhabited). The first *yoni mudrā* creates a relaxed connection with the belly so that the warmth of the palms and the fingers protects and nurtures the womb beneath. The second and third interlaced and directional *yoni mudrā*s focus that energy more powerfully and lead to the possibility of experiencing strength and power flowing into the womb, or into the direction of the fingers and thumbs (for example the forehead can rest in the *vesica pisces* shape when the thumbs rest on the third eye).

The *śakti mudrā* is described by Maya Tiwari in *Woman's Power to Heal through Inner Medicine* as a way to heal and revitalise the womb's energies and rebalance the cycles of the womb with the lunar cycles. The earth gesture (*mulādhāra mudrā*) is more generally beneficial for building positive *śakti prāṇa* in the womb.

This sequence, or indeed any of the individual *mudrā*s, can be done from a sitting or a lying position. If you choose to be lying down, then it can be a very positive and restful experience to practise this sequence of *mudrā*s in the Golden cosmic womb pose, which is itself a full-body honouring of the receptivity of the *yoni* as a cosmic gateway – a *mudrā* in the body (*kāya mudrā*) and not just in the hands (*hasta mudrā*).

HIRAṆYA GARBHA: GOLDEN COSMIC WOMB

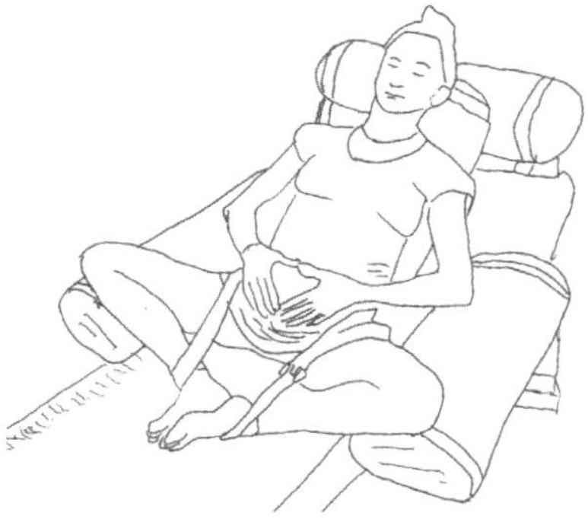

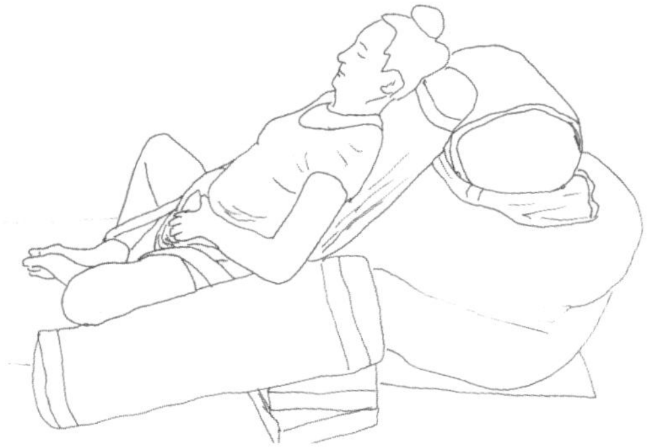

Lie on your back with the soles of your feet together and your knees relaxed outwards. Use a pillow if that is more comfortable. Place a bolster underneath both knees to support the weight of the legs. If you find your elbows are off the ground it will not be relaxing to hold any of the *yoni mudrā*s without putting a cushion, block or rolled blanket beneath each elbow to raise the upper arms up away from the floor, from shoulder to elbows. In pregnancy it is necessary to provide additional support to angle the back using further props.

In this posture of openness and receptivity, allow the exhaling breath to connect with the sacred hand gestures, and settle into whichever one feels the most appropriate for you today. Remain with the *mudrā* for as long as you are comfortable.

YONI ŚAKTI PŪJĀ: HONOURING THE POWER OF THE WOMB

Also called womb breathing, this is a gracious and spacious breath and movement practice that literally 'wafts' loving energy into the womb / womb space.

How to do it: form and flow

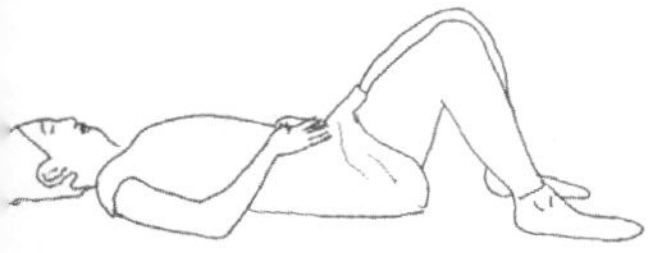

EXHALE Resting on your back, bend your knees so that the soles of your feet rest flat on the floor, about hip distance apart. Have your hands resting in simple *yoni mudrā* over your womb. Ensure your elbows are well grounded – if the elbows do not rest on the floor then support them with pillows or rolled blankets.

INHALE slowly spread the fingers and lift the forearms and hands, taking them up away from the womb and moving them out to the sides. Follow your breath slowly with the movement of the forearms and hands, so at the end of the inhale, the backs of the hands may rest

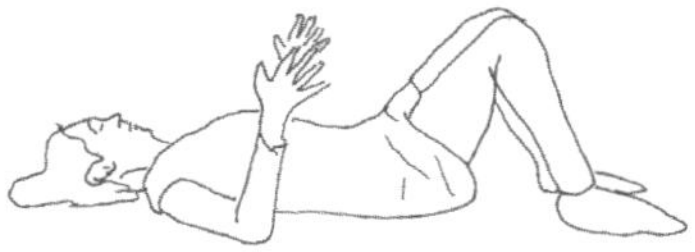

on the floor or may be up in the air. The end position is not important.

EXHALE slowly bring the palms of the hands back over to rest on your womb. Continue to breathe and match breath with movement so that rhythm of your breathing is synchronised with the opening and closing movement of the arms and hands over the womb. Repeat for nine breaths, or more if you prefer.

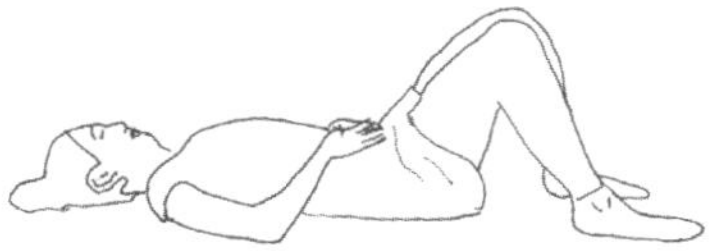

Why to do it: *bhava* or inner feeling

This practice, especially when practised at the very start of a womb yoga session, offers a restful way to honour the power of the womb: it uses movement and breath in an essentially restorative base position to heighten awareness of the possibility of moving *prāṇa* directly into the womb. As the palms of the hands rest down over the belly, literally feel the energy soaking into the womb.

SEED–FLOWER SEQUENCE

How to do it: form and flow

This sequence flows very smoothly from the previous practice, and opens out the body and breath so as to nourish the womb's qualities of creativity and growth.

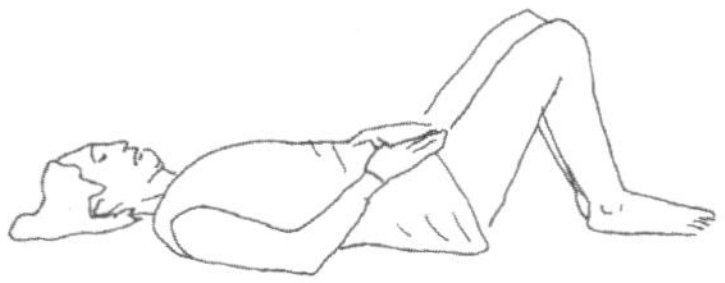

EXHALE as you settle yourself so that your knees are bent, feet flat on the floor under your knees. If you are comfortable without the pillow beneath your head, then don't use it for this practice. Let your inner knees and ankles be touching. Have your hands on your belly in *yoni mudrā* as for the previous practice.

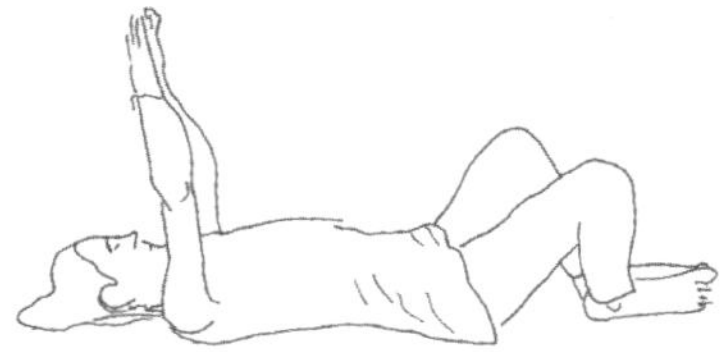

INHALE reach both arms up, hands extending towards the ceiling and then back above your head, coming to rest on the floor above your head, with the elbows bent, at whatever width is easy for your shoulders (the wider the elbows, the easier this is). At the same time as the arms move up, allow for the knees to drop wide out to the sides so that the soles of the feet turn towards each other to touch. Let the knees drop as wide as is comfortable. The position of the body at the fullness of the inhalation will be fully open: arms above head and knees wide, soles of feet touching.

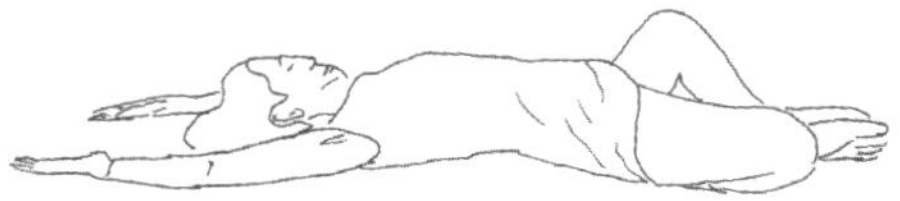

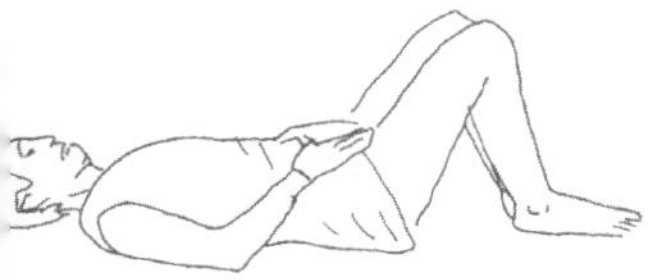

EXHALE and reverse the opening movement: bring the hands back over the body to return to *yoni mudrā*, and squeeze the legs closed so that the knees and ankles are touching again. By the end of the exhalation the body thus returns to its closed position. Continue to repeat the opening movement with each inhalation, and the closing movement with each exhalation.

The key to this practice is to synchronise the movement of the body with the breath. Move slowly. Have the palms and fingers stretched open wide. To experience a smooth flow you will need to move the legs a lot slower than the arms because they have less distance to travel. Time the movement so that the exact end of the exhalation corresponds with the fully closed position, and the exact moment of fullness on the inhalation corresponds with the fully open stretch.

When you feel that breath and movement are effortlessly synchronised then begin to pause in the open, inhalation position until your breath is ready to leave. Pause in the exhalation position until you are ready to allow the next breath in. In this way you become aware of the four components of the breath and allow the body to be nourished by the breath within it, and to rest in the fully empty, receptive place that happens when the body is awaiting the arrival of the next breath. Do not force either pause – just observe and honour the natural rhythms of the breath's passage.

Why to do it: *bhava* or inner feeling

The pair of physical poses alternates between opening and protection. The physical movements also encourage a heightened awareness of the natural flow of *prāṇa* along the river of energy between the womb and the heart. The *prāṇa* moves up into the hands as they extend behind the head on the inhalation and down into the womb as they rest in *yoni mudrā* on the exhalation. The spaciousness created in the physical body invites more *prāṇa* to move into the rivers of energy that nourish the energetic body.

WOMB ELEVATION BRIDGE SEQUENCE

This practice supports, elevates and expands the womb energy and promotes a strong connection between the energies of the well-earthed feet and the pelvic organs. There are two versions: soft and strong. The soft version is presented first and is suitable for all levels of experience with yoga. The strong version is only suitable for those women who have existing familiarity with the practices of *mūla bandha*, *uḍḍīyāna bandha* and *khecarī mudrā* (for details, see chapter twenty).

NB neither version of this practice is suitable during menstruation or pregnancy. The strong version is also unsuitable for women with endometriosis or fibroids or other growths in the womb.

How to do it: form and flow (soft version)

1

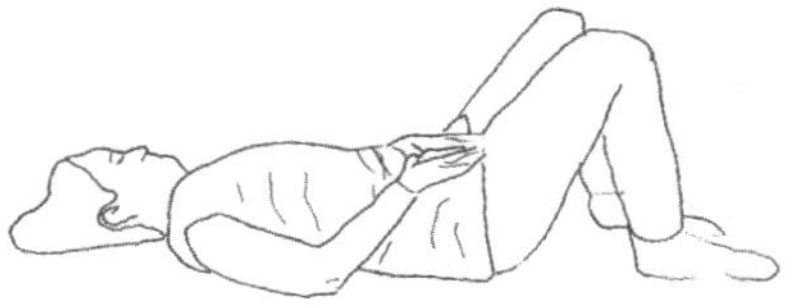

2

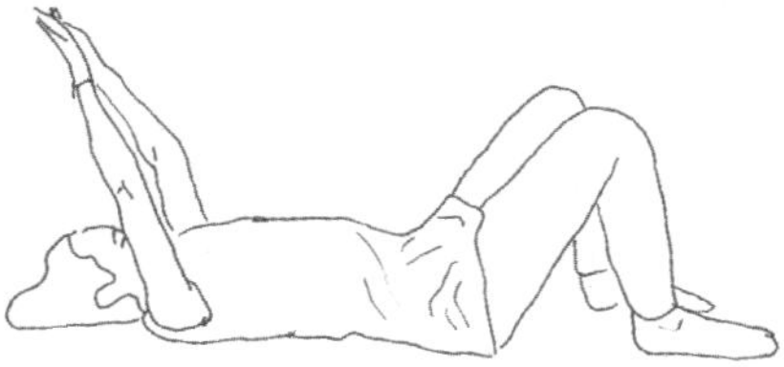

3

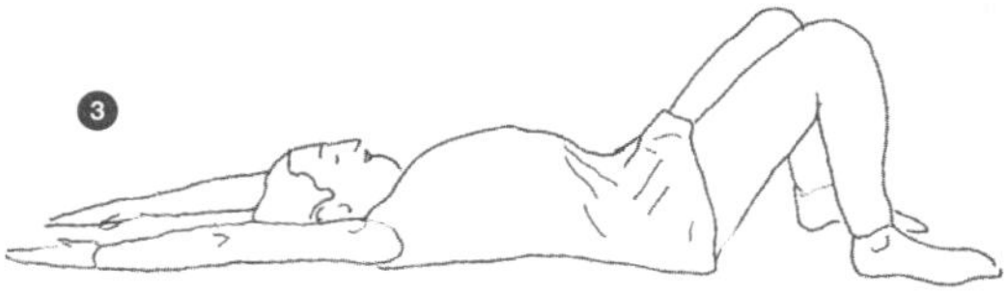

4

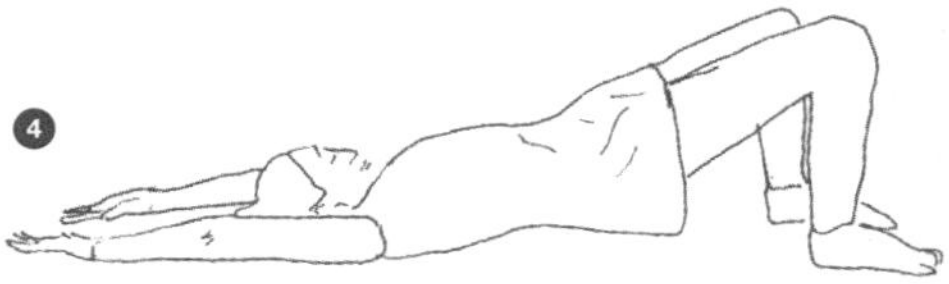

Lie on your back with the hands resting on the pelvis in *yoni mudrā* (p.150). Bend the knees and put the soles of the feet on the earth about hip-width apart. The heels should be directly beneath the knees.

EXHALE firmly, push the soles of the feet into the floor, drawing the navel down, in and diagonally back towards the spine.

INHALE straighten the arms and lift the hands up above the head, looking through the triangle of *yoni mudrā* before taking the elbows out to the sides above the head and resting them on the floor with the hands remaining open in *yoni mudrā* (2–3).

EXHALE push the feet strongly into the earth and activate the legs, lifting the pelvis up from the floor as far as is comfortable (4). Tuck the chin down into the throat and rest the tip of the tongue up and backwards on the roof of the mouth.

INHALE expand and inflate the whole abdomen and chest with a full breath.

EXHALE very slowly, lowering the length of the spine back down to earth

INHALE as you lift *yoni mudrā* back up above your head.

EXHALE lower *yoni mudrā* back onto the womb (1) and breathe freely for up to three breaths before repeating the practice up to nine times.

How to do it: form and flow (strong version)

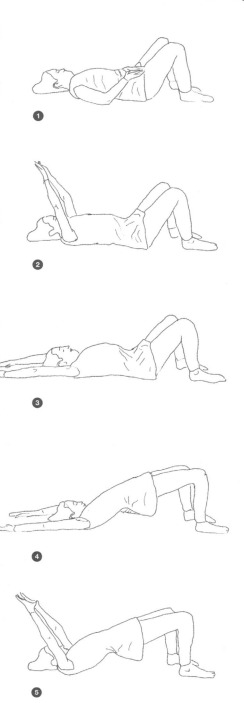

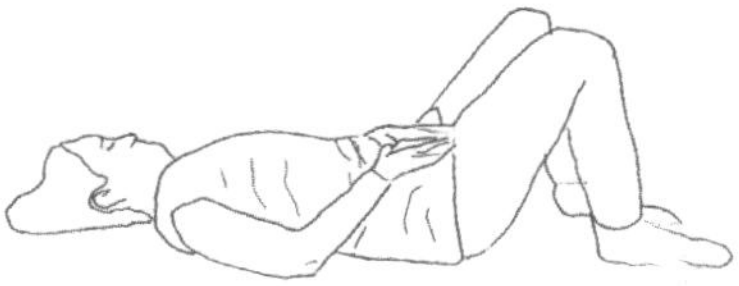

1

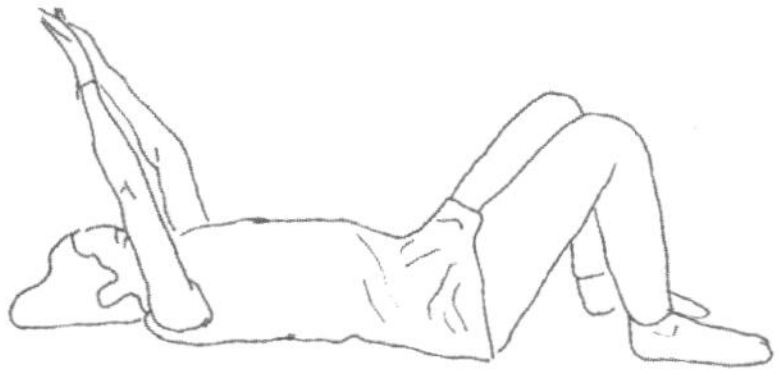

2

3

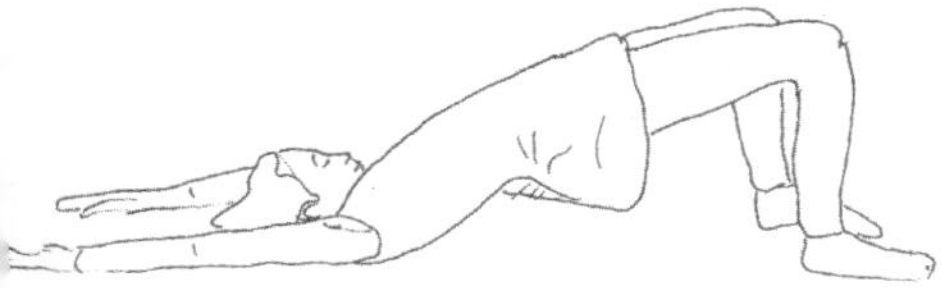

4

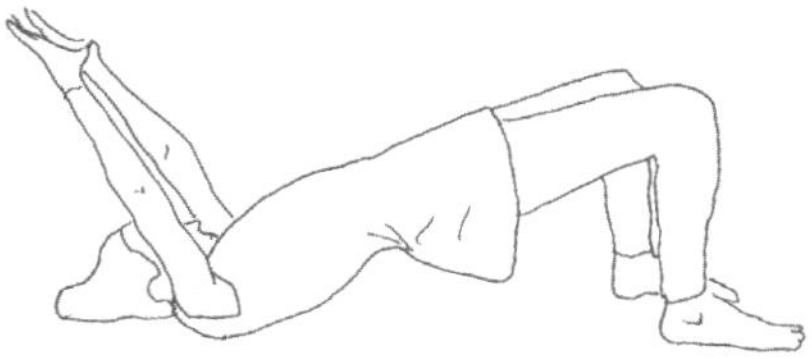

5

Lie on your back with the hands resting on the pelvis in simple *yoni mudrā* (p.150). Bend the knees and put the soles of the feet on the earth about hip-width apart. The heels should be directly beneath the knees.

EXHALE firmly, push the soles of the feet into the floor, drawing the navel up and back towards the spine.

INHALE straighten the arms and lift the hands up above the head, looking through the triangle of *yoni mudrā* (2) before taking the elbows out to the sides above the head and resting them on the floor (2) with the hands open in *yoni mudrā*.

EXHALE push the balls of the feet and the heels strongly into the earth and activate the legs, lifting the pelvis up from the floor as far as is comfortable (4). Tuck the chin down into the throat and rest the tip of the tongue up and backwards towards the soft palate (*khecarī mudrā*).

INHALE expand the whole abdomen and chest with a full breath.

EXHALE keeping the feet and elbows pushing strongly into the earth, apply *mūla bandha* (p.474). Draw the walls of the vagina inwards and upwards towards the cervix) and then, starting from above the pubic bones, allow the exhalation to suck the lower part of the abdominal wall in towards the navel and firmly up towards the point between the two shoulder blades, until the whole abdominal wall is hollow. Apply *jālandhara bandha* (tucking the chin firmly down into the throat) and maintain *khecarī mudrā*.

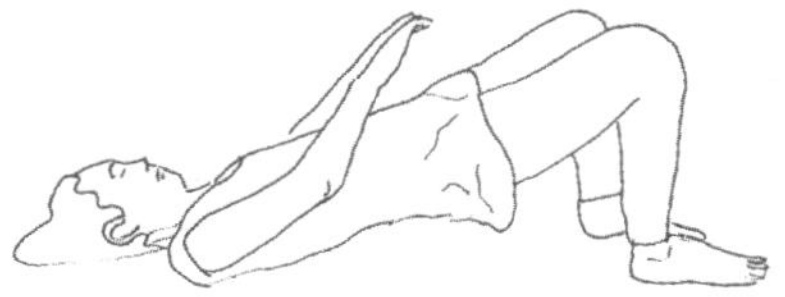

6

PAUSE AFTER EXHALE in this *mahā bandha* (four *bandhas* applied) for as long as your breath is comfortably held outside. Maintain the same physical position as you watch the breath be still.

INHALE gently releasing *jālandhara* and *uḍḍīyāna bandha* (letting go the chin lock and abdominal sucking).

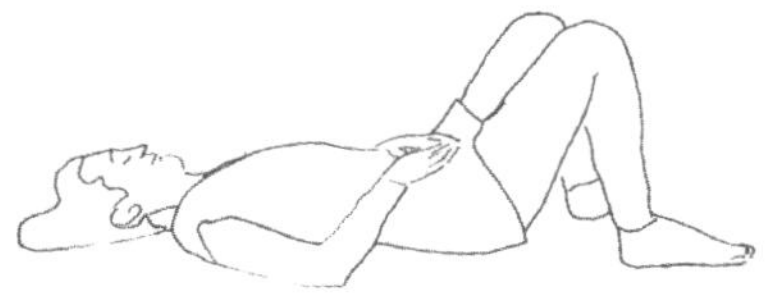

7

EXHALE very slowly, lowering the length of the spine back down to earth, maintaining *mūla bandha* until the pelvis is resting back down on the earth (5–6).

INHALE release all *bandhas*, bringing *yoni mudrā* back onto the womb (7).

EXHALE and breathe freely for up to three breaths before repeating the practice up to nine times.

Why to do it: *bhava* or inner feeling

For both soft and strong versions, the seed of this practice is classic technique from *haṭha* yoga, reconfigured to promote maximum uplift and support for the pelvic and abdominal organs. In order to practise the strong version with the *mahā* (great) *bandha* (lock), it is important to be confident and familiar with *mūla bandha*, *khecarī mudrā* and *jālandhara bandha* first (see chapter nineteen). All three of these locks work together with *uḍḍīyāna bandha* (the uplifting lock) to create a powerful synergistic uplift of the pelvic muscles and organs.

As the physical movement in both soft and strong versions creates a positive sense of support and elevation for the pelvic organs, so too do the energies and spirits lift, boosting vitality and nourishing the womb from beneath. The engagement of the feet on the floor also creates an energy portal to draw the supportive energy of the earth up into the womb to nourish and nurture her, or to heal the womb space.

EXTENDED HEART SPACE TWIST POSE

This makes a perfect gentle closure for any womb yoga practice. It affords the opportunity to bring the flow of the breath back into the river of energy between the womb and the heart.

How to do it: form and flow

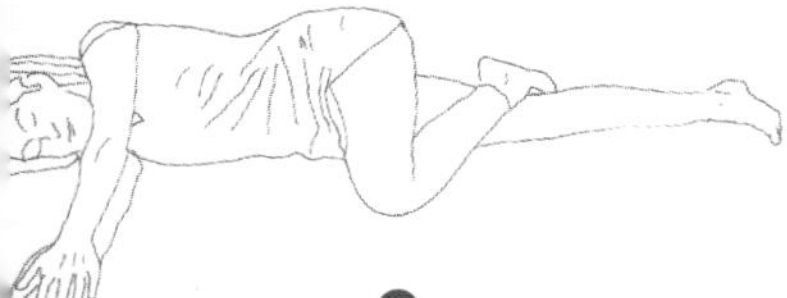

1

2

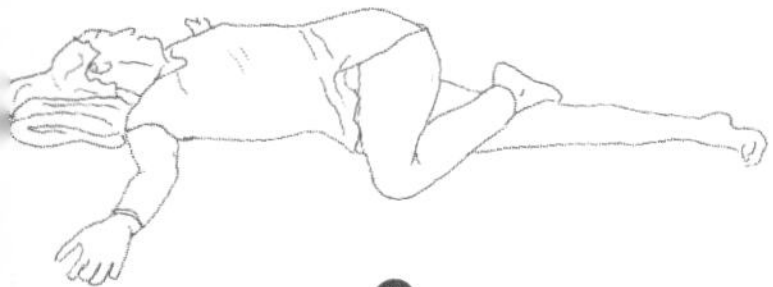

3

EXHALE lie flat on the floor with your knees and feet together. Have a pillow under your head. Bend your left knee. Draw it up towards the belly and across the body to the right hand side. Roll over so the knee settles on the floor, or rest it on a cushion. Tuck the toes of your left foot under the back of the right knee. Keep the right leg straight.

INHALE stretch the right arm out horizontally along the floor with the palm facing up. Move your left arm up across your body and place the palm of your left hand on top of the right hand (1).

EXHALE into the pose.

INHALE and lift the left arm up toward the ceiling and take it as far into an open stretch behind you as it will comfortably go (2 and 3).

EXHALE bring the arm back down again so that the palm of the left hand is resting on top of the right hand at the end of the exhalation. Repeat in time with the breath nine times. At the end of the last repetition, bend the elbow and circle the shoulder very slowly three times in each direction, in time with the breath. Repeat on the other side.

Why to do it: *bhava* or inner feeling

This sequence creates spaciousness in the heart. It relates to the quality of air, as the arc of the hand traces this spaciousness above the body. This openness invites *prāṇa* to nourish the loving energies of the heart so that they flow with generosity into the womb space. With the inhalation be aware of creating the space for gratitude and generosity. With the exhalation move consciousness down into the protected space of the womb. Direct the awareness down into the womb space to revitalise and nourish. When resting in stillness between the movements or at the end of this practice, bring consciousness to the river of energy that flows between heart and womb.

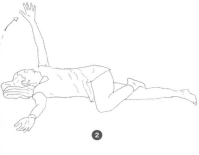

CHAPTER SIX

honouring the feminine energy of the life force: nine practices of *prāṇa śakti pūjā*

MAGICAL RIVER IN SPATE: FULLNESS FLOWING IN THE HEART-WOMB RIVER, *HṚDAYA-YONI NADĪ*

All of the practices in this chapter increase the flow of *prāṇa* in the channel linking heart and womb. They use rhythmic movement repetitions to remove physical and other blockages and entice energy to move fully and freely in this *nadī*, or magical river. Regular practice of these techniques raises the level of the pranic waters flowing in the river between heart and womb so that both energy centres (*hṛdaya* and *yoni*) are flooded with positive *prāṇa*. The benefits of removing energy blocks and allowing the river to flow into spate are experienced at many levels: there are physical benefits in terms of easier menstruations and births; delightful increases in vitality, including sexual energy; and enthusiasm and creativity, which in turn lead to a sense of well-being and contentment that guides us to experience more vividly our own sense of spiritual connection.

The foundations for the effective use of these practices are laid directly in an understanding of the flow of energy between the heart and the womb in the *hṛdaya-yoni nadī*. A full exploration of the emotional, spiritual and energetic nature of this *nadī* is offered in the preceding chapter. Whilst the techniques described in this chapter can certainly be done independently of those in the previous chapter, it is wise to acquire a sense of the healing effects of the healthy energetic flows in the heart-womb river first so that the inner feeling or *bhava* of the practices in this chapter can be fully encountered.

It can be helpful to realise that although these practices use significantly more physical movement than those in the previous chapter, they are not depleting of energy because they are not simply physical exercises. In fact, although they require movement of the body, their effectiveness rests entirely in the nature of breath, consciousness and attitude of heart, or *bhava*, that accompanies the physical movements. The most beneficial attitude is one of offering reverent honour to the feminine energies of the life force. The movement of breath with consciousness is a gentle but continual journey in both directions on the magical river or *hṛdaya-yoni nadī*: up to the heart on the inhalation and down to the womb on the exhalation.

MORE ON MUD: *YONISTHĀNA* AND THE SPECIAL PLACE OF THE WOMB

The abundant source of the magical river that flows between womb and heart is *yonisthāna*: the abode of the womb. This term is not widely used in yoga. Usually the womb is associated with *svādhiṣṭhāna cakra*, which contains the essence of water energy. But I sense also that the life of the womb and its role as the entry place of *prāṇa* has also the quality of earth. So I have sought out terms and understandings that best convey the mingled qualities of earth and water in the energies of the womb. *Yonisthāna* bridges both *svādhiṣṭhāna* and *mulādhāra cakras*. Its energies are neither solely one nor the other. *Yonisthāna* is a place of overlapping, of merging, a liminal space where the fluidity of water meets the firmness of earth. Both these qualities are present in the nature of womb energy, in literal physical terms as well as at the level of the elemental associations of the energy body. The cyclical activities of the womb during childbearing years are a flowing testimony to her fluid nature: she is the ocean in which we float as embryos, and the blood, slippery mucus and amniotic waters that pass from her through menstruating and childbearing years all carry the flowing energies of water, moving in trickles and tides and waves. The language we use to describe these experiences is the language of liquid: we speak of flooding, and soaking, or gushing and pouring, of trickling and dampness.

But the life of the womb is not all about water. We feel this when we sit firmly on the ground with an upright spine as for the first four practices in this chapter. If we engage the fluid capacity for pelvic movement even as we sit firmly and circle around the vulva, or rock along from pubic bones back to tail bone, and if we are fortunate enough to be able to do this outside sitting on the earth we can literally feel the direct connection between the opening to the vagina and the grass, mud, sand, yoga mat or whatever other earth covering on which we happen to be sitting. Similarly, when we activate our feet and legs in standing postures, especially with free pelvic movement as in the final five practices in this chapter, then the supportive and nourishing energies of the earth can flow directly into the womb or womb space.

To encounter the potency of the womb energy fully and at all levels of being–physical, ecological, emotional and spiritual –requires us to engage with the reality that she operates in two *cakras* at once: *mulādhāra* and *svādhiṣṭhāna*. The overlap between these two *cakras* creates its own special place: *yonisthāna*. This understanding of the capacity for overlap and overlay is rarely documented in the literature of *kuṇḍalinī* yoga that details the esoteric anatomy of the *cakras* and *nāḍīs*: all these centres and channels are usually separated out into distinct entities. But in my research for this book I have discovered a few helpful references that acknowledge the dual presence of both earth and water elements in relation to the womb. A brief textual diversion to explore this rarely discussed aspect of esoteric anatomy will be valuable here, so if you are not fascinated by Sanskrit textual analysis, please skip the next section and cut straight to the practices.

MUD IN THE SCRIPTURES: *YONISTHĀNA* AND OTHER REFERENCES

In his book *Layayoga*, a comprehensive survey of all textual references in Sanskrit to the *cakras*, Shyam Sundar Goswami reviews all the literatures on the subject (*Upaniṣads*, *Tantras* and *Purāṇas*), creating a comparative account that covers the terminology, position, description, and explanation of the *cakras*. He helpfully provides various different translations and variants from different textual sources on the meaning and position of the *cakras*, and his survey corroborates the general understanding in yoga of the nature of *mulādhāra* as earth, and *svādhiṣṭhāna* as water. His impressive range of reference also clearly sets out the separation of these two energetic centres and the usual placement of the womb energy as being related directly and only to *svādhiṣṭhāna*. However, he also reveals the existence in certain traditions, in particular that of the Shaivite Nāth ascetics, of an additional or alternative energy space known as *yonisthāna* (literally, 'the place of the *yoni*, or vulva') that he describes as being '...between the *mulādhāra* and the *svādhiṣṭhāna* (*Yogacūḍāmaṇi Upaniṣad* 6–7)' (Goswami 1999: 183). Goswami recognises, as does Swami Satyadharma Saraswati in her translation of this text (whose title means 'The Crown Jewel of Yoga') that in this context the *yonisthāna* is not exclusively female, but can also be understood to be the male or female perineum.

The *Yogacūḍāmaṇi Upaniṣad* clearly describes the existence of *yonisthāna* as a secondary subtle centre bordering on *mulādhāra*. In her commentary on the text, Satyadharma describes how the *yoni*, as the 'cosmic womb in which all forms that constitute the universe are developed', is rooted physically in the body in her 'headquarters', the centre of sexual desire (*kāmarūpa*). This centre borders on the earth *cakra*, *mulādhāra*, and is placed between it and the water *cakra*, *svādhiṣṭhāna*.

A similarly close relationship between earth and water is also set out in *Saundarya-Laharī*, a key text of *śākta tantra*, which is explored more fully in chapter five. In relation to the practices described below, however, it is useful to note that the ninth verse of this poem in praise of Goddess is unusual in that it describes how She is established in both earth and water, which are seen in this vision to be mingled in the first *cakra*: '*Mahīm mūlādhāre kāmapi*: As earth and water in *mulādhāra*' (Śloka 9). In all other expositions of the elemental connections of the *cakras*, *mulādhāra* is only identified with earth. However, as Swami Satyasanganda explains in her commentary on the *Saundarya-Laharī* '... according to this *mantra* [*Mahīm mūlādhāre kāmapi*], the water element is also located at *mooladhara* ... The phrase '*kāmapi*' [= also water] establishes this claim' (Saraswati 2008: 131).

Earth, and also water. The two elements are seen here in the tradition of *śākta tantra* to be mixed in the first *cakra*, and this intimate combination of earth and water within the location of a single *cakra* is not only extraordinary in the literature of the *cakras*, but also very pertinent when understanding the elemental qualities and properties of the womb, especially as we encounter them in the following practices.

Our little textual diversion into Sanskrit scriptures now being complete we can return to an experiential encounter with the mingled forces of earth and water at work in the energies of the womb in *yonisthāna*.

PRACTICES TO UNLOCK POWER AND HONOUR THE FEMININE ENERGY OF THE LIFE FORCE: *ŚAKTI BANDHAS* AND *PRĀṆA ŚAKTI PŪJĀ*

These nine core practices are all derived from a series of rhythmic postures usually referred to as *śakti bandhas* – poses to unlock power (*bandha* = lock and *śakti* = power). In yoga, *śakti* is seen as a feminine force, the dynamic creative energy through which consciousness manifests in the universe. The primary quality of *śakti* is to move, and when she gets stuck, as she often does, for example in stiff hips and a stuck lower back, then her power is limited or removed. When she can flow freely then her power is restored. *Śakti bandhas* are effective at releasing power because they work rhythmically to restore fluidity of movement in the pelvis, and build strength to support that movement through repetition. Fluidity is a quality of water and strength a quality of earth, so the practices activate both elements.

BHAVA OR INNER FEELING

The following sequence develops and refines the basic set of *śakti bandhas* from Satyananda yoga to create a womb-focused practice that I have described as a *pūjā* or ritual worship. The inner feeling to evoke in all these practices is of reverence for the life force in her home in the womb. When we greet the womb with love, and honour the feminine energy of the life force, then we are embracing the ancient truth of our cellular genesis in the primeval, fecund muddy waters: the water above irrigates the earth beneath and the earth beneath feeds the water above until their qualities merge, becoming a fertile and creative home for the nourishment and sustenance of life itself. By honouring *prāṇa śakti* in these practices of reverence and worship we acknowledge the manifestation of cosmic light in the special place of the womb: *yonisthāna* where water and earth meet for the purpose of nurturing life itself.

To sense your dominant *svara*, notice the flow of breath in your nostrils, and through which nostril the breath flows more easily. If it is your right nostril, then the right *svara* is dominant, and vice versa. For more detail, see p.466.

Prāṇa śakti pūjā: 1–4 are seated practices. If your back is uncomfortable in any of these seated base positions, then sit on the edge of a cushion or a folded mat to tilt the pelvis into an easier angle.

1 | WOMB PILGRIMAGE: MILL GRINDING (*CAKKI CALANĀSANA*)

NB Do not do this practice if you have high blood pressure, or acute lower back pain.

This rhythmic pelvic circling practice is called *cakki calanāsana* in the original *śakti bandha* sequence, which means 'grinding the mill'. The term 'womb pilgrimage' is intended to evoke the sense of the womb as an interior sacred lake. The circling movement is a respectful circumambulation of her shores.

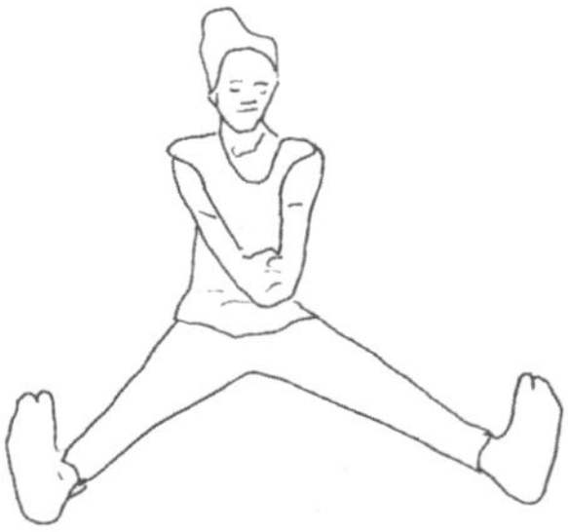

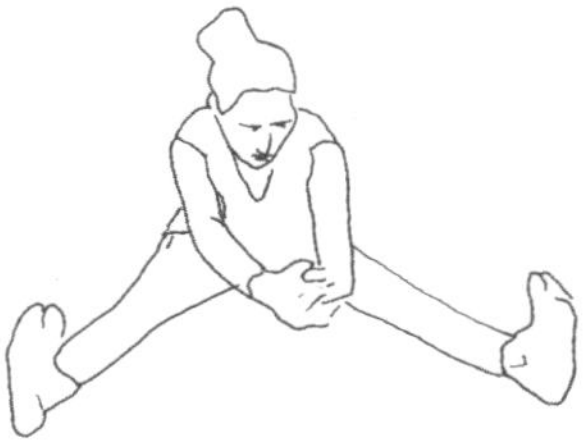

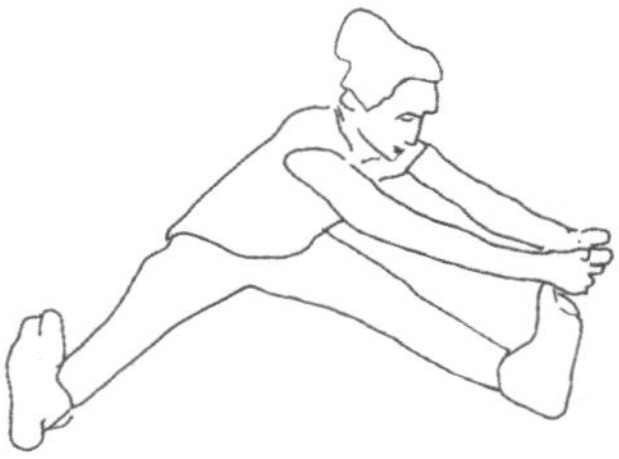

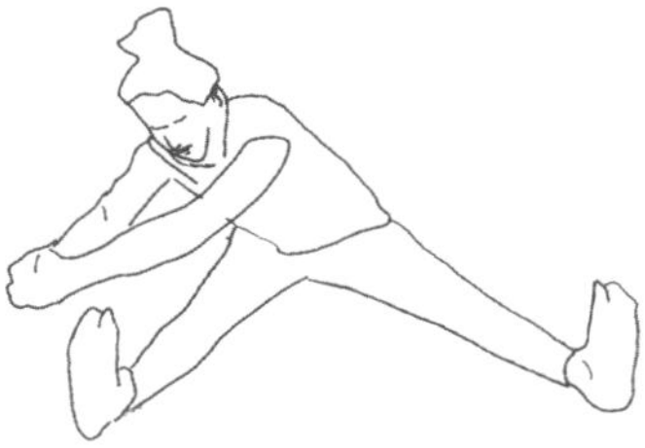

Sit with your legs straight and separate them as wide as is comfortable. Push your heels away from you and draw your toes towards you. Have your spine upright and sit forwards on your sitting bones so that your pelvis is tilted to the front. Have your arms by your sides. Extend your arms out in front, at shoulder height; your elbows can bend to allow your shoulders to slide freely down away from your ears. Interlock your fingers so that the thumb corresponding to your dominant *svara* (see p.466) is on top. Begin to circle around the womb; if your right *svara* is dominant, then you will be circling clockwise, and if your left *svara* is dominant then you will be circling anticlockwise, moving from the hips to trace large circles.

EXHALE as you move forwards and down into the circle, drawing the awareness down the heart-womb river to the womb.

INHALE as you lean back out of the circle, drawing the awareness up the heart-womb river to the heart.

One circle is one round. It takes a full breath, in and out, to complete the circle. The slower you breathe the slower the circle. Repeat nine times in the opposite direction, according to your non-dominant *svara*. Pause after the tenth round, rest the arms down by your sides. Then raise the arms back up to shoulder height, interlock the fingers with the left thumb on top, and repeat, circling clockwise. At the end of the ninth round rest the arms by the side, sit with a straight spine and observe the breath settling.

Feel that the movement comes from the hips. Keep your spine straight throughout, but let the elbows bend, and slide the shoulders down the back to let the shoulders be free.

2 | WOMB-HONOURING RHYTHM

This rhythmic pelvic rocking practice alternately embraces and frees the womb. From a structural perspective, the deep layers of the transverse abdominal muscles alternately contract and release. On the exhalation, the muscular contraction squeezes the womb in a hug, holding her tight and strong, which can be helpful for maintaining effective pelvic organ support. On the inhalation, the lower back arches and the abdominal muscles release, allowing the womb freedom and space. At a symbolic and energetic level, these two actions, of holding her close and then giving her space, create the rhythm of a healthy loving relationship in which the partners can experience intimacy and spaciousness within the safe circle of respecting each other's rhythms and needs.

1

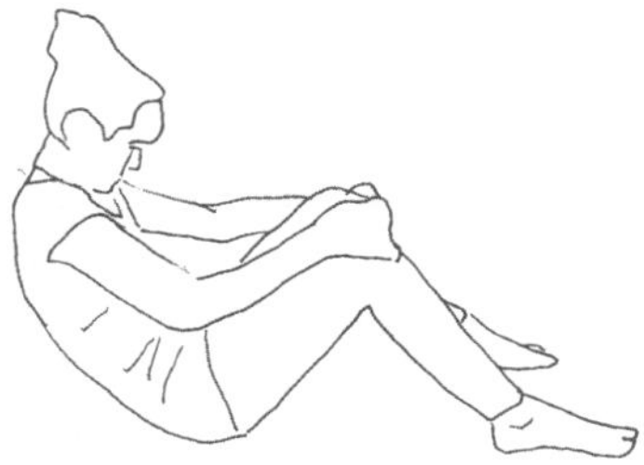
2

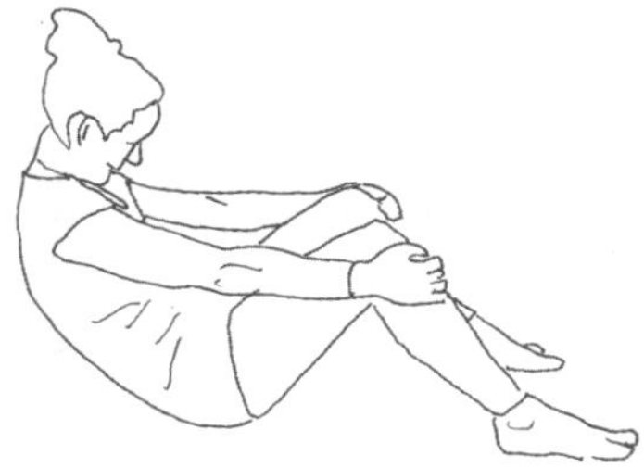
3

Sit up with your knees bent and your feet flat on the floor, as wide as is comfortable, but at least as wide as your hips. Sit forwards on your sitting bones with your spine upright. Push into the balls of your feet and heels, lifting a fine arch in the foot and spreading out the toes. Have your hands on the fronts of your kneecaps.

INHALE as you bend your elbows and draw your heart forwards and up, arching your lower back slightly, drawing the awareness up the heart-womb river to the heart (1).

EXHALE as you straighten your arms and drop back onto your sacrum. Round your lower back, contracting the abdominal muscles (especially the lowest deepest layer), drawing the awareness down the heart-womb river to the womb (2 and 3).

Repeat up to nine times or until you sense a full flow of energy in the heart-womb river.

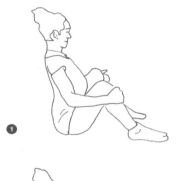

3 | LOTUS FEET BREATHING

NB This practice is particularly effective when it is used following the awakening the feet practice (pp.472–3).

In *āyurveda*, the feet are considered the 'wings of the womb' because so many of the energy channels in the feet trace directly into the pelvis. In this practice, it is as if we stretch our wings. Alternatively, the toes can be seen as the petals of a lotus opening and closing. The movement of the feet is both fluid and precise, in order to strengthen and mobilise the feet to better allow them to conduct energy up into the pelvis. Lotus feet breathing is a sister to the 'Honouring the power of the womb' (in chapter five) where the hands and arms functioned like wings, wafting *prāṇa* into the womb through the open fingers and palms. This practice uses the toes and the arches of the feet to achieve the same effect from another direction. (In fact the two practices work especially well done one after the other). The foot action is combined with the same movement of the spine in the previous practice, alternately embracing and freeing the womb.

1

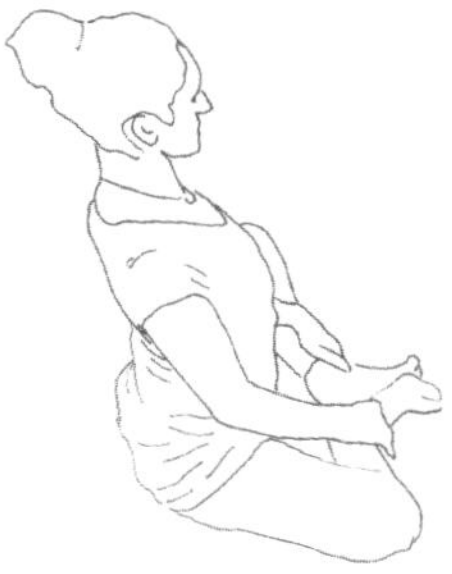

2

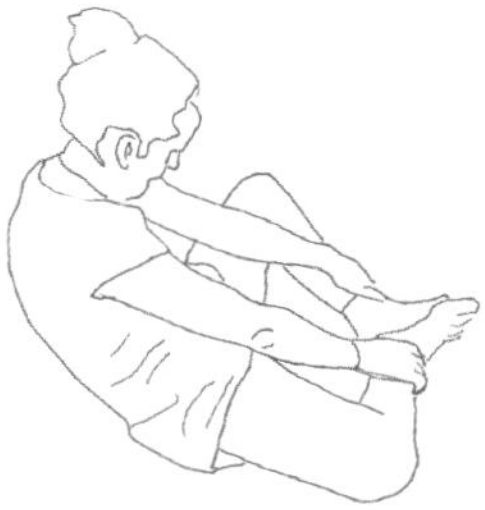

3

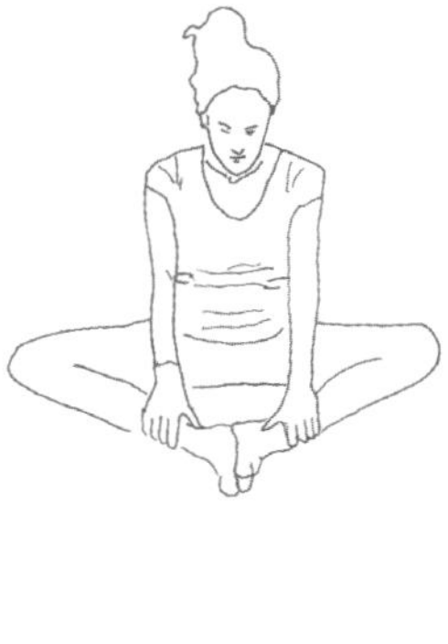

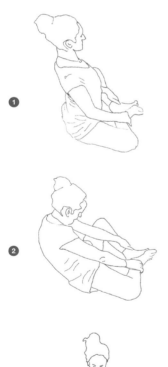

Sit up with your knees bent out to the side and the soles of your feet touching. Choose a distance between your heels and vulva that is comfortable: there should be an energising sense of openness in the thighs and groins without feeling overstretched. Sit forwards on your sitting bones with your spine upright. Push into the balls of your feet and heels, creating a fine arch in the foot and spreading out the toes. In preparation for the feet 'breathing', trace the line of the arch of the foot from the ball of the big toe to the heel back: honour the delicate shape of the *vesica pisces* created by the expression of strength in your feet. Then rest your hands on your ankles or your knees, whichever feels most natural.

INHALE as you bend your elbows and lift your heart forwards and up, arching your lower back slightly (1), drawing the awareness up the heart-womb river to the heart. At the same time, slowly open the toes one by one until a lotus blooms in your feet. Keep the balls of the feet strongly pressed against each other so that the toes can open out widely, inviting energy into the spaces between the toes.

EXHALE as you straighten your arms and drop back onto your sacrum (2). Round your lower back, contracting the abdominal muscles (especially the lowest deepest layer), drawing the awareness down the heart-womb river to the womb. At the same time, slowly close the toes one by one until the ten toes are touching. Keep the balls of the feet strongly pressed against each other so that the arches stay strong, inviting energy up from the feet into the legs.

Repeat up to nine times or until you sense warmth and strength in the feet and a full flow of energy in the heart-womb river.

4 | FULL BUTTERFLY WOMB PILGRIMAGE

This practice combines the base position of Lotus feet breathing with the circular action of the womb pilgrimages. The name 'butterfly' refers to the shape made by the two legs, spread out either side of the cunt like the wings on a butterfly.

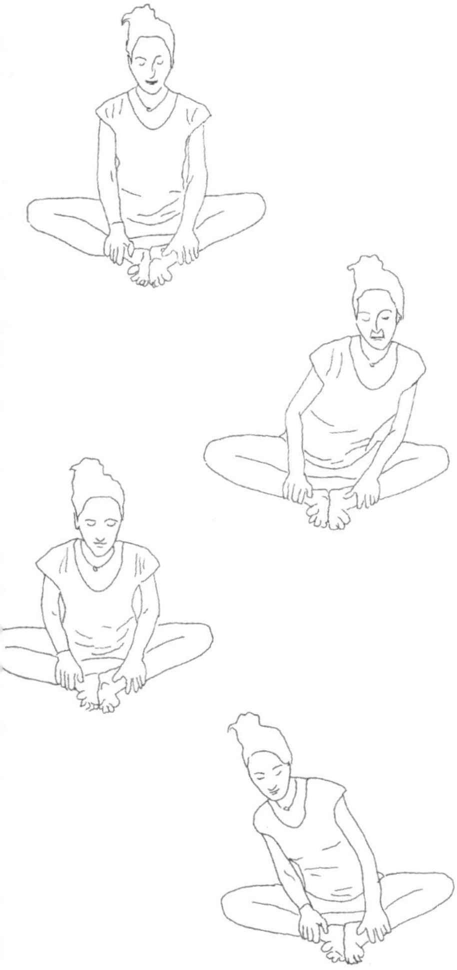

Sit as for Lotus feet breathing. Then begin very gently to circle around the womb, with the sense that the centre point of your circle is right in the middle of the womb or womb space. If your right *svara* is dominant, then you will be circling clockwise, and if your left *svara* is dominant then you will be circling anticlockwise, moving from the hips to make circles and spirals of whichever size feels comfortable.

INHALE as you move around the front arc of the circle, drawing the awareness up the heart-womb river to the heart.

EXHALE as you move around the back part of the circle, drawing the awareness down the heart-womb river to the womb.

One circle is one round. It takes a full breath, in and out, to complete the circle. The slower you breathe the slower the circle. Repeat up to nine times or until you feel fluidity in the pelvis, stability through the legs and buttocks and a full flow of energy in the heart-womb river. Then repeat in the opposite direction, according to your non-dominant *svara*.

Prāṇa śakti pūjā: 5 – 9 are standing practices. It is important with all these practices to sense that the feet are fully alive, awakened and engaged (p.472) with their function of drawing *prāṇa* up from the earth into the pelvis. It can be helpful to encourage this to happen by alternately stretching the arches and the fronts of the feet by tucking under the toes and then pushing down into the balls of the feet and the pads of the toes, bringing some weight down through each of these stretches on the exhalation and then shaking out the feet and legs, and kicking from the hips to release any tension.

Spread the toes as wide open as possible, and periodically ensure that the feet are breathing, just as they did in the Lotus feet breathing – toes up on the inhalation and down on the exhalation.

5 | SNAKE CIRCLES THE WOMB

In yoga and *tantra*, the sleeping snake is a metaphor for the unawakened cosmic energies sleeping in the earth *cakra* at the base of the spine. This sinuous and rhythmic movement is intended to move vital force up from the earth through the feet and legs and into the heart-womb river. It has the benefit of revitalising the whole body, promoting fluidity of movement and building strength in the muscles that support the whole of the spine.

Note that this practice employs *complete circles* in a full exploration of natural movement in the lower back and pelvis: arching and curling in rhythmic patterns. It is not the same as tucking your tailbone under and trying to keep it there, which is inimical to female pelvic health and should be avoided (see chapter twenty-one for a fuller explanation of why this is).

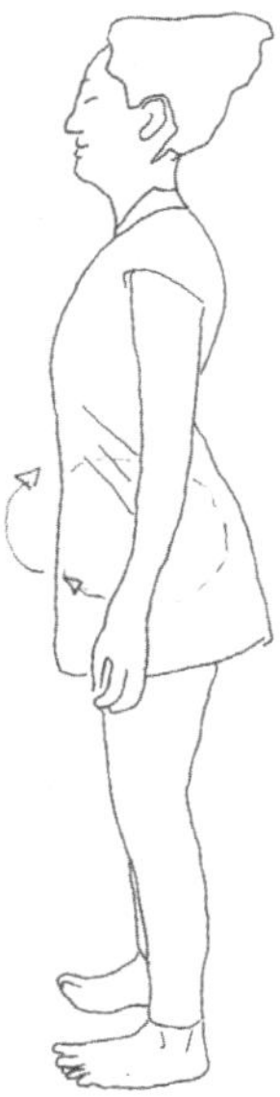

Stand with feet hip-width apart, and knees bent. Keep the arches of the feet well lifted, they support your lower back. To begin with rest the middle finger of one hand on the pubic bones at the front of the pelvis and the middle finger of the other hand on the base of your tailbone in between your buttocks. The palms of the hands rest on the belly and the sacrum, the better to detect the direction of movement and the rhythmical muscular contractions in this practice.

INHALE as you imagine that you have a long tail attached to your coccyx and extend your imaginary tail far behind you and up, lengthening and deepening the curve in your lower back as you lift your heart, drop your shoulders and bring *prāṇa* up into the heart space. Lift and separate the toes. Straighten the knees and feel the muscles either side of your lower back contracting as the abdominal muscles lengthen and stretch. The torso remains vertical.

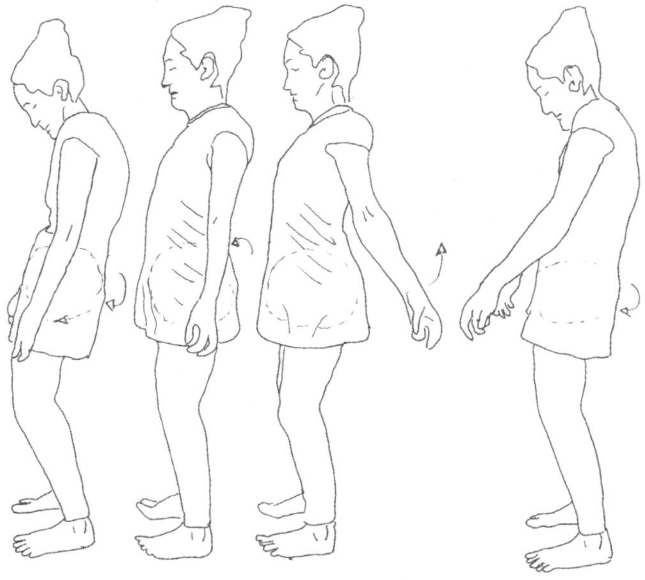

EXHALE let the imaginary tail descend, and then move it right underneath you, like a dog putting its tail between its legs. Bend your knees, and squeeze your buttocks as you move the tail forward. Feel the contraction in the deep low belly muscles, between navel and pubic bones. Bring the energy down the heart-womb river into the womb. The torso remains vertical.

Repeat until the circular movement feels fluid, strong and flowing. Release the hands as soon as you have the sense of the contraction of the deep low belly muscles on the exhale and the muscles either side of the lower back on the inhale. On the inhale have the knees straight, tail back and up, then exhaling squeeze the buttocks, move the tail under and through, as you bend your knees. Link each arc into the next like a series of little circles. Keep the breath flowing freely as you begin to link these two movements together in a continuous circular action that alternately lengthens and curves the lower back.

Sense that the rhythmic contraction and release of these large muscles builds up a warming and strengthening heat that nourishes your spine, and the pelvic organs too. If you keep with the practice you will discover the heat radiating deep inside the pelvis, healing and nourishing, whilst the movement undulates up through the spine, freeing the neck and shoulders. Sometimes it can feel as if the 'snake' of this movement is circling very centrally around the middle portion of the womb and sometimes it feels more as if the circles become ovals as the base of the snake shifts over to one side or over to the other. Allow the shifting patterns to emerge and enjoy the warmth and freedom of movement that they generate.

6 | STANDING WOMB PILGRIMAGES

These three different but related movements all combine the stance of the snake circles the womb with the *bhava* or inner feeling of the full butterfly womb pilgrimage.

Stand with your feet a comfortable distance apart and knees bent. Let your hands rest gently on your hips and let your feet breathe as in the Lotus feet breathing. For the sequence of standing womb pilgrimages it is also pleasing to let the hands rest in open *yoni mudrā* on the front of the belly as you move.

The first standing womb pilgrimage moves in circles and spirals.

Bring the focus of attention to the centre of the womb. Then begin very gently to circle around the womb, with the sense that the centre point of your circle is right in the middle of the womb or womb space. If your right *svara* is dominant, then you will be circling clockwise, and if your left *svara* is dominant then you will be circling anticlockwise, moving from the hips in circles of whichever size feels comfortable for you.

INHALE as you move around the front arc of the circle, drawing the awareness up the heart-womb river to the heart.

EXHALE as you move around the back part of the circle, drawing the awareness down the heart-womb river to the womb.

One circle is one round. It takes a full breath, in and out to complete the circle. The slower you breathe the slower the circle. Repeat up to nine times or until you feel fluidity in the pelvis, vitality through the feet and legs, and a full flow of energy in the heart-womb river. Then repeat in the opposite direction, according to your non-dominant *svara*. If you enjoy increasing or decreasing the size of the circles then let the movement spiral outwards and inwards according to what feels comfortable.

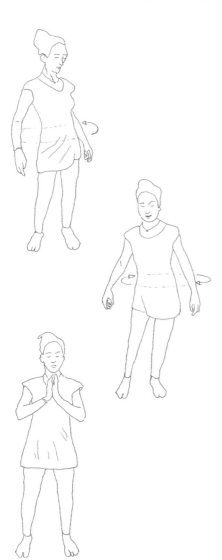

The second standing womb pilgrimage moves in upward arcs to create a 'smiling pelvis'.

Bring the focus of attention to the centre of the womb. Then begin very gently to rock from left to right, alternately shifting the weight from one leg to the other and bending the knees one at a time.

INHALE straighten the right leg and allow the hip to lift a little higher.

EXHALE as you are shifting the weight across to the left leg, and allow the lowest scoop of the arc to drop a little and deepen.

INHALE as you straighten the left leg, lifting the left hip a little higher.

These arcs create a 'smiling pelvis', with the womb in the middle of the curve of the smile and the two hips high up at either end. Continue with 'smiles' of whatever size feels comfortable for you.

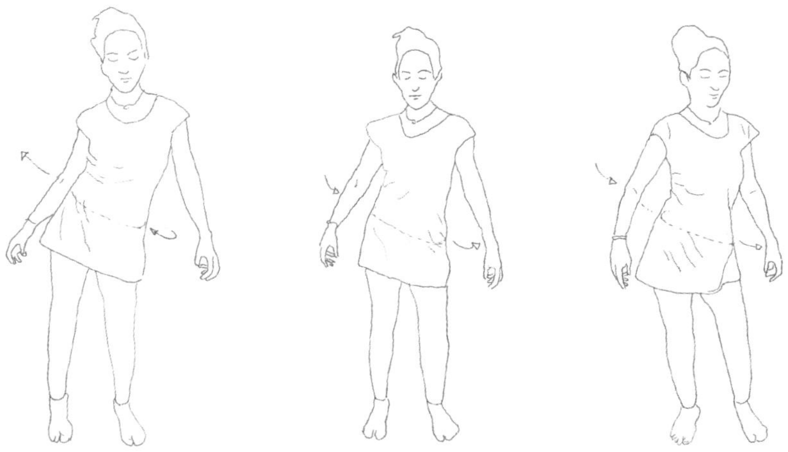

The third standing womb pilgrimage moves through a pair of opposite circles to create an infinity sign / figure of eight.

Bring the focus of attention to the centre of the womb. Then imagine that either side of this central point are two clocks. The hands of the clock on the right are moving forward into the future, travelling clockwise. The hands of the clock on the left are moving backwards into the past, travelling anticlockwise. Let your hips follow the direction of the movement of the hands of these two clocks, looping across between the two clocks to create one big infinity sign or figure of eight whose crossover point is right in the middle of the womb or womb space.

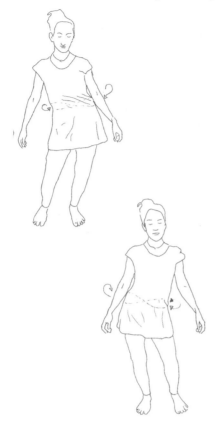

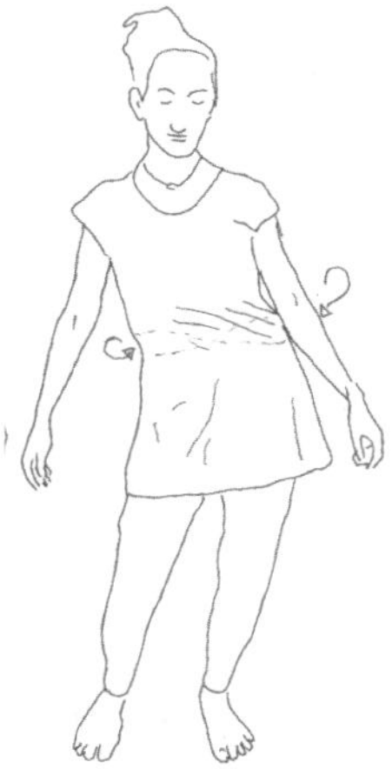

INHALE as you move around the front arc of the right circle, drawing the awareness up the heart-womb river to the heart.

EXHALE as you move around the back part of the right circle, drawing the awareness down the heart-womb river to the womb.

PAUSE the breath as you cross the central womb point in the middle of the figure of eight.

INHALE as you move around the front arc of the left circle, drawing the awareness up the heart-womb river to the heart.

EXHALE as you move around the back part of the left circle, drawing the awareness down the heart-womb river to the womb.

Continue for as many rounds as feel comfortable for you.

The suggested breath/movement synchronisation results in very slow movements, so that it can take two full breaths to complete a whole figure of eight. These practices and the other two womb pilgrimages can also be done with more rapid movements that use, for example, a single exhalation or inhalation for each circle. Allow the rhythm to alter between slow and fast if that feels comfortable, or maintain an even rhythm throughout if you prefer. My observation is that the slower approach is more amenable during menstruation or pregnancy, whilst the more rapid circles feel good at ovulation and pre-ovulation.

7 | STANDING HEART-WOMB RIVER SACRED GREETING GESTURES

This combines the fluid movements of the Snake circles the womb and the Womb-honouring rhythm with the Sacred hand gestures and *bhava* or inner feeling of the Heart-womb river greeting (ocean form) in a standing sequence.

Stand with your feet a comfortable distance apart and knees bent. Let your feet breathe as in the Lotus feet breathing (p.166).

Begin to synchronise breath and pelvic circles as for Snake circles the womb:

INHALE lengthen and extend the tailbone out and back behind you, feeling contraction in the lower back muscles and space opening in the lower part of the belly, lengthening and deepening the curve in your lower back as you lift your heart, drop your shoulders and bring *prāṇa* up into the heart space. Lift and separate the toes. Straighten the knees and feel the muscles either side of your lower back contracting as the abdominal muscles lengthen and stretch. The torso remains vertical.

EXHALE let the tailbone descend and move it forward and until it is right underneath you, like a dog putting its tail between its legs. Bend your knees, and squeeze your buttocks as you move the tail forward. Feel the contraction in the deep low belly muscles, between navel and pubic bones. Bring the energy down the heart-womb river into the womb. The torso remains vertical.

Then feel that the end point of this exhale movement leads into the start point of the exhale movement, and that the two link into each other in a continuous flow of circling.

Always keep a fluid rhythm as these circles continue and then add in the hand gestures in a progressive sequence that extends the flow of energy from inner river, to outer river, to ocean:

Lotus-river inner form:

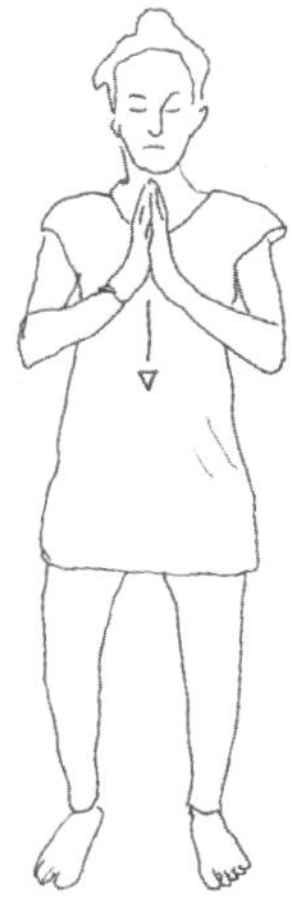

1

INHALE bring the hands palms together in *namaste* at the heart with the outer edges of the thumbs resting on the breastbone (1).

EXHALE as you keep the thumb tips touching and slide the palms of both hands outwards across the top of the breasts, until the hands rest flat and soft on the chest, with the index finger-tips touching to create an open *yoni mudrā*, the downward-pointing triangle inside the space between the outstretched thumbs and index fingers.

Continue to **EXHALE** as you slide this *yoni mudrā* down the central line of the body until it comes to rest over the womb, with the thumbs beneath the navel and the tips of the index fingers on the pubic bones. The deep

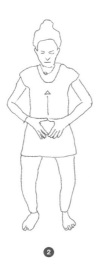

2

belly muscles will be contracted, hugging the womb as the snake circle reaches this point.

INHALE with the hands resting over the womb in simple *yoni mudrā*.

EXHALE keeping the thumb tips touching and sliding the palms of both hands inwards towards each other across the belly until the outside edges of the little fingers touch and the two hands form a lotus, ready to raise back up to the heart (2).

Continuing to **EXHALE**, point the fingers outwards and pivot the wrists until the lotus petals of your finger tips come to point upwards, and then the palms come back together as you roll the *namaste* gesture up and back into the starting position, resting on the heart. Repeat as many times as you enjoy, synchronising hand movements with breath.

Lotus-river outer form:

This simply extends the journey of the inner form described above, so that the flow of the river extends down into the earth and then up above the head before returning to the starting point; follow directions above, but then:

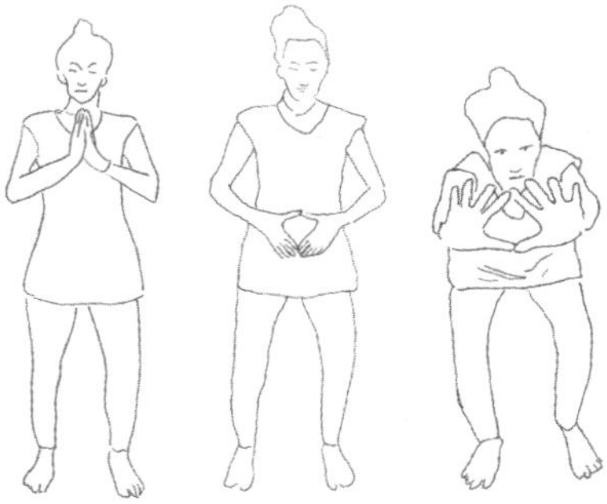

Continue to **EXHALE** sliding this *yoni mudrā* down the central line of the body, over the womb and on down towards the earth, stretching the arms and torso forwards from the hips so that the *yoni mudrā* triangle reaches down and out towards the earth, or touching the earth, whichever is most comfortable for you. Bend the knees as the hands reach forward and down so that you come into as deep a squat as is comfortable for you. Keep the heels well grounded and the feet breathing.

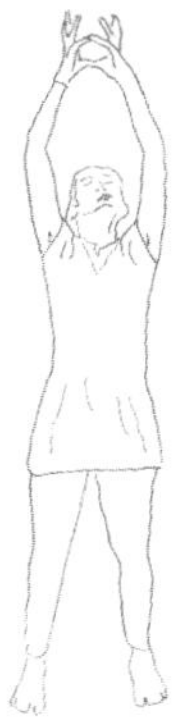

INHALE maintaining *yoni mudrā* as you reach the hands up above the head in a long arc, arms straight. Look up through the triangle into the sky. Straighten the knees as you reach up.

EXHALE keep the thumb tips touching as you bring the sides of the little fingers together so that the two hands form an open lotus above the head, and then draw this *mudrā* back down past the third eye and the nose, thumbs touching forehead, nose and chin as you draw the *mudrā* down through the central line of the body. When the hands reach the heart, press the palms back together into *namaste*.

INHALE with the palms together and outer edges of the thumbs resting on the breastbone in *namaste*. Complete the sequence with Snake circles the womb. Repeat as many times as you enjoy, synchronising the hand and arm movements with the breath. You can also alternate between the short (inner) and longer (outer) flows of this river-lotus form of the standing womb greetings.

Lotus-ocean womb greeting:

INHALE begin with the palms together and outer edges of the thumbs resting on the breastbone in *namaste*.

EXHALE keep the thumb tips touching and slide the palms of both hands outwards across the top of the breasts, until the hands rest flat and soft on the chest, with the index fingertips touching to create *yoni mudrā*, the downward-pointing triangle inside the space between the outstretched thumbs and index fingers. **SAME EXHALE** continue sliding this *yoni mudrā* down the central line of the body, over the womb and on down towards the earth, stretching the arms and torso forwards from the hips so that the *yoni mudrā* triangle reaches down and out towards the earth, or touching the earth, whichever is most comfortable for you. Bend the knees as much as is comfortable to come into as deep a squat as can be easily sustained with the heels on the ground and the feet breathing.

INHALE maintaining *yoni mudrā* as you reach the hands up above the head in a long arc, arms straight. Look up through the triangle into the sky. Straighten the knees.

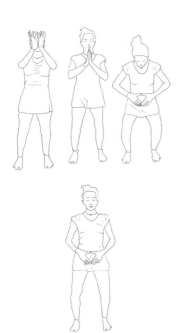

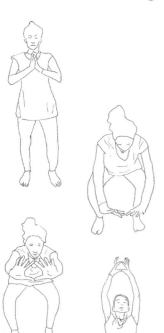

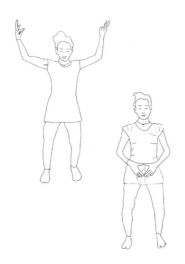

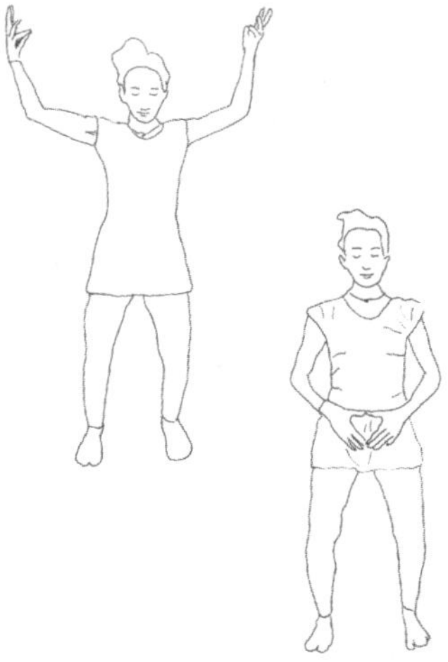

EXHALE bend the elbows, drawing them back behind you and separating the two hands so that they travel down behind the head; then pivot the forearms outwards and scoop the cupped hands back in towards the womb, starting with the palms facing upwards and ending with the palms facing in towards the body in *yoni mudrā*, over the womb.

Repeat as many times as you enjoy, synchronising the hand and arm movements with the breath and the pelvic circles. Use a transitional **INHALE** to bring the *yoni mudrā* hands back up to *namaste* so as to return to the starting point at the heart.

Why to do it: *bhava* or inner feeling

These gestures feed the flow of the river of energy between heart and womb until it grows to meet the ocean of *prāṇa* around the body. The effects of elemental connection are the same as when done seated, with the additional feeling of being grounded on the earth, connected to her power through the feet, and thus able to draw the sustaining and nurturing qualities of the earth up through the feet and the legs to nourish the womb. As with the seated forms, the experience of the practice can be deepened by resonating a hum (see *bhrāmarī prāṇāyāma* in chapter nineteen) or an Aum on the exhalation as the hands descend.

8 | FULL HANDS WOMB ENERGY PILGRIMAGE

Combining a gentle standing twist with a powerful encounter with *prāṇa śakti*, this practice flows very beautifully on from the previous standing womb greetings.

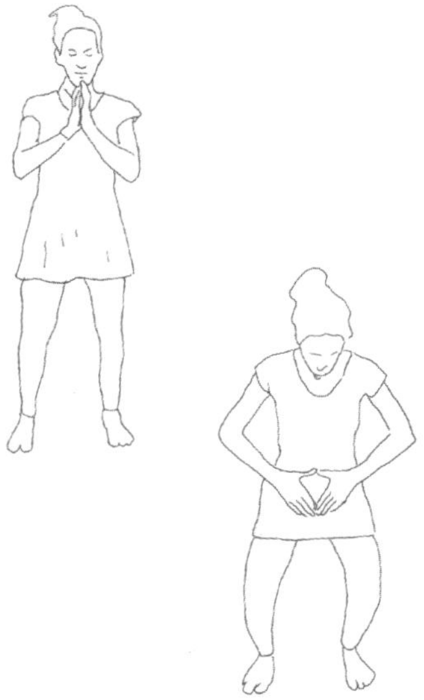

Stand with the knees soft and the feet about hip-width apart. **INHALE** begin with the palms together and outer edges of the thumbs resting on the breastbone in *namaste*.

EXHALE keep the thumb tips touching and slide the palms of both hands outwards across the top of the breasts, until the hands rest flat and soft on the chest, with the index fingertips touching to create *yoni mudrā*, the downward-pointing triangle inside the space between the outstretched thumbs and index fingers. **SAME EXHALE** continue sliding this *yoni mudrā* down the central line of the body, until it rests over the womb.

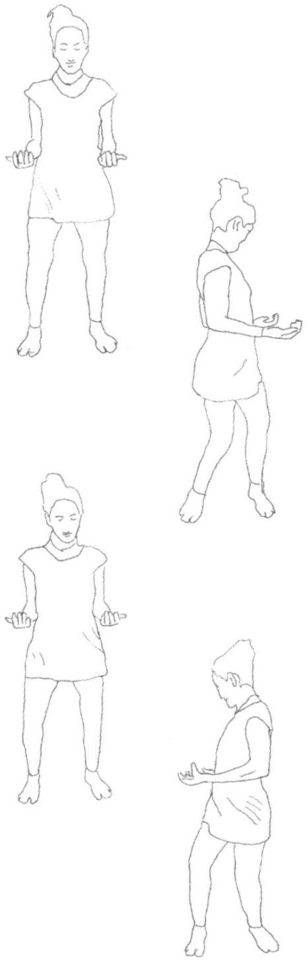

INHALE and open out the arms to the side (as in Honouring the power of the womb), keeping the elbows bent and tucked in towards the waist, and the upturned palms cupped. Send the awareness into the skin on the palms of the hands. Imagine that the cupped palms contain within them a tiny ball of *prāṇa*, an egg, or closed rosebud, a little creature such as a chick or a baby rabbit, vulnerable and intensely potent, full of life force. Carefully protect this manifestation of *prāṇa* in your hands and send your mental attention, through your gaze, into the palm of the hand corresponding to your dominant *svara*.

EXHALE as you twist, gazing into the palm of your dominant *svara* hand and turning towards it. If your right nostril has the dominant flow you will be twisting to the right and if the left nostril has the dominant flow you will be twisting to the left.

INHALE returning to centre with arms and hands in the same position.

EXHALE shift the gaze and attention to the other palm and turn to the other side.

INHALE returning to centre with arms and hands in the same position.

Repeat the twists alternating the gaze and the turn to each side at least once more, but as many times as you enjoy. At the end of the last twist as you return to centre:

INHALE deepening your squat with your heels down and extend both arms out very wide to the side, keeping the palms cupped and facing upwards.

EXHALE lean forwards from the hips and rotate the shoulders so that the palms now face forwards and begin to bring the hands palms facing together, arms outstretched in front of you in a continuous line with the spine. Interlock the fingers (dominant *svara* thumb on top), turn the palms outwards, and then:

INHALE pushing the heels of the hands away, letting the two thumb tips touch and the two little fingertips touch, stretch out the hands and arms up above you as you straighten up. Look up, and keep the little fingertips and thumb tips touching as the two hands roll into an open lotus *mudrā*.

EXHALE draw this *mudrā* down the central line of the body until it comes back to rest at the heart, or the womb, wherever feels right to you.

Repeat two or three Snake circles the womb and then repeat the arms positions and twists, changing the cross of the interlock to enable the non-dominant *svara* thumb to be uppermost.

Why to do it: *bhava* or inner feeling

The focus in this practice is on the experience of the mental powers (*manas śakti*) building the experience of the power of the life force (*prāṇa śakti*) in the palms of the hands and then drawing that power down into the heart and the womb.

9 | ETERNAL FOUNTAIN OF ENERGY INVOCATION

This practice connects to the presence of *prāṇa śakti* and sources an abundant supply of *śakti* with which to drench the energy body.

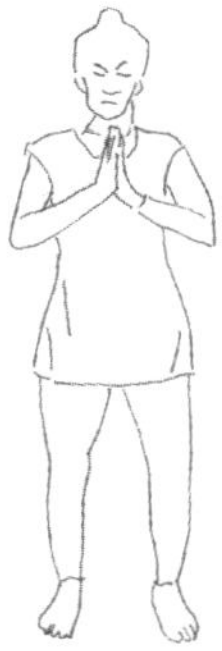

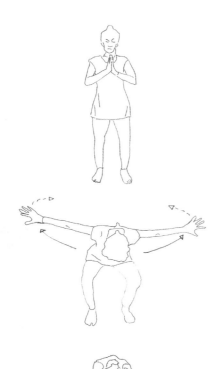

Stand with the knees soft and the feet about hip-width apart. Invite several rounds of Snake circles the womb to bring movement and warmth up through the whole body from the feet to the head. Continue to allow these circles to move as you move the arms and hands gestures.

INHALE begin with the palms together and outer edges of the thumbs resting on the breastbone in *namaste*.

EXHALE deepen your squat, keeping the heels on the ground as you reach both arms out in front of you in *namaste*.

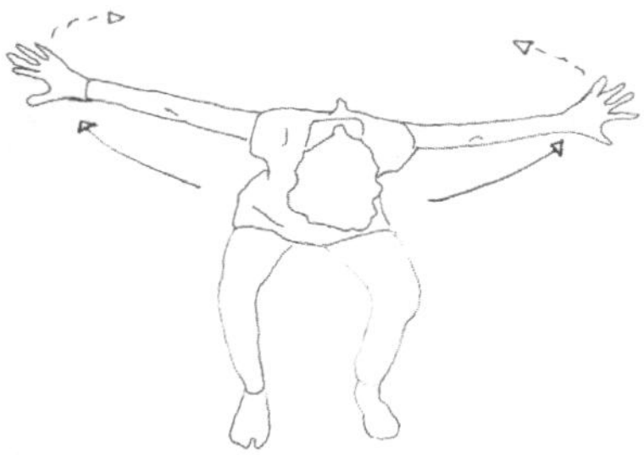

INHALE inwardly rotate the shoulders so that the backs of the hands touch, then slowly stretch the arms out to the sides and as far behind you as they will go (2).

EXHALE externally rotate the shoulders, turning the palms to face forwards and begin to bring the hands together, arms outstretched in front of you in a continuous line with the spine. Interlock the fingers (dominant *svara* thumb on top), turn the palms outwards, and then:

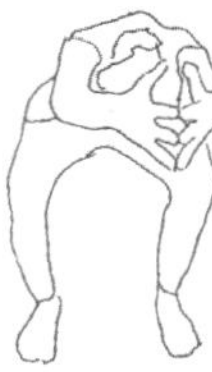

INHALE pushing the heels of the hands away, letting the two thumb tips touch and the two little fingertips touch, stretch out the hands and arms up above you as you straighten up. Look up, and shift the little fingertip on each hand to touch the thumb tip, creating a small

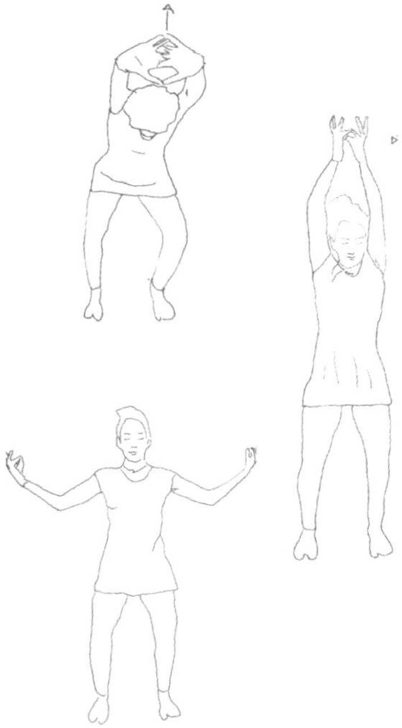

circle on each hand. Stretch out the three middle fingers of each hand and feel the spaces between the fingers.

EXHALE keep these *mudrās* in the hands as the arms stretch out and down, bringing the two *mudrā* circles back to the womb and bending the elbows. Shift the hands to *yoni mudrā*, and then the open lotus, and then:

INHALE and bring the lotus back to the heart and return to *namaste*.

Repeat two or three Snake circles the womb and then repeat the arm positions changing the cross of the interlock to enable the non-dominant *svara* thumb to be uppermost.

Why to do it: *bhava* or inner feeling

The focus in this practice is of expanding and then gathering the *prāṇa* in the palms of the hands and then bathing the body in this energy as the arms and hands lower. Because the feet are so well grounded and breathing, the experience is as if the feet have tapped into an eternal fountain of energy which bubbles upwards to drench the body with an inexhaustibly abundant source of energy.

NOTE ON *PĀDA BANDHA* AND *MŪLA BANDHA* IN THESE PRACTICES

The effect of maintaining a lift in the inner arch of the feet is to create a form of energetic lock, sometimes called the Foot arch lock (*pāda bandha*, see chapter twenty) which entices energy to flow up from the earth into the legs and the pelvis to be distributed to the rest of the body. There is a direct link between the experience of this foot lock and the more widely used Root lock (*mūla bandha*). If you are familiar with these practices and they arise naturally then please do use them. If you are unfamiliar with the practices of *pāda bandha* and *mūla bandha*, then please see the more detailed instructions in chapter twenty and gradually, as you gain confidence with them, invite them to arise naturally during these standing practices. The *bandhas* are not intended in these practices to be maintained rigidly and continuously, but rather to pulse with a rhythmic release and contraction as an expression of the expansion of energy in the movement of the breath.

CHAPTER SEVEN

embodied spirit: experiencing *yoni* *śakti* with womb yoga

ELEMENTAL CONSCIOUSNESS IN YOGA AND THE *TAITTIRĪYA UPANIṢAD*

The roots of yoga and *tantra* are deep in *Sāṁkhya* philosophy. *Sāṁkhya* is one of the earliest Indian philosophical worldviews. Its origins predate by far the first written presentation of the philosophy in the third-century text called the *Sāṁkhya Kārikā*. The earth in which the Sāṁkhyan roots grew is Upaniṣadic knowledge, and the Sāṁkhyan philosophical system recognises the *Vedas* as an authoritative source of wisdom and understanding. The *Vedas* are the earliest sources of writing on Indian spirituality, and the *Upaniṣads* themselves are considered 'Vedic', since they developed out of the *Vedas* and stand both as a reaction to them, and as the later flourishing outgrowth of their key philosophical concerns. *Sāṁkhya darśana*, or the Sāṁkhyan way of seeing the world, can be understood to be fruit of the Vedic tree.

Although the Sāṁkhyan view of the world is atheistic, in that its original structure of thought does not contain a single divine creative force, there are certainly some theistic interpretations of the system (for example in the tenth century *Bhāgavata Purāṇa*). What's more, its founding text is traditionally said to have been authored by the legendary Sage Kapila, a yogic hermit who possessed great magical powers (*siddhis*), and who is sometimes identified as the grandson of Brahma, the 'creator' god who dreamed the world from a state of *yoga nidrā* whilst reclining on a cosmic snake. In other places, he is identified with Viṣṇu, who is the supreme being for certain Hindu sects.

Sāṁkhya means simply 'about numbers', since this philosophical system literally enumerates those substances and forces from which life is understood to derive. From the Sāṁkhyan perspective, the evolution of the elements and the material substance of life on earth is perceived to derive from, and still remain part of a creative life force called prakṛti. Everything in the world is understood to be a manifestation of the relationship between spirit / consciousness (Śiva, or *puruṣa*) and matter (Śakti, or *prakṛti*). Śiva is experienced as pure being, the stillness of conscious awareness and Śakti is experienced as pure energy, the capacity to manifest and move. Śiva is male and Śakti is female. This Śiva / Śakti relationship is characteristic of Śākta (Goddess worshipping) traditions in particular, and leads to an understanding of the dynamic nature of this polarity as the cause of everything, including life itself. And so when we practise yoga with an awareness of this philosophical perspective, we are consciously embodying the sense of being literally 'children of the stars': acknowledging that our flesh and blood are in fact evolutes of these dual originating principles of pure consciousness and energy: Śiva and Śakti.

There are many complex patterns and layers in the *Sāṁkhya* way of understanding human life, and the relationships between the different dimensions through which energy manifests in the individual experience can be explained in intricate detail. But in terms of yoga practice, the simplest and most powerful way to engage with this elegant philosophical framework is to bring awareness to the connection between our multi-dimensional experiences and the five elements. I express these simply in terms of resonances, which are all laid out in the table overleaf, and which bring together the Upaniṣadic perspective on the five dimensions of human experience and the Sāṁkhyan enumeration of the five elements and their foundational relation to all of manifest creation.

For example, in the *Taittirīya Upaniṣad*, the sage Bhṛgu comes to the realisation (after much meditation and consultation with his father-*guru*) that the dimensions of human life are characterised by certain elemental qualities, and that these qualities define the nature of our experience. This begins with the physical body (*annamaya kośa*) which is a manifestation of the qualities of earth, and proceeds through an awareness of the significance of energy (*prāṇa*) as it manifests the fluid qualities of water. Bhṛgu's journey of awakening moves through the dimensions of mind and personality (*manomaya* and *vijñānamaya kośa*) which manifest the qualities of the heat of fire and the open movement of air, until he encompasses an awareness of pure bliss (*ānandamaya kośa*) which resonates at the level of space, the place in which all of the other elements exist. Bhṛgu then arrives at a final awareness that a multidimensional encounter with all of these different layers of being is possible if complete and acute awareness is brought to the appreciation of food as the sustainer of life. His final hymn acknowledges that the very process of inhabiting and nourishing the physical body with fully conscious attention is a powerful practice to develop the cosmic perspective: 'May the universe never abuse food, breath is food; the body eats food, This body rests on breath; breath rests on the body. Food is resting on food. The one who knows this becomes rich in food and great in fame' (*Taittirīya Upaniṣad* 11:7, translation in Tiwari 2011).

In relation to yoga, this means that conscious awareness of the physical aspects of our yoga can integrate with our experience of more esoteric or spiritual encounters. And so it is helpful to engage our attention both with how the body moves, and also with the *bhava* or inner feeling that the practice evokes. For example, in the practices described in this chapter, physical posture is accompanied by hand gesture and chant. The first chant comes from the *Taittirīya Upaniṣad* and the second chants are the 'seed sounds' (*bīja mantra*) associated with each energy centre (*cakra*). Additionally, the experiences of each combination of breath, posture, gesture and chant are grounded in the awareness of stability of the earth element, the fluidity of water, the heat of fire and the spaciousness of air. The poetic

PAÑCA TATTVA (5 elements)	**PṚTHIVĪ** Earth	**ĀPAS** Water	**AGNI** Fire	**VĀYU** Air	**ĀKĀŚA** Ether / Space
Tanmātra (subtle essences)	*Gandha* (smell)	*Rasa* (taste)	*Rūpa* (form)	*Sparśa* (touch)	*Śabda* (sound)
Jñānendriya (organs of knowledge)	*Ghrāṇa* (nose)	*Jihva* (tongue)	*Cakṣu* (eyes)	*Tvaca* (skin)	*Śrotra* (ears)
Karmendriya (organs of action)	*Pāyu* (anus) Excretion	*Upastha* (genitals) Reproduction	*Pāda* (foot) Locomotion	*Pāṇi* (hand) Grasping	*Vāk* (speech) Expression
Elemental nature	Heavy	Cool	Hot	Erratic	Mixed
Elemental qualities	Weight, cohesion	Fluidity, contraction	Heat, expansion	Motion, movement	Diffused, space-giving
Positive manifestation	Secure, stable	Creative, fertile, potent	Powerful, directed	Loving, giving	Authentically expressive
Colour	Yellow	White	Red	Blue / grey	Black / multi-coloured / translucent
Tattva yantra (shape/symbol)	Quadrangular	Crescent moon	Triangular	Hexagonal	Bindu / dot
Cakra (energy centre)	*Mulādhāra*	*Svādhiṣṭhāna*	*Maṇipūra*	*Anāhata*	*Viśuddha*
Bīja mantra (seed sound)	*Laṁ*	*Vaṁ*	*Raṁ*	*Yaṁ*	*Haṁ*
Antaḥkaraṇa (state of mind)	*Ahaṁkāra* (ego)	*Buddhi* (discrimination)	*Manas* (thoughts)	*Citta* (psychic content)	*Prajñā* (intuition)
Kośa layer of being	*Annamaya*	*Prāṇāmāya*	*Manomaya*	*Vijñānamaya*	*Ānandamaya*
Prāṇa vāyu (vital flow)	*Apāna*	*Prāṇa*	*Samāna*	*Udāna*	*Vyāna*
Hasta mudrā Hand gesture	*Pṛthivī* (thumb to ring finger)	*Āpas* (thumb to little finger)	*Cin* (thumb to index finger)	*Hṛdaya* (index finger to thumb root, thumb to middle & ring finger)	*Padma / Kamala* (open lotus)

multisensory visualisations of the second practice also invite other layers of being and awareness into the practice through touch, sight and smell.

This multi-elemental, poetic and multi-sensory approach to awareness in yoga practice is intended to invite a fully embodied encounter with the deep philosophical and spiritual foundations and aims of yoga practice. These practices are designed to promote a reconnection with the basic elements of life, through our senses, imaginations, body, breath and mind, and to encourage a nourishing and positive encounter with the renewed vitality that is the natural outcome of such reconnection.

TABLE OF FIVES: PENTADS IN *SĀṂKHYA* AND YOGA

(based on Swami Satyasangananda Saraswati's presentation in *Tattva Śuddhi*)
The table on the opposite page presents a way to understand connections between the five elements (*tattvas*) and human experience. Reading the table vertically reveals macrocosm within microcosm, and shows how elemental forces at play in the universe are embodied in every dimension of being, from our senses to our state of mind, from our organs to our vital energies. The colours and shapes at the bottom of the table relate to the *tattva yantra* described on p.199 (illustration p.200).

FIVE DIMENSIONS OF BEING SEQUENCE WITH GESTURE AND SOUND

The harmonious and fluid sequence that begins on page 184 integrates *āsana*, *mudrā* and *mantra* to promote an embodied experience of the elemental patterns of connection and resonance that are set out in yoga philosophy. I developed it as a way to encounter a lived experience of these philosophical patterns. There are a number of different *āsana* variations from the simplest to the most complex. The multidimensional layers of focus including *mantra* and *mudrā* are presented for each posture in the sequence. The chant is from the *Taittirīya Upaniṣad* and it simply states:

'I am food; I am prāṇa; I am mind and emotions; I am intuitive wisdom, I am bliss; I am all; I am, I am (pure being)'

Mā aham, aham annam;
Mā aham, aham prāṇam;
Mā aham, aham manaḥ;
Mā aham, aham vijñānam;
Mā aham, aham ānandam;
Mā aham, aham sarvam;
Mā aham, aham aham.

How to do it: form and flow

Stand with feet about hip-width apart and knees soft. Let the feet breathe by lifting and separating the toes. Become aware of your dominant *svara*.

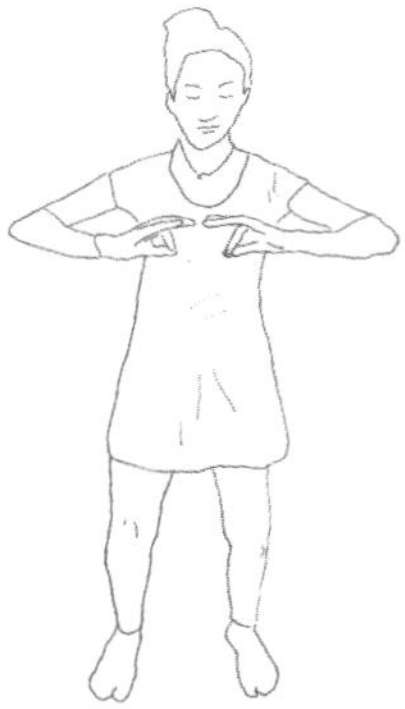

EARTH

INHALE touch your ring fingers to your thumbs (*pṛthivī mudrā*: earth gesture) and bring your hands to your heart, elbows out to the sides at shoulder height.

EXHALE bend the knees, strengthen the feet and drop a little lower in the squat.

CHANT *Mā aham, aham annam* (I am food).

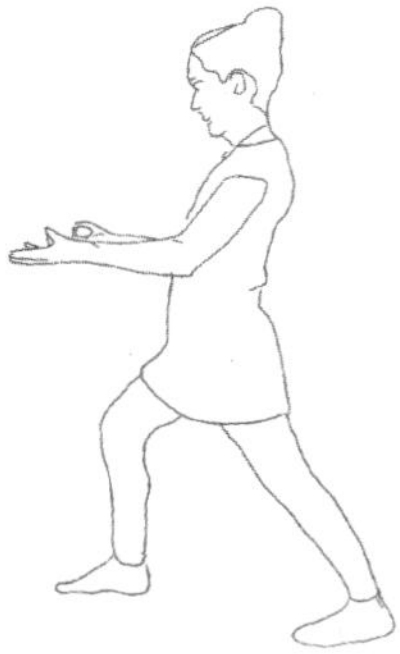

WATER

INHALE touch your little fingers to your thumbs (*āpas mudrā*: water gesture), stretch your arms out ahead of you at shoulder height with the palms facing upward and step about a metre forward with the foot that corresponds to the dominant *svara*. Have the front knee bent.

EXHALE open the arms wide out to the sides, bending the back knee and dropping your weight into it.

CHANT *Mā aham, aham prāṇam* (I am *prāṇa*).

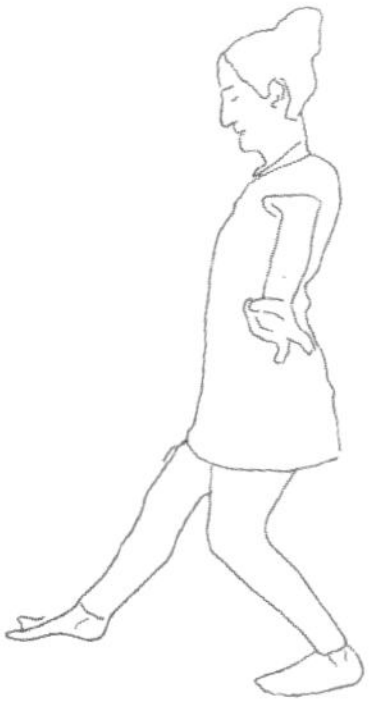

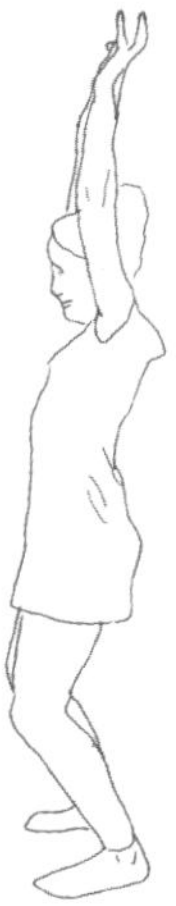

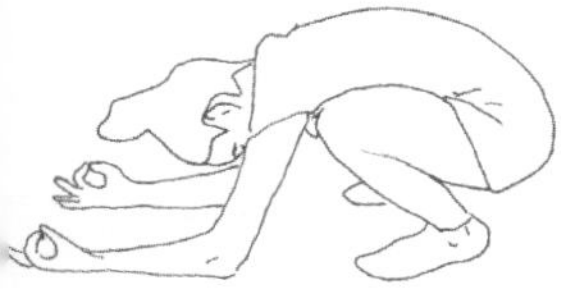

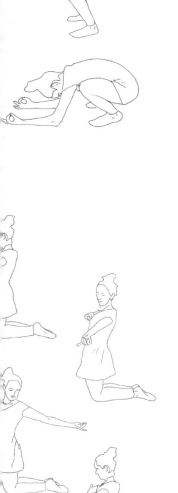

FIRE

INHALE straighten the back leg.

EXHALE bring the arms back together in front of you and drop the weight into the bent front knee.

INHALE step back to the starting position, touch the thumbs to the index fingers (*chin mudrā*: consciousness gesture) and reach the arms up above the head, as wide as is comfortable for the shoulders.

EXHALE bend the knees, reaching out and down with the arms. As you descend with the arms out in front of you at shoulder width.

CHANT *Mā aham, aham manaḥ* (I am mind).

During the chant descend further with the arms out wide in front, so that by the end of the chant either you are in a deep squat with the elbows and forearms on the ground, or you are kneeling on the ground (do whichever is comfortable, either option works).

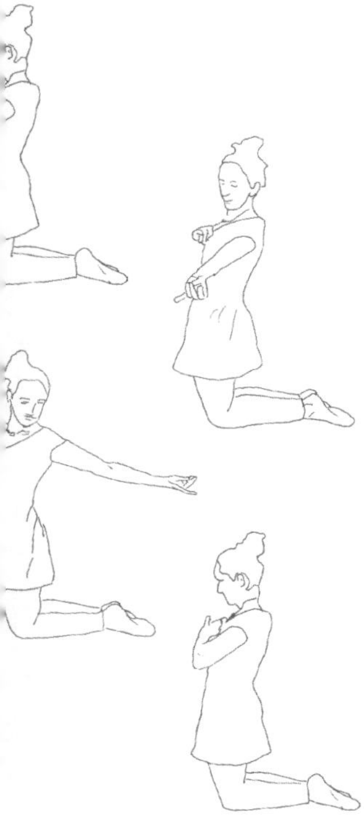

AIR

INHALE come to kneeling (if you are not already there), and lift pelvis up to high kneeling.

EXHALE bring elbows out to the sides at shoulder height and hands to the heart with index fingers tucked into root of thumb, and thumb tips touching middle and ring fingers (*hṛdaya mudrā*: heart gesture).

INHALE lengthen the spine.

EXHALE keep the non-dominant *svara* hand at the heart as you stretch out the dominant *svara* arm and move it in an arc behind you, twisting at the waist and following the hand with the gaze. **CHANT** *Mā aham* as you move into the twist.

As you move back to the centre, and return the dominant *svara* hand back to the heart, **CHANT** *aham vijñānam* (I am intuitive wisdom). Repeat the same chant as you twist to the opposite side.

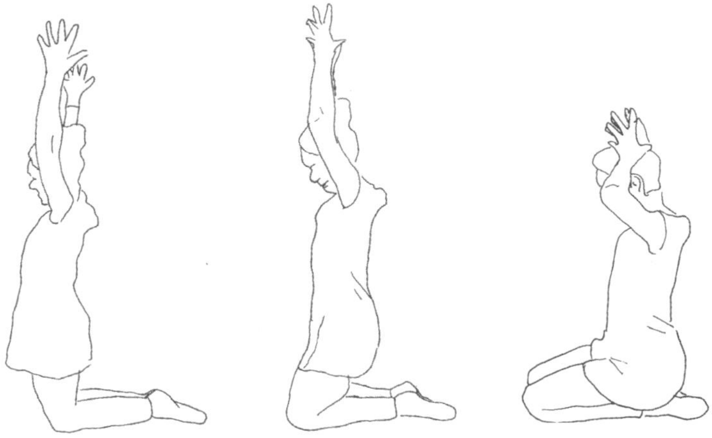

BEYOND THE ELEMENTS TO BLISS

INHALE reach both hands up above the head, with the sides of the thumbs and little fingers touching but all the other fingers stretched out (*padma mudrā*: lotus gesture)

EXHALE open up the base of the lotus, stretching the space between the tips of the touching thumbs and little fingertip, to form a 'crown', and bend the elbows to lower this crown on to the top of your head as at the same time you lower the buttocks back on to the heels.

CHANT *Mā aham, aham ānandam* (I am bliss).

AT ONE WITH ALL

INHALE separate the hands wide above the head and open the knees

EXHALE as you reach the arms and torso forward to let the forehead rest on the floor and the arms outstretched, with the backs of the hands on the ground, the palms open, all fingers stretching out and little fingers vertical (*alpapadma mudrā*: fully-bloomed lotus gesture). **CHANT** *Mā aham, aham sarvam* (I am all).

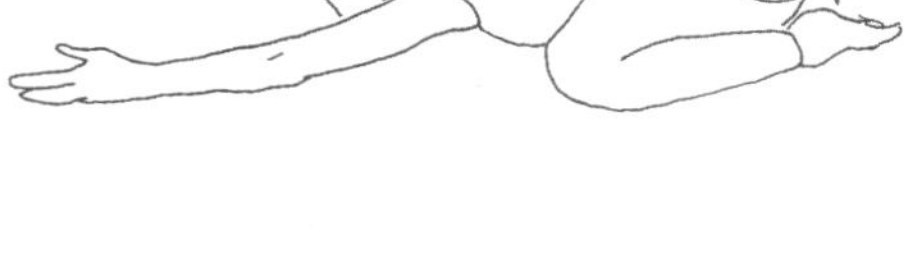

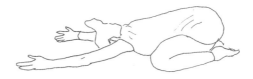

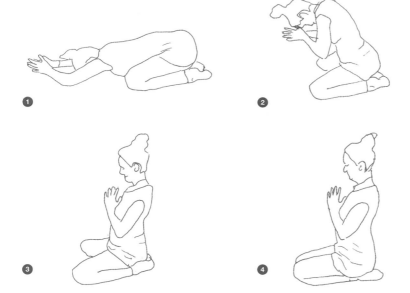

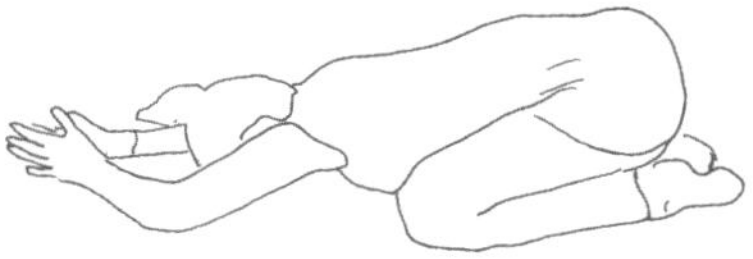

1

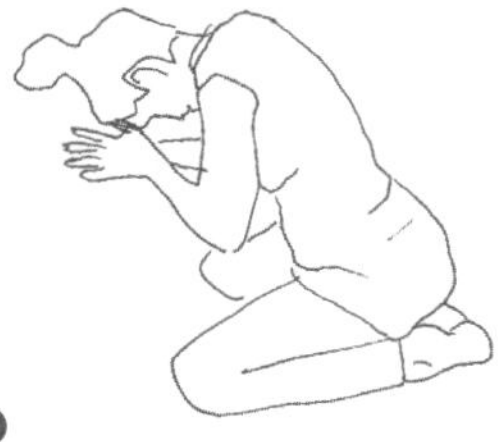

2

3

4

PURE BEING

INHALE bring the palms of the hands together on the floor (*namaste*: gesture to greet the divine light within gesture) and then, as you curl up (or sit up with a straight back), draw the hands down the centre line of the body, touching the middle of the forehead, third eye, nose and chin and coming to rest at the heart.

EXHALE sit kneeling

CHANT *Mā aham, aham aham* (I am, I am [pure being]).

TRANSITION TO START

Slowly bring the hands to the floor and push up to standing, lifting both knees together and returning to the start position to repeat the sequence with the non-dominant leg forwards with the *prāṇam* chant and the non-dominant arm arcing around behind you first in the *vijñānam* chant.

After finishing the second round of practice, you may choose simply to sit and repeat the *mantra*, perhaps with the *hasta mudrā*, or to repeat the integrated practice again with the *āsana*.

Why to do it: *bhava* or inner feeling

With each of the chants that accompanies the gestures and movement, you are affirming that dimension of your being, and the elemental resonance, sensory connections and other layers of experience associated with those aspects of being.

ŚAKTA TANTRA: THE FLOODS OF BLISS AND BEAUTY (*SAUNDARYA-LAHARĪ*) AND TEACHING ON THE WISDOM OF THE UNION OF THE INDIVIDUAL SOUL WITH UNIVERSAL CONSCIOUSNESS (*VIJÑĀNA BHAIRAVA TANTRA*)

The experience of *tantra* can be understood to be 'the process of the expansion of mind and the liberation of energy and consciousness from matter' (Saraswati 2008: 506). *Tantra* is a path of conscious integration with very many different routes and tracks criss-crossing each other. The many and various Indian schools of *tantra* often incorporate elements of the dualistic (*dvaita*) *Sāṁkhya* philosophy which, as we saw at the beginning of this chapter, ultimately divides all phenomena into consciousness or energy / matter. In other, non-dual (*advaita*) expressions of *tantra*, however, all reality can be seen as one or, sometimes, as a mysterious oscillation between unity and division. There is a huge variety of *tāntrik* philosophies and methods weaving across this span, some including a profoundly devotional element also. Central to all the many variants of the *tāntrik* vision of the world is the lived experience of microcosm / macrocosm, in which the individual body and its energies are a living blueprint of the structure and energies of the cosmos.

From within this complex web of *tāntrik* schools and approaches, comes *śākta tantra*: a Goddess-centred aspect of the Śaiva *tāntrik* traditions of India that inspires and informs the whole of *Yoni Śakti*. One of the fundamental beliefs at the roots of *śākta tantra* is that the whole of the cosmos is manifested simultaneously in the body of Goddess and in the body of the devotee, and that to worship Her is to honour the whole of creation because everything in that creation is an expression of Her *śakti* or power. In *Saundarya-Laharī* (*The Flood of Beauty and Bliss*), a key text of *śākta tantra*, each part of Goddess's body is praised. Even all the other gods in the Hindu pantheon are seen to praise Her (verse 25).

The intention of this fulsome praise and focused attention is to awaken in the practitioner a living encounter with the cosmic powers of creation which Goddess both possesses and embodies. Swami Satyasangananda Saraswati's translation and commentary of *Saundarya-Laharī* is subtitled *The Descent*, in recognition of the sense that Goddess's grace and power are Hers to send down to the worshippers who adore Her form and honour Her creative powers which have manifested the material world in which we live. In the practice below, this reverential honouring of the natural world as both the creation and the form of Goddess is united with an individual experience of elemental qualities as a bridge to a cosmic perspective that is very accessible.

The *āsana* are easy, the *mudrā*s simple and the chants just one syllable each. When practised together with a reverent inner feeling, these basic components create a rich multisensory encounter with the heart of *śākta tantra*. For the hand movements not only remind us of elements and their location in the energy body, but also relate to the *tāntrik* practice of *nyāsa* wherein the ritual placement of fingertips around the physical body literally calls the heavens to earth: '*Nyāsa* involves the human being becoming a mediator between earth and cosmos' (Amazzone 2010: 19). These integrated practices (especially *nyāsa*) make one not just a mediator, but a kind of living, harmonised map of the structure of (cosmic) reality.

HONOURING THE ELEMENTS WITH SOUND AND GESTURE

This seated flow is an inner ceremonial worship (*pūjā*) of the elements from which we are created. It combines visualisation with sound (*mantra*), sacred gesture (*mudrā*) and very simple movement (*āsana*) to create a moving meditation intended to honour our own relationship to the five elements. Each section begins with a poetic and ritual 'placing' of yourself in the scene by the river, in the water, offering light, feeling the breeze, and greeting the stars.

How to do it: form and flow

Sit on the earth or the floor with legs straight and angled out at whatever open distance feels sustainable to you. If this is not comfortable for the lower back, then have a cushion or rolled blanket under the sitting bones to create an easier curve in the lumbar spine. Push into the heels and let the feet breathe. Be aware of the flow of breath in your nostrils, and notice which *svara* is dominant.

ON THE RIVER BANK AS THE SUN SETS: EARTH

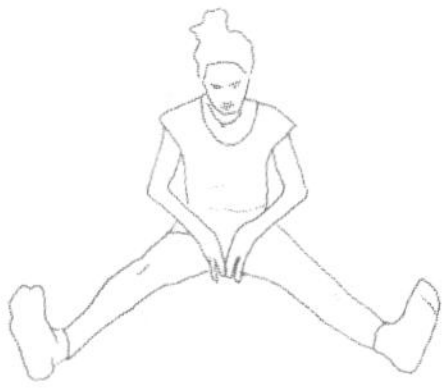

INHALE touch your ring fingers to your thumbs (*pṛthivī mudrā*: earth gesture) and bring your hands to rest just below your pubic bones so that the fingertips actually touch the earth. Sit up tall. Sense the lower body heavy, earthed and grounded, as if you are sitting on the damp earth of a river bank.

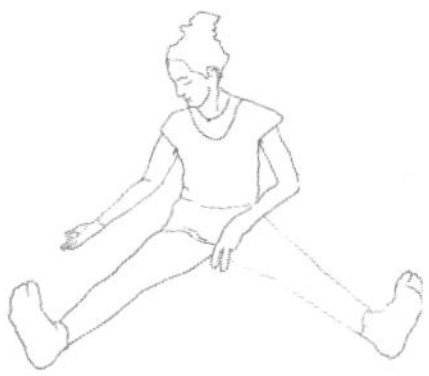

EXHALE keeping the fingertips low, sweep out in an arc the hand that corresponds to your dominant *svara*, lightly stroking the fingers over the surface of the earth. Twist all the way round until you have traced a semi-circle with your fingers and are looking behind you with the fingertips on the floor. As you move into the twist,

CHANT *Laṁ* (seed vibration for *mulādhāra cakra*, associated with the earth element).

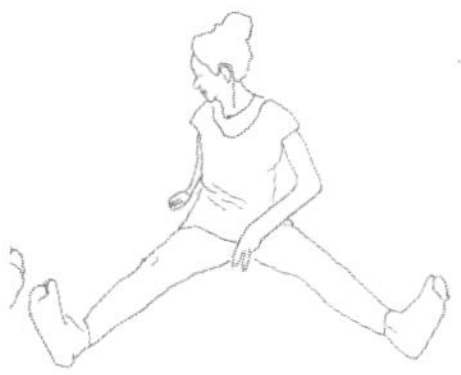

INHALE sit tall in the twist and experience the quality of stability.

EXHALE return in the same arc, tracing the fingertips over the surface of the earth and bringing the hand back to rest with fingertips on the earth beneath the pubic bones. As you move out of the twist and back to centre,

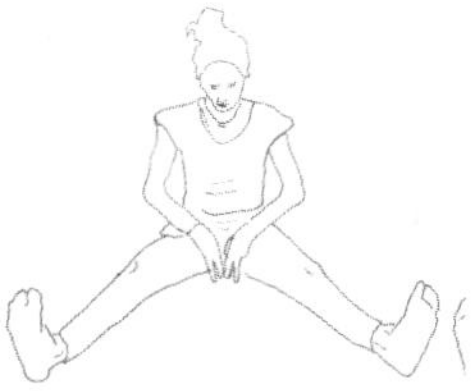

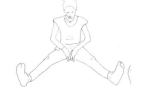

CHANT *Laṁ* (seed vibration for *mulādhāra cakra*, associated with the earth element).

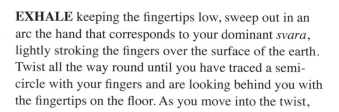

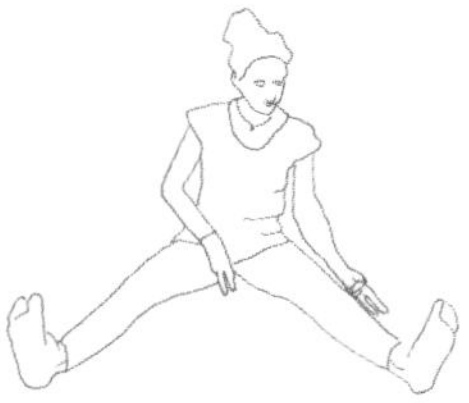

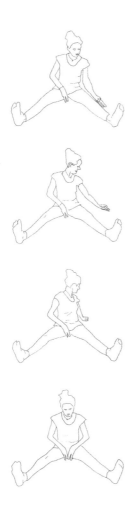

INHALE sit tall in the centre and experience the quality of stability.

EXHALE repeat the arc, twist and chant on the side corresponding to the non-dominant *svara*. Lightly stroking the fingers over the surface of the earth, twist all the way round until you have traced a semicircle with your fingers and are looking behind you with the fingertips on the floor. As you move into the twist behind you,

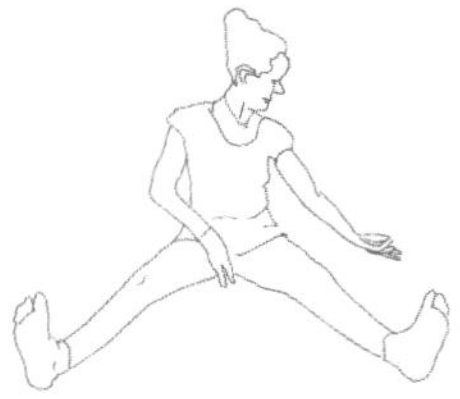

CHANT *Laṁ* (seed vibration for *mulādhāra cakra*, associated with the earth element).

INHALE sit tall in the twist and experience the quality of stability.

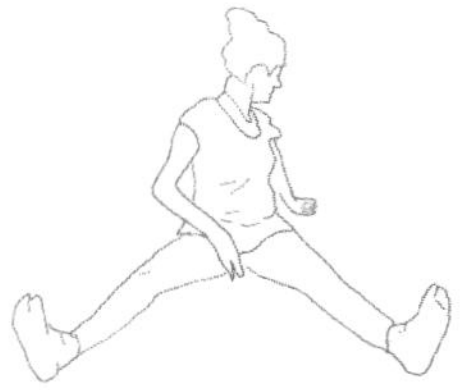

EXHALE return in the same arc, tracing the fingertips over the surface of the earth and bringing the hand back to rest on the earth with fingertips touching the earth beneath the pubic bones. As you move out of the twist and back to centre,

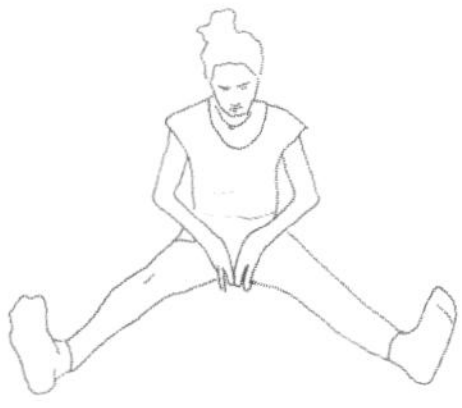

CHANT *Laṁ* (seed vibration for *mulādhāra cakra*, associated with the earth element).

INHALE sit tall with your hands just below your pubic bones so that the fingertips actually touch the earth, and experience the quality of stability.

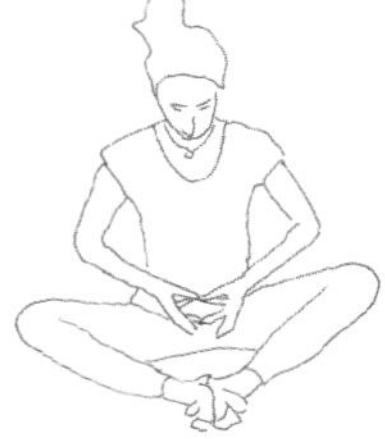

SITTING IN THE RIVER IN THE MOONLIGHT: WATER

EXHALE bring the soles of your feet together, let your knees drop to the sides and let the feet breathe.

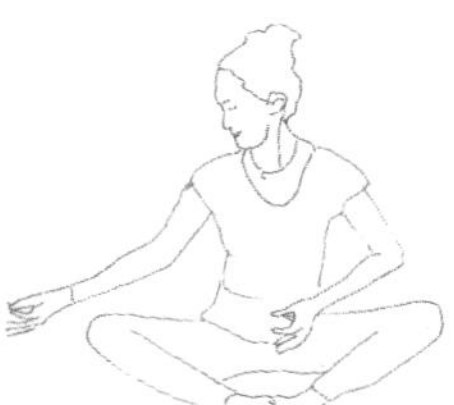

INHALE touch your little fingers to your thumbs (*āpas mudrā*: water gesture). With palms facing up, rest your hands next to your belly between the top of pubic bones and beneath the navel. Sit up tall. Sense the pelvis fluid and the lower body heavy, earthed and grounded, feel as if the waters in the river have flowed towards you and that the river bank is now awash with

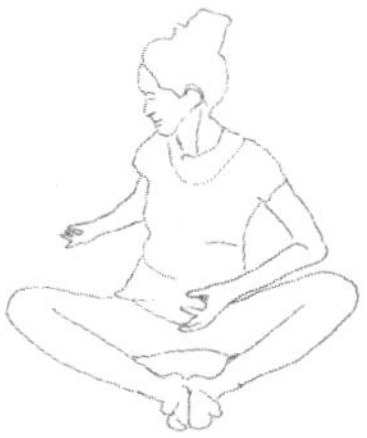

cool water. You are sitting in water up to the level of your hands. You can feel the mud beneath you. The moon is rising and shining on the water.

EXHALE maintaining *āpas mudrā* and keeping the fingertips low, sweep out in an arc the hand that corresponds to your dominant *svara*, lightly stroking the fingers over the surface of the water, creating ripples and sprinkling tiny droplets of water as you move. Twist all the way round until you have traced a semi-circle with your fingers and are looking behind you with the fingertips at the level of the surface of the water. As you move into the twist,

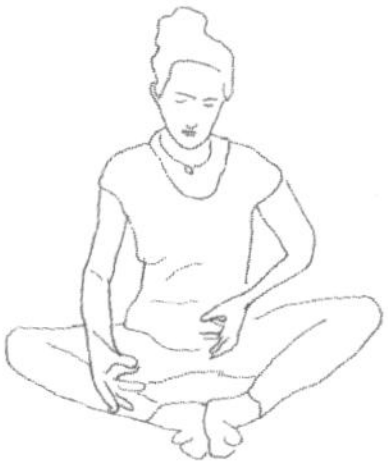

CHANT *Vaṁ* (seed vibration for *svādhiṣṭhāna cakra*, associated with the water element).

INHALE be in the twist, lengthen the spine and experience the quality of fluidity.

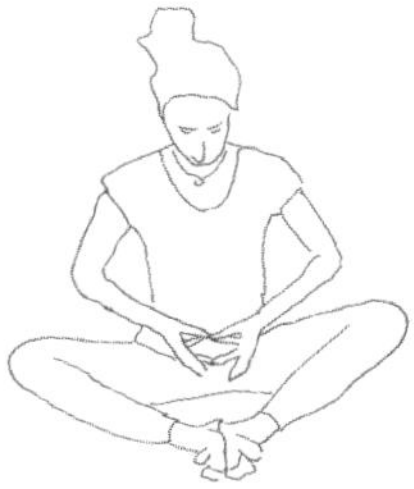

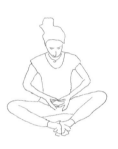

EXHALE return in the same arc, tracing the fingertips through the surface of the water and bringing the hand back to rest between the pubic bones and navel. As you move out of the twist and back to centre,

CHANT *Vaṁ* (seed vibration for *svādhiṣṭhāna cakra*, associated with the water element).

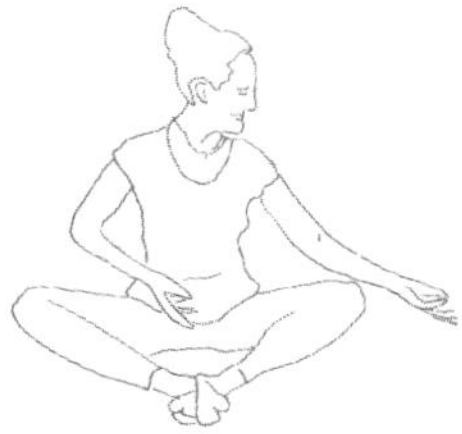

INHALE sit tall in the centre and experience the quality of fluidity.

EXHALE repeat the arc, twist and chant on the side corresponding to the non-dominant *svara*. As you move, trace a semi-circle with your fingers, lightly stroking the fingers over the surface of the water. As you move into the twist, look behind you with the fingertips at the level of the surface of the water and imagine them causing ripples in the river as they move through the water, dripping tiny droplets of water.

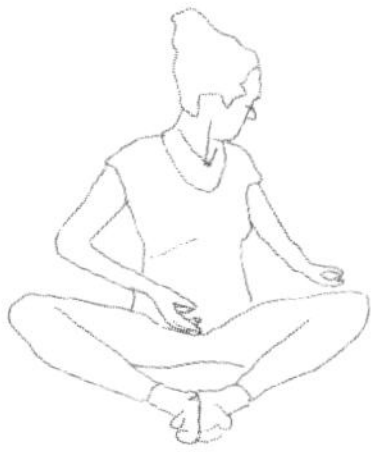

CHANT *Vaṁ* (seed vibration for *svādhiṣṭhāna cakra*, associated with the water element).

INHALE sit tall in the twist and experience the quality of fluidity.

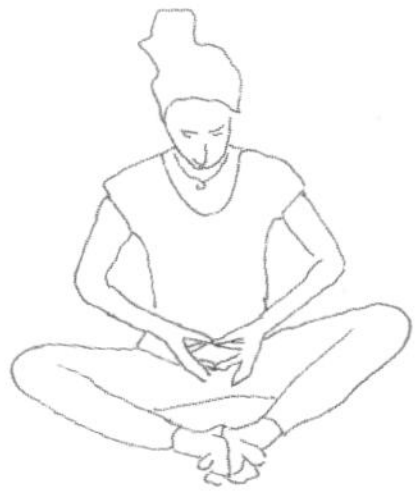

EXHALE return in the same arc, tracing the fingertips through the surface of the water and bringing the hand back to rest between the pubic bones and navel. As you move out of the twist and back to centre,

CHANT *Vaṁ* (seed vibration for *svādhiṣṭhāna cakra*, associated with the water element)

INHALE sit tall in the centre with hands resting between pubic bone and navel and experience the quality of fluidity. Feel the moonlight shining on the surface of the water.

OFFERING LIGHT TO THE RIVER IN THE MOONLIGHT: FIRE

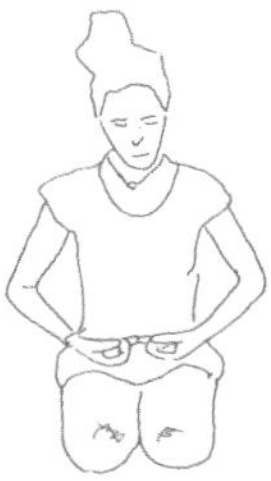

EXHALE shift into a kneeling position, either by bringing the knees over to the side, or rolling centrally across your two feet.

INHALE touch your index fingers to your thumbs (*cin mudrā*: gesture of consciousness). With palms facing up and cupped, rest your hands next to your belly at the level of the navel. Sit up tall. Sense the belly warm and powerful, feel the river waters up to the level of the pubic bones, and the mud beneath you. Imagine a little light, a flame flickering in the palm of the hand, as if it held a tiny lamp, a *dipa* with a cotton wick floating in butter or oil, burning brightly.

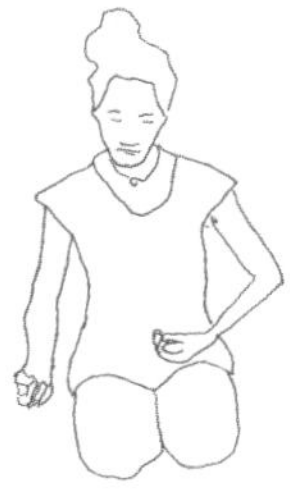

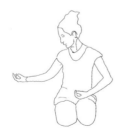

EXHALE maintaining *cin mudrā* and keeping the palms cupped, fingertips at the level of the navel, sweep out in an arc the hand that corresponds to your dominant *svara*, releasing your little light to float on the surface of the water. The surface of the water reflects the orange-gold glow of the lamplight as it floats away. Twist all the way round until you have traced a semi-circle with the back of your cupped palm across the surface of the water and are looking behind you with the fingertips at the level of the navel.

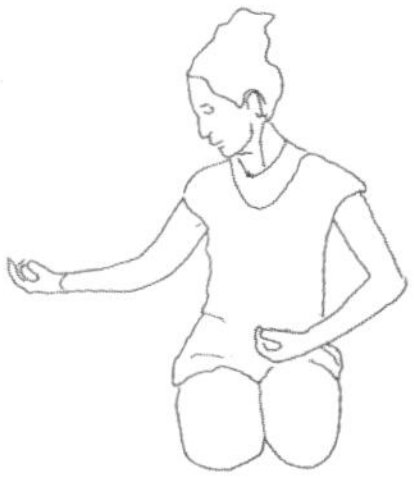

CHANT *Raṁ* (seed vibration for *maṇipūra cakra*, associated with the fire element).

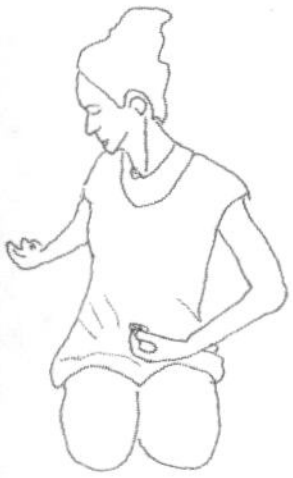

INHALE be in the twist, lengthen the spine and experience the quality of heat.

EXHALE return in the same arc, tracing the back of the cupped hand over the surface of the water and bringing the hand back to rest at the navel. As you move out of the twist and back to centre,

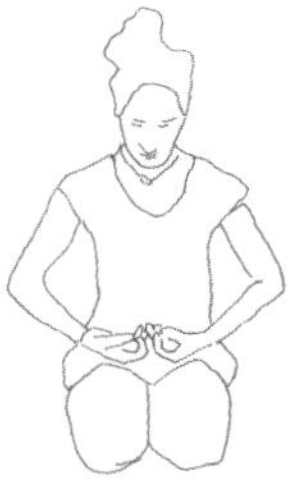

CHANT *Raṁ* (seed vibration for *maṇipūra cakra*, associated with the fire element).

INHALE sit tall in the centre with the hands at the navel and experience the quality of heat.

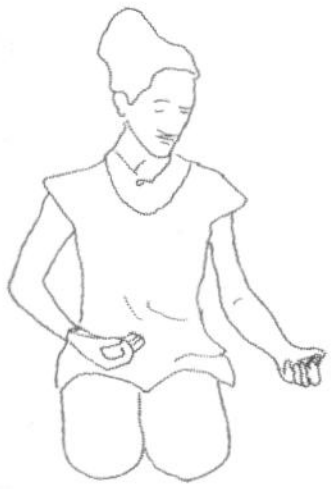

EXHALE repeat the arc, twist and chant on the side corresponding to the non-dominant *svara*. As you move into the twist, trace the back of the cupped hand over the surface of the water and look behind you with the fingertips at the level of the surface of the water, and

CHANT *Raṁ* (seed vibration for *maṇipūra cakra*, associated with the fire element).

INHALE sit tall in the twist and experience the quality of heat.

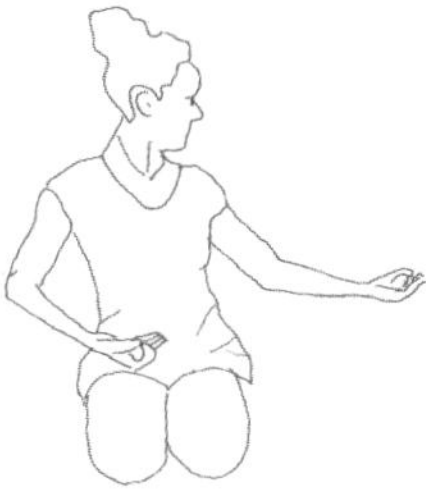

EXHALE return in the same arc, tracing the back of the cupped hand over the surface of the water and bringing the hand back to rest between the pubic bones and navel. As you move out of the twist and back to centre,

CHANT *Raṁ* (seed vibration for *maṇipūra cakra*, associated with the fire element).

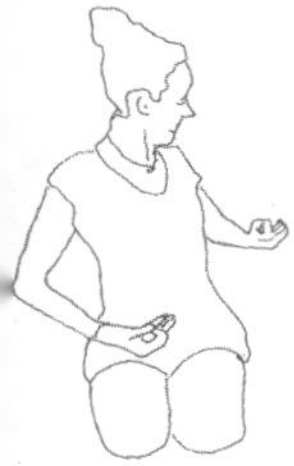

INHALE sit tall in the centre with hands resting between pubic bone and navel and experience the quality of fluidity. Feel the moonlight shining on the river and see the lights of the lamps shining as they float on the surface of the water.

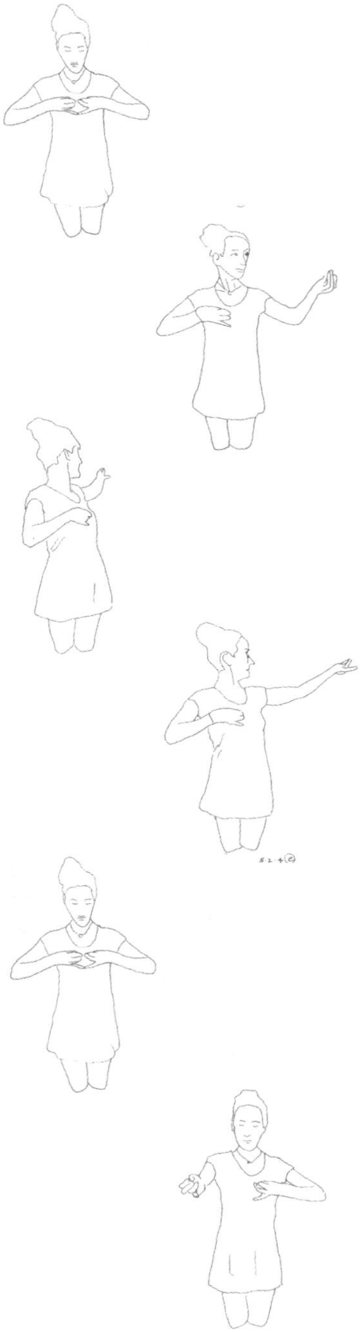

FEELING THE BREEZE BLOWING ACROSS THE MOONLIT RIVER AS THE LIGHTS FLOAT ON THE SURFACE OF THE WATER: AIR

EXHALE squeeze your buttocks and raise into a lifted kneeling position, thighs vertical with the hips above the knees.

INHALE bring elbows out to the sides at shoulder height and the hands to the heart, palms face up with index fingers tucked into root of thumb, and thumb tips touching middle and ring fingers (*hṛdaya mudrā*: heart gesture). Sit up tall. Sense the heart beating. Feel the river waters up to the level of the pubic bones, and the mud beneath you. See the flames of the little lamps you have offered to the river floating on the surface of the water and the moonlight shining on the river. Feel a slight breeze touching your skin.

EXHALE maintaining *hṛdaya mudrā* keep the non-dominant *svara* hand at the heart as you stretch out the dominant *svara* arm and move it in an arc around you, at heart level, twisting at the waist and following the hand with the gaze. Twist all the way round until you have traced a semi-circle through the air with your fingers and are looking behind you with the fingertips at the level of the heart.

CHANT *Yaṁ* (seed vibration for *anāhata cakra*, associated with the air element).

INHALE lengthen the spine and experience the quality of movement as the breeze touches your skin.

EXHALE return in the same arc, maintaining *hṛdaya mudrā* and feeling the hand moving through the air, and bringing it back to rest at the heart. As you move out of the twist and back to centre,

CHANT *Yaṁ* (seed vibration for *anāhata cakra*, associated with the air element).

INHALE sit tall in the centre with the hands at the heart and experience the quality of movement as the breeze touches your skin.

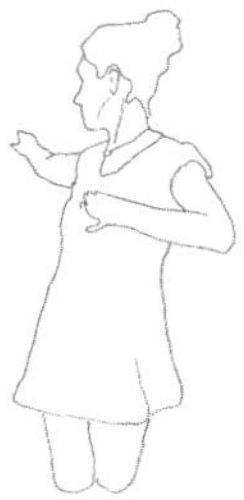

EXHALE repeat the arc, twist and chant on the side corresponding to the non-dominant *svara*. As you move into the twist behind you, maintain *Hṛdaya mudrā*, trace the hand through the air and look behind you with the fingertips at the level of the heart. As you move into the twist,

CHANT *Yaṁ* (seed vibration for *anāhata cakra*, associated with the air element).

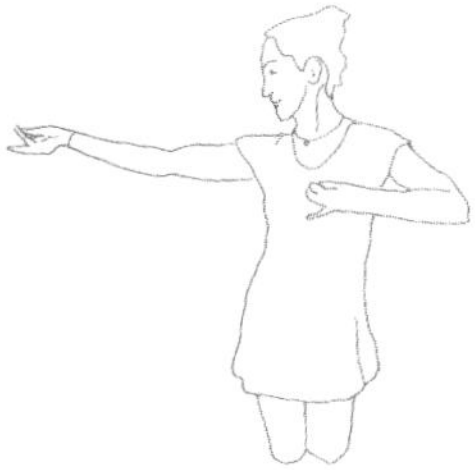

INHALE sit tall in the twist and experience the quality of movement as the breeze touches your skin.

EXHALE return in the same arc, tracing the fingertips through the air and bringing the hand back to rest at the heart. As you move out of the twist and back to centre, **CHANT** *Yaṁ* (seed vibration for *anāhata cakra*, associated with the air element).

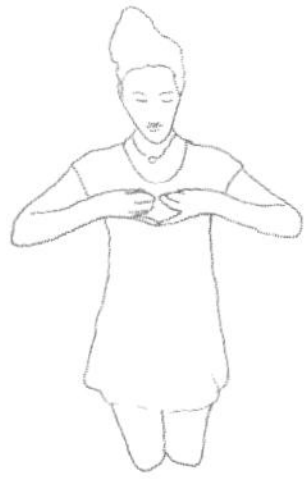

INHALE sit tall in the centre with hands resting at the heart, elbows out to the side, and experience the quality of movement as the breeze touches your skin. See the moonlight shining on the river and the lights of the lamps shining as they float on the surface of the water.

SEEING THE STARS TWINKLING IN THE DARK NIGHT SKY AS THE BREEZE BLOWS ACROSS THE MOONLIT RIVER WHERE THE LIGHTS FLOAT ON THE SURFACE OF THE WATER: SPACE

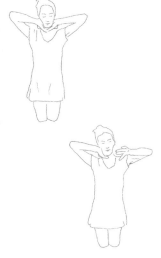

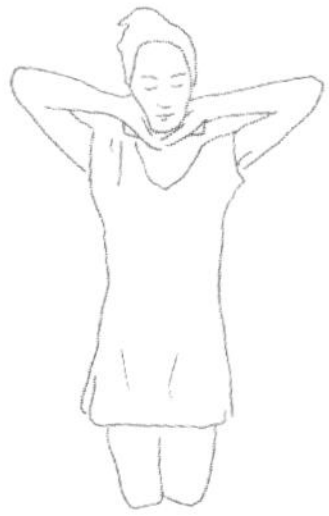

EXHALE remain in a lifted kneeling position with thighs vertical and hips above the knees. Let the middle finger touch the thumb, and all other fingers stretch out wide (*ākāśa mudrā*: the space gesture).

INHALE point the elbows up and rotate the backs of the wrists towards the shoulders so that the thumb and middle fingertips together touch the throat and the remaining fingers rest on the sides of the neck. Lift the back of the top of the head. Sense the throat open and spacious. Feel the river waters up to the level of the pubic bones, and the mud beneath you. See the flames of the little lamps you have offered to the river floating on the surface of the water. Lift your gaze to become aware of the vastness of the night sky and the stars twinkling above.

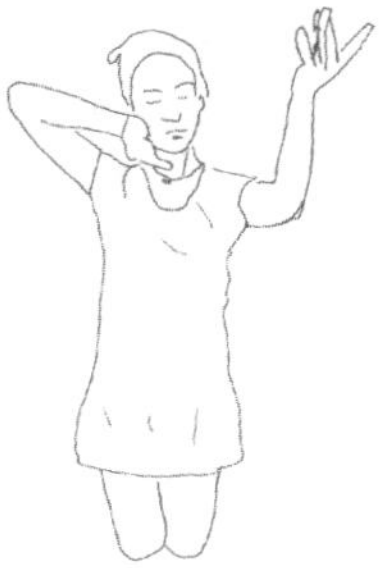

EXHALE maintaining *ākāśa mudrā*, keep the non-dominant *svara* hand at the throat as you rotate the wrist to let the fingers point upwards, slightly dropping the elbow and then stretching out the dominant *svara* arm and moving it up in an arc around and above you, twisting at the waist and following the hand with the gaze. Twist all the way round until you are looking up at the hand above your head behind you.

CHANT *Haṁ* (seed vibration for *viśuddha cakra*, associated with the space element).

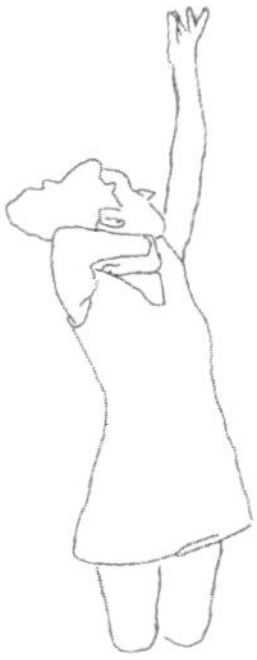

INHALE lengthen the spine and experience the quality of spaciousness as you look into the dark expanse of the sky above.

EXHALE return in the same arc, maintaining *ākāśa mudrā* and feeling the hand moving through space, rotating and dropping the wrist and pointing the elbow up to the stars so that the middle finger and thumb can come to rest back at the throat. As you move out of the twist and back to centre,

CHANT *Haṁ* (seed vibration for *viśuddha cakra*, associated with the space element).

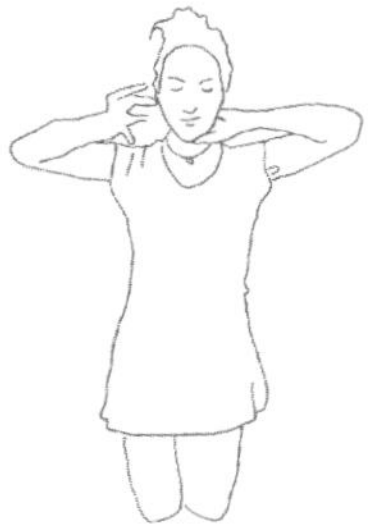

INHALE sit tall in the centre with the hands at the throat and the elbows pointing up to the stars. Let your gaze be upward and experience the quality of spaciousness as you look at the stars in the night sky.

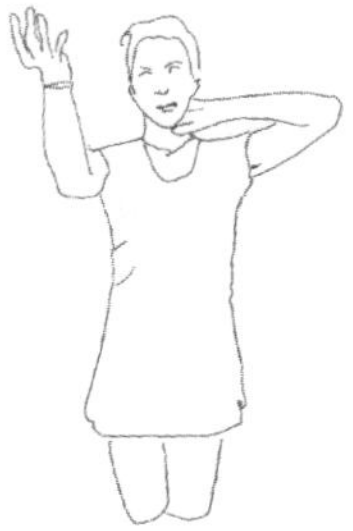

EXHALE repeat the arc, twist and chant on the side corresponding to the non-dominant *svara*. As you move into the twist behind you, maintain *ākāśa mudrā* and rotate the wrist to let the fingers point upwards, slightly dropping the elbow and then stretching out the dominant *svara* arm and moving it up in an arc around and above you, twisting at the waist and following the hand with the gaze. Twist all the way round until you are looking up at the hand above your head behind you. As you move into the twist,

CHANT *Haṁ* (seed vibration for *viśuddha cakra*, associated with the space element).

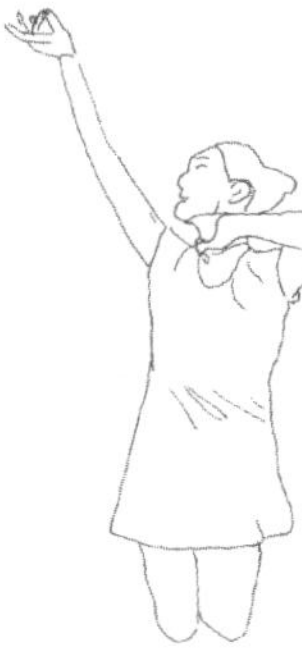

INHALE sit tall in the twist with the hand reaching up to the sky. Let your gaze be upward and experience the quality of spaciousness as you look at the stars in the night sky.

EXHALE return in the same arc, maintaining *ākāśa mudrā* and feeling the hand moving through space, rotating and dropping the wrist and pointing the elbow up to the stars so that the middle finger and thumb can come to rest back at the throat. As you move out of the twist and back to centre,

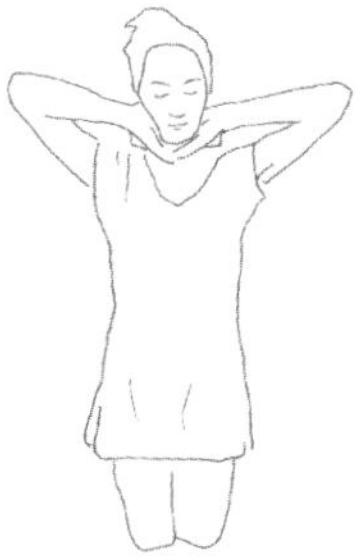

CHANT *Haṁ* (seed vibration for *viśuddha cakra*, associated with the space element).

INHALE sit tall in the centre with the hands at the throat and the elbows pointing up to the stars. Feel the river waters up to the level of the pubic bones, and the mud beneath you. Let your gaze be upward and experience the quality of spaciousness as you look at the stars in the night sky.

BEING IN THE WHOLE SCENE, CONNECTING WITH THE LIGHT FROM ABOVE: BEYOND ALL THE ELEMENTS

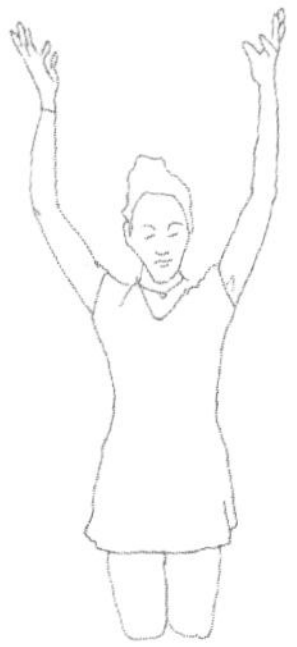

EXHALE remain in a lifted kneeling position with thighs vertical and hips above the knees.

INHALE bring the hands out either side of the head, elbows bent. Bend back the wrists and open out the palms so they face upwards, stretching all the fingers out and having the little fingers vertical (*alpapadma mudrā*: fully-bloomed lotus gesture).

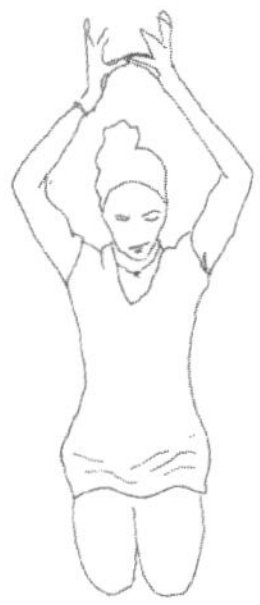

EXHALE Feel the river waters up to the level of the pubic bones, and the mud beneath you. See the flames of the little lamps you have offered to the river floating on the surface of the water.

INHALE Lift your gaze to become aware of the vastness of the night sky and the stars twinkling above.

EXHALE be in this pose and be aware of all the elemental qualities simultaneously: stability through the feet and lower legs, fluidity in the hips and pelvis, heat, in the belly, movement in the heart and spaciousness in the throat.

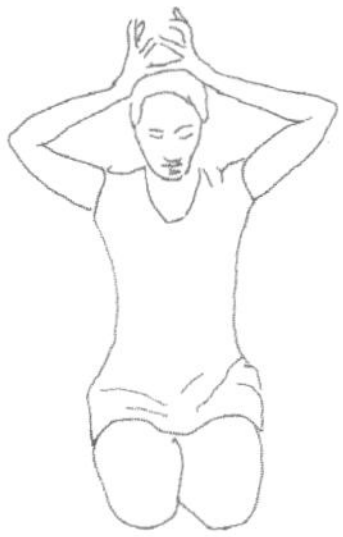

INHALE look straight up and reach the hands farther up into the sky above you, fingers and palms stretched wide. Bring the hands together and touch the tips of the little fingers and the thumbs to create an open 'lotus crown'. All the other fingers are stretched up.

EXHALE maintain the hands in this position and bend the elbows to lower this 'lotus crown' on to the top of your head as at the same time you lower the buttocks back on to the heels.

CHANT *Aum* (seed vibration for the *sahasrāra cakra* [crown energy centre] resonating beyond the elements).

INHALE lengthen the spine and experience the quality of pure being.

CLOSURE

INHALE open the knees wider and separate the hands wide above the head, still keeping the palms open and facing towards each other with all the fingers stretched out.

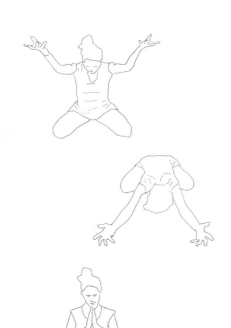

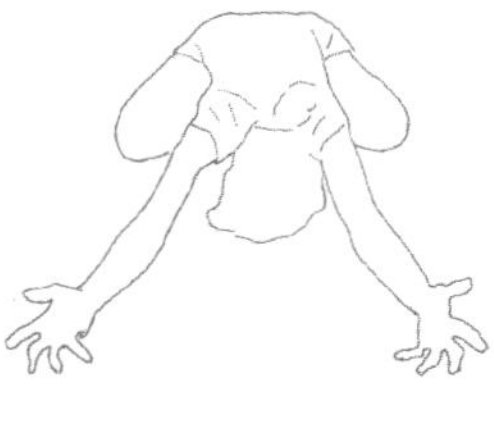

EXHALE as you reach the hands, arms and torso forward to let the forehead rest on the floor with the arms outstretched. The backs of the hands are on the ground and the palms face upwards, with all the fingers stretched out and the little fingers vertical (*alpapadma mudrā*: fully-bloomed lotus gesture).

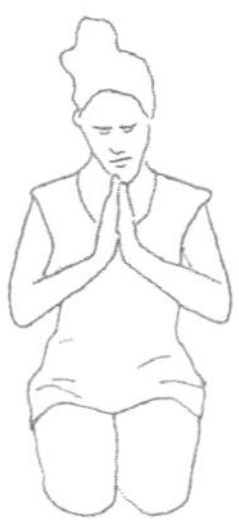

INHALE bring the palms of the hands together on the floor (*namaste*: gesture to greet the divine light within) and then, as you curl up (or sit up with a straight back), draw the hands down the centre line of the body, touching the middle of the forehead, third eye, nose and chin and coming to rest at the heart.

EXHALE sit kneeling or cross-legged, whichever is more comfortable for you, with your hands palms up, fingers outstretched on your knees. As you sit,

CHANT

Pūrṇamadaḥ pūrṇamidam pūrṇāt
Pūrnamudacyate pūrṇasya pūrṇamādāya
Pūrṇameva-avaśiśyate
(Īśa Upaniṣad)

Everything in this, our inner world, is whole, complete and perfect. Everything in that, the outer world, is whole, complete and perfect. Everything that is whole, complete and perfect comes from wholeness, completion and perfection itself, and the original source of all this perfection simply remains always perfect, even though the entire, complete and perfect world, and everything in it, emerges from it.

In a more poetic rendering, as shared by Mukunda Stiles, this meaning can be expressed thus:

Thou art ever one, and ever whole.
From you this perfect world was born.
Yet should all this world disappear from view.
You would always be the same.

TATTVA YANTRA

The *tattva yantra* (see illustration overleaf) provides a visual connection with the five elements in this practice. Each symbol resonates with the qualities of the element with which it is associated, and by 'placing' these symbols at the different energetic points associated with each element, the whole body becomes a yantra or sacred geometrical form in which the elements of creation are literally seen to be present in the human body itself:

Golden, glowing yellow square (from feet to pubis) symbolises *pṛthivī tattva*, the element of earth, representing stability, the capacity to nurture, nourish and protect.

Silvery, luminous white crescent moon (at pelvis) symbolises *āpas tattva*, the element of water, representing fluidity, the fertile capacity to create, imagine and desire.

Flaming, bright red downward-pointing triangle (at chest) symbolises *agni tattva*, the element of fire, representing heat, the directive capacity to assimilate, digest and illuminate.

Celestial sky-blue hexagon, or set of six spheres (at neck and head) symbolises *vāyu tattva*, the element of air, representing the open capacity to experience compassion, empathy and connectedness.

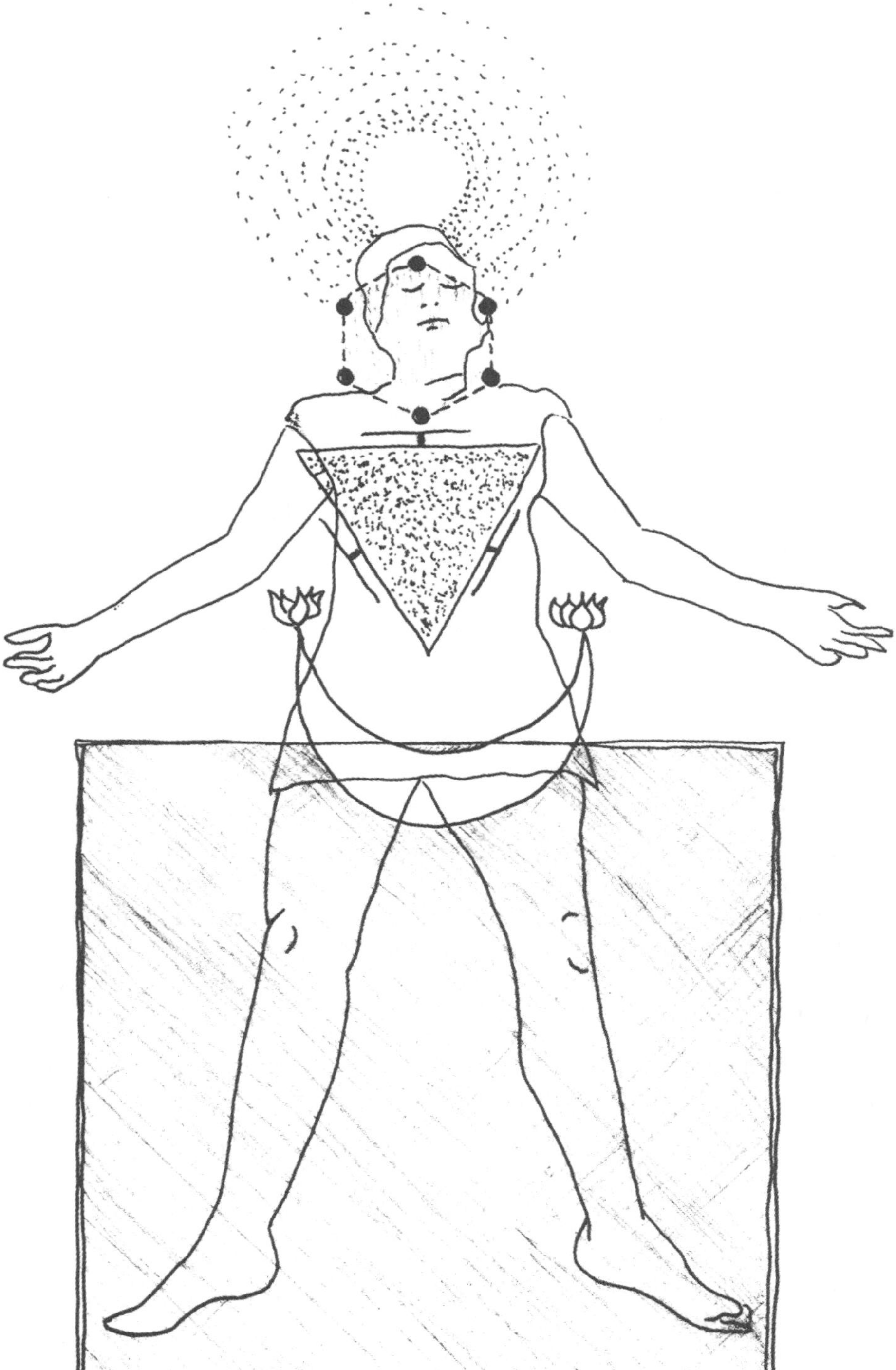

Infinite dark blue / black midnight sky (above crown) strewn with scraps and twinkles, stars and squiggles of every colour imaginable to symbolise *ākāśa tattva*, the element of space, representing the limitless capacity to experience pure being.

Why to do it: *bhava* or inner feeling

With each gesture and chant, and visualisation in this sequence, the awareness is brought to the qualities of each element in turn. At the end the awareness rests in the consciousness of pure being. The feeling the practice evokes is of a tender and respectful connection with the beauty of each elemental manifestation: the stability of the earth, and the flowing waters, and the shining lights which float on the waters, the soft touch of the breeze on the skin, and the vast openness of the sky above. At the end, the practice brings you to rest in a state of pure being, and the closing chant resonates an experience of everything in the inner and outer worlds unfolding as it should. This *bhava* or inner feeling is a vital experience in the process of creating an inner harmony, especially in the world of the womb, and relating the elements of this inner state of harmony and balance to the natural world outside. It encourages a lived experience of the yoga of connection and being at one with the world we inhabit.

The powerful ecological effects of sensing how our physical body, and especially our womb, is a microcosm of the world outside is explored more fully in chapter twenty-seven which considers the resonance between personal awareness and planetary evolution.

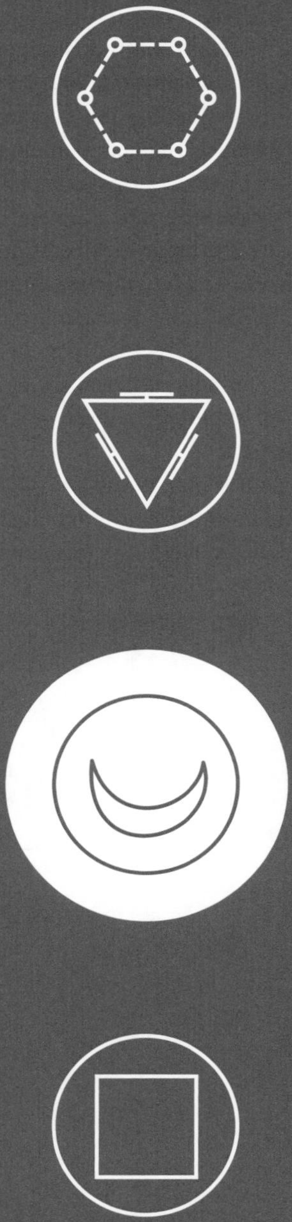

PART TWO

LIFE CYCLES & THE WISDOM GODDESSES

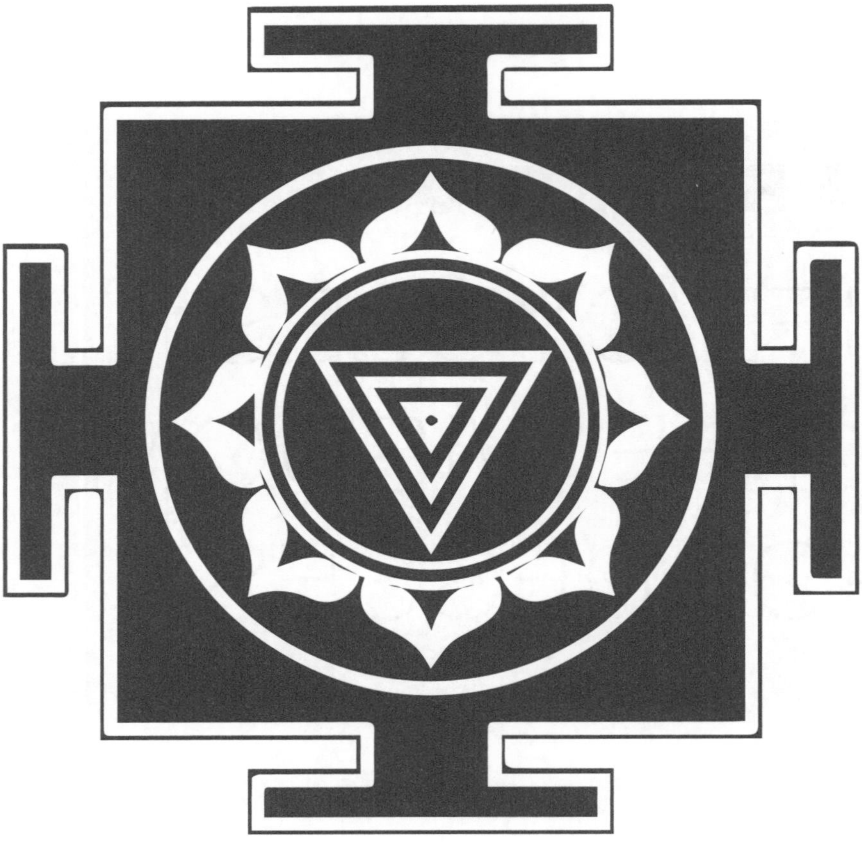

CHAPTER EIGHT

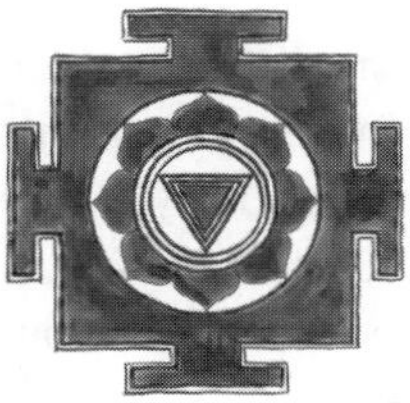

Kālī

Cycles and circles of female *siddhis*

In the previous chapter I proposed understanding the apparently biological functions of women's bodies as a series of powerful manifestations of the capacity for insight and deep wisdom: the female *siddhis*. I invited you to consider that the biological occurrences that signal potential *siddhis* are a cycle of female, embodied yogas that punctuate our lived experience, and whose spiritual and initiatory capacities may be so profound as to have inspired a whole technology of spiritual endeavour in the form of the *haṭha* yoga project.

These female *siddhis* do not exist independently of each other. Women's lives move in interconnected cycles and rhythmic spirals. Encounters with the female *siddhi*s mark initiatory transitions from one cycle to the next, and the response a woman brings to her encounter with each *siddhi* can have a profound resonance with every other *siddhi*. These resonances operate at physical, emotional and spiritual levels. The life cycles and their attendant *siddhis* circle around each other so that the cycle of a woman's whole life experience contains within it many interconnected circles where themes and variations characteristic of each *siddhi* overlap with each other, overlaying resonance and pre-echoes of previous and future cycles. For example, the nature of a woman's encounter with her menarche and monthly periods can set the tone for her own response to the onset of perimenopause. The degree to which a woman has fully engaged with the depths and heights of her own sexuality and menstrual life can determine her capacity to meet the experiences of labour and birth with courage and openness. For the powerful oxytocin surges that are present during orgasm are also crucial to the management of pain during birth, and the pain and visionary intensity of menstruation can pre-echo the other-worldly experiences of early labour. The confusion and anger that often accompanies menarche and adolescence may find a later echo in the disquieting uncertainty of perimenopause. The extreme hormonal shifts and exhaustion of the postnatal period can raise a range of challenges similar to those experienced at menopause. There is a direct match in terms of emotional and hormonal dynamics between the experiences of premenstrual and menopausal women. There are so very many parallels and overlaps, such a range of echoes and resonances across and between these different cycles as they unfold throughout a woman's life.

These echoes and overlaps spiral out beyond the life cycle of an individual woman. Indeed, because the hormonal and emotional experiences of menstruation and menopause are so powerfully communicated between women's bodies and hearts, there are profound inter-generational overlaps and interconnections between the different *siddhis* occurring at the same time in different women: for example, in the potentially challenging nexus of a daughter reaching the peak of her fertility at precisely the time her mother begins to enter menopause (Shuttleworth and Redgrove: 278); or the synchronous 'sympathetic' encounters that often arise between one woman's labour and her sister's (or birth companion's) menstruation. The quality of feeling that accompanies the *siddhi* of lactation can likewise invite sympathetic or synchronous consciousness of deep *karuṇā* [compassion, mother-love]. For example, I have had the honour over the past thirteen years of facilitating many yoga groups for postnatal women who are often all breastfeeding their babies together in the class, and I can testify to the remarkably powerful meditative ambience that such group feeding creates. Indeed, it can be very valuable to welcome in the sensory experiences of feeding a child (whether breast or bottle feeding) through a practice of inner silence (p.460).

Synchronous menstruation is a common experience in households where a number of women live and bleed together, and in the intense focus of energy on a yoga retreat, for example, similar effects often occur. I have witnessed, on a number of occasions in women's yoga training courses, the powerful effect that being in a group with many menstruating women can have on women whose cycles have apparently stopped: after not having menstruated for over two years, one *yoginī* in her late fifties who was attending an intensive pregnancy yoga training in Antwerp announced with astonishment on the third day that her period had returned. The same experience occurred also in London to a woman who had not menstruated for over eighteen months.

Such is the power of these female *siddhis* that synchronous experience of any given female *siddhi* creates a tangible force that impacts not just on other women, but on whole communities. The impact of synchronous menstruation, for example, is so tangibly powerful that radical anthropologist Chris Knight has elaborated (in *Blood Relations: Menstruation and the Origins of Culture*) a convincing theory that synchronous ovulation and menstruation are in fact the key factors that triggered the 'human revolution' at the origin of our species. In chapter twenty-nine I return to consider the future applications of these and other powerful forces that can be created by circles of women.

In terms of an individual woman's life cycle, there are, circling around all of the interconnecting series of *siddhis*, the two great sisters, the '*mahā*' [great] cycles of the moon above and the moon within. It is the menstrual cycle, and its heavenly accompaniment the lunar cycle, which teaches the wisdom necessary for a woman to engage consciously with the experiences of all the other *siddhis* in her life. From a consciously honoured experience of menarche can grow a positive and respectful encounter with menstruation. It is upon this foundation that a woman builds her capacity to grow and change through pregnancy, and to fully embody the initiatory challenges of labour and birth. This initiation, in turn, opens her heart to embrace the unfathomably deep and demanding *sādhanā* of mothering, including the physical embodiment of unconditionally generous giving and surrender that is lactation. And all of the circles of initiation and spirals of power through which a woman has passed in her life are revisited through the perimenopausal period when the initiatory test is to question and reconsider all that has been done, to re-encounter regrets and griefs, scars and longings. At menopause, this process of questioning is tested again, for some kind of clear resolution is required in order to pass through menopause with honour and without bitterness at anything that has been left unconsidered or overlooked.

In the crowning times of a women's life, it is the quality of her previous responses to these initiatory *siddhis* and challenges that determine the nature of her later years: as if the energy which she planted in the earlier initiations, and the consciousness with which she was able to embody the power of the female *siddhis* both give harvest. We can only reap what we have sown, but the magic of the female life spiral is such that resonances and harmonic convergence of different *siddhis* do offer many opportunities for us to heal, mend and re-sow these initiatory experiences in our cycles. The heightened awareness we develop through appropriate yoga practice supports us in this 'repair work'. For example, a woman who has had negative experiences of menstruation and menarche may well approach birth with less emotional inner preparedness than a woman who has a fully developed consciousness of her menstrual power, but the experience of birth itself offers an opportunity to transform menstrual disempowerment. Likewise, a woman whose experience of labour and birth is distressing or disappointing for any reason, or a woman who is adopting a child, may feel she has 'missed' the chance of the initiation of birth as a gateway into motherhood, but positive experiences of lactation and conscious mothering can offer her other routes to encounter the powers of this *siddhi*, and to appreciate the perhaps more subtle transmission of power that has occurred. The opportunities to revisit and recreate experiences of menstruation are offered every single month during a women's menstruating years, and once periods have ceased, and the moon inside no longer waxes and wanes, then a conscious engagement with lunar and other cycles presents monthly opportunities to honour and reform the understanding of cyclical wisdoms.

In this section, the female *siddhis* are set out in their usual chronological order, and they are accompanied by recommended yoga practice to support our conscious encounter with these experiences. It is this chronological progression of initiatory spirals that offers the most straightforward openings from one form of encounter with power to the next chance to face up to our potential *siddhis*. But as the spiral structure of the circles folds back on and into itself, there re-emerge many opportunities to re-embody different engagements with power throughout our lives.

A TWENTY-FIRST CENTURY NOTE ON WOMEN'S RHYTHMS AND CYCLES

> *... women living now represent the first generations to ovulate thirteen times a year for most of their adult life. Our ancestors spent more time pregnant and lactating than they did otherwise.' (Greer 1984:185)*

> *[Amenorrhoea is]... the reproductive state that was the norm of our ancestors. (RV Short 1976)*

Recognising the cycle of our experience of female *siddhis* can create for contemporary women a powerful connection with female experience over thousands of years of history, a 'direct encounter with the continuous substratum of women's reality existing behind the patriarchal foreground all over the world.' (Noble 2007). This can be a very positive aspect of female spiritual re-empowerment because it reconnects women with the source of our inner wisdom, validating our own experiences, for example in relation to menstrual or menopausal mood shifts, by seeing them as part of a widely shared truth of women's ways of being: 'an atlas for inner exploration' shared by women of all ages over time, and which 'arises spontaneously today in women who take their dreaming and their menstrual cycle seriously'. (Shuttleworth and Redgrove: 268). But before setting out the cycles of a woman's life just as if twenty-first century women were replicating exactly the rhythms and patterns of all the women who have ever lived on this planet, it is needful to sound a quiet note of caution.

It is important to recognise that the overall pattern and number of women's menstrual cycles has changed very dramatically in the past sixty years. Contemporary women, in particular those in western industrialised nations, now have more periods than any other women in history because our current life experiences frequently tend not to include multiple pregnancies, miscarriages, or extended breastfeeding and resultant years of lactational amenorrhoea (cessation of periods during breastfeeding). Today's western women have proportionately less exposure to these other cycles of reproductive life than our female ancestors. The present common experience of continuing menstrual cycles throughout the whole of a woman's life from puberty to menopause is in fact a very unusual experience in the broader context of women's womb life cycles over history. It certainly has not been 'the norm' for women to have continuous monthly cycles throughout their lives, and now that this is happening widely, there are a number of health and other issues that can give contemporary women a different perspective on the relationships between their different life cycles, in particular the menstrual cycle.

This is my experience: I have had five pregnancies, two miscarriages, and breastfed three children. These activities have created in my life three prolonged periods of lactational amenorrhoea. This means I've spent roughly two and a half years of my life pregnant and seven years breastfeeding. This experience places my menstrual cycle awareness in quite a different context than a woman who has not had children or breastfed for years. It is not the same context as the experience of amenorrhoea due to anxiety or illness because I've had those experiences too and can tell that they are quite different. In the context of pregnancy and lactation, the absence of periods is not a problem, it's a naturally arising state of being 'out of cycle', and its length varies from woman to woman. I explore these variations in more detail in chapter fourteen. Having begun menstruating at sixteen, and been childbearing and breastfeeding through my thirties and early forties means that out of a possible thirty years of menstrual cycles, I have in fact experienced about twenty years of cycling, which amounts to two thirds of the maximum that might have been experienced had I not been pregnant or breastfeeding.

When I look back to my maternal grandmother Eileen Dinsmore née Waters, I see a different pattern of cycles. Eileen began menstruating at seventeen, gave birth to eight children (between the ages of twenty-eight and forty-two) and breastfed them all, had a relatively early menopause in her mid forties and was dead by the time she was seventy-two. Out of her possible maximum of thirty years of menstruating years, she probably only had regular periods for ten years, or one third of that time. Eileen's pattern of amenorrhoea is pretty typical of a working class Catholic Irish woman in Dublin during the 1930s and 40s, although possibly because of her exceedingly light frame and low body weight, she may even have menstruated less often then I am estimating. And I can make an educated guess that my maternal great-grandmother and her sisters, who all had more children then Eileen, probably had even fewer periods.

From the experiences I have had, and the patterns I see through my female ancestors, I observe that this present situation, where hundreds of millions of western women are well fed enough, and not pregnant or breastfeeding for long enough, to menstruate now sometimes for their whole lives, is totally unprecedented. This is a big shift that has happened, this shift that can create the circumstances where continued cycle awareness over decades is a possibility for any woman.

The widespread and continuous menstrual cycling throughout a woman's life that is considered the norm now is not only an unprecedented experience for women when we look at our patterns of life over the past few thousand years, but it has somehow happened without anybody thinking that it matters. I have been directly involved in women's health and menstrual awareness work now for many years and even in these pro-menstrual worlds there is very little explicit recognition of the unusual nature of our current patterns of cycles. And certainly, if nobody in the worlds of menstrual health education is speaking about this, I can't imagine that it has suddenly become a hot topic down the local boozer.

This remarkable shift in the menstrual patterns and experiences of women deserves some kind of wider acknowledgement. We now have a critical mass of menstruating women who are, for the first time in thousands of years of patriarchal suppression and oppression of women's blood wisdom, living in a supportive enough cultural environment to be able to collaborate on the project of conscious menstrual cycle awareness. In the past we would most of us have been pregnant or lactating most of the time, and so repeated unfolding of the menstrual cycle and respect for its cyclical wisdom would not only have been a very uncommon experience but also something perhaps, I conjecture, that would have attracted unpleasant censure like being called a witch, or an old maid, or a barren hag or some other such title of esteem. I feel positive about the potential for wisdom and healing which all this menstrual blood brings with it. At the same time I am aware that we should integrate consciousness of the rhythms of other cycles surrounding and suspending the monthly cycle with our attention to the menstrual cycle herself.

For if we do not hold all these different cycles and the historical uniqueness of the current menstrual moment clearly in our minds, then we are really missing the big picture: the picture that may well be still unfolding in the lives of women who do bear and feed a few children (like me), and the picture that we get when we draw back from the present moment to see our place in the stream of history that flows from our ancestors. Context like this really matters. It also matters that we engage intelligently with those in the medical establishment who correlate the rising age of mothers and the increasing number of menstrual periods with a rise in gynaecological disorders such as endometriosis, fibroids and ovarian and uterine cancers. 'Since natural selection has always operated in the past to maximize reproductive potential,' runs this argument, 'women are physiologically ill-adapted to spend the greater part of their reproductive lives in the non-pregnant [menstruating] state' (Short: 20). There is only a tiny step between accepting the socio-biological conservatism of such a statement, and agreeing that we'd all be better off permanently suppressing our menstrual cycles by synthetic hormones, in the manner advocated by the anti-menstruation Brazilian gynaecologist, Dr Elsimir Coutinho. Co-author of *Is Menstruation Obsolete?* Coutinho promotes Depo-Provera implants and other long-term hormonal suppressions of menstrual cycles.

But whilst we may argue vociferously for the benefits of a naturally arising menstrual cycle as the key to tapping women's wisdom and embodied intelligence as a force for spiritual evolution, healing and heightened consciousness, we must also be prepared to acknowledge that our current situation is very new indeed: our womb lives are not the same as those of our grandmothers', and patterns of reproductive life have changed not just massively but very quickly. Clearly there have been other changes at work too, for example, the impact of environmental pollutants, hormonal contraceptives, stress levels, new working and eating patterns, the widespread use of computers and many other aspects of twenty-first century life that make our lives very different from our grandmothers' in ways that are not just about menstruation. But part of this change in reproductive patterns is also an evident increase in the occurrences of fibroids, endometriosis, ovarian and uterine cancers and subfertility. From a pro-menstruation point of view we can see that a lot of these health issues may well be rooted in the cripplingly painful embodiments of shame, guilt and suffering visiting the wombs of women now, and that we have the collective consciousness and ability to achieve much healing through cycle awareness. I see this kind of healing happening every day. Christiane Northrup's work on holistic health also really bears this out, and her ideas are explored throughout this chapter in relation to different cycles.

Whichever explanations we accept for the causes of the epidemic in women's health problems, and however we choose to respond, it is important to acknowledge historically just how unusual all this menstruating is. Part of that acknowledgement is to look at what changes may be occurring as a result of spending so many more years of our lives menstruating than our grandmothers did. When we make active acknowledgement of the unprecedented nature of the 'shift to menstrual critical mass', then we bring a sense of historical perspective and context to the value of menstrual cycle awareness, as a powerful source of guidance through the whole of a woman's life cycle.

There have clearly been, and continue to be, other cycles at work throughout women's lives that surround, suspend and relate to the menstrual cycle. The experience of leaving the menstrual world and then returning to it (perhaps on several occasions) can create, at the level of menstrual cycle awareness, great opportunities to develop fresh perspectives and appreciation for the treasures of the cycle's wisdom. At this time in the history of women's health, the vast number of women menstruating for the majority of their reproductive years offers a remarkable opportunity for wide-scale engagement with this powerful '*mahā*'[great] *siddhi*, consciousness of whose rhythms and experiences develops the cyclical wisdom crucial to our positive engagement with the other potential *siddhis* in our life cycles.

The trouble is that, for many contemporary women, the idea of female *siddhis*, in particular menstruation and menopause, offering positive opportunities for spiritual growth is totally inadmissible. For some women this can be because they are no longer experiencing the naturally arising forms of these *siddhis* (for example because they are on the contraceptive pill or HT [hormone therapy]), but this is only part of the problem. It is not that women have stopped doing these things, because they have not: evidently there are still many girls and women all over the world who are starting periods, menstruating, having orgasms, being pregnant, miscarrying, giving birth, lactating and experiencing menopause every day of the week. The issue is not that female bodies have stopped performing these feminine functions, it is that even the women whose bodies perform these functions have to a very large extent lost the awareness and respect of these bodily functions as anything more than physical experiences. And this is why their capacity to be experienced as *siddhis* has all but disappeared.

The most crucial aspect of feminine understanding, the *mahā siddhi*, the great mother *siddhi* of all the other *siddhis*, is intuition. Without intuition, or rather, to be more correct, without the acknowledgement and respect for intuition as a true guiding light in a woman's life, as her blood wisdom, upon which rests her *yoni śakti*, then all the female *siddhis* can easily be experienced as purely physical phenomena that bring much discomfort, pain and difficulty into women's lives. It is intuition that enables a woman to fully encounter the nine *siddhis* as sources of power, portals to spiritual ascent, and as experiences which demand huge respect and attention. A woman who is connected to this intuitive understanding is able to see that these physical experiences are powerful signals to guide her spiritual growth. Intuition enables us to recognise that the very foundations of our spiritual authority are rooted deep in the acknowledgment of these feminine experiences as the key to full connectedness with the rhythms of the cosmos.

The problem here is quite complex. It is not even as simple as saying that intuition is needed for a woman to experience her biological and hormonal life as the material evidence of her spiritual connectedness, because even if there is an insight of this kind, then that doesn't necessarily change a woman's real experience of herself, all it does is provide an intimation of how things might have been once. No, what has happened is at a much larger and more alarming scale: because even if individual women have retained their intuitive capacity to recognise that these female experiences are doorways to an experience of soul, that special knowledge and embodied understanding can hardly thrive for long, if at all, in a culture where intuition is denigrated and reviled to the extent that even women who can somehow get a whiff of it are taught to believe that it smells bad. This is why, when I assign protective goddesses to each of the *siddhis* in the next section, that I align the most powerful of all the goddesses to the task of minding the '*mahā siddhi*' of intuition.

The intention of this chapter is to explore these cycles in their relationship to each other, and to the *mahā siddhi* of intuition, whilst holding clearly the understanding that we have right now a menstrually unprecedented and precious opportunity to do this work, and that the key to engaging with the blood wisdom of our life cycles is conscious menstrual awareness. This awareness is the royal road to freedom.

Having sounded my uncharacteristically cautious note on the topic of the importance of historical menstrual context, I now invite you to embrace with me wholeheartedly the many cycles of women's lives within the circle of our life.

THE WHOLE CIRCLE: A PATTERN OF INTERCONNECTION

Since yoga offers us an holistic approach to self-healing and the cultivation of conscious awareness, its practice encourages us to regard the whole of our lives as a pattern of interconnection. This is very helpful, especially for women who live in a culture where there is such profound disconnection, not only from our rural ancient roots and the natural world, but also from each other, across generational lines. Ageism and consumerism combine to promote attitudes of deep fear and disrespect for ageing: the powerful multimedia message is that only youth is valuable, and only youthful beauty is visible in most of our movies, TV shows, advertisements and magazines. In the context of these media creations, which in turn shape the consciousness of every girl and woman who sees them, ageing women are laughable, frightening, invisible or non-existent. So there develops amongst women a desperate scrabbling resistance to any signs of change or physical age, an obsession with potions and pills and programmes of exercise and diets that promise to keep us young, apparently fertile, and desirable forever. Truly this resistance to change is utterly inimical to women's mental and spiritual well-being, for our whole lives are marked out by cycles of continuous change and shift. With the holistic impetus of yoga then, it is both a comfort and a challenge to face up to these changes and understand that each part of a women's life experience is of its own intrinsic worth and value, and that all these separate 'roles': the girl, and the sexual woman, the mother, the creative powerhouse, the middle-aged woman of confidence and the wise crone, all these are part of the whole.

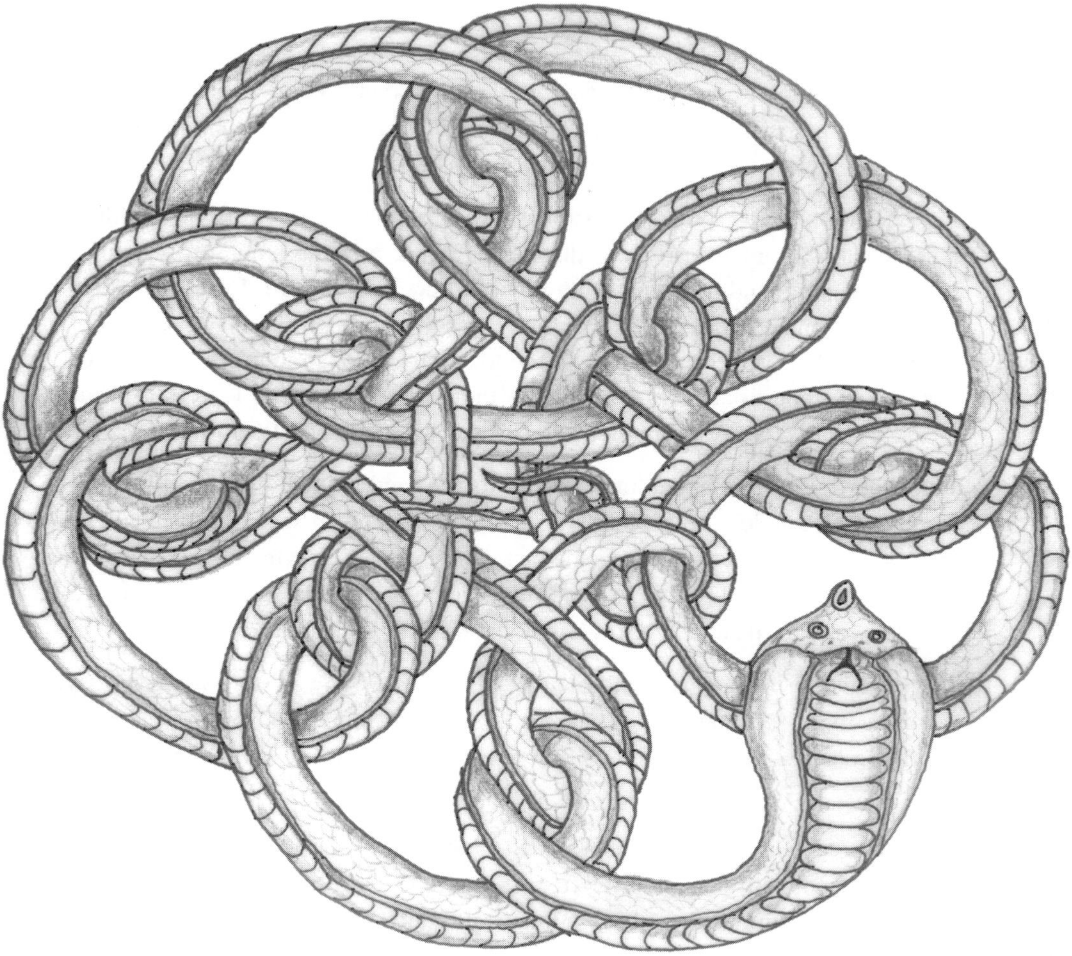

Intertwining, spiralling and circling snake, representing the interconnecting cycles of a woman's life

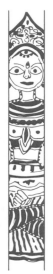

FROM BUD TO SEED: CYCLES AND CIRCLES

One of the most helpful metaphors I have encountered in relation to this understanding of the interconnection of our life cycles is the image of the woman's life cycle as a full circle of continuous transition.

There are key points of stillness within this circle: it begins with the closed bud of girlhood, that opens out to the blossoming of young womanhood, and then moves through into the fragrant full flowering of the mature woman, and into the fruiting of her life, through the manifestation of her *śakti*, her capacity to create in the material world, in the form of children, or poems, pots, paintings, or any of the myriad projects of work, spiritual endeavour, creative expression and sustenance that may fill our middle years.

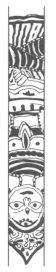

Once the fruit is ripe, it has the capacity to feed and nourish us, delighting all the senses. It also holds the promise of the future. For deep inside the fruit lies the seed. It is the seed that represents the experience of later life: the potentised wisdom and knowledge of a lifetime of experience contained in the seed case, ready to be planted to grow and nourish the next generation.

The seed is the metaphor for the crone: a woman of power and knowledge, with the capacity to seed her wisdom for the benefit of a future she will not see but can intuit. This metaphor reveals the beauty in every stage of life, within the context of the whole cycle.

The closed buds and the seeds equally have their own perfection, as do the flowers and the fruits. All grow from the earth, and the cycle of their unfolding connections brings them back home to the earth at the end. There is neither sense nor beauty in preventing the bud from flowering, nor in holding back the flower in a perpetual state of open bloom so that it may never fruit. To attempt to prevent these cyclical unfoldings is to pour our energies into a fruitless endeavour that eventually depletes and disempowers us.

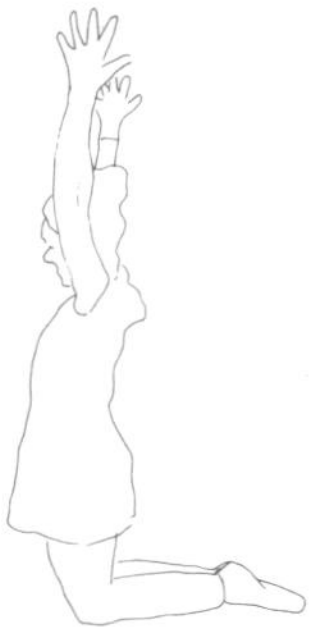

There is simply no point in trying to hold on to the blooming fresh petals of the blossom when it is time to fruit, for just as the seasons of the year create the perfect opportunities for growth, and blooming and harvesting, so too do the inner seasons of our monthly and life cycles create a rhythm that moves through us.

The yogic perspective on presence and acceptance teaches us that grief and sorrow reside in resistance to the cycles of change, just as much as joy arises when we accept the invitation to dance to the rhythm that moves us now.

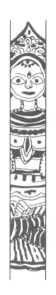

It can also be helpful to understand this bud-seed circle from the shamanic perspective of initiations and power: from this angle we can perceive that menarche provides an initiatory opening into the monthly moon cycles, and that each menstrual cycle offers the opportunity to practise the power that was shown at menarche. If we embrace this practice through our menstruating years as a kind of *sādhanā* or spiritual practice of unfolding conscious awareness of our own cycles of feeling and insight, then we prepare ourselves through these repeated encounters with the *siddhi* of menstruation for the *mahā siddhis* of powerful initiations such as the experience of birth, and we can then arrive at the gates of perimenopause fully prepared for the grandest passage to power of them all, the 'great change' of menopause.

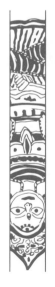

Menarche initiates us into the power, menstruation provides the opportunity to practise that power, so that by menopause we are able to inhabit the power we have been practising all these years: to step into it and discover that we have become the power we once practised.

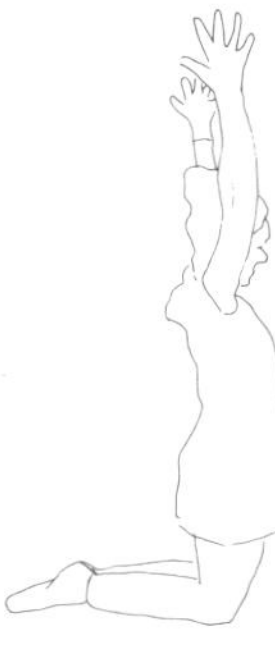

WOMBS / ROOMS

A final helpful image to assist in our understanding of the unfolding of the *siddhis* in a women's life is offered by Christiane Northrup. In *Mother-Daughter Wisdom* she sets out the cycles of a woman's life as a series of wombs / rooms. She presents the metaphor of our life as a house, with the basement representing our experience as babies during labour and birth, and the ground floor taking us through thirteen chambers of development from babyhood and girlhood to maturity. In this house, after we climb the stairs of the perimenopause we enter into the first floor, which holds the rooms of our experiences from menopause to death. The attic of the house is the spiritual realm. Northrup uses a set of seven-year cycles to distinguish between different times in a woman's life, and different 'rooms' in her house of spiritual growth. 'Based on tradition and my own experience, I have assigned seven years to the passage through each room in the house of life. This however, is not meant to be a straitjacket of 'shoulds' that you must follow to be healthy and successful. It is meant rather as a broad framework to give you an idea of the terrain you or your daughter will be covering in your unique journey through life' (Northrup 2005: 26).

SIXTEEN CYCLES

A similar set of seven-year periods is also set out by Clarissa Pinkola Estes, but she adds five extra cycles (from age seventy-seven to one hundred and five!) that pick up where Northrup leaves off, at age seventy-seven:

00–07	age of the body and dreaming / socialisation, yet retaining imagination
07–14	age of separating yet weaving together reason and the imaginary
14–21	age of new body / young maidenhood / unfurling yet protecting sensuality
21–28	age of new world /new life exploring the woods
28–35	age of the mother / learning to mother others and self
35–42	age of the seeker / learning to mother self / seeking the self
42–49	age of the early crone / finding the far encampment / giving courage to others
49–56	age of the underworld / learning the words and rites
56–63	age of choice / choosing one's world and the work yet to be done
63–70	age of becoming watchwoman / recasting all one has learned
70–77	age of re-youthanization / more cronedom
77–84	age of the mist beings / finding more big in the small
84–91	age of weaving with the scarlet thread / understanding the weaving of life
91–98	age of the ethereal / less to saying, more to being
98–105	age of pneuma, the breath
105 +	age of timelessness

These phases are not meant to be tied inexorably to chronological age, for some women at eighty are still in development at the young maidenhood stage, and some women at age forty are in the psychic world of the mist beings, and some twenty year-olds are as battle-scarred as long-lived crones. The ages are not meant to be hierarchical, but simply belong to women's consciousness and to the increase of their soul-lives. Each age represents a change in attitude, a change in tasking, and a change in values (Estes: 447).

GODDESSES AND *SIDDHIS*

In this chapter, I have chosen to group women's life experiences into a set of nine headings corresponding to experiences of female *siddhis*. My intention is to heighten awareness of the overlaps and continuities in a woman's life, rather than to parcel it out chronologically. So these nine headings often contain many more than one of the seven-year cycles proposed by Northrup and Estes.

The first section, **Celebrating menarche** gathers the experiences of roughly the first fourteen years of a girl's life and reviews them from the perspective of entering into womanhood. The second section, **Honouring the cycles of the moon within** covers an unspecified number of years from fourteen until menopause, with the exception of time spent in the experience of other *siddhis* like pregnancy and breastfeeding. The third section, **Freeing the śakti** again is not limited to a particular set of seven-year cycles, but instead takes a yogic perspective on the manifestation of the full spectrum of sexual energies throughout the whole of a woman's life; the fourth section, **Manifesting the śakti** is about expressions of creativity and is also presented as a life-long adventure, closely related to sexuality, because from the *tāntrik* yoga perspective, creative and sexual life are fed by the same forces. The fifth section, **Nourishing the golden womb** is specifically about creativity in the form of childbearing, which activity could be located in multiple rooms of Northrup's house, or extend across many of the seven-year cycles proposed by Estes. The sixth section **Thanksgiving and healing** relates to postnatal recovery, including recovery from miscarriage and stillbirth, and treats the ongoing *sādhanā* of mothering, from breastfeeding to the departure from the home of grown children, which means that it could extend on until the end of a woman's life. The seventh section **Stepping into the unknown** covers the time of the perimenopause, whose beginning is only known in retrospect, and which can extend over a number of years. The eighth section **Embracing our power** deals with the menopause and the fourteen years (or so) immediately following it, whilst the ninth and final section **Living our wisdom** explores the remainder of the postmenopausal period, which, when enjoyed in good vitality and health, may well extend, as Estes suggests, to one hundred and five years. My own model for the expansive nature of these crowning years is that of my paternal grandmother, who lived happily until she was a hundred and four. I have chosen to place experiences of grandmothering across the last two sections, even though it is clearly possible for a perimenopausal woman to be a grandmother.

As we move through these interlinking life cycles and engage with the initiatory challenges of the *siddhis* appropriate to each one it is helpful to become aware of the changing attitudes and values which attend our journey. To assist us in these transitions from one state of awareness to the next, I have chosen a set of ten wise goddesses from the *śākta tantra* tradition to accompany us on our journey.

THE TEN GREAT WISDOM GODDESSES (*DAŚA MAHĀVIDYĀS*) AND THE FEMALE *SIDDHIS*

> *... the goddesses are the Mahāvidyās or great forms of knowledge because they signify wisdom that arises through the cosmic energies of life, not the knowledge found in books. (Frawley in Chopra)*

In *śakta tantra*, there is a powerful set of goddesses called the *Daśa Mahāvidyās* – the ten great wisdom goddesses. By integrating their presence into this chapter I symbolically call upon these ten goddesses to protect our well-being and to support the spiritual re-empowerment of women that we invite as we bring conscious awareness to our encounter with the female *siddhis*. The *Daśa Mahāvidyās* are clear guides to illuminate the unfolding cycles of *śakti* in action in our lives because they represent, in feminine form, different aspects of consciousness, wisdom and power. Their names, in the order in which they most usually appear, are:

1. **Kālī** [the black goddess],
2. **Tārā** [the goddess who guides us through troubles],
3. **Ṣoḍasī** [the sixteen-year-old] also known as **Tripura Sundarī** [beauty of the three worlds],
4. **Bhuvaneśvarī** [she whose body is the world],
5. **Bhairavī** [the fierce one],
6. **Chinnamastā** [the self-decapitated goddess: consciousness beyond the mind],
7. **Dhūmavatī** [the widow],
8. **Bagalāmukhī** [the paralyser],
9. **Mataṅgi** [the outcaste poet, the utterance of the divine word],
10. **Kamalātmikā** [the lotus goddess of delight].

The *Mahāvidyās* are first described in the *Purāṇas*, the spiritual folktales of India which were composed as written texts between the fourth and eighth centuries CE, although it is very likely that the stories and the deities within them, including these goddesses, were present in oral tradition for a very long time before they were written down. The origins of the ten wisdom goddesses as a group could therefore be traced to the beginning of the Common Era, and their roots may be even older than that. The *Mahāvidyās* are an especially popular focus of worship in Bengal. There are few temples dedicated to them as a group, but they appear singly and also in places of honour in temples dedicated to other deities, for example in the Sankata Morchan Hanumān temple in Vārānasī, where they are placed around the ceiling in the front of the porch in front of the main deity (Kinsley: 37). They exist independently of each other, but are often grouped together. They certainly appear together in the *Devī Māhātmya* (c.750) and feature prominently in *tāntrik* and *puranic* texts such as the *Mahānirvāṇa Tantra* (c.300) in which a hymn to Tārā observes with reverence the awesome power of even thinking about the goddess: 'Wrathful Ḍākinī, great birds, tigers and other dreadful creatures / Forthwith take flight at but the remembrance of thy name, / And are powerless to do aught of evil' (Woodroffe 1913: 44 [29]). In the third *patala* of the *Yoni Tantra* (c.350) a slightly different listing that includes most of the *Mahāvidyās*, locates each goddess as part of the *yoni*, with Kālī and Tārā in the '*yoni cakra*' [wheel or outer lips], Chinnamastā in the pubic hair, Bagalamukhi and Mataṅgi on the rim of the *yoni*, and Bhuvaneśvarī and Ṣoḍasī inside the vagina. More usually, the *Mahāvidyās* are seen to be powerful agents of the great goddesses, fighting demons and destroying the enemies of ignorance and egoism.

Wherever these *tāntrik* goddesses appear, they are powerful, often frightening and usually very violent. As a group entity or as individuals, the *Mahāvidyās* are always implicitly linked to *siddhis*: magical, meditative or yogic powers (Kinsley 1998: 37). They wield astounding magical powers, which are often destructive. For example, depending upon which origin story you choose, the goddesses are manifestations of the power of Satī (Śiva's first wife) in the *Mahābhāgavata Purāṇa*, or Pārvatī (Śiva's second wife), or Durgā, the ultimate warrior goddess who slays the buffalo demon Mahisha in the *Durgā Māhātmya*. In the first two stories they are the forces of resistance manifested by an offended wife and daughter. The awesome powers of the *Mahāvidyās* manifested by Satī, Pārvatī and Durgā embody with full force the *siddhis* of the great goddesses who call them into being to help them defeat their enemies, or to frighten their husbands into letting them follow their instincts. In these contexts the *Mahāvidyās* are '...embodiments of female fury precipitated by male neglect and abuse' (Kinsley 1998: 26). They show their full force because the goddesses have been neglected or disrespected. They are destructive because the *Mahāvidyās* need to re-establish respect for the goddesses who manifest them.

The powers of the *Mahāvidyās* thus offer us direct parallels to the current state of awareness of the female *siddhis*: these uniquely female forces of spiritual growth have been neglected and abused, and so, like the great wisdom goddesses, they now demonstrate their innate transformatory power on a truly grand scale. The great initiatory and wisdom-bestowing powers of these female experiences have been so systematically disrespected, disregarded, oppressed and suppressed by the attitudes and values of the patriarchal possessing entity which has been our consensus reality for the past five thousand years that they are now manifesting with immense destructive capacity as a global epidemic of women's health problems. Lara Owen puts this beautifully in her study of menstruation, *Her Blood is Gold*, where she likens menstrual energy to pure power: 'Power is strong energy, and whenever strong energy is not focused and utilized it will act unpredictably. Energy is information: it will always surface somewhere, and if it is not allowed out through the life force, the creative drive, then it will surface in the body as symptoms or in our emotional lives as relationship problems' (Owen: 55).

At an individual level, each woman embodies the ancestral and karmic effects of the suppression and neglect of women's cyclical wisdom and naturally arising potential for realising the *siddhis* that are her birthright as a female. Many of the experiences of menstrual, perinatal, postnatal and menopausal sufferings can be directly relieved by open acknowledgment of their status as potential *siddhis*. Many more manifestations of women's deep health challenges, for example osteoporosis, fibroids, or breast and uterine cancers, can be understood as the effects of these ancestral and karmic suppressions and disrespect manifesting as a desperate, embodied call for the healing balms of full attention and respect. At a global level, the *siddhis* of the planet earth's disrupted cycles, in the form of her capacity to create tornadoes, hurricanes, floods, tsunamis and earthquakes, are manifesting with great destructive force as responses to the continued abuse of the natural rhythms, cycles and resources of her delicate ecosystems. The relationship between an individual women's body and the planet we inhabit is intimate: the world is our womb. Chapter twenty-seven explores this relationship in detail.

The forces of the female *siddhis*, as modelled by the often terrifying and always powerful forms of the ten great wisdom goddesses, have the capacity to defend and empower the women who honour them, just as the *Mahāvidyās* are able to protect the great goddesses from disrespect by revealing the astounding power of female wisdom and instinct. I have 'appointed' a *Mahāvidyā* as a symbolic guardian for each of the female life cycle stages presented in this part of the book, invoking their protective and empowering presence as a source of inspiration and understanding of the *siddhis* associated with each part of our lives as women.

The *Mahāvidyās* are often divided into two camps, the 'fierce' and the (relatively) 'benign', but they can be grouped in very many different ways, including as representatives of the different phases of the moon, or as grouped manifestations of the three *gunas* or qualities of life. In the order they are usually presented, they can be seen as *tāntrik* symbols of progressive spiritual development, with each goddess conferring a certain type of *siddhi*, a 'perfection, blessing or awareness', with Kālī as the most completely unfettered knowledge of self and of ultimate reality, and the other goddesses demonstrating various stages of spiritual enlightenment, unfolding in descending order through the usual sequence of Tārā, Tripura Sundarī (Ṣoḍasī), Bhuvaneśvarī, Bhairavī, Chinnamastā, Dhūmavatī, Bagalāmukhī, Mataṅgi and Kamalātmikā. This sequence is the most usual presentation of the ten goddesses, and the unfolding order they present can be seen to reveal a variety of interrelationships within the group. For example, David Kinsley (1998) identifies thirteen different perspectives on the nature of the relationships between the *Mahāvidyās*, including seeing them as sisters, as forms of the great goddess, and as stages of creation and destruction. Kinsley considers the 'stages of a woman's life' explanation of their inter-relationship to be 'unsatisfactory as the key to understanding the interrelationships of the group' because he understands there to be '... little or no emphasis on the motherhood of the *Mahāvidyās*... they are not shown with infants or children, and their independence from male consorts is stressed... The married and motherly aspects of the female life cycle are minimised in the mythology of the *Mahāvidyās*' (Kinsley 1998: 41). His conclusions seem perfectly logical, but only if one views the stages of a woman's life from outside, from a male perspective that interprets motherhood primarily in terms of a mother's visible relationships with her children and partner. As a mother, and as a *yoginī* with a close relationship to those aspects of consciousness manifested through the *Mahāvidyās*, it is perfectly possible to view the experiences of motherhood as an expression of those transformations that occur to the consciousness of a woman. From this perspective, for example, although Chinnamastā may not be outwardly depicted as suckling infants or caring for children, the graphic image of her as the self-decapitated goddess can speak directly to the profound shifts in consciousness that occur during the postnatal period. And whilst Kinsley is right to observe that the 'married and mothering aspects of women's life stages are minimised' in terms of the outward depictions of the *Mahāvidyās* as female figures with no consorts or family around them, this does not mean that as a group they cannot effectively resonate with the whole of a woman's life: in the first place, marriage and motherhood is not part of every woman's experience, and in the second place, even if it is part of our experience, then from the perspective of our inner world, those *siddhis* associated with the experiences of motherhood are in fact profound spiritual experiences or inner transformations that do not need to be represented by the presence of suckling babies or protective partners. Often the intense emotional and physical states of these experiences are more effectively represented by the symbolic empowerments of the *Mahāvidyās*, their capacity to destroy, or to awaken us to astonishment and delight.

So for the purposes of expanding our awareness of *yoni śakti*, the most helpful way of considering the *Mahāvidyās* as a group is to regard them each as aspects of consciousness that relate to certain stages of women's lives. Instead of presenting them as a hierarchy in the traditional order or sequence, I have chosen here to regard each goddess as giving access to the *bhāva* or feeling associated with the different aspects of consciousness that match the chronologically unfolding cycles of women's lives. This is certainly not a very orthodox or scholarly reading of the symbolic function of the *Mahāvidyās* (but then most of the scholarly appraisals of the *Mahāvidyās* have so far been written by men: cf. Frawley 1994 and Kinsley 1998), so in breaking up the usual sequence and linking each *Mahāvidyā* to those aspects of consciousness that evolve through different female life experiences, I can be seen to have played rather freely with these goddesses. I feel however, that my deliberate disruption of their usual order of appearance is in the service of guidance

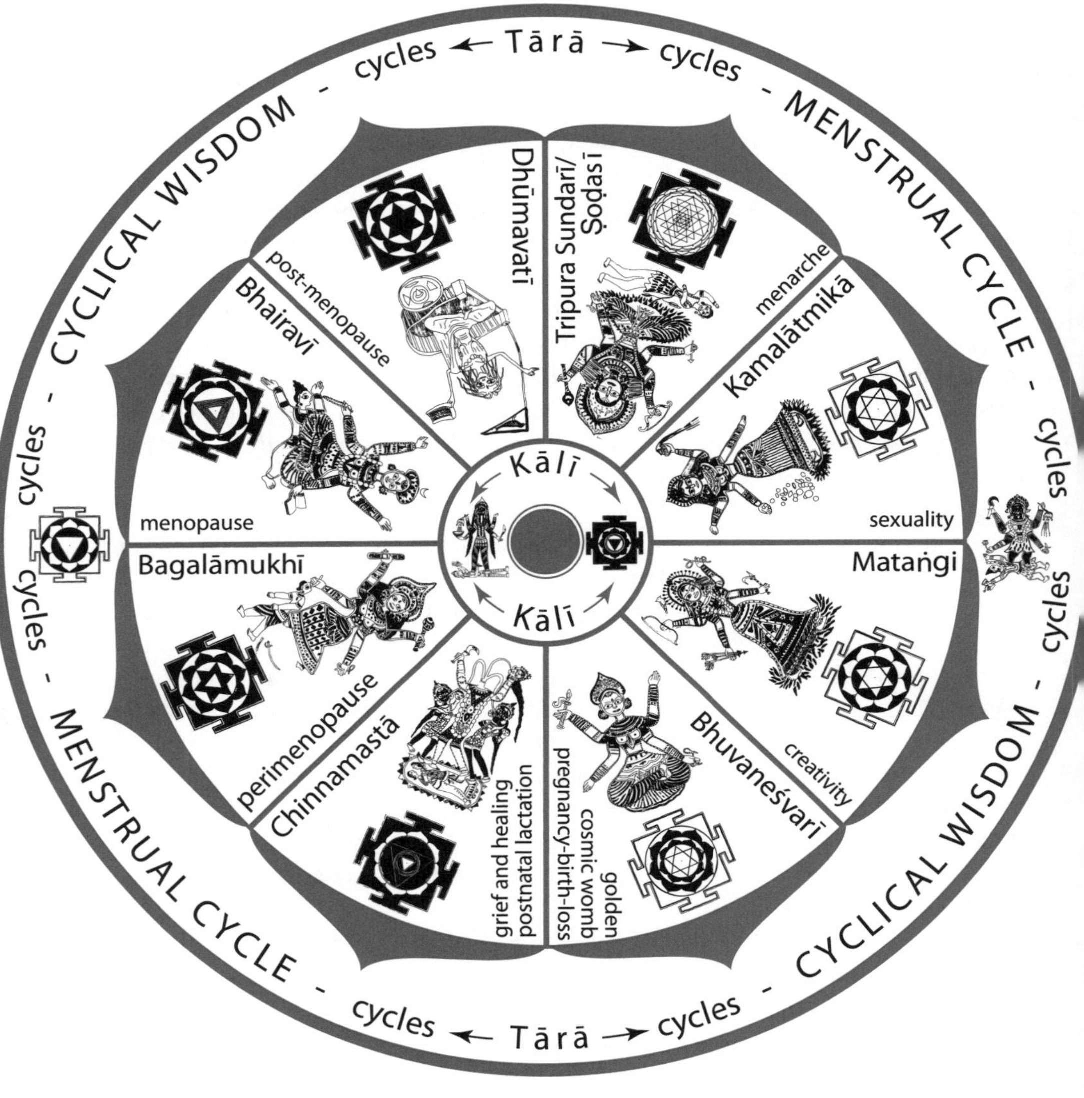

Ten wisdom goddesses and female *siddhis* wheel of information and assistance for many women, and I trust that the liberties I have taken with these powerful *tāntrik* goddesses will be forgiven.

In the chapters that follow in this part of the book, the symbols and descriptions of each goddess's particular *siddhi* or power are presented in detailed relation to the life cycles over which they preside. As an introductory guide, the wheel beneath sets out the fundamental qualities associated with each goddess in the constellation. Just as the female *siddhis* themselves can be seen to be a serpentine flow that contains circles overlapping within circles around a central point, so I place the black goddess Kālī at the central point of the whole series of interconnecting life cycles. Like the sun, her presence is central to the constellation of all the other goddesses who circle around her, held in their orbits by her powerful force. So whilst she remains as the central principle and guiding force of the whole life cycle, the power of her influence creates a protective circular boundary to the whole dance of all the life cycles, containing within her presence the whole of all the changes and shifts represented and guarded by each of the other goddesses.

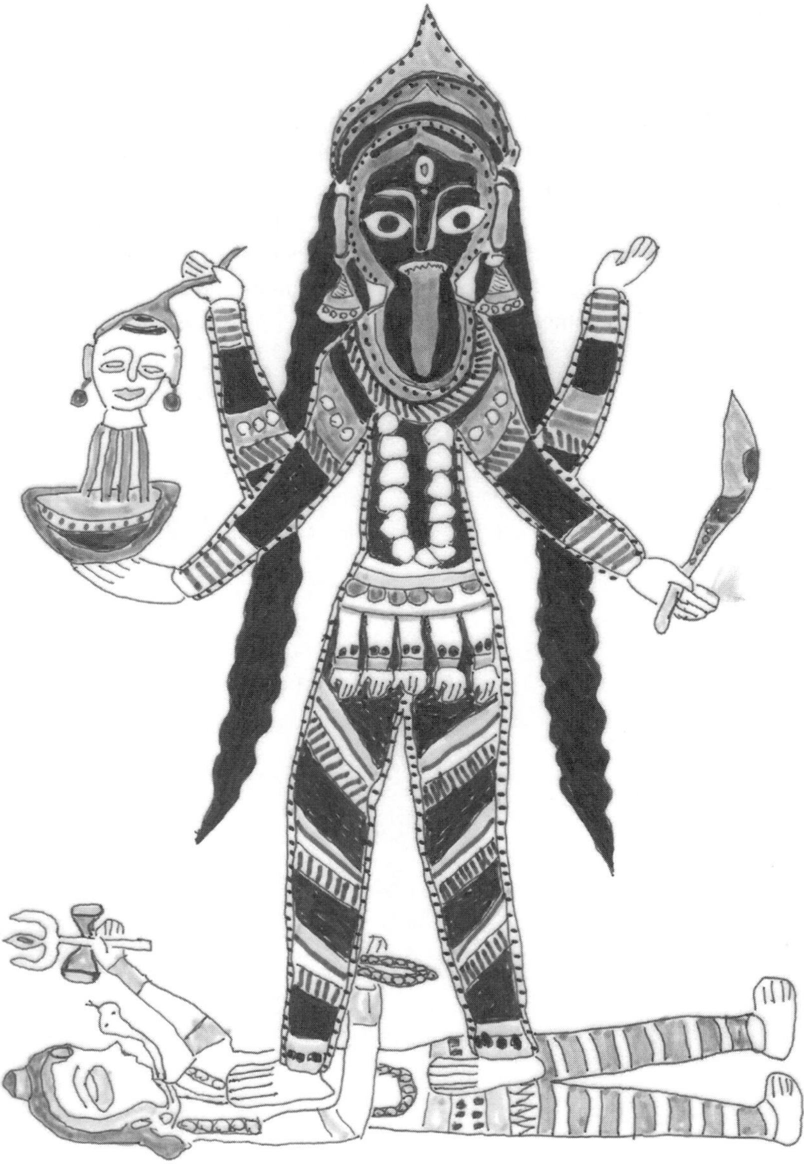

The fierce goddess Kālī is time itself; she stands for change, transformation, liberation and destruction

MAHĀVIDYĀ AND *SIDDHI*

WISDOM AND POWER

Queen amongst the wisdom goddesses, Kālī acts here as a central holding force with a powerful sphere of influence that contains the whole circle of *siddhis* within the peripheral reaches of her power. Kālī stands in this context for the inevitability of change, and an empowered acceptance of yogic transformation. She is the *Mahā-mahā-siddhi* (the greatest of all great powers) whose powers of transformation, liberation and destruction both contain and permeate the whole life cycle. She is depicted as a dark blue-skinned goddess, standing or dancing triumphantly with her feet on the body of the dead Śiva, wearing a garland of severed heads and a skirt of human arms. In the first of her four arms she carries a severed human head by its hair, the neck dripping blood; in the second she wields a bloody chopper; whilst the fourth and fifth hands display gestures to dispel fear and to grant wishes. As she laughs, her long tongue rolls right out and her eyes stare. She is the image of immense power, with the murderous capacity to terrify. Her gory accoutrements, in particular the severed heads, all signify her capacity to separate us from the limitations of our 'I-am-this body' ego identifications, in order that we might live in freedom.

The literal meaning of the name Kālī is time. Time is the power of change that forces all living things to grow and to develop. 'Why should we look on time as a goddess or a feminine form?' asks David Frawley in his book on the wisdom goddesses: '[because] Time is not a mere abstract continuum in which things occur, it is a living field, a conscious energy, a matrix and a vortex. Time is the great womb … Time is the working out of the cosmic intelligence, it is the very breath of the cosmic spirit … the very stuff of experience, the rhythm of our lives. What are we apart from time? Time is our mother and origin as well as our final abode.' (Frawley 66).

Kālī teaches us about time as an inescapable power. Kālī is also time and change from the perspective of cyclical knowledge; for the way that time is measured out in women's lives is through the repetition of cycles, each one the same yet different from those before and afterward. When we place this powerful goddess as the protective entity around the cycles of our lives, we embrace the inevitability of change as a potential for great wisdom and understanding. Kālī, in her closeness to death and darkness, shows us the necessity for self-acceptance and surrender. Her *mahā-siddhi*, or great power, is the power that comes with acceptance of change, and the willingness to let go in order to grow.

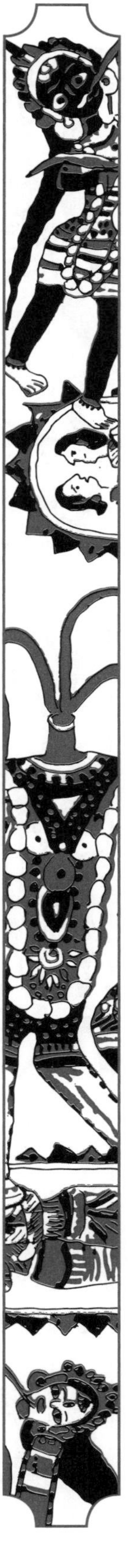

At its most profound level, Kālī's *siddhi* empowers us to drop the limitations of who we think we are in order to encounter the limitless potential of what we can become. Kālī invites us to surrender completely any ideas that come from a desire to fix or define our sense of identity. To access the unlimited powers of her *siddhi* requires that we allow a part of us to die, the part that most strenuously asserts that it is the very source of our identity: our idea of who we are.

From a woman's perspective the source of this 'identity' is frequently founded on limited and self-denying behaviours and patterns of understanding. Our ideas of what it is to be a woman have been twisted and stunted by thousands of years of patriarchy. Especially limiting is the sense that women are worth less than men, that the cyclical functions of female bodies are somehow wrong, or at least need to be controlled, and that older women are worth less than those possessed of youth and beauty. These ideas disempower women by damaging our self-image and fixing set limits on our potential. Even so, these ideas are the cultural basis of who we think we are, and we cling to them. Even if the origins of these beliefs are toxic, it still may comfort us to believe that there is something about who we think we are that remains stable and secure, which is why perhaps we invest so much energy in efforts to remain identified with the outward signs of femininity (youthful beauty perhaps, or sensuous fertility, or nice hair, or whatever) in an attempt to ward off any signs of change and growth.

Proportionately more energy goes into the futile efforts to fight off the signs of ageing and maintain the outer shell of ourselves in response to cultural norms of beauty and value, than is put into the inner work that would empower us to meet Kālī's *siddhi* of the acceptance of change. Whilst it is deeply frightening to let go of the idea that we can always appear to be a certain way, with the passage of time it is absolutely inevitable that Kālī's power needs to be faced. Such is her power, that if we choose not to engage with its effects through conscious acceptance and willing surrender, it will get us in the end through suffering, grief, bitterness and regret. In relation to the cycles of a woman's life, what Kālī's *siddhi* offers us is the immense power to recognise that the only constant is change itself. In our youth, our menstrual cycles teach us this lesson over and over again, and the sooner we wake up to what we are to learn, the sooner we are able to embrace our own limitless power and potential to live life in freedom.

Kālī's power is heavy. And so in the interpretative diagram of the dancing constellation of goddesses (see overleaf) she occupies the central point, so that the weight of her power can spiral out to influence the movement of every cycle, and to create an outer boundary that contains the whole dance. Kālī, or the power of change and time, is the only true constant. As with the stars in the sky, which appear to occupy fixed positions, but are in fact wheeling around in a constant heavenly dance of shifts and change, so too it appears from the diagram that the individual *Mahāvidyās* are placed in stillness. In fact, what the diagram represents is one moment of potential pattern in an endlessly unfolding dance of spirals and circles.

In this diagram, Kālī's presence at the centre is surrounded by an interlocking circle of three goddesses who are associated with the changes that occur in the earlier part of a woman's life: menarche, pregnancy, birth, postnatal recovery including pregnancy loss, and mothering. These experiences are represented by the girl goddess Ṣoḍasī, Bhuvaneśvarī (the mother of the world) and the self-decapitating Chinnamastā. The three circles that form this inner circle are surrounded and connected to a double circle of interwoven snakes representing the twin forces of sexuality and creativity. Sexuality is represented by Kamalātmikā, the goddess of delight, whilst creative expression is under the protection of Mataṅgi, the outcaste poet goddess. Within a downward-pointing triangle that overlays and interconnects with these twin snakes are the three goddesses who correspond to the wisdom and power of later life: the experiences of perimenopause are represented and protected by the paralysing goddess Bagalamukhi; the fierce clarity and freedom of menopause are presented in the form of Bhairavī the warrior goddess, whilst the grandmother spirit Dhūmavatī rests at the base of the triangle. Spiralling from Kālī's centre point and influencing all of the other goddesses is the guiding grace of Tārā, the protectress.

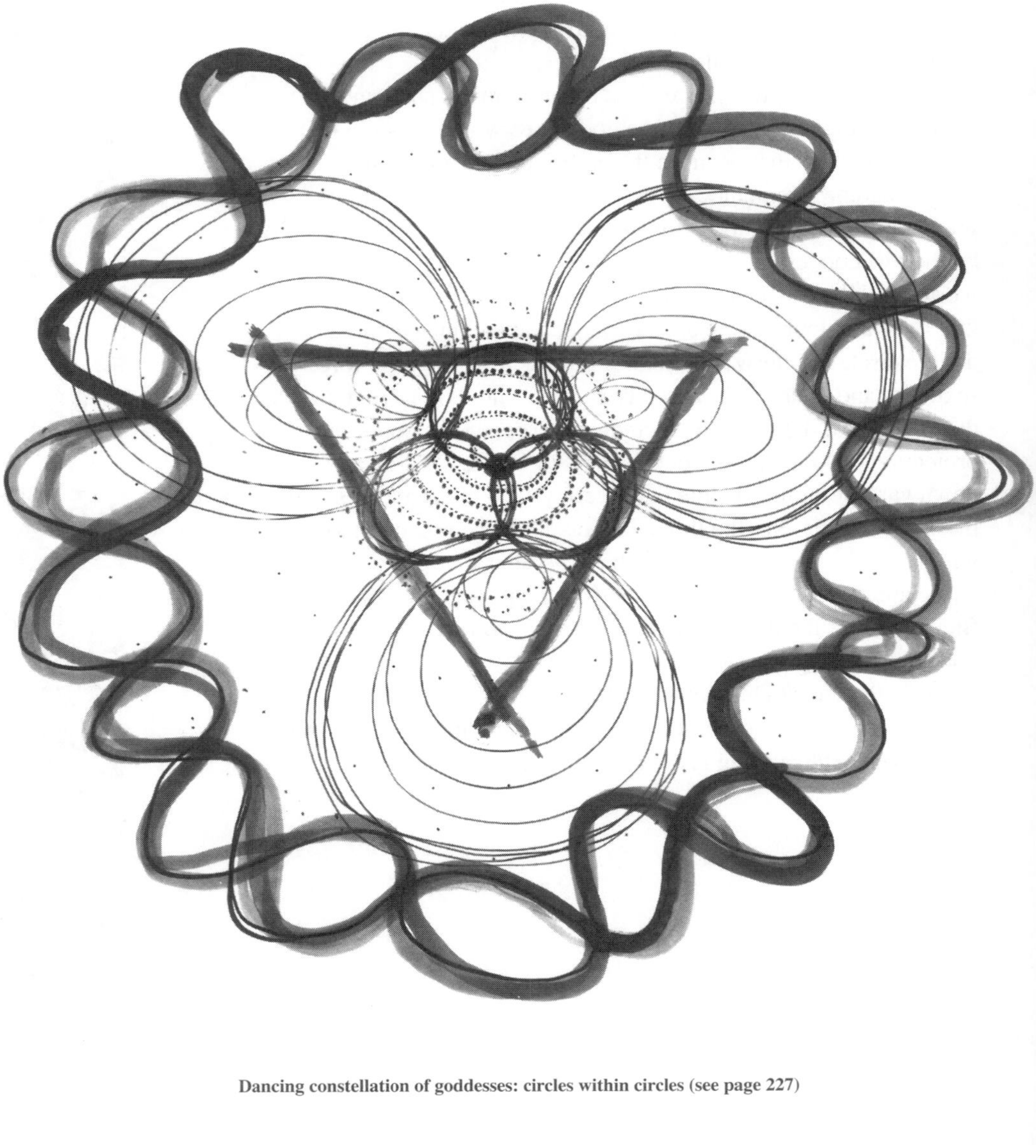

Dancing constellation of goddesses: circles within circles (see page 227)

MAHĀVIDYĀS IN THE CYCLES OF WOMEN'S LIVES

1 **Kālī** [the black goddess] is the spirit of time herself, embodiment of change and cyclical shifts.

2 **Tārā** [the goddess who 'guides through troubles'] is known as the 'saving word'. She has a similar relation to change and transformation as Kālī, so I have offered her the task of the guardian of the *siddhi* of the menstrual cycle – the *mahā siddhi* that forms the preparation for all the other *siddhis*.

3 **Ṣoḍasī** [the sixteen-year-old] or **Tripura Sundarī** [the beauty of the three worlds] is associated here with the *siddhi* of menarche. She represents an innocence and unknown power, and is the only one of the *Mahāvidyās* without fearsome attributes.

4 **Kamalātmikā** [the lotus goddess of delight] is traditionally associated with abundance and she is linked in this scheme with the creative range of full spectrum feminine sexuality.

5 **Mataṅgi** [the outcaste or 'untouchable' poet], is associated here with the experiences of manifesting the *śakti* in creative expression.

6 **Bhuvaneśvarī** [she whose body is the world] is also known as the queen of the universe. She holds the power of love, and I have linked her to the section on the *siddhi* of pregnancy, birth and pregnancy loss: nourishing the golden cosmic womb.

7 **Chinnamastā** [consciousness beyond the mind] is the self-decapitated goddess whose own blood feeds her devotees and herself. I have assigned her to the section on postnatal recovery: thanksgiving, grieving and healing (also nourishment and lactation).

8 **Bagalāmukhī** [the paralyser] who has the capacity to stop a person in their tracks by the hypnotic power of her gaze is associated in this chapter with stepping into the unknown, encountering perimenopause.

9 **Bhairavī** [the fierce one] is a warrior goddess associated closely with Kālī, and I have invited her to stand guardian over the section on menopause: embracing our power.

10 **Dhūmavatī** [the widow] is the grandmother spirit whom I have placed in relation to the final section on postmenopausal life: living our wisdom – yoga and the crowning of a woman's life.

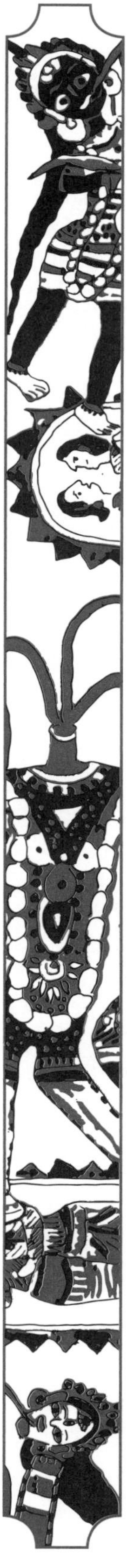

LIVING WITH THE *MAHĀVIDYĀS*

At a personal level, these ten goddesses have been speaking to and through me since 1996, ever since I bought a copy of David Frawley's Tantric Yoga and the Wisdom Goddesses *in the shop at the Sivananda Ashram in Val Morin, in the Laurentian mountains of Quebec. I read the book avidly by torchlight every night in my tiny tent pitched precariously at the top of the hill beneath the recently completed temple. I wanted to know more about the goddess Uma, whose name I had received in an initiatory ritual as part of a yoga teacher-training course. The book is partly dedicated to Uma as the Divine Mother and 'bestower of knowledge,' and is prefaced by a quote from Gaṇapati Muni's* Uma Sahasranam. *Muni was a disciple of Ramana Maharshi, and a* tāntrik *adept and scholar upon whose studies Frawley bases his understanding of the goddesses. Other than her honourable mention in the dedication and a beautiful illustration, the goddess Uma herself does not put in much of an appearance, since the book is devoted to an explication of the history, symbolism and worship of the* Daśa Mahāvidyās. *So instead of finding out about Uma (thereby hang a number of other interesting tales), I learnt instead a lot about a set of mostly very scary goddesses whose significance I did not fully understand at the time.*

But the seed of a connection with these astonishingly powerful forms of wisdom was planted deep, and in surprising ways began to inhabit my consciousness and to fill my home and working environment. Without any special seeking on my behalf, within a short time of my return from the Canadian yoga aṣram *where I had first encountered the great wisdom goddesses, I found myself totally surrounded by* Mahāvidyā yantras. *I received a beautiful Kālī* yantra *on a birthday card from a Swami at the yoga centre in London where I taught, and for the whole of my PhD studies, this* yantra *hung directly in front of my desk space in the postgraduate centre where I worked. Every time I looked up, I came face to face with the visual form of the greatest* Mahāvidyā. *Every time I took a break from writing my thesis, I stared up into this* yantra. *It was no wonder my life began to move in astonishing cycles of yogic change and transformation. This* yantra *was the beginning of a flood of* Mahāvidyā *imagery and teachings that eventually engulfed me and has now created the structural framework for Part Two of this book.*

Over a period of thirteen years I was brought into direct contact with śakta tāntrik *teachers who truly understood the powers of the* Mahāvidyās, *foremost amongst them Swami Satyasangananda Saraswati, Peetasdishwari of Rikhiapīth, who includes a vivid description of the* Mahāvidyās *as a protective psychic shield in the introduction to her translation of* Saundarya-Laharī. *Later, trainings with Mukunda Stiles and his wife Chinnamastā brought other aspects of devotional response to the* Mahāvidyās *into focus. But at the outset, it was the vision of my husband Nirlipta Tuli, whose* Mahāvidyā yantras *and drawings illustrate this book, which brought the* Mahāvidyās *alive.*

Nirlipta's experiences with Chinnamastā had manifested in his painting of countless different versions of her yantra, *big and small, so that our home was filled with geometric embodiments of the self-decapitated goddess who represents consciousness beyond the mind. Later, over a period of seven years, Nirlipta produced ten full-colour* yantras *for the first Śakti Rising, a women's yoga retreat event near Glastonbury that I created together with Wendy Teasdill, in 2005. These* yantras *appear in the full-colour appendix to this book, Ten* Mahāvidyā Yantras*: for meditation and contemplation* (p.641–56).

In the present part of the book you will find full-page black and white drawings of the ten wisdom goddesses. The intention with these images is to convey a vivid visual sense of the powerful energies associated with each of the Mahāvidyās. *The goddesses are not simply presented to observe as figures external to us, but as expressive of qualities and experiences that are found within ourselves. The images are stylised and the figures are sometimes striking or fierce, because the power of the experiences they present are gateways to the female* siddhis, *and the purpose of the goddesses in this context is to honour and protect those encounters with our deepest powers that have too often been dishonoured and disregarded.*

The drawings are done in pen and ink, in a graphic style inspired by the women artists of Madhubāni, a village in Bihar in the north east of India that is well known for its folk art. Nirlipta created these images especially for the purpose of communicating directly the qualities of the wisdom goddesses described in each of the following chapters.

The style Nirlipta adopted in making the images is partly traditional Madhubāni, and partly inspired by a connection with the goddesses themselves that he developed over a fifteen-year period of focused tratak *on the* Mahāvidyā yantras *which are presented in the appendix.*

Swami Satsangi's vision of the ten wisdom goddesses as protectors of spiritual endeavour puts them in place as the guardians of our journeys to other states of consciousness. In the context of women's spiritual empowerment, these goddesses can be invoked to provide safe passage through states of being that lead to a rediscovery of feminine spiritual authority. As protectors, these goddesses need to be fierce because feminine spiritual authority has been so very greatly suppressed and denigrated by our culture. Women who had access to their own deep knowing, for example the millions of European women healers who were murdered as 'witches', were seen as threats to the patriarchal value system. This is because when you are following your intuitive guidance you do not need to look outside for affirmation and approval: women who have found their own inner guide can live outside of the control of social expectations and so tend to upset the existing patriarchal power balance. Their freedom offers a different perspective that can disrupt the conventional order of values and priorities.

In relation to the material focus of contemporary culture, one practical aspect of such disruptive freedom is that women who are connected to their own spiritual authority are quite likely to become skeptical of the motivations of media advertising, and this is likely to make them 'bad consumers'. If you are happily at peace in your freedom, then you don't need to buy any of the things that our culture says women need to have in order to be happy. Women who truly rest in their own inner power are not likely to believe that certain kinds of expensive cosmetic surgeries or glamorous outfits or uncomfortable shoes are actually necessary to their sense of well-being or self-worth, and neither are they likely to believe that it is right and proper for women to continually starve themselves on slimming diets, or to be paid less or disrespected in the workplace if they don't wear the right make up or carry the right handbag. When the presence of inner power and guidance is acknowledged then there is no need to look outside for joy. Such people are free. And this is so unusual, and regarded as so very dangerous to the precarious balance of our current set of consumer values, as to require some fairly powerful protection.

This is where the *Mahāvidyās* come in. For these goddesses can awaken our inner guidance, and so are often regarded with the kind of awe that expresses deep fear of their potential capacity to destabilise social structures and value systems. People who really know about the *Mahāvidyās* recognise this. David Kinsley, for example, who has been studying and writing about the *Mahāvidyās* for over twenty years, says: 'These goddesses are frightening, dangerous and loathsome. They often threaten social order. In their strong associations with death, violence, pollution, and despised marginal social roles, they call into question such normative social 'goods' as worldly comfort, security, respect and honour…' (Kinsley: 251). The *Mahāvidyās* need to be powerful because fundamentally what they offer is support for any spiritual awareness that allows the power of the highest force to shatter conventional behaviours and limitations. Kinsley gets to the heart of this when he describes the *Mahāvidyās* as 'social antimodels' who offer us 'The perspective from the cremation ground (Kālī, Tārā, and others) or the perspective of a polluted, culturally peripheral person of low caste (Mataṅgi)' (251). Dhūmavatī, for example, the grandmother goddess, is a socially ostracised widow, who is avoided like the plague, and shunned as a bringer of bad luck. So to worship such a figure is to subvert our usual cultural norms, and to break from accepted patriarchal frameworks of meaning. If we make a connection with these goddesses, we are inviting big change to occur. By seeking freedom in this way, we are stepping outside of the priorities of the belief systems in which we may have been brought up, and become free to move beyond the boundaries of expected behaviours for women.

In *Yoni Śakti*, I invite you to consider that many of the beliefs and behaviours that have defined how we should respond to the experiences of being a woman are in fact a kind of cage. To live inside this cage is no longer helpful to anyone, men or women. It is not our real home. Living in a cage like this is to be locked out of our real home, our own deep peace with who we really are. To live in a cage of limitations not only constrains our social behaviours, it cripples our consciousness. I invite you to consider that it is profoundly limiting to regard menstruation as an inconvenience, or to see birth as a potential medical emergency to be managed, or to believe that menopause is something never to be spoken of. These attitudes cage our consciousness and cause us pain and suffering because they disconnect us from the spiritual depths of our own experiences. Instead, we can recognise that conscious encounter with these experiences of being a woman gives us access to a powerful spiritual authority of self-acceptance that empowers us to live freely by the lights of inner guidance.

To escape from the cage of existing attitudes and to travel to this more expansive acknowledgment of the feminine foundations of deep spiritual insight can be a long and difficult journey. It can also be very scary. There's a huge and terrifying chasm lying between the sense that life would probably be better if you didn't menstruate at all, and the experience of every bleed time as a spiritual gateway to visionary guidance and cosmic connection, an opportunity to 'call in the vision'. Even to take the first step on this pretty wild trip may invite conflict and opposition, both internal and external. It is likely to frighten us, and it may make a lot of people angry. This is why I have called upon the *Daśa Mahāvidyās* to accompany us.

WHAT TO EXPECT IN THIS PART OF THE BOOK

Every chapter in this part of the book could well have expanded to fill a book of her own, and indeed the material in the sections on pregnancy, birth, postnatal recovery and mothering is explored in much more detail in my previous books, *Mother's Breath* and *Teach Yourself Yoga for Pregnancy and Birth*. Thankfully there are loads of other marvelous writings out there on all the other life cycle topics too. So part of the job of *Yoni Śakti* is to bring together much existing material that gives good guidance on these topics and to share these resources at the end of each section. The main body of these sections presents a rich practical digest of yogic approaches to the stages of life and the wisdom of female *siddhis*. The intention is to set out both the limitations and the potential for freedom in each section and, by keeping things brief, to show how each section relates to every other section, so that we never lose the full picture of the potential of a woman's life lived at every stage in freedom.

Each section in this chapter begins with a brief reflection on the 'wisdom and power' of a particular life stage in relation to the *Mahāvidyā* chosen to represent the consciousness of the *siddhi* associated with that aspect of a woman's life. The goddesses are represented by pictures and by their *yantras*, or geometric designs that embody their energies. The nature of each life stage is presented in the form of the powers or challenges for each phase, for example: the *siddhi* of birth is to bring us 'face to face with creation', and the *siddhi* of menopause invites us to 'grow or die'.

Next follows a summary of the 'limitations' associated with that life experience, and the corresponding 'freedoms' that may be encountered through the practice and perspectives of yoga appropriate to that aspect of being. For each life stage there are stories and experiences that illuminate the particular qualities, gifts and challenges which accompany that cycle in a woman's life. The sections end with a selection of yogic techniques and awareness practices, including *prāṇāyāma*, *āsana*, meditations and rituals that are appropriate for each section, including some radical suggestions about how to feed the wild *yoginīs* under whose protection the life cycles have been placed. Following these recommendations, which are yoga practices to support the general spirit of each life cycle, follows a more specific list of yogic remedies and responses to common challenges associated with that stage of life. As with all the other chapters in this book, each section of this chapter closes with some questions and pointers to reliable sources of further reading and research. Towards the end of chapter ten, centring on Tārā, you will find one of the egg-shaped 'fairy stories' that occur throughout the book. I placed this one with the intention of creating a link between the '*mahā* menstrual' cycle described in the Tārā chapter, and the rest of the *Mahāvidyās* – the aim was to share a story that puts the emphasis on the menstrual cycle as a central point of orientation for women's well-being.

One of the biggest compliments I have ever been paid by a yoga student was offered by a Dublin teacher at the end of a weekend retreat in Burren Yoga in the west of Ireland, where I had presented many of the techniques of womb yoga, wrapped up in the stories, reflections, *mantras*, and poems that nourish the heart, mind and soul even as the physical body is engaged in the practice of the poses or *prāṇāyāmas*. 'What I like about your teaching,' she said at the end of the weekend, 'is that you can be so "up there" and so "down here" at the same time. It makes the philosophy and spirituality of the yoga completely accessible and practical, so that we can actually use it every day.' This is the intention of the sections in this chapter: to present the deep spirituality of yoga and *śākta tantra* as practical assistance for living daily life in a state of freedom. Follow the page references to read detailed instructions for all the practices recommended in these sections.

QUESTIONS AND REFLECTIONS

I invite you to consider now the cycles of *śakti* in your own life by asking yourself some (or any, or all) of the following questions:

1. What rhythmic patterns do I see in my life?
2. What rhythmic patterns do I see in my mother's and/or daughter's life/lives?
3. What links might there be between my current stage of life and the experiences of the other women close to me now?
4. What does the idea of a female '*siddhi*' actually mean to me?
5. How have I welcomed my female *siddhis* in my life so far?
6. How have I neglected my female *siddhis* in my life so far?
7. How has yoga supported me in the experience of my female *siddhis* so far?

FURTHER READING AND RESEARCH

On the subject of women's life cycles and the development of awareness of interrelated circles that can help us to heal, **Christiane Northrup**'s books are the gold standard, especially *Women's Bodies, Women's Wisdom*. *Mother-Daughter Wisdom* is especially helpful on the relationship between different generational attitudes to femininity and the legacies of physical and emotional challenges these can create. *The Female Brain* offers a neuro-psychiatrist's fascinating perspective on the hormonal changes that influence a woman's thoughts, emotions and perceptions of reality at different stages in her life.

On the subject of the Wisdom Goddesses, **David Frawley** (1994) and **David Kinsley** (1998) have both written fascinating books: Frawley's is more geared towards practice, and includes *yantras* and beautiful clear drawings of each goddess, whilst Kinsley's is more scholarly, with many fascinating stories gathered firsthand in India from pandits and devotees about the origins and symbolism of the goddesses.

For an enthusiastic expression of the ten great wisdom goddesses as 'ten fundamental aspects of the Supreme Cosmic Mother's personality' and their application to personal development and spiritual growth as utilised in a Danish *tantra*-yoga camp, see: **www.nathayogacenter.com/category-blog/88-yoga/142-maha-vidya-yoga-ten-great-cosmic-powers**

For images and articles about the *Mahāvidyās*, Exotic India, **www.exoticindiaart.com** is a helpful and inspiring resource. For contemporary worship of the *Mahāvidyā Bhairavī* on a very grand scale, see *Linga Bhairavī*: **www.lingabhairavi.org**

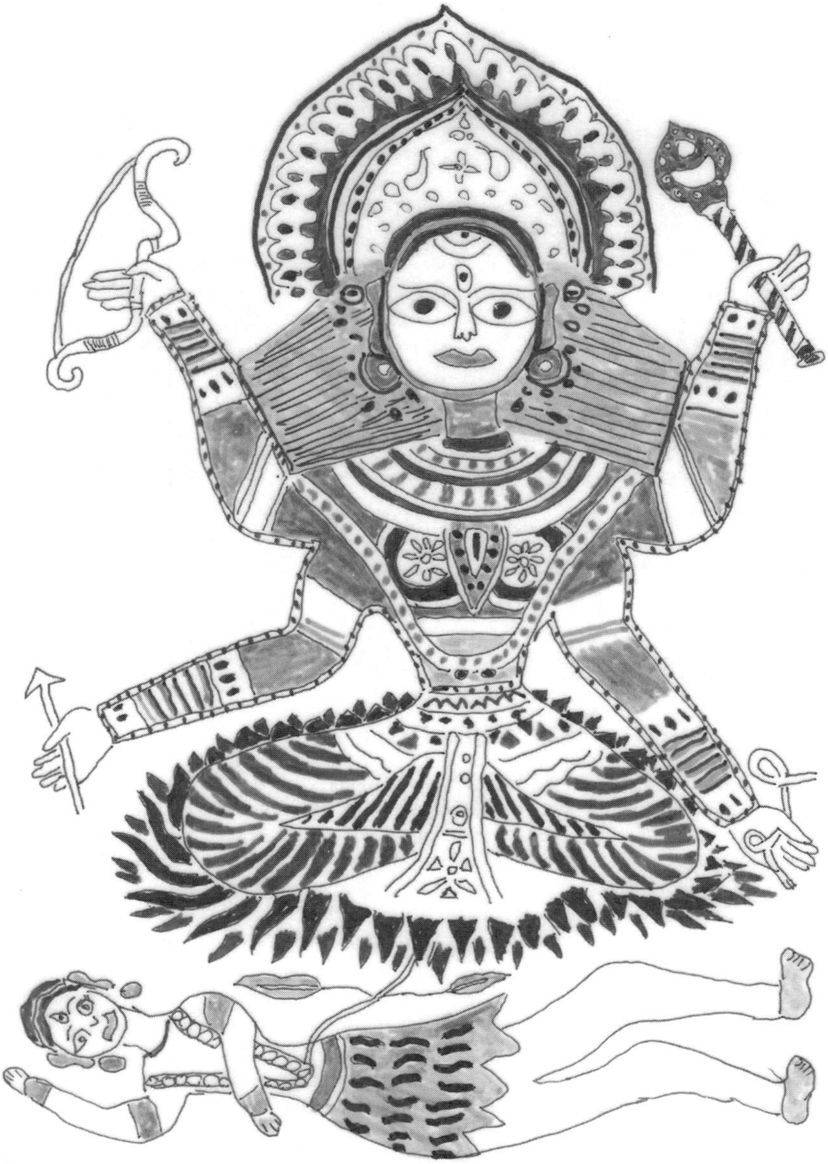

Ṣoḍasī / Tripura Sundarī holds the immense power of innocent beauty: clarified and illumined perception

CHAPTER NINE

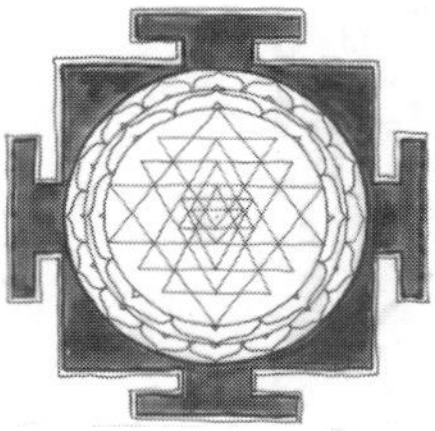

Ṣoḍasī

Celebrating menarche: yoga and girls' initiation into womanhood

> *When women are first introduced to the research on young girls and their fall from self-confidence ... in a rush of recollected pain, women remember their own silencing. They remember the bright, strong, vibrant girl they had been before the lights went out and feel ... Grief at first, but then ... something more empowering. A profound determination to break the cycle of silencing ... When women go to the assistance of young girls who are colliding with this culture's expectations of women, they often make a discovery for which nothing has prepared them. They meet themselves – the parts of themselves they'd left behind, believing they had to, when they were eleven or twelve. (Flinders 1998: 302–5)*

MAHĀVIDYĀ AND *SIDDHI*

WISDOM AND POWER AT MENARCHE

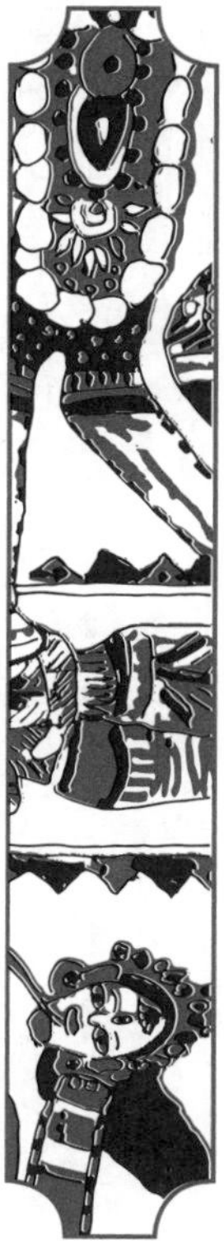

Ṣoḍasī is the *Mahāvidyā* I have associated with menarche, the onset of menstruation. Ṣoḍasī means 'the sixteen-year-old', for she is seen as an eternally youthful beauty of sixteen years old. Uniquely amongst the ten wisdom goddesses, she is without any fearsome attributes, save for the pair of sugar cane bows and arrows that she holds in her hands. She is also sometimes called Tripura Sundarī, 'the beauty of the three worlds'. She is utterly gorgeous, the '... giver of great compassion, who has wide eyes and wanders free...' (Frawley 1994: 86) and can be understood as the beauty of pure perception that allows for the light of consciousness to shine.

Ṣoḍasī's beauty rests in this purity of illumined perception, her innocently wide eyes give her a clarity of understanding that is based on openness rather than experience. She embodies the power and wisdom of innocence and trust. Accompanying this trust is an immense natural power, symbolised in traditional images of Ṣoḍasī by her sitting on a lotus that rests on the supine body of Śiva, the lord of the *yogis*. Śiva's body in turn lies on a throne whose four legs are formed by the four chief gods of the Hindu pantheon: Brahma, Viṣṇu, Śiva and Rudra. The placing of these deities beneath the form of Ṣoḍasī indicates that the pure beauty of her innocent perception gifts her a power that is irresistible. Ṣoḍasī may be unaware of this power, but its force is of cosmic proportions.

The special quality of this time in a woman's life is the sensitive awareness that comes with the vulnerability that awakens us to delight. The literal translation of Sundarī is 'beauty', but in the case of Tripura Sundarī, this is not an external beauty of form, but the beauty of clear vision, of delight and astonishment. Both her beauty and the roots of her *siddhi* or cosmic power lie in her absolute openness and receptivity: these are the qualities that shine through a positive experience of menarche, and which are, sadly, and to the detriment of our girls and young women, systematically closed down during adolescence.

There are rituals and attitudes in *śākta tantra* that are helpful in creating awareness of the precious energy of a young girl. For example, in the *tāntrik* festival of Sat Chandi, as it was observed in recent years at Rikhiapīth by the late Swami Satyananda and by Swami Satyasangananda, every ritual is presided over by a '*kanyā*', a 'lass' or a young girl. These girls are accorded great respect and honour because they are seen to be physical embodiments of the goddess. They are in charge: 'This is the most ancient concept of *Śākta Tantra*, where a young girl is regarded as the embodiment of divine energy, and there are replicas of the goddess everywhere'. The girls are the hostesses of every ceremony, chanting the *Sundarya-Laharī*, the *mantras* for the fire ceremonies, and leading the devotional singing. The luminous power and energy of the young girls are worshipped as embodiments of the divine mother Goddess. As an occasional visitor to the villages close to the site of these ceremonies over a period of fifteen years, it has been astounding to me to witness the practical impact of this spiritual practice upon the status and personalities of young girls in the region where the ceremonies are held. Girls' levels of confidence, their self-assuredness and delight in their own powers are palpable. In practical support of their ritual status as replicas of the Goddess, the programmes for girls' education established by the ashram have further empowered these young women, so that as they approach menarche they enter into womanhood conscious of their own strengths and powers, fully prepared to embrace the *siddhi* of menarche.

LIMITATIONS: CULTURAL EXPECTATIONS

Menarche has a profound and lasting impact on a woman's experience of menstruation. It can illuminate. It also has the potential to cast a very long shadow. Cultural context and social expectation determine the degree to which menarche can be experienced by a girl as a coming into the power of Ṣoḍasī, of the vulnerable but powerful experience of pure openness of perception. If negativity, shame or discomfort surround the first bleeds, or if the attitudes of those around the young girl are not positive and encouraging, then the experience of menarche can be not simply upsetting, but can utterly undermine a girl's confidence in herself.

Secrecy, shame and embarrassment frequently colour the experience of menarche and early menstrual cycles. These constricting and disempowering emotions are the opposite of the clear open perception and trust which Ṣoḍasī symbolises. When a culture of secrecy surrounds menarche and the early years of menstrual cycles, then the possibility of encountering these experiences as an initiation into the power of trust is replaced by feelings of shame and embarrassment. The language that is used to describe menarche sets the scene for a girl's first period, and this has an impact on her attitudes to menstruation for the rest of her life. If we tell a girl she has 'the curse' or 'women's troubles', then she is unlikely to be positive about her menstrual cycle. If we have no language to affirm her experience then it will be difficult for her to view menstruation as anything other then negative.

For example, in Denmark there is no direct translation for menarche. It takes a whole Danish sentence to explain the single term used in English (which isn't English at all, but a Greek import that literally means the first, or beginning, moon). So at the first womb yoga intensive in Copenhagen, when we came to discuss the experience of first periods, we realised there was literally no word to use to describe this initiation into womanhood. Without language to express it, the experience can remain a darkly hidden secret: and girls can only gauge how to respond to it by the attitudes of those around them. One young Danish *yoginī* explained that on the day of her first period, her mother simply said 'So you've got that shit now too.' For her, the Danish for menarche, and for all the years of menstrual cycles that followed, was 'shit'. 'It's not a very pleasant memory' she said. Tears welled in the eyes of the woman sitting next to her, and she offered her own recollection: 'The day I reached menarche [she used the English word] my mother gave me a special amulet, a pendant in the shape of a womb. It was beautiful. My older sister had worn it when she got her first bleed, and then when my younger sister got her period I passed [it] to her. We still have it. If I have a daughter I plan to pass it on to her.'

The first Danish *yoginī* had encountered menstruation as a source of suffering and shame in her life, and the second had entered into womanhood with a sense of pride. These two contrasting experiences show very clearly the power that language has to create the nature of our experience of ourselves as menstruating women. When the language of a culture does not explicitly praise or value menarche or menstruation (for example in the way that *śākta* tantrist texts refer to menstruation poetically as the *yoni puṣpam*, or flower of the womb), or indeed, if the language lacks any word to describe it, then menarcheal girls in that culture are powerless to claim the experience on their own terms: their attitude to the natural functioning of their own maturing female bodies is entirely dependent on the language of their families and friends. Clearly, in such a culture, it is entirely possible to create a positive experience for girls, as the story of the menarche amulet demonstrates, but it is not easy. Such open welcome celebration of menarche is rare. This rarity means that it is very unusual for girls to receive a positive affirmation that they can trust the wisdom of their own bodies: for if the girl learns that what is happening to her is 'shit', then nothing that her body has to teach her will be heeded. The girl is shut out of her own body. She needs to look elsewhere for wisdom and power.

When other sources of externally acquired wisdom, for example knowledge of popular culture or academic learning, are valued more highly than the emerging wisdom of a girl's own body, then shame and embarrassment obscure the experiences of menarche and early menstruations, hiding this powerful source of wisdom from view.

For example, between the ages of twelve and eighteen, I resided daily inside an academic pressure cooker disguised as a girls' high school in Buckinghamshire. Perched at the top of a hill, and housed in a huge glass and metal building that resembled an elegant cruise liner, each year's cohort of girls were gathered together in clusters of classrooms at the top of turning staircases in different parts of the building. The youngest girls were housed out in a set of portakabins on the edge of the playing fields far from the road, and the eldest girls had a special red brick building close to the school entrance, with a common room, special laboratories and a library encircled by a balcony opening onto study rooms. The sole purpose of the school was for each student to gain as many grade A examinations as possible before she left. As the girls grew older, each year group moved into a different part of the building, gathering exam results and various stress-related eating disorders and anxiety-driven skin problems until they acquired the full set of neuroses and academic achievements considered necessary to gain places at top universities around the country.

About one thousand girls attended this school. Assuming most of the girls had reached menarche at around fourteen, at least two hundred of us would have been menstruating in any given week of the month. In practical terms, that makes for an awful lot of blood. It also means that there were very many feminine hygiene products to dispose of, which created an occasionally intolerable pressure on the infrastructure of the ageing plumbing, with alarming results that I shall describe shortly.

With that number of girls, there was a vast range of different menarche and menstruation experiences: there were the anaemic girls whose flow was so heavy and their pains so intense that they were carried fainting and moaning from chairs smeared with menstrual blood and laid on the beds in sick bay to await collection by their distressed parents, who were advised to 'sort something out' so that their daughter's academic success would not be hampered by future embarrassments; there were the girls whose hormonal cycles were so unpredictable, with such flooding and cramping and flaming acne that they were prescribed contraceptive pills by their family doctors to 'even things out'; there were voluptuous, full-breasted girls with womanly curves and perms and tights, whose cycles had been a familiar part of their regular monthly rhythms since they were ten, and then there were the thin bony ones, so light and sparse that their periods had not arrived by the time they reached sixteen.

Amidst this landscape of bloody richness and academic pressure, where menstruation was the lived experience of around at least one quarter of the student body at any given time, one might imagine that there would be a very visible and evident culture of knowledge, support and practical facilitation of the processes and experiences of menarche and menstruation. But this was not the case. For periods were the enemy of academic prowess and therefore were inadmissible. Other than the muffled suggestions from friends or form teachers to go down to the basement, where one of the younger games teachers was rumoured to keep a small cardboard box of samples of various sanitary protection products which she would give out (behind closed doors), in cases of urgent need, menstruation was, quite astonishingly in such an environment, an entirely hidden phenomenon.

Menstruation was literally an underground activity. Girls and staff together conspired to render the blood flows of two hundred girls weekly all entirely invisible, and menarche was never mentioned. Clearly this was a remarkable act of consensual repression. Menstruation was a source of severe embarrassment and shame. No girls would even dream of willingly allowing anyone other than (possibly) her closest bosom friend to know that she was menstruating. Sanitary towels were hidden inside gym bags, and hung on pegs in the corridor, or tucked inside secret pockets in the business-like briefcases that were the preferred carrier for our seriously heavy stacks of books and homework. Girls would pretend to have business with their gym kit or briefcase in order to secretly retrieve the towels and hide them up sleeves, inside blouses or in pockets before skulking to the toilets to equip themselves for the next flood.

Elegant as the boat-shaped building was, and efficiently as the corridors and turning stairs directed the flow of girls through their years of academic development, the girls' toilets were woefully inadequate. They simply did not provide enough disposal units for the sheer number of towels and tampons that two hundred bleeding girls could soak through during the school day. In the long lines of cubicles, only one ever contained a disposal unit. So of course, when crowds of girls filled the toilets, any girl who entered the far cubicle with the disposal unit would clearly be advertising the fact of her current menstruation. Since menstruation was a secret, it wouldn't do to be seen to enter that cubicle. And if you entered the other cubicles, without the disposal unit and discovered the need to change a towel, then where would the soaked towel go? This was in the days before towels were slim and lightweight, with bags and packets to camouflage them. Some dutiful girls would roll them up and bring them home. But some would not. And so the toilets carried an invisible burden of blood-soaked towels and tampons.

But the tides of blood flowed, no matter how hard everyone tried to pretend that they did not. Outside of a sound academic grasp of the graphs and diagrams of the female reproductive systems copied from the board in biology lessons in order to be able to make intelligent responses to examination questions about the functions of oestrogen and progesterone in the monthly cycle, menstruation simply had no place to live in the consciousness of anyone at the school.

And so, homeless and denigrated, the wild and secret menarcheal blood power occasionally threatened to engulf the entire school, girls, buildings and all. One memorable morning, the deputy head, a portly Welshman, addressed the assembled thousand with a very serious complaint about the vast expense which menstruating girls had caused the school by flushing sanitary towels down the toilets in the main building. A shocked ripple of horror rolled through the rows of girls as he gave the gory details of the numbers of plumbers who had been involved, and the numbers of them who had inspected the state of the plumbing and then refused to take on the job of clearing the bloody blockages. The only plumber who would consent to take on the disgusting task was clearly in a position to charge a hefty premium for his services. Because of this, the deputy head informed the girls, the school's maintenance budget had been massively overspent, and severe restrictions would need to be put in place in order to recover the cost. It was, he told us clearly, all our fault, and we should feel ashamed of ourselves.

Such an overflow was inevitable. Ignore something that is flowing, or leaking or dripping for long enough and it does not go away, it merely finds some other surprising escape route. At some point the mess has to be cleared up, and if there is no attempt made to address the root cause of the mess, then similarly alarming blockages are bound to occur again and again. This is what happened at the girls' school I attended, and I have a feeling, from conversations with women who attended similar establishments, that my school's attitude to menstruation was not unusual. What was quite remarkable about the deputy head's blaming of the girls for the blocking of the pipes was not that he somehow expected that the girls could just stop menstruating and then the mess would never occur again, but that the heart of his complaint really concerned the deep embarrassment which the girls had caused the male plumbers involved in the clear-up. The shame which he desired we feel was not really about the shame of having created the mess in the first place, but about the deep discomfort, disgust and embarrassment which it had caused the plumbers (and the deputy head himself) to experience. This was the truly reprehensible aspect of the whole menstrual blocking of the plumbing. The preferred solution offered by the deputy head was that girls should be mindful of how they disposed of their feminine hygiene products, not because they might block the toilets, but because it would be embarrassing for the plumbers to unblock the toilets.

I remember at the time of this event being very surprised that the job of breaking this news to a thousand girls was given to a man. The deputy head was usually concerned with timetables and issuing warnings about falling behind with exam revision. But on reflection, I can see that it was in fact a strategic choice to have a man voice the complaint. It was the men who were most troubled and disgusted by the process of menstruation, and as girls we were asked to contain, repress, hide and dispose of our bodily fluids and the products we used to soak them up, in such a way as to render the whole process invisible to men who might be embarrassed by the sight of our blood.

This story is not extraordinary or unusual. It is the logical outcome of a culture that suppresses and dismisses menstruation, and denies the significance of menarche as a *siddhi*, as an encounter with power and wisdom. This is the culture in which many young girls enter menarche. This is the culture that shapes young women's attitudes to menstruation.

FREEDOMS: YOGA PERSPECTIVES, TECHNIQUES AND AWARENESS FOR BREATHING, MOVING AND BEING

Twenty years after I left my girls' high school, I found myself back in a very similar environment, sharing yoga practice with the bright young women of an academically successful convent school in South London. The project was part of a three-year initiative to bring 'healthy living skills' to Lambeth schools by offering, amongst other things, yoga, tai chi and nutrition workshops in schools all over the borough. I set up for a whole day's teaching in the school chapel, where classes of girls between the ages of thirteen and eighteen arrived throughout the day to learn about yoga for stress management and positive health. I shared a range of practices like those recommended at the end of this chapter. In order to ensure that the girls had good information about what practices were suitable at different points in the menstrual month, I spoke openly and matter-of-factly about menstruation; in order to teach the practices accurately I also described the anatomy of the female pelvis and encouraged the girls to practise yoga with an understanding of their own physicality and how it was affected by the movements and breath. The language I used was clear, simple and direct. The girls' responses to their experience of yoga revealed that the culture of shameful secrecy surrounding my own early years of menstruating was still, twenty years later, shaping girls' attitudes to themselves and their bodies. What was inspiring to see was how the limitations of this culture could be melted away by the practice of appropriate, womb-friendly yoga.

The girls thoroughly enjoyed the mixture of yoga postures, breathing and relaxation that I shared, but even as they began to re-inhabit their bodies with conscious awareness, there were giggles and blushes in response to the word menstruation itself, and there was much alarm and confusion about the effects of certain of the pelvic muscle awareness practices. 'Will we still be virgins if we do this?' How does the blood get out anyway? Are you sure this doesn't move things about into the wrong places?' Mostly, what struck me about the girls' attitudes was how a culture of secrecy had locked them out of knowing basic truths about their own bodies, and how a simple encounter with yoga was showing them a way back home to themselves that was healthy and empowering: 'I feel great! I feel different, I feel kind of more, somehow in myself. It's totally fabulous. Love it! Can you come back and do this everyday with us? – I feel totally chilled out.' When the girls practised yoga with respectful attention to their own bodies, they could feel that it was shining light into places that they had hitherto been exploring in darkness and shame: 'Nobody here talks about this stuff. Nobody tells us about this. They don't want us to ask questions. They want us to pretend like nothing is happening. We have to behave like we don't bleed: nobody asks us how we feel about it.' The questions all bubbled up after the final relaxation. I was mobbed at the end of the class by girls who wanted details of local yoga teachers, so they could continue to practise what they had learnt just because 'it felt so good'. Most of all, what really lit the girls up was a feeling of relief that they had been given permission to access language and experiences that helped them understand who they were and what was happening to their bodies. This is how yoga can help us to remove the limitations that our culture has created around menstruation because of the way we teach girls to respond to menarche.

In contrast to the shame and disgust with which many girls are taught to regard menstruation in western industrialised societies, a girl's first menstruation is often a cause for celebration and delight amongst people who live in cultures that are earth- and body-positive. There are, for example a number of ceremonies and rituals in the Cherokee and Iroquois nations of the native American peoples that welcome the girl's first menstruation as an arrival into great strength and power. Similarly, in South India, ceremonies to mark the girls' entry into womanhood are occasions of much delight, and the girl's menarche is welcomed by the whole village as a sign that her '*śākti*' has arrived (Owen: 2001). The more earth-friendly the life of any given human culture, the more girl-friendly its response to menarche is likely to be: people whose world-view includes a respect for the sacred feminine are people who welcome menarche as a positive initiation for a young woman into an intimate relation with her own maturing femininity.

Knowing about other attitudes to menstruation inspires women in cultures that are not so menarche-positive to create their own ceremonies to support a change in girls' attitudes to the onset of menstruation. Sometimes this happens first at the level of the imaginary, and then seeps down into the lived experience of real live girls. For example, the magical menarche ritual imagined in Ntozake Shange's novel *Sassafras, Cypress and Indigo*, celebrates the first bleed of the young heroine, Indigo, by letting her be cared for by Sister Mary Louise Murray, an older women of spiritual standing in her community who encourages the girl to step proudly into her womanhood and acknowledge the multi-dimensional initiation of menarche by calling on her to '… raise your voice so that the Lord May Know You as the Woman You are…'

The newly-bleeding Indigo is bathed, decked in flowers and given a sacred space among the roses: '"There in the garden, among God's other beauties, you should spend these first hours… Take your blessing and let your blood flow among the roses. Squat like you will when you give birth. Smile like you will when God chooses to give you a woman's pleasure. Go now, like I say. Be not afraid of your nakedness." Then Sister Mary shut the door. Indigo sat bleeding among the roses, fragrant and filled with grace.' The beauty and power of this welcoming of the first bleed is inspiring. It celebrates every aspect of the girl's initiation, as Carol Flinders' appreciation of the passage reveals: '… puberty is presented as an awakening to a whole range of feelings and capacities, all at the same time: sexual desire and the ability to give life and nurture it, but also, unequivocally, spiritual power and spiritual hunger. Courage and joy. Sister Mary invites her young friend to recognise all of these feelings in herself simultaneously and welcome them.' (Flinders 1998: 303). This multi-dimensional welcoming of all aspects of the womanly self that arrive around menarche and mature through the first menstruating years is a very yogic response: it recognises all elements of our being and enables us to encounter them in freedom.

Such welcome, open celebrations of the first period may seem very alien in a culture where much of the energy around a girl's first period is directed to the avoidance of embarrassment by the secure establishment of secrecy and invisibility for the bleed. It is not widely acceptable in most conventional circles to talk openly about the arrival of menarche. Yoga classes especially for teenage girls can help to create a safe environment where this can happen, and where girls can discover simple practices for self-care that support healthier attitudes towards their menstruations. There are also many encouraging signs that conscious women are bringing a newly positive attitude to menarche into the lives of our daughters. The work of Sushann Movsessian, Amrita Hobbs, Janet Lucy, Terri Allison, DeAnna L'am and Jane Bennett are all empowering girls to feel supported and affirmed at the time of their first menstruations, by co-creating with their mothers some powerful means to counter the prevailing negativity around menarche. Details of this work are provided at the end of this section in the resources paragraph.

Much of this wonderful and heartening work is focused around creating a positive experience of menarche that supports girls as they encounter the first months and years of menstruation and grow to understand the unique rhythms and experiences of their own menstrual cycles. It is important to make every effort that we can to support the positive experience of menarche and early menstruation for our daughters by sharing wisdom and understanding that assists girls in embracing the *siddhis* of openness and trust, the power of Ṣoḍasī's open-eyed vulnerability and potency that is characteristic of this special time of life.

But whilst it is crucial to offer this support to girls and young women, there is also a great need for women who have been menstruating for years to reconnect with the spirit of menarche for healing purposes. There are many women who have never had the opportunity to encounter menarche feeling fully supported and informed, and there are also many women whose natural cycles have never become fully established since menarche. For example, sometimes, the culture of suppression and shame around menarche can lead very young women (and their worried parents) to seek to control or eradicate through synthetic hormones the natural challenges which may be experienced with menarche and early menstruation. The prescription of contraceptive pills to teenage girls for the purposes of menstrual management to eradicate heavy bleeding, erratic cycles or extreme menstrual pain is very widespread indeed. Often the Pill is seen as the first option for a young woman to consider. It is quite usual for the first few years of natural menstrual cycling to be anovular and erratic, or to include episodes of heavy bleeding or pain, experiences which usually settle down if the cycle is given an option to establish its own rhythm and the girl is encouraged to welcome and understand her own cycle.

> *For example, when Nikki started her periods at the age of fourteen, her bleeding was so heavy and she needed to change her sanitary towels so frequently, that the family budget was stretched to afford the cost of the many packets of towels she required each month. Her money-conscious stepmother was concerned about these seemingly unstoppable tides of blood, and brought Nikki to the family doctor for a solution. Contraceptive pills were prescribed within the first five minutes in the doctor's office. Alarmed by the idea that somehow her newly arrived natural cycle would be controlled by synthetic hormones, Nikki refused to take the Pill, contacted her mother, and together they visited a doctor with a more holistic outlook. Shocked by her colleague's rapid recourse to synthetic hormones for such a young woman, the second doctor strongly advised against the Pill, pointing out that it can take around six years for a cycle to get established, and that during that time, the delicate balance of a girl's own rhythms can be thrown right off course by synthetic hormones. 'I sensed that first doctor had wanted to take my body's own power away from me,' recalls Nikki, 'she didn't want for me to have the experience of my body figuring it out by herself. She didn't have the patience for it, and neither did my stepmother. It was inconvenient for them. They wanted to take charge of my cycle.'*

Nikki was fortunate to get a second opinion on the matter, but for many teenage girls, the wisdom of taking contraceptive pills within the first few months of menarche is never questioned. The long-term effects of such early encounters with synthetic hormones can be to suppress the development of a natural menstrual cycle, so that although the girl reaches menarche, the establishment of her own menstrual rhythm is hijacked, and she never actually experiences an authentic cycle. In the long term, as Susan Rako's overview of the research into the effects of the suppression of menstrual cycles clearly reveals (Rako 2003), bone density is significantly reduced, risks of cardiovascular disease are increased, and young women are put at risk of developing other problems, including a suppression of libido and early menopause symptoms. At a level of self-knowledge and self-aceptance, girls whose menstrual cycles are suppressed by contraceptives over many years miss the opportunity to get to know the nature of their own cycles and how they can support subtleties of self-understanding: as young women they are cut off from an entire dimension of their being.

This is what happened to Janet, who had first been prescribed contraceptive pills for the management of menstrual pain within five months of her menarche. When Janet first arrived in a womb yoga class, she was in her early thirties and she was seeking to conceive. After two years of unprotected regular sexual intercourse she was not yet pregnant, and was beginning to worry about infertility. Medical tests had revealed no problems, either in terms of herself or her husband's sperm-count. Confused, and rather desperate, Janet had read about yoga as a support for healthy conception, and that is why she had turned up at a womb yoga class. Although her motivation for attending the class was concern about fertility, it transpired that it was her experience of menarche that lay at the source of her difficulties.

As Janet described her menstrual history, she repeatedly spoke about how she had been menstruating for only two years. She described her cycles over the previous couple of years as her 'first cycles,' and clearly regarded this time as the start of her menstruation, which was strange because she also had identified that her periods had started when she was fifteen. When I encouraged her to speak more about her experience of menarche, Janet told how her first period had coincided with a very difficult time in her family. Her older brother had become terminally ill, and her parents had done their best to hide the seriousness of his illness from Janet. She had sensed that something was very wrong. Her brother died, and Janet began menstruating shortly afterwards. Her recollection of the place of her menarche in this sad situation was that it was 'just one more thing' for her parents to have to deal with. From menarche on through the first few monthly cycles, Janet experienced pain on the first day of her cycle. She described it as severe enough to require her taking the day off school once a month. She had been attending a good school with high academic standards, an establishment not unlike the girls' school whose menstrual plumbing issues I described earlier. In the context of her family's natural desire to protect their recently bereaved daughter from any further suffering, and the school's concern for her continuing positive academic performance, Janet was prescribed hormonal contraceptive pills. The Pill changed her experience of menstruation to the degree that she no longer really noticed it and had no need to take the rest and time out that the menstrual pain had prompted.

Janet continued to take the contraceptive pill regularly for the next fifteen years. It was only when she decided that she wanted to conceive that she stopped. At that point, she experienced genuine menstrual cycles for the first time since her menarche. And so, in her consciousness, menarche for Janet in fact only really happened at the age of thirty, in the sense that it was not until she reached this age that she was able to welcome the experience. The circumstances of a sibling death around the time of menarche were distressing and had a specific impact upon Janet's encounter with her first menstrual cycles, but Janet's experience with contraceptive pills shortly after menarche is not unusual. Once she began to realise that the Pill had not been 'regulating' a natural cycle, but had in fact suppressed her own menstrual rhythms, Janet became interested in the idea of menstrual awareness. It was as if a light went on in her consciousness, and she fully embraced the powerful siddhi *of menarche that had been inaccessible to her in her adolescence and during her twenties. Janet's womb yoga therapy programme was simple and effective: she rested and breathed in the supported 'womb breathing' restorative postures (pp.550–5), practised* yoga nidrā *with visualisations of lunar phases, and charted her menstrual cycle, not simply with the mechanical interest in the numbers that revealed her fertile period, but with an open-hearted desire to learn from the changes in moods, dreams and emotional states that signalled the poetic wisdom of her menarchic powers of trust, innocence and pure love.*

The ritual and yoga practices I share below are all intended to promote confidence and comfort for girls in the early stages of menstruating years. They can also be used by women who feel that they would benefit from a re-encounter with the energies and power of that time in their lives, perhaps by performing a symbolic 'retrospective' menarche ceremony, or by 're-starting' menarche by bringing conscious awareness to the processes of menstruation, as if for the first time. These practices use the conscious awareness of the *siddhi* of trust, innocence and potency to create a positive context for menarche, to establish a supportive practice to empower girls and women to build (or re-establish) a sense of excitement and pride at the gifts of inner wisdom which are given as we enter into womanhood.

WRITING A LETTER TO YOUR YOUNGER SELF

The following simple practice can help forge a link back to the girl we once were: we can write a letter to ourselves to celebrate our own menarche. The process of writing a letter to the girl we were at the time of menarche can invite us to hold the memory of that girl with tenderness. Expressing the kindness or sadness that we may feel for who we were when we experienced our first menstruation can help us to heal our present menstrual challenges. For example, we may be able to help our younger selves to see how so much of the suffering we may have experienced has a wider cultural base. Write the sort of letter you feel that the girl you were would have been delighted to receive. In the interests of helping this practice come alive, here's the text of a letter that I know my sixteen-year-old self would have been pleased to read:

Dear sixteen-year-old self,
I know you are feeling pretty rubbish today. It's not easy right now. And you're tired and confused and just want to stay in bed. It's not even just that you're in pain, although I can tell that you are coping with the cramping so bravely. It helps to keep warm and breathe out. Sigh out the pain. And it helps to know that this has a real meaning. It's not just an inconvenience, it's something huge that is going on here now inside you.

I'm writing because I wanted you to know that what's happening to you **is** *really important. Nobody has said that. And it's true. Just because everyone around you seems to want to keep it a big secret doesn't mean it doesn't matter. Bleeding is a big thing, and I know you can feel that. I know you can sense this is an exciting time, and I know you'd begun to think that it would never happen to you. It's not just about being embarrassed for the bloodstains on your knickers, or worrying about where to put the bloody sanitary towels when you're in someone else's house, or whether you'll bleed on your friend's bedsheets when you stay for a sleep-over. It's actually bigger than all of that.*

Listen, it's a spiritual thing. I know you thought it might be, and it **is**. *It's about how you feel, and how much energy you have, and how you dream and what kind of stories you can write. This bleeding is a sign to you that you've got the key now: to understanding more about who you are in the world, and what it means for you to be a young woman. This bleeding is a part of who you are. It's a way to connect with being more yourself, being truer to your real self. Deep inside. If you listen to what your body is telling you then this whole thing can show you a deep magic. Honestly.*

It's natural to feel a little more tired around this time of the month, and it's good to pay attention to how you feel. If you need to rest, it's probably because you need some space to get in touch with the deep feelings that are unfolding. This is a time to connect with those visions you've been having. You might not quite understand exactly what they are yet, but I know you can feel this is something magical and absolutely crucial. It matters, so make notes! You can write about this too. You can be proud that you're a woman now. And that doesn't mean you have to do it just like everybody else. Being a woman who is true to herself means being in tune with your whole world of feelings and meanings. It's your own special vision. You've got the key – turn it in the lock and step right into yourself. It's been a long time coming and you are ready for it now. Welcome!

YOGA PRACTICES

The following yoga practices are especially useful to help young women positively connect with the experiences of their first menstruations. They are also valuable for older women who want to re-connect with their earlier experiences, or re-vision how they experience menstruation, especially after a time without a natural pattern of monthly cycles. Like the process of writing a letter to the girl you were at menarche, or the placenta stone ritual (pp.252–3), these practices can help women who have been menstruating (or not) for years, to re-inhabit some of the youthful innocence and excitement that may have been lost or eradicated by negative cultural attitudes to menarche.

Heart-womb river meditation (p.147) This and all the womb greetings develop a tender and nourishing way to relate to the presence of the womb and her cycles.

Being in the cycles (pp.517–21) This is a very helpful practice for embodying the experience of being part of a wider pattern of cycles and flows. It is especially powerful when practised as part of a group, either in circle or grid formation.

Spiritual warrior dance (pp.536–8) Especially when practised with a partner, this flowing practice promotes strength and the celebration of connection and support between women and girls.

Seed-flower sequence (pp.154–5) This is a beautiful and tender practice to honour the cycles of the womb and bring a loving kindness to yourself.

Rising snake series (p.543) For times in the cycle when there is abundant energy, this practice helps to keep energy flowing freely, and to prevent the stuck, stagnant pooling of energy that can exacerbate menstrual cramps and other pains.

Hare pose with fists and blankets (p.553) This can be a highly effective remedy for menstrual pain. It is comforting and warming.

Surrender and worship (p.555) To promote an easier acceptance of the fluctuations in the cycle, especially during the first menstruations or the first menstruations after a long gap. It's an embodied surrender to the power of the earth, and of cyclical wisdom.

Menstrual root lock (p.475) The releasing of the pelvic muscles in synchronisation with the out-breath is a really helpful way to encourage an easy menstrual flow and to relieve pain.

YOGIC REMEDIES AND RESPONSES

Perhaps the most common negative responses to menarche are fear and resentment. The physical difficulties associated with the first periods can exacerbate both of these responses, and so yoga practices that offer pain relief can be a helpful starting point to deal with other emotions.

Menstrual cramps: The menstrual *mālā* (pp.560–3), a circle of practices to do at different times of the month, will help to heighten your awareness of your needs at different times in your cycle. Developing respectful awareness of the whole cycle is a crucial first step in healing pain and suffering associated with the bleed time. During bleeding, Hare pose with fists and blankets (p.553) and Golden thread breath (p.462) make a powerful combination of pain management techniques. Explore which Restorative pose (chapter twenty-five) works for you, and settle into that pose if there is pain: use Peaks and valleys breath (p.463) and listen to the Cyclical wisdom *yoga nidrā* (pp.443–4) or the New beginnings *yoga nidrā* (p.442) to carry you through the intensity of your experiences. At the opposite side of the cycle, using practices such as the Moon salutes (pp.522–31) that promote full range of movement without depleting your energy, can help to minimise or prevent menstrual pain later in the month.

Resentment of menstruation: Yoga offers us some powerful techniques to welcome and transform emotions. The practice of being in the cycles (pp.517–21) can genuinely shift deep-seated resentments through an embodied practice of re-connection with the meaning and deeper significance for menstruation. Using the poses of deep surrender such as *praṇāmāsana* (p.555) and restorative poses such as In the golden cosmic womb (pp.552–3) can also help to free us from these feelings.

Fear: Connecting to our own power, both physical and mental, is a powerful antidote to fears we may experience at this time. Outside of menstruation, pumping breaths like the Essence of fire cleansing (pp.515–6), Shining skull breath (p.516) and the Spiritual warrior (pp.536–8) are effective ways to build our own strength and inner fire. The New beginnings *yoga nidrā* (p.442) is also a helpful practice to enable us to experience that allowing ourselves to be moved by the cycle of flow is in itself an encounter with power and strength that is a good antidote to fear, but it also enables us to encounter our fear as an expression of a vulnerability that is an important aspect of who we are as women, and to see this as a part of our inner strength. Opening the lotus to *prāṇa śākti* (pp.136–9) can also foster this understanding.

FEED THE WILD YOGINĪ

A RITUAL TO RECONNECT THE PLACENTA WITH THE EARTH AND A RITUAL TO RE-VISION YOUR OWN MENARCHE

There are many complex and beautiful forms of ceremony that mark menarche. If, like most of us, you have not been fortunate enough to have experienced a celebratory ritual for your own menarche, then I can recommend the following practice as a very healing re-connection to the energies of that time. This practice was shared with me by Alexandra Pope as part of the preparation for her Women's Leadership Apprenticeship, and she in turn learnt about the ritual during her time in Australia. There is a fuller description of the ritual in Jane Hardwicke Collings's *Ten Moons: the inner journey of pregnancy* (Appletree House, Roberston, 2010, p. 51). The teaching for this ritual is from Australian Aboriginal Elder woman Minmia, who explains that at menarche, the mother earth 'feels' the grown presence of the newly emerging young woman, and begins to guide the individual on her life journey. This link to mother earth is connected to an earlier ritual—the burial of the placenta after baby's birth. It is said that on the surface of the placenta (the side connected to the mother's womb) is the Miwi print. The Miwi is the spirit or soul and holds all the information about that person's life journey. The placenta is buried with the Miwi print face down into the earth. This activity alerts mother earth to this person's life journey and when the girl reaches puberty mother earth will begin to guide her in that journey.

So if that first ritual was absent from our lives, as is very likely if we were born in hospitals where most women never get to see the placentas of their newborns, then somehow our menarche is 'ungrounded'. The idea is that mother earth does not know we have arrived, because our placenta is not buried face down in the earth. Without this ritual announcement of our origins on the planet, according to this wisdom tradition, then the earth is unaware of a young woman's approaching menarche. As a way of establishing this connection, to enable guidance for the womb wisdom to flow from the earth into the womb of the young woman, there is a simple re-connection ritual. In her description of this ritual to me, Alexandra reflected 'It's a ritual I did myself when I was in Australia and I remember how after that for the first time I had a sense of belonging to a physical place, it was as though my spirit had finally landed on the earth. It was rather special... It's wise as with any ritual to do [it] when the timing is right for you. Have a special place to do it in, ideally outside and in privacy, but if that is not possible anywhere that's private and safe and can be made to feel a little sacred'. You will need some of your own blood, so either practise this ritual when you are menstruating, or keep a little of your menstrual blood until you are ready.

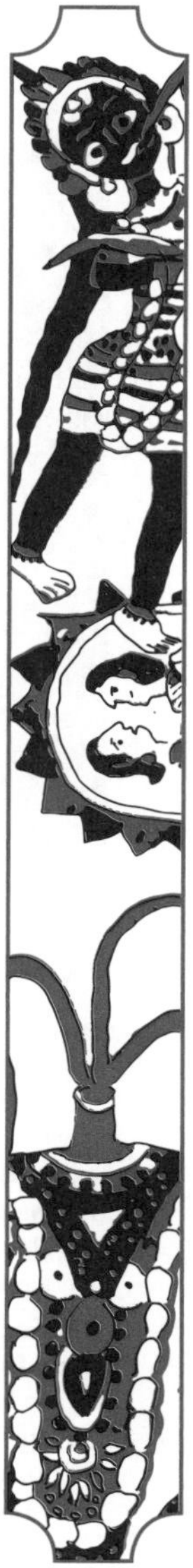

1 Find a stone (this will be your 'placenta'). Decide which is the 'face' of your stone.
2 Burn some of your hair over the 'face', rub the remnants into the stone, and then smear with some of your blood.
3 Bury the stone 'face' down in the earth. If you don't have your own garden, or patch of ground, is there a bit of wild parkland or countryside near you? It's not important that it be a place close to where you live. It's about connecting you to the earth.

Once this ritual is complete, you are ready for your menarche (or menarche re-visioning) ritual, which can be a creative adventure of your own, or can be as simple as this: choose a friend with whom you feel happy to share your menarche experience. Make two dates to meet. On the first meeting, simply tell your friend all about your menarche. Then tell her how you would have loved it to be. Write a script that includes all the things you wish your mother/guardian had said to you back then. Swap over and do the same for your friend. At the second meeting, each bring a gift for the girls you were at menarche. Let your friend welcome you with open arms and tell you all the things you have written into your script. At the end, she can give you the gift you would have loved to receive at your menarche. (This is a simplified version of the very beautiful multiple menarche ceremony conducted on the first module of Alexandra Pope's Women's Leadership Apprenticeship. For further details of this training see p.614).

QUESTIONS AND REFLECTIONS

I invite you to explore your own experience of menarche and how it may be supported by yoga by asking yourself some (or any, or all) of the following questions:

1 What do you remember about your menarche?
2 What is the relation between your memory of your internal emotional response and the outer circumstances of your first bleed? i.e. how did the emotions you experienced 'match' the responses of those around you?

3. How do you feel about the idea of a menarche ritual for yourself, your daughters or other young women in your life? If the idea appeals, what form might such a ritual take?
4. If the first menstruations were painful experiences, or if there has been difficulty in re-establishing a pattern of natural menstrual cycles after a time of cessation (e.g. after having been on the Pill), consider which yoga practices you may wish to include in a daily practice that changes through the month to support a more comfortable experience of menstruation that may be easier to welcome into your life.
5. How do the powers and wisdom of Ṣoḍasī, her innocence and trust, and her capacity for delight and astonishment, play out in your experience of menarche? How much of her power and beauty remains in your life now?

FURTHER READING AND RESEARCH

There is a truly encouraging range of positive work around menarche, both in terms of supporting girls to celebrate their entry into womanhood, and also for older women to re-claim or re-invent their own first encounters with menstruation. A generation of conscious, feminist mothers and aunties together are finding ways to create positive cultures of menarche for their young daughters and nieces. From the illuminating anthropological studies of a range of ritual welcomes for menstruation worldwide, to the tender creation of contemporary ceremonies and workshops for mothers and daughters to attend together, there is much in this global grassroots movement to give delight and great hope that menarche is beginning now to receive honourable and loving recognition as a precious initiatory *siddhi*.

For some beautiful stories and suggestions for mothers and daughters to share around a girl's coming of age, **Janet Lucy** and **Terri Allison**'s *Moon Mother and Moon Daughter* is a fabulous resource. **DeAnna L'am**'s *Becoming Peers – Mentoring Girls into womanhood* (2007, Red Moon Publishing) is a guide for mothers, grandmothers, step-mothers, aunts, and all women who wish to nurture a girl through her menarche. For a girl-focused approach to the experience of puberty, **Sushann Movsessian**'s *Puberty Girl* is accessible and fun. **Lara Owen**'s *Her Blood is Gold* includes some beautiful descriptions of menarche rituals to give inspiration. **Christiane Northrup**'s *Mother-Daughter Wisdom* puts the experience of a daughter's menarche in helpful context. For a scholarly perspective on menarche rituals, *Blood Magic* is a treasury of anthropological accounts from around the world. **Susan Rako**'s *No More Periods?* provides the scientific background research on the health risks of menstrual suppression, especially for young women.

Amrita Hobbs' work on menarche focuses on mother-daughter workshops and rituals: **www.amritahobbs.com**

Jane Bennett's 'girltopia' workshops and resources provide support for conversations with girls and their families about puberty and fertility: **www.janebennett.com.au/events/workshops**

Jo Macdonald offers support, ideas, books and workshops to celebrate first periods and the health benefits of cycle awareness. The letter-writing ritual is Jo's idea: **www.jomacdonald.com**

To hear the Kannyas of Rikhia chanting the *Sundarya-Laharī* at the *tāntrik* celebration of Sat Chandi Yagna visit **www.rikhiapeeth.net**

Natural fertility sites worth visiting include:

www.nfmcontraception.com

www.gardenoffertility.com

www.fertaware.com

CHAPTER TEN

Tārā

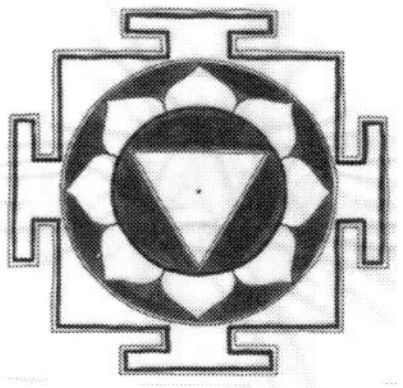

Honouring the cycles of the moon within: yoga, menstruation and fertility

> *Tampering with the hormonal climate of healthy menstruating women, including teenage girls whose lives stretch ahead for decades, for the purpose of 'menstrual suppression' is, in a word, reckless. (Rako 2003: 85)*

> *Synthetic hormonal contraception impedes the normal function of a woman's ovaries, thereby interfering with their beneficial effects ... and the production and action of a woman's natural hormones. [The pills] replace her natural rhythms and hormones with synthetic hormones and imposed rhythms. (Welch: 73)*

MAHĀVIDYĀ AND *SIDDHI*

WISDOM AND POWER

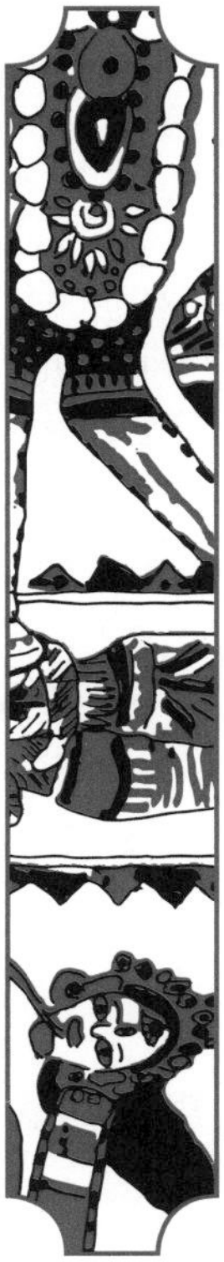

Tārā is the great wisdom goddess with whom I have associated the *siddhi* of menstruation. Her name literally means 'star'. Tārā is a luminous reminder of the yogic dimensions of our ultimate direction and meaning. She provides us with stellar perspective and guidance for conscious understanding of the journey of monthly bleeds and accompanying cycles. She invites us to place these experiences in the broader cosmic context. In the Buddhist pantheon there are a number of different forms of Tārā, each with a different quality and colour. In Buddhism her most widely recognised quality is that of beneficence and compassion, but within the Hindu *tāntrik* context of the *Mahāvidyās*, Tārā also has a fierceness and capacity for violence that is very similar to Kālī. In fact, in terms of their external appearance, Tārā is so similar to Kālī that it can be very hard to tell them apart.

Like Kālī she carries deadly weapons, and like her she stands triumphantly upon the dead body of Śiva. Tārā has a paler complexion, but she is every bit as fierce. I understand this

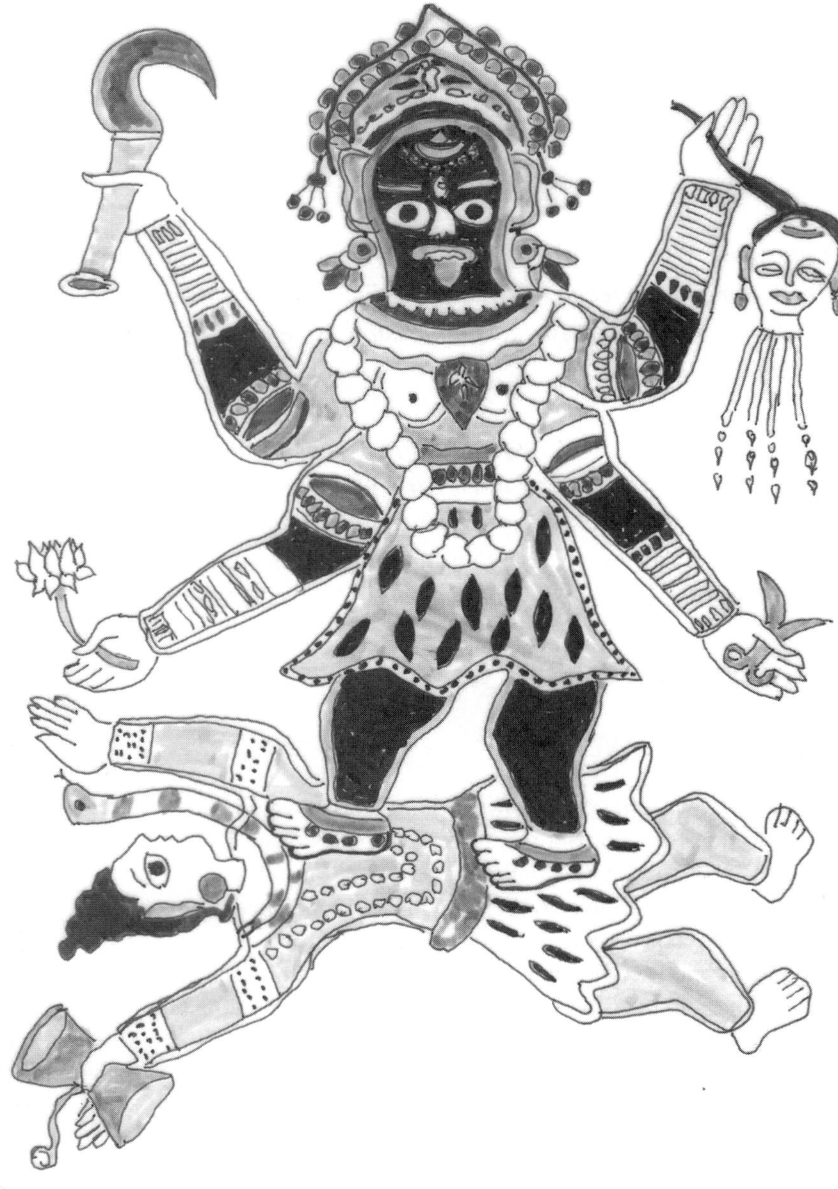

Tārā provides us with stellar perspective and guidance for the journey of our monthly cycles, and by extension leads us through all cycles of change in our lives fierceness to be a strong compassion, a love that has the capacity to bestow deep liberation. In the context of the range of female *siddhis*, menstruation is the *mahā* (great) *siddhi*, for the circle of monthly journeys gives access to a deep wisdom, which is the key to understanding all the other *siddhis*.

The *siddhi* associated with Tārā is the *siddhi* of trust in change as a way to be carried through difficulty. The root syllable of Tārā's name, *tṛ*, means to take across, and the feeling of her power is that it can carry us over and through challenge, but only if we give ourselves up to it. This is the central revelation of menstrual cycle awareness: that if we honour and respect the forces of change that work within us through the menstrual cycle, then what we learn about this cycle carries us through the challenges of all other cycles of change. Meeting the challenges of our experience of the menstrual cycle supports our capacity to embrace change in all the other dimensions of our lives.

Tārā's *siddhi* has the capacity to carry us through the mire and confusion of suffering and difficulty to reach the solid ground of wisdom and knowledge. Tārā is also, like Kālī, a great goddess of transformation. She is the first transformation of Kālī: the primary manifestation of the force of change at work. The notion of transformation is central to a spiritualised understanding of the power of the menstrual cycle: for, it is through an acceptance and understanding of the rhythms of our own monthly cycle that we are able to accept the transformative wisdom which each of these experiences has to offer us. If, however, we do not take the opportunity (or are denied the awareness that makes such acceptance and intimate knowledge possible), then the great gift of cyclical knowledge and its capacity to transform us becomes a curse. Without the *siddhi* of understanding and acceptance which Tārā offers us, then the greatest female *siddhi* of them all becomes nothing but a heavy burden. For to encounter menstrual cycles without awareness of the capacity for deep wisdom that resides within them becomes an experience of difficulty and challenge that seems to have no point: a focus of resentment, annoyance, embarrassment and shame.

Tārā is sometimes also called the 'saving word'. The sound of her *mantra* – *oṃ* – is the sound that can carry us across the difficulty and challenges that we may experience at menstruation or through the menstrual cycle. Tārā helps us to understand the intensities of menstrual suffering as opportunities to develop that state of awareness that enables us to clearly understand our own internal challenges and shifts. By understanding the *siddhi* of transformation that Tārā brings, we may better access the vast potential power which conscious menstruation offers us.

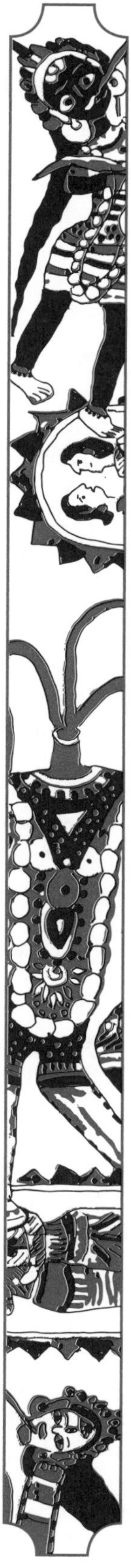

LIMITATIONS: CULTURAL EXPECTATIONS

> *Going against natural bodily rhythms can create stress... Imagine a doctor telling you to ignore your circadian [daily] rhythm. Ignore the natural inclination to sleep at night, just keep going til you drop. Not only would it be difficult to order society, it would be madness for your wellbeing. But in essence that's what's happening to women when we're told to ignore the rhythm of the menstrual cycle. (Pope 2001:76)*

In a deeply unfortunate turn of events, most women have never been encouraged to develop conscious awareness of their menstrual cycles. It is rare to meet women who have a deep acceptance of their menstrual cycle as a source of spiritual guidance. For the most part, it is shame, embarrassment and annoyance, or fear and resentment of menstruation that shapes many women's encounters with this potential *siddhi*. As a result, many women simply endeavour to live their lives as if they did not menstruate at all. Attitudes to menstruation in patriarchal industrialised cultures do not foster respect and attention for women's cycles. Those brave and remarkable women who have, in the face of huge cultural opposition, been able to honour and accept the guidance of the menstrual cycle as an authentic and intimate source of wisdom can offer us great gifts. These women have re-discovered that practising awareness of menstrual cycles, in the form of shifting dream worlds, emotional states and the physical changes that accompany monthly cycles, is a form of feminine meditative consciousness. This consciousness is a powerful connection to deep wisdom at an elemental level, for it awakens understanding of our own menstrual rhythms and cycles as a microcosmic echo of cosmic patterns: evidence of the universal patterns of creative cycles in our own bodies. When we become aware of how our cycle connects us to the influence of wider rhythms, for example when we discover ourselves bleeding at new moon and ovulating at full moon, or in response to our own natal moon cycle, or perhaps also in time with the rhythm of our sisters and housemates, then we can begin to understand how the rhythm of the cycles of our inner world may hold within them the wisdom to unlock the conscious awareness of the rhythms of the cosmos and our place within it: we literally experience 'yoga' because we see our connection to these wider cycles. This is an expansion of consciousness beyond our selves: it is a spiritual teaching of menstruation.

Awakening to the spiritual teaching of the menstrual cycle has been prevented by identifying menstruation as a 'curse'. So long as the experiences of the menstrual cycle are regarded in this negative light, it is not possible to welcome menstruation as a spiritual teacher. The cultural legacy of patriarchy has created a painful toxic overlay of ancestral and karmic patterns of suffering and shame around menstruation. Because women have been taught to be ashamed of menstruation, we collude to render our cycles invisible. This shame, and the related desire to hide the fact of menstruation, is at the root of the capitalist economic exploitation of women's practical menstrual needs: the global multi-billion dollar 'sanitary protection' industry has us by the short and curlies, selling women the disposable products that can make menstruation invisible, as our culture demands that it should be, and then charging us value added tax on these items because they are defined as 'luxuries'. It's big business because the products are disposable, and so we need to buy more every month. Over a lifetime's use, that adds up to approximately 150 kilos of towels and tampons for each woman (the massive environmental cost of such products is explored in chapter twenty-seven). The unique selling point of these products is their capacity to enable us to carry on life 'as normal' during our bleeds, as if we were not menstruating. The Pill, in addition to its contraceptive uses, carries the same attraction: the capacity to 'even out' the peaks and troughs of monthly cycles so we (and the people with whom we live and work) are not troubled by the sometimes intense rhythms and changes of a naturally occurring menstrual cycle. The sanitary protection industry and the pharmaceutical corporations make a lot of money out of women's desire to eradicate all evidence of natural menstrual cycling.

Ironically, even though so much of our culture is geared towards eradicating evidence of menstrual cycles, deep down in the darkest recesses of the belly of the patriarchal beast is a primal acknowledgment of the power of the cycle: it is manifested in the economic reward of women in the fertile phases of our cycles. In strip clubs (and you don't get much deeper into the belly of the patriarchal beast than a strip club), topless lap-dancers earn more when they are ovulating, and less when they are menstruating. Although the entire edifice of our culture is built on the desire to eradicate all evidence of women's menstrual cycles, when it comes right back to basics, and a man in a strip club gets the chance to stuff bank notes in a topless dancer's knickers, he invariably gives her a way bigger tip in the fertile part of her menstrual cycle. This is not because the dancers tell their audience what day of their menstrual cycle they are on, because they don't. It's simply because, even if this information is hidden from conscious awareness, it has a power to affect the fiscal responses of the men on whose laps the women sit when they dance.

Researchers from the University of New Mexico spent months studying the earnings of dancers in Albuquerque's strip clubs to discover this. They concluded that financial rewards for being a topless lap-dancer are far greater during the fertile part of the menstrual cycle, with dancers earning nearly twice as much at peak ovulation time, for example $335 per five-hour shift, and only fifty-five per cent of this during menstruation. Interestingly, the effects of the contraceptive pill, which eradicates peak ovulatory sexual response for women, was also evident in the earnings of the topless dancers in the strip clubs: women taking the Pill consistently earned on average $80 less per shift at all points of their cycle than the women who were not taking the Pill (Hallinan: 47). This evidence corroborates previous research conducted with waitresses in truck-stop café-diners who earn markedly more tips at ovulation than during the rest of the month. All these women, whose work puts them directly in touch with the way the men in our culture value certain aspects of women's cycles and devalue others, can testify to the fact that a fertile woman simply earns more tips. This economic valuation of fertility pans out across our lives, and is reflected in the denigration of older women (see chapters fifteen to seventeen). In terms of its effects upon our own responses to the menstrual cycle, our culture has a clear message to us: that we are rewarded for ovulating and devalued for menstruating.

In the case of the lap dancers and diner waitresses, these rewards are purely monetary, but the evidence of such financial rewards reveals how deep cultural structures of value convince us that menstruation is worthless to men, and thus should be disregarded and rendered invisible.

This causes us big problems. The deep suffering, pain and resentment experienced by many women in relation to their menstrual cycle is rooted in a disrespectful disregard of women's experiences that has disconnected us from the source of our own spiritual wisdom. Medical science has pathologised cyclical openings to wisdom as 'premenstrual syndrome', and has developed drugs to alter our relationship to our cycles, or even to eradicate natural menstrual cycles altogether. Hundreds of millions of women who take synthetic hormones for contraceptive purposes do not experience menstrual cycles at all. Implants, patches, and intra-uterine contraceptive devices secrete synthetic hormones that ursurp the delicate and constantly self-adjusting balance of a naturally occurring hormonal cycle so that many women have no opportunity to realise that the rhythms of their own bodies have an intimate connection with the phases of the moon, with the pull of the ocean tides. The feminine hygiene industry makes billion-pound profits from selling women products that soak away our blood before it can flow free (desiccating our vaginal juices and rubbing trace fibres of bleached fabrics into the delicate tissues of the vaginal walls in the process), in order that we might pretend we are not bleeding. The cumulative effect of all this is to have disempowered a whole generation of women who never experienced directly the rhythms of their own natural menstrual cycles, and who thus live a life disconnected from the very source of their own embodied spiritual wisdom. Additionally, not to experience the natural highs and lows of a naturally unfolding menstrual cycle is also to be out of touch with the intensity of sensual and sexual response that is characteristic of peak natural ovulatory experiences; so the artificial regulation of menstrual cycles also denies access to an encounter with the full spectrum of female sexuality (see chapter eleven). This in turn has a limiting effect on our creativity (see chapter twelve), for these two aspects of our being dance to the rhythm of our inner cycle during our menstruating years.

When menstrual cycles are artificially regulated or eradicated, when our menstrual experiences are denigrated and resented, then women are denied access to a source of great freedom, pleasure, creativity, peace and power. This leads in turn to a separation from any true inner knowledge of our own fertility. Lack of respectful understanding about our own fertility is profoundly disempowering: it leads us into ignorance and confusion about effective means of conscious conception and contraception. Without awareness of our menstrual cycle, we have no access, for example, to forms of contraception that can work in harmony with the natural cycles of our bodies. This can lead women to make desperate decisions around fertility support or unwise choices about contraception, simply because we are unaware of the existence of other options. Conscious and respectful management of our own fertility is like taking delight in a beautiful garden. But the gate has been locked shut. Only women who have the key of menstrual cycle awareness can open it. Everybody else is locked out of the garden, scrabbling around to find whatever options for fertility support and contraception that have been developed outside the gates of ourselves, by a medical industry that regards women's fertility as a danger to be controlled rather then as a garden to enjoy. Out of fear of unwanted conception, women are prepared to accept all kinds of intrusive devices and drugs, and to live shut off from our own rhythms. Believing that these forms of contraception give us sexual 'freedom', women's sex lives are in fact curtailed and diminished, for the artificially created 'fake pregnant' states that replace a natural menstrual cycle eradicate the peak sexual experiences of heightened desire and deepened response that accompanies natural ovulation. Sex on the Pill or on Depo-Provera is like watching a movie out of focus. Sex in response to the natural intensities of the consciously experienced menstrual cycle puts the whole experience into vivid focus: there's no comparison.

But out of fear and ignorance, women willingly spend decades of their lives swallowing contraceptive pills or using implants that not only diminish our sexual response, but cause many very serious long-term health problems, including bone density loss, weight gain, migraine, susceptibility to stroke, deep vein thrombosis, heart attack and breast cancer, not to mention compromising natural fertility. Out of fear of not being able to conceive, and often in ignorance that many natural methods to assist fertility are available, women willingly undergo all kinds of painful and unpleasant procedures, and hijack their natural cycles with massive doses of synthetic hormones. These are all desperate choices born out of fears that there are no other options. But with the key of menstrual awareness, the fears that prompt such desperate choices largely disappear, as women unlock the gates of their own fertile gardens and enter the fecund spaces of delight with confidence, knowledge and power.

Without the key of menstrual awareness we dismiss the great *siddhi* that Tārā has to offer us. To deny this inner wisdom is to dishonour ourselves and to live disconnected from our source of wisdom and power. When we live with such deep disrespect for the rhythms of our own bodies, we need to seek other rhythms and values to validate the nature of our experiences. Locked out of our bodies, we look outside ourselves to media-created images of what it is to be a woman or how it is to live as a female on this planet. We accept the limitations of these images of women's lives because we do not know the expansive powers of other ways of being. Disconnected from the original source of our own spiritual authority, we cannot live freely.

FREEDOMS: YOGA PERSPECTIVES, TECHNIQUES AND AWARENESS FOR BREATHING, MOVING AND BEING

But there are places now where Tārā's guiding star has been observed. There is a global grassroots movement to reconnect women to the power of Tārā's *siddhi* of conscious menstruation. Thankfully, many women now are lifting 'the curse', and embracing conscious menstrual experience as a route to a spiritual wisdom that liberates feminine experience from the limitations of patriarchal cultural expectations. We can use the practice of womb yoga to address ancestral repetitions of suffering and shame around menstruation, and we can use breath, movement and awareness practice to embrace the flow of the bleed, to alleviate the physical and emotional pain and suffering that may be associated with our experience of menstruation.

The first step towards freedom, and towards a full encounter with the powerful *siddhi* of conscious menstruation, is to develop respect and honouring for the rhythms of our cycles. Fortunately at this point in the evolution of human consciousness, a number of women have offered methods for developing such cycle awareness, and the details of their different but related approaches to this form of developing cycle consciousness are presented in the further reading and resources section at the end of this chapter. There are as many different routes to encountering consciousness of menstrual cycles as there are women in the world. Charting and journaling, ritual observance of the bleed, keeping track of the cycle in calendars and diaries, using phone apps and text reminders and wall charts, can all help to grow an inner understanding of the particular rhythms of one's cycle. All these means serve to honour the cycles of womb-life, and to create a state of self-awareness that fosters a deep sense of self-respect. This self-respect is the foundation for growing confidence in one's capacity to live in freedom.

One of the simplest and most effective ways to grow one's own sense of cycle awareness is to become attentive to the unfolding of the inner seasons of the menstrual cycle with the same spirit of observance and delight that we may bring to the turning of the cycles of the year. Alexandra Pope describes this as the 'inner yoga of women'. Her guidance for encouraging this form of awareness is to sense the quality of feeling during the pre-ovulatory time as an inner springtime, to recognise ovulation as an inner summer, to see that the pre-menstruum corresponds to autumn, and to understand menstruation itself as an inner winter. More detailed descriptions of how such seasonal awareness can be practised, and the understandings that it may bring are described below, but at this point it is sufficient to note that the dynamics of the seasonal circle as a whole are finely balanced, and that any disturbances or insufficiencies in any part of the cycle have an impact on the balance and harmonious flow of the cycle as a whole. At the level of living in freedom with one's cycle, awareness of the importance of inner balance provides opportunities for self-care. Cycle awareness empowers each woman to attend to her own needs and enjoy her own unique powers at every point in the cycle.

This can be a liberating discovery: it enables us to acknowledge the particular experiences, challenges and gifts at each point in the cycle, thus helping us to recognise pattern and rhythm instead of despairing at what appears to be chaos and unpredictability. Getting in tune with the inner rhythms of our own cycles helps us to create a powerfully nurturing sense of nourishment and rightness in the unfolding of each monthly cycle and also to see clearly how these cycles are foundational to our experiences of the interlinked energies of sexuality and creativity (for more details see chapters eleven and twelve). At times when the regular patterns of the menstrual cycle gives way to other rhythms, for example during pregnancy or lactation (see chapters thirteen or fourteen) or during perimenopause (see chapter fifteen), then our capacity to adapt and adjust to different patterns and cycles is enhanced by having developed an intimate and easy familiarity with our 'usual' pattern of menstrual rhythms. Overall, cycle awareness makes it possible for us to see that the remedy for any imbalance lies within and not without, and to realise that the source of inner harmony and optimal balance rests with the capacity of our own conscious awareness to respond to the needs of our own cycles.

Womb yoga is of powerful assistance to this process of self-discovery and empowerment. The practices of greeting the womb with love, and honouring the power of the life force within our womb cycles (as described in chapters four to seven) are very helpful ways to foster deep respect for menstrual life. This can be a healing experience, especially if our attitudes to menstruation have been shaped by suffering and difficulty. Such suffering and difficulty can be mental and emotional, or it can be physical. In my own case, I spent my first fifteen years of menstrual cycles believing that I was totally bonkers. Any amount of counselling, psychotherapy, homeopathy and Prozac did nothing to relieve this sense. Regular haṭha *yoga helped to some degree, but the intensity of the problem only lessened when I began to discover that the intense sensations of murderous rage and general craziness that prompted me, amongst other things, to get into fights on the road with van drivers, and dive into dizzying vortices of black depression, were in fact manifestations of extreme premenstrual challenges. The fights and misery disappeared when I began to practise the 'inner yoga' of cycle awareness and self-care, and to adapt my yoga practice to support the naturally arising wisdom of my menstrual cycles. At the point when I discovered the simple truth, that paying respectful attention to the whole of my menstrual cycle was the key to mental health, I felt an overpowering relief, combined with a sense of regretful sadness that life had felt so difficult for so long. 'Why did no-one tell me this before?' is a cry I have heard frequently from women whose menstrual cycles have caused them intense emotional or physical suffering.*

Thankfully, though, as younger women connect to this inner yoga, then it doesn't take decades to find the key to mental and physical well-being, even if mistakes are made early on.

For example, Alison, a social worker in her late twenties, was recommended long-acting injections of Depo-Provera for contraceptive purposes. 'All they said was "You just won't have any periods, and you won't get pregnant". It sounded good to me. It wasn't until later I realised how unpleasant the side effects were. Now I want to conceive, I can't. My cycles are so screwed up that I bleed every two weeks. It's like I'm in early menopause. I don't know where I'm at. If I'd known what harm I was doing to myself then I would never have taken it.' Alison came to womb yoga to help her make peace with the disturbances she had experienced in her womb life, and even after the first week she found the womb-centring movements and meditations really nourished her vitality and assisted her in the devlopment of compassionate 'inner yoga' that helped her to feel her way through the deep challenges of severely disrupted cycles and compromised fertility, and to begin to feel balance and understanding growing with every cycle.

For other young women, the challenges of a heavy painful bleed have led them into a space of despair to which they feel there is no solution but to go on the Pill, even if they feel that's not right for them.

For example, at nineteen, Gilda was the youngest woman attending a womb yoga retreat, and for her menstruation had become a great burden of physical suffering and pain. Typically she experienced more than eight days of bleeding with debilitating cramps on at least three of these days of her period. She said that she had come on the retreat because she was fed up with her period being a source of deep misery and she wanted to learn ways to help herself to heal her menstrual pain. She had done some yoga before but found the womb yoga greetings opened up a new healing dimension in yoga practice because they helped her to feel positive about herself, and gave her really simple and practical things to to accept and embrace her womb life. Her experiences on the retreat connected her to effective yoga and cycle awareness practices to begin her healing. She headed off on her journey of cycle awareness.

A year later, Gilda began attending regular womb yoga classes, sharing astonishingly beautiful tales of her deep healing and empowerment with the other women in the group. Since the retreat, she had developed an intimate understanding of her own rhythms, using womb yoga greetings and restorative yoga sequences to ease menstrual cramps, which she found had lessened dramatically since practising womb yoga. She had also used the Deer exercise (pp.496–7) with positive results, reducing her eight-day bleed to five days. One of the most healing aspects of Gilda's journey was her pride and delight in establishing herself in her own wisdom, and in having her experiences acknowledged by the other women in the group.

One morning during the ovulatory time of her cycle, Gilda shared a vivid dream she had the night before, commenting with a relaxed assurance: ' I know I always dream like that when I'm ovulating'. A woman on the other side of the circle gasped and laughed: 'Thank you so much for that – I've just been having some very crazy dreams and was wondering if there was a pattern to them: I couldn't figure it out, but what you've said shows me my hunch was right. You're so wise!' 'Not me' said Gilda, pointing lovingly to her womb, 'it's her. I just listen to her, and she tells me what I need to know.' Gilda was glowing with confidence: by attending to her womb cycles and finding practices that supported her experience of menstruation she had tapped into a profound wisdom: her periods no longer depleted and overwhelmed her, her bleeds no longer caused her suffering, and the wisdom she had gained on her healing journey was acknowledged and affirmed by other women. She was in her power, and yoga had helped her to get there.

In Gilda's case, the practice of womb yoga had helped her to honour her own cycles and rediscover freedom and joy in being a young woman. In Alison's case, dealing with the shocking and depleting effects of menstrual suppression and the two-week cycles and infertility that followed, womb yoga was like a healing balm to help her recover balance and clarity. For both these young women, womb yoga was nourishing and empowering. For yoga to act in this healing manner, it is important for it to be appropriate and supportive to women's needs. Sadly, this is not always the case.

For example, Della discovered haṭha *yoga in her early twenties and dived deep into the wonderful world of* mudrās *and* bandhas *and inversions and powerful practices that lifted and toned the pelvic muscles with abdominal pumps and breath retentions, '... and then my periods stopped. For about ten months they just disappeared. I got spotty and crabby and felt really weird. But I was so into the practices I just carried on, all through my cycle. It took me a while to realise that it was the yoga that was causing the problems. When I realised what was going on, I eased up, and gradually the periods came back. I didn't like that feeling when they'd stopped. It was like I had let the yoga completely disconnect me from where I was really at. In the end it didn't really feel like yoga to be so cut off from myself.'*

Della's experience was briefly unpleasant, and soon remedied. But for other women the trouble lasts longer.

Lynne had been an avid practitioner of aṣṭaṅga vinyāsa *yoga for many years. She had attended intensive trainings and retreats with top teachers around the world, and had landed a wonderful job at a tropical retreat centre where she got to live her dream, teaching and practising* aṣṭaṅga vinyāsa *yoga every day. Ever since she had begun menstruating, Lynne had experienced severe menstrual cramps and very erratic cycles. She found her yoga practice seemed to help to ease pain, but after a while she began to notice that her cycles were becoming more and more erratic. There was no rhythm to them. Her pain on menstruation was increasing. She was diagnosed with polycystic ovaries and possible endometriosis. The pain got worse, and the spaces between her bleeds got more erratic. And through all of this she continued to practise every day. 'I was convinced that my yoga practice would help me heal,' she explained when she arrived to do a pregnancy yoga teacher training course, 'I was absolutely rigid about my practice schedule. In the end it took me ages to realise that part of the problem was my refusal to adapt the practice to my cycles. The cycle was screaming at me to stop – causing pain. And so when I refused to listen, the cycles just stopped altogether. That was when I decided I had to pay attention.'*

Lynne went to her doctor and got a referral to a gynaecologist. The appointment she was given was almost nine months later. So she decided that in the meantime, she would take her healing into her own hands and see what happened. She began to adopt a softer yoga practice. She rested more. She took time to notice changes that were signs of her cycle returning. She invited through her change in attitude to her practice, a change in attitude to her cycle. 'I realised I had been in denial about the whole thing for decades. My problem wasn't my menstrual cycle. My problem was my attitude to my yoga practice. I practised like I didn't have a cycle and so I ended up with problems. When I admitted that I needed to make a change, things improved.'

When she finally arrived in the gynaecologist's office, the first suggestion the doctor made was to put her on the contraceptive pill: 'We'll need to get your cycles regular before we can do anything about the polycystic ovaries and endometriosis'. When Lynne explained that over the past nine months, her change in diet and lifestyle had brought her cycles back to regularity, the gynecologist looked at her in amazement. 'She looked at my medical notes and she looked at me and told me she couldn't believe it and wanted to know what I'd been doing.' For Lynne, it was the discovery of a more feminine, womb-friendly approach to yoga that empowered her to reconnect to the presence of her menstrual cycle. With this reconnection came health and wisdom: 'I can look back now at what I was doing and realise I was kidding myself that it was yoga. It was just a way for me to hide from myself. That approach to yoga practice didn't help me be well, it cut me off from what I knew was really good for me and my menstrual cycle.'

Lynne's experience enabled her to discover an approach to yoga practice that helped her respond to her own cycles and to restore her menstrual health. Her motivation had been her desire at some point in the future to have children, and that it would be better to sort out the menstrual problems now, rather than to leave it until it was too late. The desire to conceive is often a powerful motivating force for women to reconnect with their menstrual cycles. Menstrual health is the foundation of positive fertility. So yoga that supports healthy menstruation is yoga that promotes optimum fertility. When women come looking for yoga therapy to support their fertility, I suggest womb greeting and honouring practices like the ones described in chapters five and six, and also a responsive programme of breathing and moving that honours the different phases of the menstrual cycle. For full details of this programme, please see the menstrual *mālā* in chapter twenty-six.

There is a delicate relationship between yoga, menstrual health and optimal fertility. As Lynne and Della's stories show, a very intense practice of *haṭha* yoga can adversely effect menstrual cycles. On the other hand, as both Lynne and Della discovered for themselves, optimal menstrual health often arises in yoga practitioners simply because a moderate practice of womb-friendly *āsana* (yoga postures), and relaxation has a generally beneficial effect on all aspects of health, and can often serve to balance the functioning of the endocrine system. A sensitive and responsive approach to yoga practice can also help a woman to develop her own 'inner yoga' of cycle awareness, and this can positively support her physical and emotional health because it enables her to treat the rhythms of her inner world with respect. When this respectful awareness is combined with the practice of womb yoga, then positive menstrual health can result.

> *Poppy, for example, came to womb yoga because she had suffered with endometriosis since her early twenties. She was seeking support for her desire to heal the endometriosis and to conceive a child. Because of the difficulties with her menstruations over the years, Poppy was using IVF (*in vitro *fertilisation, an assisted reproductive technology), for conception, but was doubtful that it would actually work. A combination of acupuncture and womb yoga daily practice, using the womb greetings and gestures from chapters five and six, helped her to re-connect with the link between her heart and womb, and supported her through the first cycle of IVF which resulted successfully in a conception. As she had feared, Poppy miscarried a month later. Initially distressed at the loss, Poppy then realised, as she got her period after the miscarriage, that in fact something very positive was occurring. Her eyes were shining and she oozed positive energy and well-being as she explained 'Usually, with the endometriosis, I had so much pain, and the blood was always dark, and very stagnant. This time was totally different! I had my first pain-free period. I can't ever remember having a period without pain in my whole life. And it was fine. And the blood was bright red. It was fresh, and flowing free. I had a healthy period. The womb yoga worked!'*

Menstrual health is a positive foundation for optimal fertility. Often when women of childbearing age devote more time and energy to their yoga practice, for example by enrolling on a yoga teacher-training course, they discover they conceive fairly rapidly. I have noticed remarkably high numbers of pregnancies on certain of my yoga teacher-training courses, for example on the pregnancy yoga teacher training, where many of the women have an active desire to conceive, sometimes as many as one third of the trainees are pregnant by the end of the course. At the first meeting of one training course group in London, five out of twenty-four students were pregnant, but by the final meeting of the course four months later, there were four further pregnancies, including one student who had conceived after the first weekend of the course, then miscarried and re-conceived, bringing the total number of pregnant women on the course to nine.

There is a lot of subsitute teaching available in pregnancy yoga because the field is full of teachers on maternity leave who are looking for cover: women who work with other pregnant women seem to get pregnant a lot. Obviously this is partly to do with the fact that they may be choosing to teach pregnant women because they are planning to have a family themselves, and it is partly to do with the beneficial effects of being in the relaxed company of lots of pregnant women who might make a person feel 'broody', but I am convinced that at least part of the reason for the high rate of pregnancy among pregnancy yoga teachers has to be down to the womb-friendly yoga practice which they are doing regularly.

> *The feminine spirals and circles and sensual pelvic movements that are at the heart of pregnancy yoga all serve effectively to support and nourish womb health, for example in the case of Bodil, an Aṣṭaṅga yoga teacher from Copenhagen who had been told by her doctors she had only a one in ten chance of conceiving naturally. She had struggled through six IVF cycles before conceiving her first child and then four more IVF treatments to conceive her second child. But when she began to shift her previous yoga practice to the sequences she learnt to support womb health on a pregnancy yoga teacher training course, Bodil discovered that she had conceived a third child with no medical intervention of any kind. She attributed the ease of the third conception to heightened fertility supported by the yoga practices she was learning to teach to pregnant women. Because the pregnancy yoga breath, movement patterns and relaxation support the womb's activities in their most demanding and challenging phase, they also support menstrual health and optimal fertility. This is why the pregnancy yoga repertoire is the wellspring for practices of womb yoga.*

YOGA PRACTICES

All of the **womb greetings** in chapters five and six use breath, movement and awareness to open up to the possibility of welcoming the cyclical wisdom of womb life as a source of inner peace and spiritual guidance.

The **Cyclical wisdom *yoga nidrā*** (pp.443–4) is a profound and easy way to awaken to an awareness of the inner world of cycles and the qualities of feeling and understanding that accompanies each phase of the menstrual cycle.

Menstrual *mālā* (pp.560–3) this provides a simple but effective programme of yoga poses that resonate with different stages in the menstrual cycle, and can help to support an awareness of natural fertility, for the purposes of conscious conception and conscious contraception.

Restorative poses (chapter twenty-five) are helpful to create the deep quality of ease and comfort that is often hard to achieve if menstruation is painful. These poses are also useful to practise during the rest of the cycle, to ensure sufficient rest and quiet time to support health and well-being, especially if you have a tendency to 'overdo it' and find it difficult to give yourself permission to slow down.

FEED THE WILD *YOGINĪ*

MENSTRUAL BLOOD *PŪJĀ*

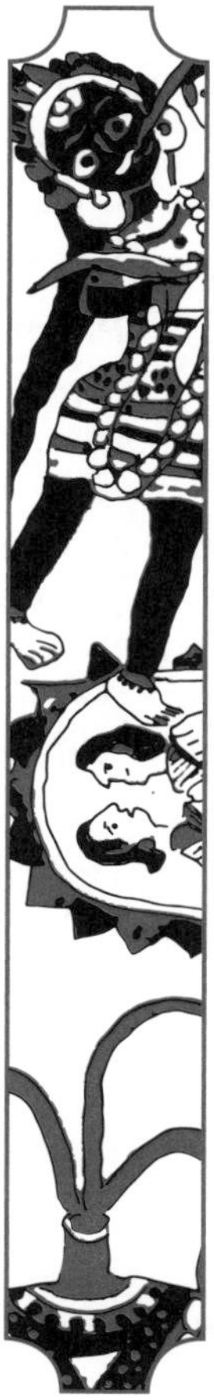

Pūjā is a form of Hindu, Buddhist and/or *tāntrik* worship that uses ritual items such as flowers, incense, water, light and food offerings to invoke and celebrate the living presence of deities. In certain sects of Hindu *tantra* menstrual blood is described as *yoni puṣpam*: the flower of the womb, and is a prized substance in certain rituals and sexual yogas. It can be a very healing freedom to treat one's own menstrual blood with sacred reverence, by offering it as a *pūjā* to the living presence of the Mother Earth in the form of plants and trees. This can be done metaphorically, for example, by feeling the downward flow of blood as a way to return attention to the presence of the living earth and the plants rooted in her, or it can be done literally by bleeding directly on to the earth or collecting menstrual blood and returning it to the earth. If a literal offering appeals to you then it is easiest to collect the menstrual blood in a moon cup (see Further reading and research section, below) and decant it into a bowl or cup kept especially for menstrual *pūjā*. Offer the blood directly into the earth at the foot of a chosen tree or plant with an attitude of reverence and connection, or dilute it with water and pour the water into your houseplants and watch them grow. Trees and pot plants that are fed by offerings of menstrual blood thrive.

YOGIC REMEDIES AND RESPONSES

Specific guidelines for particular difficulties are outlined below. Please bear in mind that a regular practice of the womb greetings and honourings in chapters five and six is of especial value in establishing the free flow of loving and respectful energy to the womb that can help to eradicate menstrual difficulties at source rather than treating sympotoms.

Menstrual cramps: some comforting yoga poses that can be of assistance in the relief of menstrual cramps are the Hare pose with fists and blankets (p.553) and the Golden cosmic womb (pp.552–3). *Praṇāmāsana* (p.555) is also helpful for some women. It is worth trying them all to see which one provides relief for you. As a preventive, the *śakti bandhas* in chaper six can help to promote free circulation of energy throughout the rest of the cycle so that the bleed itself is less painful.

Ovulation pains: for some women these can be very severe. Relief can be found sometimes through the use of lying twists: the Supported side-lying (p.551) or the more open Heart space twist (p.159). The Rising snake series (pp.543–4) may also be helpful. As with menstrual cramps, prevention is often the better strategy than symptomatic relief, so it is wise to include some free movement such as Being in the cycles (pp.517–21) as a means to relieve any congestion or tension that may exacerbate the pain.

Premenstrual tension: It can be very helpful to bear in mind that many of the most severe experiences of tension and difficulties at the pre-menstruum are associated with imbalance or over-doing it at other points in the cycle. For example, if you routinely tend not to grant yourself the permission to take time out to slowly recover and re-group after your bleed, but instead return immediately to everyday activities, you may discover that there is a sense of deep exhaustion and frustration by the time the pre-menstruum comes around. If you tend to really over-stretch yourself during the energetic, 'out in the world' summer time of ovulation, you may enter the autumn with a feeling of total burnout. The best way to avoid premenstrual tension is to practise restorative yoga poses (chapter twenty-five) as a regular part of your yoga practice throughout the month, and especially during the pre-menstruum. *Yoga nidrā* can also be very helpful (see chapter eighteen).

Heavy bleeding: It can be helpful to make use of some of the restorative poses recommended above for menstrual cramps, but also as a preventive measure to practise the Deer exercise (pp.496–7), which can help to reduce the length of your bleed time.

Off the Pill and where's the baby? If you have recently come off the contraceptive pill or have ceased using other contraceptives such as a coil, an implant, or a patch, and have been hoping to conceive but have not yet done so after two years, then it will be helpful to invest some energies in a detailed charting of your cycle, to develop familiarity and trust with the unfolding monthly rhythms. Deep relaxation such as the Cyclical wisdom *yoga nidrā* (pp.443–4) or the New beginnings *yoga nidrā* (p.442), and restorative yoga poses such as In the golden cosmic womb (pp.552–3) may be very helpful in re-establishing healthy menstruation.

It is valuable to develop an awareness of your cycle in relation to the lunar cycle, without any expectation or intention to 'get it right'. A pleasing way to establish this connection is to practise some moon salutations (pp.522–31) in tune with the phases of the moon. Follow the menstrual *mālā* of practices (pp.560–3) to explore how different yoga practices can support your experience of different aspects of the monthly cycle. Instead of just pinpointing 'the window' when conception is most likely to occur around ovulation, explore also the time of your natal moon to become conscious of other times in the cycle when conception may occur as a result of spontaneous ovulation. Any good astrologer will be able to calculate the time of your natal moon given the date, time and place of your birth, and this then provides a guide to your natural lunar fertile phase throughout your menstruating years. For helpful websites, see the references at the end of this chapter.

PARAMPARĀ, OR THE YOGIC TOWER

Imagine for a moment that you are a young woman, a *yoginī*, climbing up a steep spiral staircase inside a beautiful wide round tower.

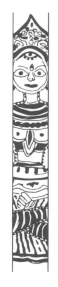

The stone steps are narrow and old but the tower and the stairs are secure. Every step is well worn by the countless feet that have ascended this way before you. Something drew you here and you are not quite sure what, but the pull was strong and now you feel powerfully compelled to ascend the tower. It is a beautiful structure, ancient and elegant; you are happy to have found it. You are heading determinedly for the light open space at the top.

The steps are built into the outer wall of the tower, and in the centre of their spiral there is an open stairwell. At ground level, where you have entered the tower, this circular space is stuffed with rubbish. It smells bad. There are rusting pushchairs and the internal workings of broken washing machines, and all kinds of domestic detritus. Even, if you dare to look a little closer, there are used sanitary towels and tampons, dirty underwear and stained sheets screwed up and rotting.

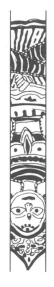

There is no handrail to grasp on the inner edge of the steps and you have a fear of falling back down to the bottom of the stairs, or into the stinking heap in the centre of the stairwell, and so you press your back against the stone walls of the tower for support and focus intently upon ascending sideways, one step at a time. You are hoping that if you get up high enough you will reach the top of the heap and the smell will be less bad, but for the moment it provides a powerful olfactory incentive to speed your ascent.

After a few crabwise steps with your back to the wall you begin to feel something sticking sharply in your shoulder blades. And so, fearful of falling back down the stairs or into the smelly void of the stairwell's rubbish, you turn slowly to face the wall. There hangs a portrait of a benevolent old *yogi*, smiling kindly and pointing the way up the next turn of the stair. Grateful for the reassurance and happy to have some guidance, you follow where he points, keeping your gaze on the walls of the tower where

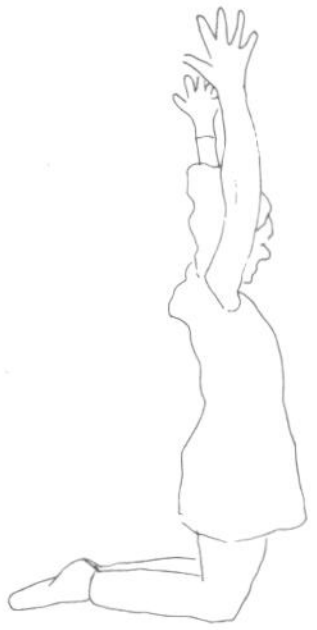

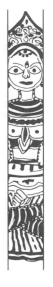

you are glad to see
hanging many portraits
of other wise *yogi*s, all teachers of
wisdom, and all pointing the way up the
spiral stair towards the brilliant sunlight that is
shining down the stairs from the top of the tower.

As you ascend you begin to notice the signs of others who have climbed the stairs: the notes they have carved into the wall, little guidebooks they have deposited on the stairs. Reading these notes and guidebooks you realise that some are very helpful, warning you of pitfalls on the steps ahead, or suggesting that you pause to admire a particularly beautiful fossil trapped in the stone of the tower walls. In fact, you are quite astonished to discover that the guidebooks cover almost every aspect of your experience in the tower, describing precisely your feelings and struggles. It as if the texts had been written especially for you. But then again, some of this guidance is so esoteric as to be totally mystifying. It makes no sense, and offers no help, so you simply ignore it and continue to follow the smiling and pointing faces of the old *yogis*.

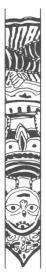

Fortuitously, morsels of tasty food appear on the steps above you whenever you feel hungry, and fresh water pours freely from spouts in the walls whenever you feel thirsty. It is as if, having entered the tower, that the very edifice itself, and all the *gurus* who reside within and the seekers who have passed before, are conspiring to support your efforts to ascend. Even the mystifying esoteric nonsense does not dampen your enthusiasm or deplete your energies.

Periodically, as and when you feel the need for a brief rest, you come across a window in the tower wall, and you admire the beautiful views of the wooded countryside below. These pauses to take in the views are very welcome, and the land below looks increasingly beautiful the higher up you go.

The journey goes on. This is a fairy-tale imaginary, and so you need not be alarmed to know that you have by now spent several weeks or dream years inside this tower. At a certain point you pause to look up towards the bright light shining down from the top of the tower, and it is only then you begin to realise what a long and arduous journey you have ahead. You sit down on the steps and recognise that you are extremely tired already. It is then that you begin to feel the familiar cold dull ache of a menstrual cramp, and you know that you

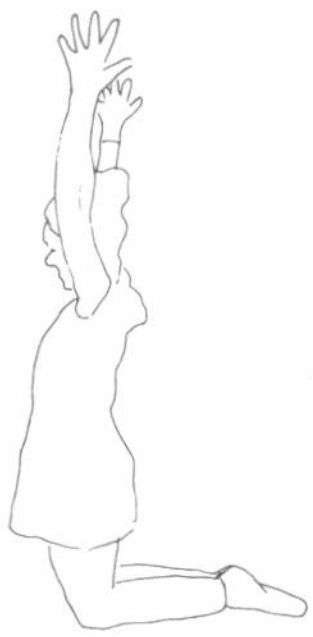

cannot continue right
now. You are beginning to
feel a little bit alone, sat there on the
stairs by yourself in the tower with only the
old *yogi*s on the walls for company.

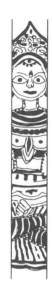

You are also feeling as if you had let the side down. After all, these helpful *yogi*s and the people who had passed this way before had really done their very best to offer all the guidance and encouragement and sustenance you might need to get to the top of the tower. And it is then that you sense they might not really understand how you feel right now, as you sense your womb's blood getting ready to flow, and you feel so tired and irritable. 'What is to be done?' You sense no answers are likely to be forthcoming from the *yogi*s on the walls. 'Come to think of it', you reflect, looking back, 'None of the guidebooks said anything about what to do in case of a menstrual emergency'.

In fact, now you think about it, you've been in this tower for weeks or years and you have only very rarely found any mention of menstruation in all the guidance that you have read. This now begins to strike you as a little strange. 'Some of those *yogi*s in the portraits were women', you think, 'and all that I ever read about menstruation was how to adapt the poses and / or what breathing practice to avoid. In fact, I am sure some of the guides told me that I should not even be allowed in the tower if I was menstruating'. Those were some of the ones you had ignored. You begin to have doubts. 'But perhaps I really should not even be in here at all?' you wonder. And then you feel very alone, and deeply confused. To make it worse, the smell from the rotting garbage in the centre of the stairwell is now worse than ever.

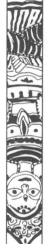

You rest against the walls of the tower and decide that it is probably best to try and overcome the tiredness and the pain and keep climbing. After all, most of the guides had stated that diligence and perseverance in practice would be rewarded. Perhaps there would be some sanitary towels at the top of the tower, thoughtfully provided in case of menstrual emergency. You doubt it.

You are just beginning to gather your energies to stand when you hear a rustling from far away, down at the bottom of the tower, and you are not very sure whether to be afraid or relieved. You can hear voices too, women's voices. They sound loud and old, but it is hard to make out what they are saying.

So you wait, to see what happens next.

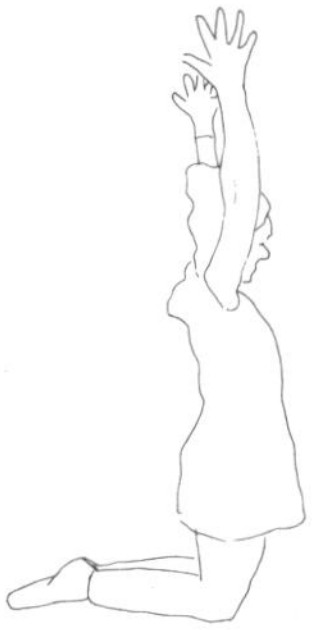

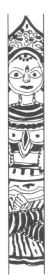

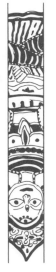

And then you notice that the heap of stinking rubbish is beginning to shift and sink. At first this seems unimaginable, since it is so high, and so huge, but you watch carefully and notice it happen again. You can still hear the old women's voices, and begin to make out what they are saying. 'Give us a hand love!' They are calling up the stairs. 'We'll clear from the bottom and you chuck it out from the top.'

You are astounded. Here you are, nearly at the top of the yogic tower of ascension and some old crone is shouting at you to clear the rubbish out the window. You had carefully managed to avoid even touching just one of those bags on your way up, and having got this far without getting your hands dirty you are not now inclined to start grabbing armfuls of garbage. So you ignore the calls of the old women below.

Instead you pause on the stairs, feeling the cramps in your belly and beginning to feel very sorry for yourself. You watch the smelly heap of rubbish shifting, and little by little it starts to descend. 'What are they doing? What am I doing?' You withdraw your awareness from the tower and the rubbish behind you, and, separating your senses from your surroundings, you surrender to the dragging sensation just hours before the blood begins to flow.

You slip effortlessly into a state of deep meditative awareness and stay there. You are not sure how long you remain in this state before the sound of the women's voices grows louder and more insistent, and you awaken with a profoundly renewed understanding of the nature of your situation. The light dawns. Literally, a light seems to be shining right inside the very top of your head. And you have, for the first time since you entered the tower, absolutely clear conviction, based not on any external guidance, nor anything you have read in the books, but on a profound sense of knowing that comes from deep within yourself.

You now understand what the old women are asking you to do. You heave up a bulging sack of rubbish and throw it out of the window. Down below, at the bottom of the tower, you hear an appreciative yell of thanks: 'About time too.' Looking out of the window you see that in a clearing in the woods, a vast team of older women are sorting through the rubbish: one has cut away turf and started a fire to burn what can safely be burnt, and the others are creating neat heaps of

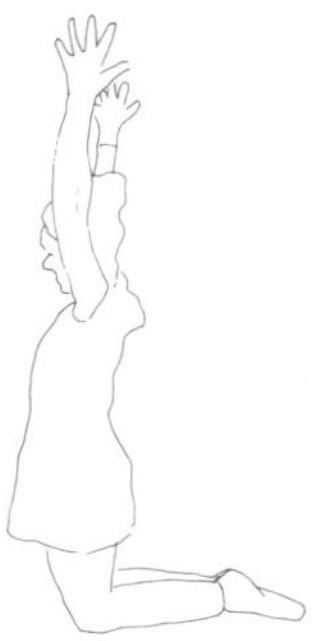

materials for recycling. They look up and gesture for you to send more rubbish down, and so you set to work.

By the time your blood is about to begin flowing, the whole heap of rubbish has been cleared from the tower, and outside the old women have created a remarkably organised collection of items, ready for recycling and re-use.

At the very bottom of the tower, in the foot of the stairwell that was once piled high with stinking rubbish, is now a pure clear circular space of bare earth. In exhaustion and relief you run all the way down the steps, lay your body down on the earth and gaze directly up at the sunlight streaming through the opening at the top of the tower. As you surrender to the feeling of the earth beneath and feel the soft breeze across your cheek and the warmth of the sun shining on your belly, you know that your blood is beginning to flow and you feel it sinking directly into the earth beneath. At that moment, in a powerful surge of energy, as if you were being borne up by the the earth herself, you are carried straight up through the centre of the staircase, higher and higher, far swifter than ever you could have climbed. Passing all of the friendly *yogi*s on your ascent, you come to rest in a state of exalted connection and heightened awareness in mid-air at the very top of the tower, bathed in light.

You rest in that state.

Not sure for how long you have been there, you awaken to more everyday consciousness by acknowledging a quiet but insistent voice inside your head. 'So there is a direct route I could have taken to get up here. Why did no one tell me?'

Sitting up, and looking about you, you find yourself once again at the side of the tower, next to the walls. The bleeding has stopped. You look over the parapet. Below there remains no sign of the impressive clean up job done by the old women in the woodland. The stairwell is clear and free from rubbish. The air smells sweet, and you slowly descend the steps of the tower, mindful not to disturb the neatly placed guidebooks and notes for aspiring ascenders, and respectfully greeting all the friendly *yogi*s on the way down. At the bottom of the tower, in the clear space of bare earth, you notice the faint imprint of a human form, and a dark circle at the centre where your blood had soaked into the ground. Looking

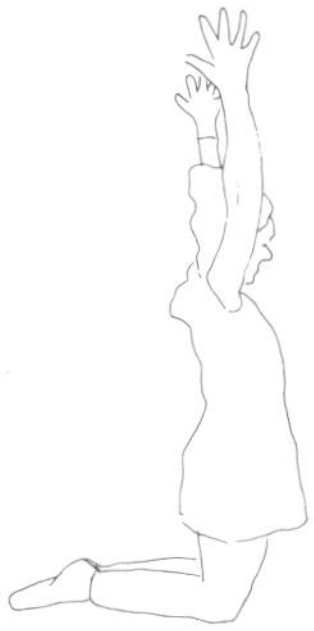

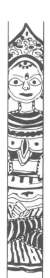

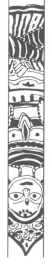

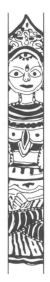

a little closer you become
aware of a complex network of
triangular forms, some pointing upwards
and some pointing downwards. The network of
interconnecting triangles fills a circle about the size
of the human body shape imprinted in the earth. The
triangles criss-cross the figure, with a central downward-
pointing triangle at the level of the pubic bones. The structure of
this network shines in fine lines of sunlight.

You begin to track the lines of light with your fingers, and one by one discover forty-three triangles mapped on and around the bodyprint in the earth. You recognise *Srī Yantra*: the geometric embodiment of unified consciousness and energy together. Her perfection and beauty takes your breath away, and you are drawn to sit in meditation over the centre point. Here you re-experience the clarity of focus and illumined awareness that you had encountered at the top of the tower, but this time you are seated on the earth, hearing the birds, feeling the breeze and the warmth of the sun: fully conscious of all around you.

As you leave the woodland tower, you know that you now carry within yourself the clarity and direction of your own deep inner teacher. Within your heart you feel the presence of this guide and hear the words 'With great respect and love I honour my heart, my inner teacher'. Welcome home.

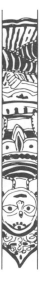

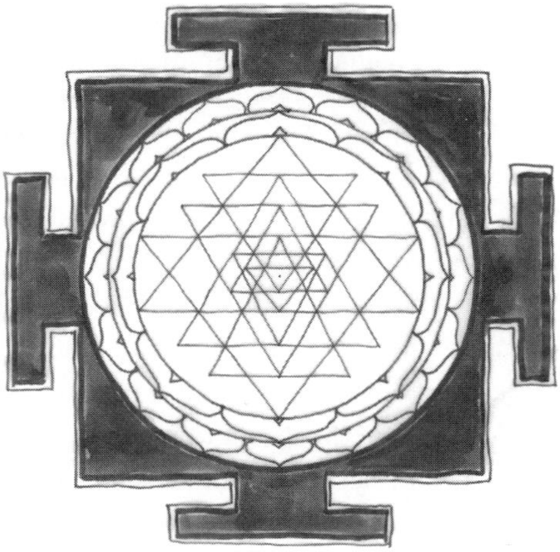

Srī Yantra

EXEGESIS

Paramparā is a Sanskrit word describing the lineage of a *guru*. It tracks the direct transmission of teachings from student to pupil, sometimes for hundreds or thousands of years. Often, a yogic *paramparā* will seek to establish a connection, through the *ṛśis* or seers, to the primary yogic teacher, Śiva, the god of yogic asceticism and transformation. To connect to a lineage through a teacher with *paramparā* is a source of great power, strength and security. It acts as a guarantee of the authenticity and clarity of the yogic teachings that are being transmitted. Most of the current schools and forms of yoga endeavour clearly to establish their own *paramparā*, and this way students within a particular lineage are connected to the long chain of respect and honour in which the teachings they are practising have been held and preserved. A yogic text, such as the *Yoga Sūtra* or the *Haṭha Yoga Pradīpikā* can also be part of a *paramparā*. Discussion of the effects of these lineages and texts upon contemporary practitioners of yoga, in particular female practitioners, was set out in chapter two, so here, it suffices to say that the lineages are largely male, and that it is right and proper for contemporary *yoginīs* and *yogis* to be immensely grateful to all the *guru*s and *paramparās* for their effective preserving, protecting and transmitting of the traditions of yoga for over three thousand years.

That is why the *yoginī* in the tower respectfully thanks all the friendly *yogis* whose portraits she finds on the tower walls, and ensures that the written guides and notes (metaphors for the yogic scriptures), are carefully replaced on the steps as she descends for others to find. She does not disrupt, disturb or disrespect the *paramparā*, for she knows from her own experience that it has an important role to play.

Neither the guidebooks, nor the helpful *yogi*s were able to show our imaginary *yoginī* the direct route to the top of the yogic tower, because they simply did not know that it existed. The knowledge of the direct route is within.

In the story, and in this book, you are invited to engage with the very real possibility that a conscious encounter with the guiding power of menstruation (and/or other female *siddhis* including orgasm, childbirth, lactation and the hot flushes of menopause) is potentially a path to profound and powerful spiritual experience.

But this possibility is simply inadmissible in many yogic towers. As in the tower in the story, centuries of cultural conditioning, religious baggage and fears of pollution, witchcraft, and other feminine evils, have been piled up in the stairwell of the tower of yogic *paramparā*. The rubbish has blocked the sacred central passage to the light. With the space so heaped with myths and prejudice, and shame and guilt, and fear and disgust, it becomes not only unattractive, but utterly inaccessible.

The crones in the story represent those women whose wisdom and power grants them clear sight and willingness to clear the heritage of misogyny and fear around menstrual blood that permeates even the tower of yogic *paramparā*. It is not until she listens to their voices that our *yoginī* can begin to realise that beneath this heap of garbage is a portal to spiritual power. She only gains this perspective when she has respectfully ascended the tower under the guidance of the smiling *yogis*, and it is only the efforts of the wise old women below who draw her attention to the need to clear this passage to her own power.

Once she gains this awareness, significantly at the point when she is conscious that she is just about to begin to menstruate, and is therefore entering a time of heightened awareness that has huge potential for spiritual transformation, then she engages with the effort of her older sisters and between them they clear the way for her rapid ascension to the top of the tower. The dumping ground becomes a launch pad for this ascent, affording a direct route to the light above. It is through her willingness to clear away the stinking garbage that has filled this passageway that our *yoginī* is able to embrace the powerful guidance of her inner teacher.

The womb yoga presented in *Yoni Śakti* points the way back home to the wisdom of the body's rhythms. It offers direct routes to the illumined space of pure conscious awareness, so that in future other women who enter the yogic tower will see immediately that there are choices to be made about how to get to the top: whether by the stairs, with guidance and pointers from those *yogis* of the *paramparā* who have gone before; or by the direct route of conscious awareness that opens up to a woman at certain special times and experiences in her womb life. When we have awareness and respect for these special times we are invited to return to an ancient place of knowing, or an embodied experience of feminine spiritual power. She is naturally arising, deep and powerful. She is your own inner guidance, and she has been waiting for you to turn and greet her. She says 'Welcome back home to yourself'.

QUESTIONS AND REFLECTIONS

I invite you to explore your own (current or previous) experience of the menstrual cycle and how yoga may support that by asking yourself some (or any, or all) of the following questions:

1. How interested are you in your cycle? How does it relate to the phases of the moon? How does it influence your choice of yoga practice?
2. How do you prefer to keep track of your cycle? If you don't enjoy keeping notes, have you considered using a phone app (e.g. period tracker) or some other means to create your own menstrual calendar?
3. Which are the most enjoyable parts of your menstrual cycle? What aspects of yoga practice do you most enjoy during this part of the cycle?
4. Which are the most challenging parts of the menstrual cycle? What strategies do you have in place to help you through this time, and what yoga practices have you found to be the most helpful at this time?
5. Looking at your cycle as a whole, how far do you sense that it has some balance? For example, are there certain points within the cycle whose energy drags you down, or when you feel buoyed up by abundant vitality? How does your yoga practice relate to these experiences?

FURTHER READING AND RESEARCH

There are now many resources that support self-help of menstrual difficulties. Each author has her own perspective, so the following suggestions highlight the qualities of each approach to assist you in finding what resonates. **Alexandra Pope**'s *The Wild Genie* takes a broad spiritual perspective on the power of menstruation, offering insight and inspiration through vividly retold case studies, and sensible lifestyle advice (**www.wildgenie.com**). The same author's *Women's Quest Workbook* provides practical guidance on how to chart your cycle for self-healing, spiritual empowerment and freedom from suffering (**www.womensquest.org**). **Miranda Gray**'s *Red Moon* connects the spirituality of cycle awareness to a pagan-Celtic mythology and metaphors drawn from the Tarot (**www.mirandagray.co.uk**). **Lara Owen**'s *Her Blood is Gold* combines a personal story with a sensitive reading of the cultural issues that can shape our experiences of menstruation (**www.laraowen.com**). Other women who have produced valuable material to support menstrual awareness include **Jane Hardwicke Collings** in Australia and **Lucy Pearce** in Ireland.

For detailed guidance on diet and lifestyle changes that can support menstrual health, the work of two US medical doctors provide superb resources: **Christiane Northrup**'s *Women's Bodies, Women's Wisdom* and **Susan M Lark**'s: *Heavy Menstrual Flow* and *Anaemia: a Self-Help book*. Lark's book includes solutions for fibroid tumours, endometrial hyperplasia, bleeding due to hormonal imbalance, and low blood count, founded on diet, exercise, lifestyle and self-care. The same author's *Menstrual Cramps: Self-Help Book* brings a similar approach to menstruation pain and PMS.

Jane Bennett and **Alexandra Pope**'s *The Pill: are you sure it's for you?* presents all the major concerns related to the use of the contraceptive pill in a most accessible format. *The Baby Making Bible*, by acupuncturist and fertility specialist **Emma Cannon**, brings together suggestions to support healthy menstruation as the key to optimum fertility (**www.emmacannon.co.uk**). Her guidelines are applicable both for natural conception and assisted reproductive technologies. For general practical support and information on natural fertility, the work of **Francesca Naish** is invaluable, in particular *Natural Fertility*. For alternatives to disposable sanitary products, see **www.mooncup.co.uk** and **www.moontimes.co.uk**.

A popular fictionalised account of the red tent experience, where women gathered during menstruation to share stories and support each other is **Anita Diamant**'s *The Red Tent*. The documentary film *The Moon Inside You* brings together some fascinating interviews and information from around the world.

All of this work rests on a bedrock of feminist scholarship that effectively exposes our culture's negative attitudes towards menstruation. For example, **Janice Delaney**, **Mary Jane Lupton** and **Emily Toth**'s 1976 classic feminist reference *The Curse* provided a radical cultural history of menstruation that was revised and expanded in 1988 at the time when *The Sanitary Protection Scandal* (Costello, Vallely and Young) first presented the evidence of the global ecological crisis that had been caused by the disposal of 'feminine hygiene' products, and **Sophie Laws**' *Issues of Blood* (1990) explored the politics of menstruation. **Penelope Shuttleworth** and **Peter Redgrove**'s 1978 book *The Wise Wound* assembled an astonishingly broad set of cultural references to menstruation from Greek myths to horror movies, and its recent reissue (2005) testifies that there is still a hunger for this information.

The profitable business of making and marketing sanitary protection for women is examined by **Elizabeth Arveda Kissling** in her study *Capitalising on the Curse* (2006) and menstrual hygiene technology is explored by **Sharra L Vostral** in her historical exploration, *Under Wraps* (2008). For a lighter, funnier and beautifully illustrated popular history, I warmly recommend *Flow: the cultural story of menstruation* (2009) by **Elissa Stein** and **Susan Kim**; it contains a fascinating collection of vintage (and not so vintage) adverts for douches, sanitary pads and tampons that are by turns astonishing and alarming.

For reliable links to conscious menstruation sites, I recommend **Belinda Garcia Reyes' www.meztlicihuatl-english.blogspot.co.uk**. For online English translations of the menstrual blood worshipping tantrik texts see **www.shivashakti.com**

An increasing number of smartphone apps now exist to help you track your menstrual cycle and engage in fertility awareness.

The following websites offer services that not only calculate that time of your natal moon, but also provide guidance on using menstrual lunar synchrony for conscious conception or contraception:
www.menstruation.com.au/menstrualproducts/basiclunar.html
www.nfmcontraception.com/index.htm

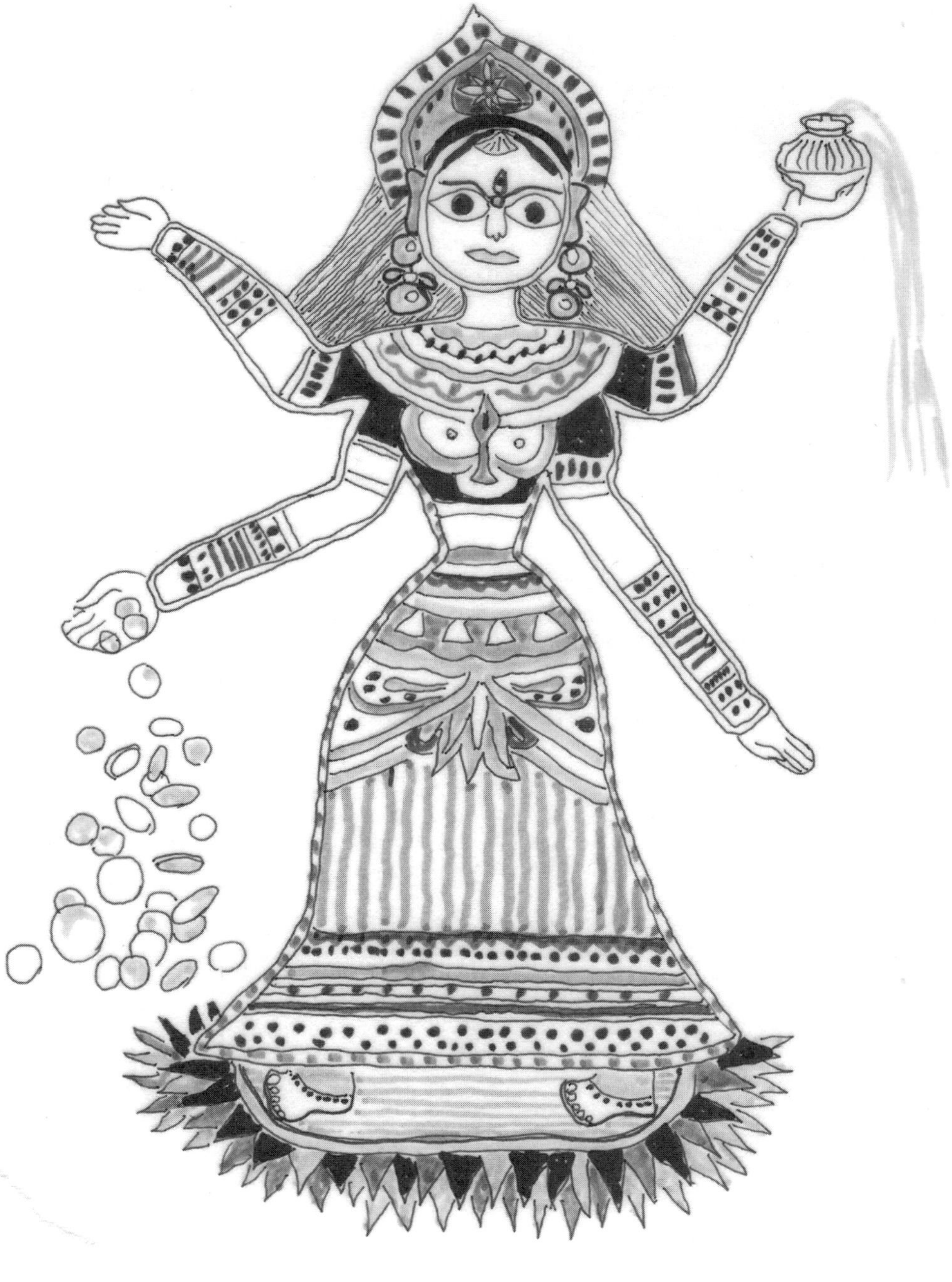

Kamalātmikā is associated with abundance, love, pleasure, delight and beauty

CHAPTER ELEVEN

Kamalātmikā

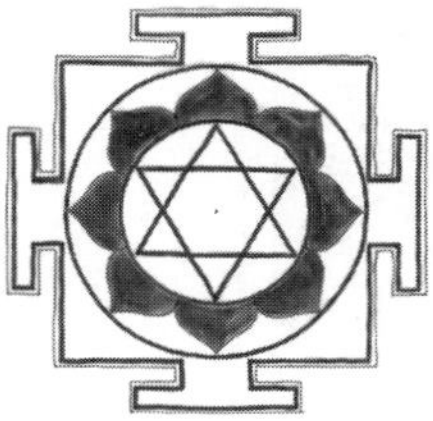

Freeing the *śakti*: yoga and full spectrum feminine sexuality

Our sexuality is not only something that can be used for the enhancement of intimate relationships, for physical pleasure, or procreation. It can also be used for personal transformation, physical and emotional healing, self-realization, spiritual growth and as a way to learn about all of life and death. An honest, sexually knowledgeable woman, or group of women, is a divine and extremely powerful force that not only can inspire other women, but also have the potential to contribute to the well-being of all life on earth. (Annie Sprinkle, in Foreword to Sundahl 2003)

MAHĀVIDYĀ AND *SIDDHI*

WISDOM AND POWER

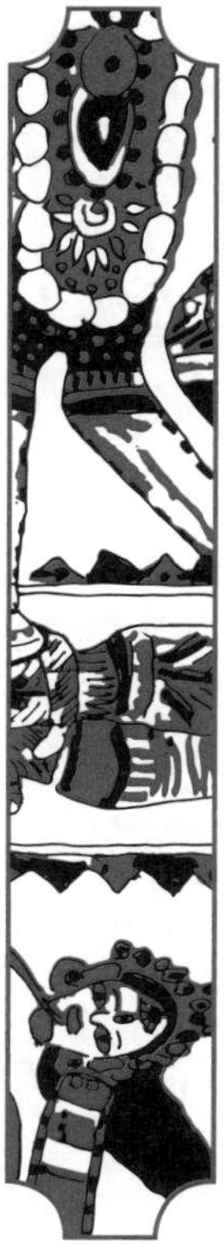

Kamalātmikā, the radiant golden goddess of delight, is always associated with abundance, love and beauty. She is linked in this section with the deep beauties of full spectrum feminine sexuality. Her *siddhi*, or special power, is the capacity for experiencing pleasure and delight in abundance, and her name literally means the goddess who originates in the unfolding nature of the lotus (*kamala*). She is depicted on a lotus flower, with one of her four hands holding a full pot of water, another pouring an endless shower of golden coins, and the last two hands offering gestures that grant wishes and dispel fears. She is generous. Everything about her image shows this: for, the lotus is the symbol of the precious beauty of spiritual unfolding, whilst the water represents the communion of love and spiritual grace. The endless shower of golden coins that pour from her hand represents the absolute and continuing abundance of spiritual and material wealth. Of all the *Mahāvidyās*, it is only Kamalātmikā who is always beneficent: all the others, even the gorgeous Ṣoḍasī, who carries sugar cane bows and arrows, have weapons or fearful aspects. It is Kamalātmikā alone whose abundance and grace is always generous and giving.

In relation to sexuality, Kamalātmikā's radiant beauty and abundant generosity reveal the deep and continuous capacity for delight that experiences of conscious sexual fulfilment can bring throughout our lives. Hers is a powerful *siddhi* that connects us with the power of pleasure as a spiritualising force. When we explore the full spectrum of female sexuality, then the experience of the spirit of sexuality not only includes pleasures we bring to ourselves and those we share with others, but may also include periods of celibacy. Kamalātmikā's generosity extends to these celibate times, because as a counterpart of sexual activity, the experience of celibacy also contains within it the abundant energetic charge of delight, free to manifest in different forms.

There is a very special and intimate relation between the *siddhi* of sensual delight represented by Kamalātmikā and the *siddhi* of creativity represented by Mataṅgi. Both are powers that connect us directly with the experience of abundance through the free flow of *śakti* or powerful energy. The focus is confined to sexuality in this section on Kamalātmikā, and the discussion about creativity follows in the next section on Mataṅgi. It has been very challenging to separate sexuality from creativity in this way, because in my experience of these manifestations of *śakti*, sexuality and creativity are essentially one and the same force at work in different ways. To be honest, in practice, it makes little sense to consider sexuality as a force separate from creativity, which is why Kamalātmikā and Mataṅgi appear as twin snakes in the image of the dancing constellation of goddesses (p.228).

In more orthodox presentations of the *Mahāvidyās*, Kamalātmikā is usually placed as the final wisdom goddess, representing 'the full unfoldment of the power of the Goddess into the material sphere' (Frawley 1994:149). As the tenth goddess, she thus stands alongside Kālī, and is often understood to be a form of Kālī. The relation between Kālī and Kamalātmikā is deep: for if Kamalātmikā is the beauty and delight unfolded into the physical and material realm, Kālī is the beauty of the void from which everything manifests. It is only by absolute surrender to Kālī that the true grace of Kamalātmikā can shower upon us.

The radiant golden beauty of the generous and beneficent Kamalātmikā who supports us in the fulfilment of physical desires only manifests once we have let go of all attachment and surrendered to the powers of Kālī. If we are attracted to the power of delight and pleasure at a superficial level—for example if we pursue sexual experience for the gratification of unconscious needs or the acquisition of status and power—then, inevitably, the lotus goddess of delight will show us her other form, and the hands that shower down the golden coins and abundant water will become the hands that hold the bloody chopper and the severed head. The immense power of pleasure is, when pursued without consciousness of its spiritual dimension, a potentially destructive force that can deplete, demean and/or disempower us.

As well as her intimate relation with Kālī, Kamalātmikā also has a resonance with Lakṣmī, the goddess who confers spiritual and material wealth. As one of the *Mahāvidyās*, Kamalātmikā is that form of Lakṣmī which is particularly related to the practice of yoga, and so her connection to pleasure and delight carries a special yogic quality. To connect with the powers of Kamalātmikā is to bring our consciousness alive to the perception of earthly beauty and delight, including sexuality in all its forms, and to embrace the possibility that the fulfilment of material and physical desires can in fact be a part of a soulful unfolding of our spiritual evolution. Such is the immense power of the fulfilment of our desire for pleasure that it has the potential to enhance every aspect of our being. In particular, and when approached from the perspective of yoga *tantra*, conscious experiences of the deep beauty of our sexuality can hold the keys to a truly vivid encounter with spirituality.

As the goddess who represents the great wisdom that we experience through pleasure and delight, Kamalātmikā shows that there is an intimate relation between material, bodily bliss and the capacity to perceive the existence of a cosmic higher force, through encounters with transcendent states of unified consciousness. The power to feel and enjoy those aspects of sexual pleasure that enliven and awaken us to an experience of pure love can be a very clear path to spiritual awareness. When encountered with a certain consciousness, such as that embodied by Kamalātmikā, the joyful beauty of sexual pleasure can be experienced as a delightful manifestation of one aspect of the bliss of pure being.

The healing power of sexual delight can also be a central support to the healthy and positive experience of being a woman at all stages in our lives because it literally can 'free our *śakti*' or unblock our power, allowing it to flow where it is needed. The free flow of our power in this way brings many benefits to all dimensions of our being. Its obstruction is inimical to our health and happiness, separating our vital energies from their home at the very foundations of our energy system. If our relationship with the *siddhi* of Kamalātmikā becomes distant, if we lose connection for whatever reason with the true nature of our sexuality, then we become exiled from the source of our identity and vitality.

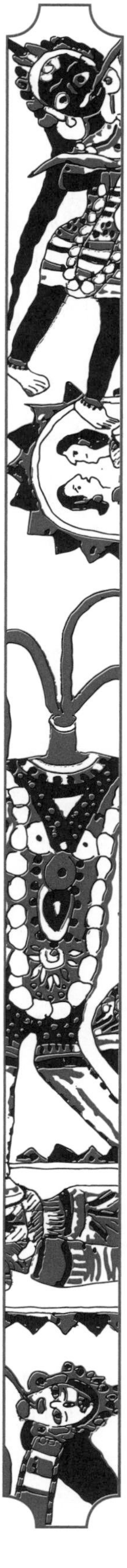

LIMITATIONS: CULTURAL EXPECTATIONS

> *There is nothing in you that is of value; everything of value is outside you and must be acquired. (hooks 1996: 291)*

We have long been exiled. The deep freedom of loving sexual expression as women is our motherland. But we've been away so long we don't even know what it feels like to come home.

Our cultural expectations around the nature of female sexuality are so profoundly limiting, but so deeply ingrained in general understanding, that we may not even notice them. It is only in recent years that anything like a freely expressed, genuinely women-centred account of female sexuality has even begun to be heard. And still, even as these voices whisper of other possibilities, what most of us believe makes women really feel sexy and vital and fabulous is total nonsense. Growing up as girls in a culture that teaches us that menstruation is shameful and should be invisible, we grow into women who have been taught to ignore natural cycles so effectively that we have trouble feeling any kind of authentic connection to the ebb and flow of our naturally arising cycles of sexual desire. For many women who are on the Pill or using long-acting contraceptive implants and injections, there exist no such naturally arising cycles of sexual desire, or at least, the peak experiences of sexual responsiveness at ovulation are suppressed. For young women encountering their first sexual experiences without any subtle or empowering guidance about the relationship between their menstrual cycle and its impact on fertility, emotional life and sexuality, then the fear of unwanted pregnancies can cast a shadow over their sexual awakening that can utterly disconnect them from any practical, inner understanding of the links between menstrual cycles, fertility and sexuality.

> *For example, Jinny, a fifteen year-old girl who got pregnant the first time she had unprotected intercourse with her boyfriend, was so disconnected from the natural rhythms of her own cycle that she did not detect the pregnancy for nearly four months. Her experience of abortion was upsetting and physically very difficult and depleting. Shocked and embarrassed by the whole experience, Jinny was immediately brought to her family doctor by her worried father, who was looking to safely control the alarming consequences of his daughter's evidently awakened sexuality. In the midst of her grief and distress about the pregnancy and the abortion, Jinny was in no place to make informed decisions.*
>
> *And so, out of fear of the apparently uncontrollable effects of her own cycles, and from a place of total disempowerment, Jinny agreed to have a long-acting contraceptive injection. She believed she had no other choice.*

The fear of future abortions, the pressure to be sexually available at all times without danger of getting pregnant, and the cultural pressure to behave as if the menstrual cycle does not exist is a potent combination of forces that leads many young women like Jinny to make decisions about their own bodies that do not respect the subtle cycles and rhythms of women's sexual and emotional lives. This combination of forces does not just affect young women; throughout our sexual lives, our encounters with our own sexuality are often confined, limited and determined both by cultural pressures and by the effects of synthetic hormones. And so, whether these cycles have been eradicated by contraceptive drugs, or whether we have simply been trained to disguise and disregard them, we can become disconnected from the inner source of guidance to our own wellspring of delight: fear and ignorance have locked us out of our sexual selves, and so we look around outside for help.

And what guidance does our culture have to offer us on the subject of women and sexuality? Not much. Even if we feel free from the medical and social control that disempowers young women like Jinny, we are still impoverished by our culture's lack of positive images and role models for women who seek genuine sexual freedom. The guidance our culture offers us is mostly to do with how we look and what cosmetic, depilatory and surgical activities we should undertake to render our bodies glamorous and sexually attractive to men according to standards set by porn-stars. Not only is this utterly separate from the joyous experience of an authentic encounter with the energies of our own unique sexuality, but we have to pay for it.

The sale of glamorous availability in place of the true beauty and spiritual power of loving sex is all bound up with patriarchy and capitalism. It is also, in many ways quite literally, deadly to women: the Pill and all the long-acting contraceptive drugs have very serious side-effects that are damaging to our health; the surgical alterations of labia, clitorises and breasts damage and degrade female sexual response; under-wired bras, those crucial components in the armoury of sexed-up glamour, have been the focus of debates about whether or not wearing them can cause breast cancer; the processes of repeated under-arm depilation and the application of certain kinds of deodorants can expose vulnerable skin to toxins and possible carcinogens; most make-up is also full of these nasties; the habitual wearing of high-heeled shoes cripples women's feet and causes long-term lower backache and other unpleasant pelvic and spinal problems that reduce mobility; and repeated experiences of conventional thrusting hetero-sex that involves rhythmic friction between penis and vagina without prior adequate female sexual arousal, such as that practised in most bedrooms and aggressively promoted on every porn channel / internet site in the world, causes long-term damage and desensitisation of female genitalia, to the point where many women are unable to experience vaginal, uterine or G-spot / blended orgasms. Tied into any expression of women's sexuality is also a deep fear of the dangers to which it makes us vulnerable: the dangers of verbal and physical abuse, of public humiliation and rape. Our culture permits hardly any safe spaces for the genuinely free exploration and expression of female sexuality.

In a culture that thus separates women from the true sources of our own inner knowing about sexuality, what are sold back to us are empty shells: glamorised versions of conventional sex acts intended to gratify men as and when they desire, with no respect or reverence for the unfolding cycles of sexual response and desire that a woman in tune with her menstrual cycle can clearly perceive. At the heart of many of these empty shells of female sexuality is the profound paradox that the contraceptive pill and its long-acting sisters, the Depo-Provera implants and patches, which have been almost universally welcomed by women as a key to sexual freedom, in fact lower libido and reduce our responsiveness to sexual pleasure. The 'sexual freedom' of being on the Pill / patch / implant is really the freedom to disconnect from the cyclical nature of our own sexual reality.

Our culture's conventional definition of female sexuality truly is an empty shell, a poor shred of tat, packaged and sold back to us as if it were the beating heart of our sexual being. What we are persuaded to believe to be sexy and pleasurable has been reduced to the creation of this outer shell: our make-up and clothes, our hair and shoes, our underwear, the fashionably depilated absences of our pubic hair, our surgically altered labia and breasts, and the fact that, because we are on the Pill, we are sexually available at all times: all of this is what we are led to believe will really make us desirable. To be a sexual woman in our culture now is to be a woman who looks a certain way in order to elicit sexual desire in others. It has nothing to do with the inner arising of our own feelings and experiences. With all this focus on cosmetics and depilation, on surgical remodelling, on primping and preening, and on the consumption of synthetic hormones to render us easily available without the need to recognise our own cycle of sexual responsiveness, the true source of the inner power of female sexuality has been utterly neglected. It is as though we have re-painted the front door of the house whilst inside the whole place is falling apart, derelict, neglected and cold, with no fire in the grate.

Perhaps the most alarming evidence of how completely women have accepted the profound limitations which our culture places on our experiences of sexuality, particularly in relation to our feelings about our own breasts and genitals, are the rapidly rising rates of plastic surgery to alter the shape and form of our cunts and breasts. Implanting silicone gel to augment breast size is the most popular cosmetic surgery procedure in the UK and the US. Nine and half thousand women in the UK had breast augmentation surgery in 2010, a ten percent increase on the previous year. In comparison to the steady growth in breast surgeries, the rapid increase in the numbers of cunt surgeries is astounding: there has been a three hundred per cent increase in labiaplasty (reduction or alteration of the labia) in the UK over the past five years, including a seventy per cent increase in labiaplasties carried out on the NHS. Labiaplasty is the fastest growing field of cosmetic surgery in the UK.

There are complex reasons surrounding the choices women make to have these surgeries, but especially in relation to the dramatic rise in the number of labiaplasties, there is an evident link to the unrealistic portrayals of women's genitals in pornographic media: these images, of hairless cunts with surgically reduced and removed labia, have a powerful impact on the self-esteem and self-image of women, especially young women. As radical sexual health activist Lady Cunt Love writes, 'The porn that the majority of these young people are watching is the hard and fast free stuff on Red Tube, Porn Hub etc. and these videos objectify women, ignore the clitoris and depict unrealistic portrayals of sex. They make us feel inadequate... Many men and women are now trying to be like porn stars and act like porn stars. Sex becomes about performance, not about pleasure. Young, impressionable teenagers are watching porn in substitute for sex education and this scares me to death.'

In a world where our young people see hardcore pornography as a source of information about sexuality, and where women voluntarily submit to surgical removal of their labia to create utterly unnatural cunts that degrade their capacity to experience sexual pleasure, it isn't easy for women to feel good about ourselves and our sexuality from the inside. Even women who feel that they are 'in tune' with their own sexual needs, and who believe that such surgeries will augment their orgasmic capacity, are in fact depleting their range of sexual pleasure, for example through surgeries that pump collagen into the G-spot and thus render it utterly unresponsive, or through breast augmentations that reduce breast sensitivity and the capacity to experience sexual arousal.

It is hard to fathom how we could have become so astonishingly disconnected from an aspect of ourselves that is so intimately intrinsic to our well-being. It is beyond the scope and intention of this book to fully address this massive question, but if we seek to free ourselves from the profound cultural limitations that constrain our sexuality, then it's helpful to consider briefly what may have set them in place at the start. From the perspective of a feminist *yoginī*, the basic premise is this: that the fearful patriarchal impotence and sense of inadequacy that accompanied men's failure to understand or control female sexuality and other female *siddhis* led to a resentful devaluing of women's sexuality in the spirit of: 'If we can't have it, neither shall you'. This resulted in a forcible removal of women's sexual power and spiritual authority over centuries that extended right through to every aspect of women's autonomy in other spheres too. You know the rest of the story: until the 1880s in the UK women were not legally permitted to own property, nor were we allowed to attend medical school or university, or to vote; in other countries around the world still we are not permitted to drive, or to learn how to read. Even though massive changes have occurred in the past generation, and women in industrialised nations are free to live our lives in ways that our grandmothers would have found unimaginable, the stranglehold on female sexuality has never really been fully released. The increase in labiaplasty surgeries, the numbers of women on the Pill or the contraceptive implant, and the massive growth of the international porn industry are all testimony to its grip.

The most vigorous attempts to free us from this stranglehold have come from feminist women's health debates and sexual activism. The work of women like Deborah Sundahl and Betty Dodson has raised awareness of the full spectrum of female sexuality through encouraging open discussion and information sharing. This has done much to help us to hear women's erotic experiences. But the trouble with this work is that it has ended up in a kind of ghetto. It has not really been joined up with other aspects of women's experiences. Many (not all) previous feminist attempts to address issues of female sexuality have focused on gender politics, sidestepped the relationship between sexuality and spirituality, and thus missed the opportunity to explore freely the limitless expanses of full spectrum female sexuality as an expression of our spirit. And even when this connection is made, then the links to other aspects of women's *siddhis* have not always been forged. This is a pity, because it helps us to understand the amazing scope of our sexuality when we see how sexual energy manifests in many different forms throughout our lives.

It is helpful to parallel what has happened to our understanding of female sexuality with other expressions of primal female power, for example the visionary state of consciousness at menstruation and the experience of birth as orgasmic gates to spiritual awareness. Both of these *siddhis* can be seen, like our sexual response, to transform women's everyday consciousness into portals of unified awareness that invite consciousness of cosmic rhythms and waves of energy. However could such immense power have been taken from women? Could it be that the sheer vastness of the potential for women's spiritual authority and deep insights at these times have seemed to men so impossible that they simply could not believe it could happen, and have thus endeavoured to remove these burdens from us, to give us contraceptive pills to eradicate the peak experiences of our menstrual cycles, and epidurals to take away the potential pain caused by awakenings of labour and birthing, and thus reconfigure and control these powerful initiatory experiences along the lines of a more limited male model? The remodelling has been so remarkable and shockingly effective that even the women ourselves believe the stories told to us by the men. We believe that we're better off not menstruating, and that we cannot give birth unaided by narcotics or episiotomies.

So too with the stories we believe about female sexuality: it is as if the scale and depths of the intense pleasures and spiritual insights which women can access through female sexuality in its full expression of profound spiritual connectedness have seemed so unimaginable to the patriarchal psyche that men and women have worked together to reduce and reframe the nature of women's experience into a more manageable, partial form that men can handle, and that helps the good daughters of patriarchy feel safe because we know what we need to do to be well-behaved. What this means is that all those books on female orgasm and female ejaculation and understanding women's pleasure, even if they have been written with the intention of increasing women's pleasure, and even if they have been written by women, are mostly missing the point, and denying women access to our birthright: the fully spiritualised experience of our sexuality. Because the ordinary male sexual response has been the template for all of our culture's understandings of sexuality – the rapid drive to climax of the male orgasm in its most limited form – it has created a sadly limited model for sexuality in our culture that actually damages women's capacity for full spectrum female sexual response.

So instead of the truly fabulous cosmic expressions of our naturally arising female sexual nature, what do we have now? A few rags and tatters, and some grotesque fakery. It is as if we've arrived at the human sexuality party bedecked in our own naturally arising splendour, and traded it all in for some truly uncomfortable underwear, a surgically remodelled cunt with reduced capacity for sexual response, no pubic hair, gigantic silicone tits that can't feel a thing and shoes we can't even walk in. It's grotesque, and it's very disempowering, for 'Sadly, when women choose to stay with conventional sex – which is a distorted form of male sexuality – we give away our unique feminine magic and power' (Diana Richardson: 3).

There's nothing left to lose here. We've been so securely locked out of our sexual selves for so long that any sign back home is worth following, even if we're not sure we can read it. Yoga gives us some clear directions to follow.

FREEDOMS: YOGA PERSPECTIVES, TECHNIQUES AND AWARENESS FOR BREATHING, MOVING AND BEING

And so, if looking to the culture outside for guidance about female sexuality has exiled us from our home in our sexual selves, then what we need to do to get back in touch with the great *siddhi* of Kamalātmikā, with our own naturally arising sexual power and capacity for pleasure, is to turn our backs on that culture and redirect our attention back inside. Kamalātmikā is generous: she gives abundantly, and the range of delightful pleasures she offers in relation to our sexuality is limitless when our *śakti* flows freely. To liberate our *śakti* is to gain access to the full spectrum of sexual delight. This is one of the fabulous side effects of yoga. It's absolutely liberating. The practice of yoga gives us free passage home to ourselves. Yoga clears our way back to our own inner knowing. By freeing the flow of our *śakti*, we create the possibility for full expression of female sexuality. It offers us supportive practices that empower us to recognise the cycles of our own desires, and to explore and enjoy this wonderful manifestation of *śakti* in our lives.

A woman who is directly and happily in contact with the true nature of her own sexuality is a woman who is genuinely in touch with her greatest power. Yoga can help us to make this contact. The practice of yoga heightens our awareness of our inner rhythms and patterns, and puts us back in touch with the guidance of our inner teacher. There are so many ways in which positive experiences of sexuality can improve women's health that an empowered encounter with this powerful manifestation of *prāṇa śakti*, the life force, can be foundational for a woman's well-being, whether she is single or partnered, celibate or sexually active, young or old, homosexual, bisexual or heterosexual, a mother, a maiden or a crone. At all stages of life, positive experience of our sexuality can enhance every dimension of well-being. An exploration of how experiences of each life stage can be supported by a positive experience of female sexuality is set out under the 'Yogic remedies and responses' at the end of this section. What follows below are some stories and reflections that illustrate the yoga perspective on female sexuality, the relation between *tantra* and love.

> *I first began to link my understanding of the effects of my yoga and meditation practice with an awakening sense of my own sexuality as a young woman. I made the connection out of necessity because I found that the kinds of experiences I encountered in a state of sexual arousal were nothing like any of the images or descriptions I had come across in relation to female sexual response. I was looking for some other explanation that described my own experiences. As an adolescent in the 1980s, I learnt most of what I knew about sexuality from films and books and popular music and television, so the images I had of what sex was like for women were based on what media had to offer me.*
>
> *I could see from all this that the experiences women were depicted as having did not match up with what was occurring to me. What I saw on the telly that passed for images of female sexual experience seemed mostly to be gorgeous woman lying about and writhing, making groaning noises and then stopping when the man involved*

ejaculated. There was a lot of interest in the removal of these women's bras, and shoes, and a fair amount of focus on the wildness of their hair and the openness of their very red mouths, but to be honest, I was confused, because none of this really matched up in any way with the experiences I was beginning to encounter as a sexually awakening young woman.

There were no men involved at this stage, and what was quite overwhelming to me was the degree to which the power of inner experiences of sensual awakening could create astonishing and multi-dimensional experiences of bliss that involved physical sensations as well as powerful emotions and pulses of energy through every part of my body. This happened in meditation, and in the particular state of conscious visionary half-waking that I later understood to be a precursor to the state of yoga nidrā. *In the most intense encounters with these awakened sexual energies, the sense of melted union with the universe was so palpable and real that I would actually feel as if I had entirely disappeared and was literally at one with the cosmos.*

As my meditation practice deepened, and as I began to encounter sexual partners with whom to explore these experiences, I realised the potency of these astonishing sexual experiences lay in their completeness: every single aspect of my being was lit up by the state of arousal. This was definitely not just something that happened to genitals. It was not about removing my bra in an enticing manner or gyrating in a certain way. It was a portal to a whole other universe of experience that was truly transcendent. I thought I knew about transcendental experiences because I had learnt Transcendental Meditation (TM) from a man in Marylebone during my first term at college and I practised every day. I'd been totally fired up to learn the TM method after persuading a college mate to come with me to a public talk on meditation at Swiss Cottage library, and whilst she had remained deeply unimpressed – 'Naah! If it's that simple, then why isn't everybody doing it?' – I had glimpsed something precious and went haring after it as rapidly as I could. TM gave me a formal practice to ensure repeat entry into the state of awareness that I had continually dropped in and out of as a child. Now I could go back in there whenever I meditated. Things happened in that state that helped me understand the roots of the sexual experiences I was encountering.

Fortunately for me, at the time of my early discoveries about the links between meditative states of bliss and complete sexual arousal, I was happily inhabiting the multi-sexual world of a London college full of drama students and radical political activists for whom sexual (re-)orientation was an ongoing daily adventure. There was no shortage of willing friends and partners with whom to explore these experiences, at the level of intellectual discussion (Foucault's History of Sexuality *was the big topic), at the level of intimate sharings, and at the level of sexual partnerships. But in the midst of all this what I discovered about the link between yoga and sexuality simply blew everything else out of the water.*

Whilst it was great to have a whole team of friends who happily called their rented house 'The Closet' simply because 'people were always coming out of it', and whilst I rapidly acquired a clear 360-degree vision of every possible sexual orientation, as various of my close circle discovered that they were lesbian or gay or bisexual, or transgender (or some combination of all of the above), none of this really resonated with what actually went on for me during sexual awakenings. For sure, I broadened my experience and understanding of the living reality of a full spectrum of possible sources of sexual pleasure and gender-identity, but none of it really seemed to match up to the endless reaches of energetic flow and aliveness that was happening in other dimensions in my inner world.

The intensity of these experiences began to increase dramatically when I started practising yoga and meditation with a little more attention and discipline. Although my earliest memory was of adjusting my mother's bow pose in front of a television yoga programme that she enjoyed to watch, and through my childhood I had 'invented' certain kinds of movement sequences that were clearly yogic in origin, it was not until after the TM encounter at college that I had begun to practise meditation and āsana *more regularly. This had an immediate and remarkable effect upon my experiences of sexuality as a multi-dimensional awakening.*

Part of the potency of the yogic influence upon sexuality is not simply that it opens us to the fullest flow of *śakti* in the physical body, but also that it supports a total shift in attitude. Initially, whilst practising daily some simple *āsana* and meditation on a student tour of South East Asia, for example, I discovered that even a glance or a kiss could awaken profound sexual response and release. When conscious breath is directed with attention into the sensations of the lips, then a long deep snog is breathtakingly exciting. One practical application of the *tantrik* yoga attitude is to fully inhabit the nature of the experience rather than to see it as prelude to something else. Joyful delight can be a focus of meditative awareness, as described in verse seventy-one of the *Vijñāna Bhairava Tantra*, which presents the *dharana* (meditative concentration) on joy: 'When great joy is obtained… one should meditate on that with one-pointedness, until the mind becomes absorbed and the bliss ever arises'.

The heart-stoppingly exquisite evening-long kisses and embraces I shared with the sweet-breathed proprietor of the wooden holiday shacks on a Thai island that I visited in my early twenties were essentially *dharanas* on joy, or 'kissing meditations'. These meditations were openings to a wider state of consciousness of pure love. Intercourse or other conventional sex acts were not necessary to consummate this experience, the glances and kisses alone were enough to create powerful surges of energy throughout my body, that returned in other forms during periods of meditation, dream yoga and *āsana*. It was not until I began to learn about *kuṇḍalinī* and *tāntrik* philosophy that I found any way to make sense out of the intense levels of these experiences. When I found out about the esoteric anatomy of the body and the *cakra* system and the flow of energy through the body in channels of energy called *nāḍīs* (for a fuller explanation of these terms please see chapter five), then everything started to make sense. I realised then why it was that certain kinds of yoga practice could engender certain states of consciousness, and how it was that these states of consciousness were at play in the intense experiences of sexual arousal I had encountered. Recently, William Broad's review of scientific studies of yoga has demonstrated that 'yogasm' is indeed a physiologic state of arousal comparable with sexual orgasm. A number of postures and breathing practices raise testosterone levels (the hormone associated in women and men with sexual arousal) and create orgasmic responses that are scientifically measurable.

Of course it is one thing to explore these very pleasant side effects of yoga practices alone or with a friendly person who is up for interesting sexual explorations, but it is of a different order of intensity to discover a partner who has an understanding of these dimensions of being. The paradox was that those people who were teaching me about esoteric anatomy were either dead (they wrote their books before they went), or celibate. And few of the books that I am now in the happy position to recommend to other women had been written back then. So it took me some years to locate a sexual partner who had a living understanding of these esoteric matters that matched my own experience. When I found him, I married him. Three times (once in secret in London; once in front of seven thousand people at the Sita Kalyanam festival organised by Swami Satyananda in Rikhia; and once in a ruined Cistercian abbey in the west of Ireland at a ceremony presided over by the Celtic mystic, priest and poet, John O'Donohue). In the meantime, though, I discovered that the combination of meditative practice, fluid *āsana* and dance was an effective means to channel the potency of sexual energies into abundant healthful vitality and the possibility of cosmic union at the point of sexual arousal (alone, or in partnership).

Heightened sexual response and deepened sexual pleasure can be a very pleasing side effect of yoga practice. Kamalātmikā's generosity in this regard is quite astounding. Up to a certain point, it can seem that the more yoga that is practised, the greater the degree of sexual arousal and response that becomes possible.

> *My own experience in my late twenties, of beginning to practise yoga and meditation far more intensely then I had during my college years, seemed at the time to coincide with a sexual awakening that was accompanied by the arrival in my life of a series of delightful encounters with unlooked-for lovers. In hindsight of course, this was not a coincidence, but one of the effects of yoga practice upon my experience of sexuality. After nine years of monogamy, I left to live on my own with the intention of devoting more time to my practice of yoga, and to my doctoral studies. Pretty much all I did, when I was not studying for my thesis, or teaching at the university, was to meditate, chant, practise yoga (including karma yoga), and dance.*

The daily practice of yoga and meditation began to create an expanded field of intense energy that seemed to attract remarkable sexual experiences. For example, after meeting the man who became my lover for over a year, I inhabited a state of fully expanded sensory awareness that was so intense I didn't need to sleep or eat. The first night we met, the sexual experience created a soul opening so profound that my energy levels were elevated for two months. Similarly, an experience of sweet intimacy with a lesbian friend shifted my consciousness into an altered state of awareness that created an open-hearted melding with life that persisted for weeks. Wherever I danced, a magical sense of excitement and delight pervaded every dimension of my being. The expansion of energy frequently led to experiences of profound arousal and orgasm whilst meditating and moving, dancing, or even whilst working.

Something about the quality of awakened awareness at the level of energy had somehow amplified my sensitivity to sensual pleasure, and others around me who were in tune with this picked up on this and gravitated towards it. And this, as I began to be aware, was absolutely nothing personal: many yoga practitioners experience heightened sexual pleasure as a result of the physical, energetic and emotional awareness that is cultivated through the practice of yoga āsana *and* prāṇāyāma. *Numerous* yoginīs *of my acquaintance have since corroborated that this heightened awareness can also function as some kind of magnetic attraction that is noticed by others with similar levels of awareness and sensitivity: 'When I got back from my intense one-month yoga retreat,' confided a North American* yoginī *in her mid thirties, 'somehow I just seemed to be exuding some sort of sexual magnetism; everyone I met wanted to fool around with me, in the most delicious and intimate way. It was a pretty weird yogic side effect. I didn't expect it. But I enjoyed it.'*

In the newly solitary domestic life I embraced after I left my partner, I continued to practise prāṇāyāma, āsana *and meditation daily, and the quality of sexual arousal that I was experiencing increased. Odd things began to happen. At around this time, I discovered that merely being in the same room as a young colleague of mine with whom I had experienced pleasurable sexual intimacy was sufficient to elicit a state of total sexual arousal. Just knowing he was somewhere on campus sometimes had the same effect. This was a delightful experience, but somewhat distracting, since I was at the time supposed to be directing energies towards the completion of a doctoral research project. By the time I met my husband, the flow of* śakti *was so utterly free and the levels of pleasure and delight experienced in sexual intimacy were so profound and exquisite that they began to be indescribable and almost perpetual. It was an intensely pleasurable and creative, productive time (the doctoral thesis was completed within two-and-a-half years), and it gave me clear insights into the intimate relationship between sexuality and creativity that I explore in the next chapter.*

The huge advantage of discovering sexual partnership founded on a shared experience of the transcendent possibilities of the arousal of sexual energies is that it facilitates a conscious connection through the breath with the movements of energy and awakenings around the body. When two partners engage in this awareness together then their link doubles the intensity of the encounter, and makes it possible to experience sustained encounters with energetic levels that can literally transform consciousness. Such transformations create powerful ripple effects so that shifts in awareness can be felt in every dimension of everyday life at the level of continued vitality, good health and positive creativity and radiant being. My experience of this double-strength awakened *śakti* extended into the the first ten years of our married life, when our love for each other and our work literally generated a thriving family yoga centre out of nothing: hundreds of students and many teachers were attracted to the work we were sharing around yoga, pregnancy, birth, fertility and early years parenting. The development of our yogic partnership, Sitaram, was rooted in the awakened *śakti* that nourished our capacity to live in a state of loving connection. We were able to give and share so much, because we could feel absolutely that none of the energy was ours, it was simply the *śakti* flowing through us, free.

This free-flowing *śakti* is a manifestation of the defining characteristic of Kamalātmikā: her abundant generosity. There are literally no limits to the range and depth of sexual pleasure that a free-flowing *śakti* permits. When writers and researchers attempt to codify experiences of female sexuality they run into difficulties because it is impossible to encompass the full range. For example, even the most enthusiastic, radical and free-spirited of writers on female sexual pleasure, Deborah Sundahl, has blind spots. Whilst she provides, in *Female Ejaculation and the G-spot*, possibly the best and most useful detailed practical explanation of the relationships between different types of female orgasm across the whole spectrum, from clitoral, through vaginal and uterine, to G-spot, and 'blended' orgasms, her focus, in theory and in practice, is almost exclusively genital, and there is simply no listing for breasts or nipples in her extensive index. Which is a bit of a pity really, since the depths of orgasms she describes can for many women be super-enhanced by attentive breast stimulation. On the other hand, when Diana Richardson, the literary queen of writings on *tāntrik* orgasm for women, considers the spectrum of female sexual experience, she pays very little attention to the G-spot information Sundahl so very usefully sets out. When one's intention is to live in the freedom of the full range of all of these experiences, then it's best to keep the options open. In my experience, this is what yoga can do for us: it literally frees our *śakti*, enabling us to resonate, at every level of our being, with depths and heights of sexual pleasure, as the stories I have told reveal.

A NOTE ON SEX IN NEO-*TANTRA* AND *TĀNTRIK* YOGA

Scholars of *tāntrik* history have spent years amassing the evidence to prove conclusively that western neo-*tantra* is 'an invented tradition' (White: xii) and that it has very little to do with the original rituals described in the texts of medieval (and earlier) *tāntrik* sects in South Asia. It's certainly indisputable that the original focus of these tenth-century *tāntrik* ceremonies is not preserved in most current neo-*tāntrik* 'sacred sexuality' workshops, for example those that promise bigger orgasms or *tāntrik* sexual 'intiations'. The main difference is that whilst the original focus of South Asian *tantra* was sexualised ritual, what most neo-*tāntrik* practitioners now engage in is ritualised sex. In the original contexts of South Asian *tantra*, the purpose of sexual congress was to collect sexual fluids, including menstrual blood, semen and the clear fluid ejaculated from the female prostate, in order to make ritual offering of these fluids as food for the fearsome *yoginīs*, to propitiate their anger, and to secure worldly power for their devotees and their patrons. Because this particular understanding of the function of sexual fluids has largely been lost, the intention of contemporary neo-tantrists is quite different from the original practitioners whom they often claim as their spiritual ancestors. Historically speaking, it is important to recognise that the 'neo-*tantra*' popularised in the west by teachers of workshops on 'sacred sexuality' is not in any literal way perpetuating the living traditions of South Asian *tāntrik* forms of worship. The focus is less on the worship of the *yoginīs*, and more on the massaging of the egos of those involved in the '*tāntrik* sex'. Many so-called '*tāntrik gurus*' have little clue about the original basis of what they claim to practise.

However, it is also helpful to acknowledge that although there are many dodgy *tāntrik* sex charlatans and smutty videos that have taken the name of *tantra* in vain, there are also many dedicated and authentic practitioners who are sharing forms of *tāntrik* awareness that clearly provide great and joyful empowerment to many people. The living essence of the *tāntrik* world-view has not entirely disappeared. Certainly it is alive and well in the work of thousands of *tāntrik* practitioners in contemporary India, as the writings of David White, William Dalrymple, Laura Amazzone and Shambhavi Lorrain Chopra all testify. And the powerful teachings of *tāntrik* yoga consciousness have also been preserved and maintained in living lineages whose authentic teachers have shared their experience with students from all over the world, so that the genuine practice of *tāntrik* yoga is thriving in the West. My own deep debt of gratitude is to Swami Satyasanganda Saraswati, disciple of Swami Satyananda Saraswati, whose translations of *Tattva Śuddhi*, *Sundarī Lahari*, and the *Vijñāna Bhairava Tantra* in particular have brought these authentic *tāntrik* understandings alive for me and for many thousands of *yoginīs* around the world. The essential message of the *tāntrik* world-view communicated in these meditations – recognition and honouring of the elemental constituents of the cosmos within human dimensions of being, and reverence for *śakti* as the energy present in all life, including the creative and sexual urges and cycles of women – is indeed living and thriving in the authentic transmission of genuine teachers. Such teachers include some of those associated with the Satyananda yoga lineage, and also Mukunda Stiles in the US, Jewels Wingfield in the UK, Diana Richardson in Switzerland, Daniel Odier in France, and Laura Doe Harris in Australia. Womb yoga is also informed by an embodied experience of the essential philosophy of *śakta tantra*. The practices shared through these teachings, and others like them, promote a *tāntrik* attitude to living and loving that honours *śakti* as a manifestation of the life force in every aspect of human experience, including sexuality, and that positively celebrates and embraces women's freedom to express the full spectrum of female sexuality.

Having said that, it's important to recognise, from the *yoginī*'s perspective, that even some of the explorations of the most authentically open-hearted and spiritually connected contemporary *tāntrik* teachers are limited by a tendency to see sex as intercourse, and to focus attention on a particular understanding of 'sex' in the terms that have usually been defined by men. If this definition marks the boundaries of possible sexual experience, then female sexual response is bound to be limited: 'The normal male orgasm is an act of violence against the woman. It's an expression of male impotence, using this brief pleasure like a knife to take a stab at all that's hidden deep within her infinitely capable body' (Odier 1997: 135). If the authentic ground of *tāntrik* experience is to honour the power of *śakti*, then it means honouring experiences of sexuality from a feminine perspective. This is well expressed by Devī, the female *tāntrik guru* whose teachings are described in Daniel Odier's *Tantric Quest*: 'When the *tāntrika* discovers that his pleasure is no longer bound up with coming as quickly as possible, too quickly to satisfy a woman, he discovers all the richness of his feminine side. And discovering that, he rises to the power of the woman ... The male body is numbed by the localisation of pleasure in the penis alone, while most women know overall pleasure without doing any apprenticeship' (Odier 1997: 135).

The point here is that Odier, the willing male *tāntrik* apprentice, having devoted years of his life to meditative and spiritual quests, spends several months as the direct disciple of a female *tāntrika*, undergoing intense austerities and initiations of fearful terror in order to reach the place of sexual and sensual sensitivity which the female teacher acknowledges most ordinary woman naturally experience simply by virtue of being female. The kind of sexual and sensual experience that Devī creates for her apprentice is a fully engaging spiritual quest for a man, but a naturally occurring experience for a woman. It is not, as she points out, that there are no exercises for a woman to engage with the innate power of her own sexual experiences, but that these exercises are intended to heighten and refine what is already existing, whereas for the man, the process of the initiation enables him to discover experiences of sexuality which were previously entirely unknown to him. Most women have a natural, albeit vague sense of the potential of this full spectrum sexuality, if only because we may experience a lingering sense of disappointment that male sexual partners may well seem to be completely unaware of our needs and utterly unaware of the full spectrum of our capacity to experience sexual pleasure.

For example, during his initiation, Odier describes an entirely 'new' range of sexual experience: that of orgasm without erection, orgasm without ejaculation and orgasm that enabled the localised sense of pleasure in the penis to become instead transformed into the experience of 'waves of excitement spread into every hidden recess of my body' (Odier 1997: 133). He also expresses amazement that it is possible for him to experience orgasm with no direct physical contact whatsoever. That such a sensitive and highly conscious spiritual man can consider these experiences to be strange (for this is how he describes this range of sensations), clearly indicates how different the experience of sexuality may be for men and women. For such experiences, in particular full body orgasm and the capacity to orgasm with no direct physical contact, are simply natural expressions of the fullest spectrum of female sexuality. Any woman who has experienced any kind of sexual arousal prompted by emotional or mental imaginings would not regard any of Odier's hard-won *tāntrik* initiations as being in the least bit unusual. From my experience, and from the reports of the *yoginīs* who have shared their stories with me, and with the teachers who celebrate full spectrum feminine sexuality, it would seem that this capacity to engage in the free flow of *śakti* through every dimension of our being is a characteristic of female sexuality that can bring women great freedom and joy.

To discover this freedom is to reconnect ourselves to the pulse and power of the whole of creation. For from the *tāntrika*'s point of view the woman's body (indeed each human body) is literally the embodiment of all the elements, the building blocks of the universe. Because we literally embody the powers of the universe within us, then our capacity to experience pleasure and bliss is truly cosmic. Through the embodied consciousness of our sexuality we find it is possible to encounter this unlimited undifferentiated experience of cosmic time in which all is one and all is love: 'Orgasmic moments transpire when essential elements align themselves' (Richardson: 53). The *tāntrik* understanding is that this embodied experience of elemental alignment is our birthright, that it is available to men and women, but that it is more accessible to women because we have the good fortune to inhabit a female form, whereas for men, this experience usually needs to be accessed through conscious effort.

It is not to say that this experience of timelessness or absolute love is not available to men, rather that the experience of inhabiting a female body can bring women more readily into a fully embodied understanding of what this actually means. For example, many women who have had the opportunity to experience normal physiological labour and birth report this clear sense of 'timelessness' as the intensity of the experience demands their absolute attention; and those women who have made the efforts required to honour and respect the natural rhythms of their menstrual cycle, especially the exquisite heightened visionary awareness of menstruation itself, develop a sensitivity to this experience that provides a very vivid monthly reminder of the quality of yoga or union with cosmic rhythms. Relating these experiences of our blood wisdom to our experiences of female sexuality can give us a sense of coming home, a profound relief to be back in touch with ourselves. When we unlock our *śakti* we re-connect with our capacity for inner joy and peace with ourselves: all our experiences begin to join up and make sense. Freeing our *śakti* in this way gives us the key back to our sexual selves, so that we may inhabit our whole being with authenticity and joy. Welcome home!

YOGA PRACTICES

The following section presents positive yogic means for women to encounter those deeply spiritual sexual pleasures that open into encounters with pure love. It shares experiences that map direct paths to our own experience of pleasure, power and delight, practices to encourage wonder and astonishment and bliss. The intention of all these practices is to heighten our awareness. It is this heightening and refining of our awareness that brings women straight to the heart of a rediscovery of what was already ours and has never gone away – the discovering of our own *śakti* as an expression of pure energy that can align with ultimate love. To engage in these practices is to cease searching for the sexed-up glamour that everyone wants us to buy, and by turning our attention instead to our inner world, to discover there the immense wealth of a hidden inner treasure: the freedom we find within our own sexual selves.

Pretty much all yoga practices have positive relevance to the sexual dimension of our being, but the most significant are practices that bring **consciousness into the breath** (for example the *prāṇāyama* practices pp.127–35), and heighten awareness of sensory input (for example *antar mouna* pp.460–1). Whilst it is beyond the scope of this section to give detailed examination of every practice that has value in relation to female sexuality (there are tips for further reading and research at the end of this section), what I offer below is a selection of recommended practices that are of proven value in the development of those states of consciousness that enhance experiences of full spectrum female sexuality and encounters with pure love.

Of primary usefulness in this respect is any practice that makes us fully conscious of the potency of each breath. Breath awareness practices such as the **Circle of flowing breath** (pp.128–31), and the others described in chapter four are positive ways to access this consciousness. Breathing with awareness enables us to experience the reality of each breath as a both a portal to the inner world of sensation and a conduit for cosmic energy to inhabit the body and expand consciousness.

Practices such as the ***śakti bandhas*** in chapter six that liberate and enliven the energies of the pelvic region are also very helpful, because the rhythmic movement patterns focus a liberatory release into the energy centres relating to earth and water, and these centres initiate the arousal of the sexual energies. It is important to note, in terms of accessing the more heavenly reaches of cosmic union through love, that pelvic stillness (not tension or restriction, but stillness) may sometimes be the more effective route.

The Deer exercise (pp.496–7), a well-known Taoist practice that I have co-opted to the yogic repertoire, is of particular value in cultivating female sexual energy. It works well to awaken our sensitivity to the nourishing energies of the breasts in relation to the whole of our sexual and hormonal response systems. When the Deer exercise, which uses direct touch stimulation to the breasts, is combined with a sensitised feeling into the breasts from inside, using pure awareness, then this can heighten our capacity to experience loving cosmic union through sexual pleasure. This is because such practices enable us to become aware of the channels of energy that feed downwards from the arousal of the breasts into the vagina and clitoris and then flow back up again: '...there is a circular movement in the female energy system that flows down first and then upward. Following polarity, the sexual energy awakens initially in the breasts and then overflows to the vagina before returning upward again to return to the heart. Any intensification of touch or awareness at the breasts at any time will create further overflow and intensification of experience...' (Richardson: 78). Awareness of this triangular pattern of energising and awakening from the breasts down to the vagina is valuable for women of all ages, but it becomes especially significant at times when the cunt's ready production of juices is compromised, for example during postnatal recovery or menopause. Shifting the focus of attention to the upper points of the triangle of sexual energy generation in the breasts can be a practical and delightful means to support re-connection with juicy arousal responses.

The **Womb elevation sequence** (pp.155–8) is an effective *āsana* series to awaken the consciousness of the connection between the energy pathways from the toes and feet, up through the legs and into the pelvis and the spine. This is a positive foundation for the free movement of energy throughout the entire body during sexual arousal.

Fierce goddess and lord of the dance *vinyāsa* (pp.539–40) is a practice that awakens us to the paired Śiva / Śakti energy of male and female qualities. This is especially valuable in cultivating a sense of balance in our sexual energies.

Extended heart space twist (p.159) is an extravagant and leisurely opening pose which liberates free flow of energy through the body and optimises the conditions for the experience of multi-dimensional pleasure and cosmic union.

There are two different breath synchronisations that can be used with the **Vaginal root lock practices** (pp.474–5), the first is a version of the standard classic *haṭha* yoga practice and the second is for use when the womb is 'full' i.e menstruating or pregnant. Practising either version of this technique for women not only improves the muscle tone of the vaginal walls but also increases circulation to the whole of the vagina, cervix, vulva and clitoris. Because the physiology of female sexual arousal involves the engorgement of the blood vessels of this area, good circulation can enhance sexual pleasure. The yoga approach to these practices involves an integrated, full body awareness including the response of the breath and mind, which makes the authentic practice of vaginal *mūla bandha* unlike the more genital-focused 'Kegels' which merely contract and release the pubo-coccygeal muscle in isolation, often thereby creating tension. The holistic, multi-dimensional nature of this yoga approach to the pelvic muscles ensures that the enhancement of sexual pleasure is not merely located in the genitals, but can freely extend throughout the whole of the physical, mental and emotional bodies also. Sustained grip or rhythmic pulsing of the vaginal squeeze during intercourse is not simply a tool to focus pleasure around the genitals, but can be combined with a psychic circuit of breath and energy awareness that circulates the flow of *prāṇa* around the body. In particular, a more sustained level of steady arousal can be maintained by using a vaginal squeeze in synchronisation with the breath as the focus point of the bottom of a downward-pointing triangular flow of energy that directs energy between the clitoris and the nipples.

The practice of both the squeeze and release elements of the vaginal root lock can over time enable women to bring conscious awareness and feeling high up in the vagina around the cervix. This is important in relation to the expansion of sexual pleasure into the reaches of cosmic love, because it is in this area of the vagina that we are able to encounter exquisite experiences: '… it is here that the feminine electro-magnetic pole is most negative and most receptive. This is where a woman is more likely to experience quite heavenly sensations and access altered states of consciousness.' (Richardson: 73).

The other yoga practices which relate to the sphincters in the pelvic muscles are also helpful in developing the holistic awareness that enhances sexual pleasure. The **horse gesture** (anal squeeze) and the **psychic gesture** (urethral squeeze) described in chapter twenty are practices that both develop a healthy tone and function for these sphincters, and, crucially for the experience of full spectrum sexual arousal, also enable us to learn to release and let go completely in these areas in order to permit the free flow of sexual energy around the whole of the body. In particular, the capacity to consciously release the urethral squeeze and to turn it into a 'push' is crucial to the capacity for female ejaculation. For detailed instructions of how to develop and enjoy this aspect of female sexual experience, I highly recommend Deborah Sundahl's *Female Ejaculation and the G-Spot*.

Wild garden *yoga nidrā* (pp.445–6) is a remarkably powerful practice to explore the wilder reaches of experiences of sexual pleasure and cosmic union. For this application of *yoga nidrā*, use the introductory stages of *yoga nidrā* as a fundamental practice of awareness (pp.435–40) or the invocation to *yoni śakti yoga nidrā* practice (pp.17–19) to enter into a state of altered consciousness with the intention of inviting encounters with experiences that may guide or illuminate your experiences of intense sexual pleasure and love. In this practice, the experiences you invited can be imagined, recalled or actual. You can use this altered state of consciousness to expand your awareness of the spiritual dimensions of sexuality, either by practising alone, or by entering into the state together with a sexual partner. This can be practised prior to, or instead of, other forms of sexual engagement. If the state of *yoga nidrā* is accessed prior to sexual intercourse, or other partnered sexual activity, the deeply relaxed mode of response which it encourages enhances our capacity for sexual pleasure and experiences of deep love and union.

YOGIC REMEDIES AND RESPONSES

At each stage of our lives, every dimension of our health and well-being can be supported by a positive experience of our own sexuality. Yoga practice can help us to discover the true nature of this great healing power. As a foundational practice, the core techniques of womb yoga, especially the loving greetings to the womb as set out in chapters five to seven, can help us to re-open the channels of energy between heart and womb. In relation to a positive experience of sexuality, what this makes possible is a flowing energy of love from heart to womb and vice versa, that enables us to heal and nourish the creative sexual energies of *yonisthāna*.

Sexuality and fertility

When we are seeking to conceive, it is important for the river of loving energy to flow readily from the heart into the womb. Combined with a positive energetic irrigation of the womb, a happy and fulfilling experience of sexual intercourse with the intended father of the desired child is an absolutely crucial ingredient in optimising fertility. The trust and intimacy that is nourished by a positive experience of sexuality at this time is equally important in lesbian couples who are seeking to conceive, and in heterosexual couples who are using assisted reproductive technologies such as IVF, for the foundational relationship between the mother to be and her partner, regardless of how the baby is conceived, form the ground of being into which new life is invited: this 'ground' is the nourishing energy that connects our heart to our womb, linking our capacity to love with our abilities to create and nurture. Unfortunately, this loving connection is often the first casualty when the desired conception does not happen as planned. For all kinds of reasons, not least because of the pressure that turns spontaneous love making into a scheduled baby-making task, the loving link between *anāhata* and *yonisthāna* can be severed. This severance can cause deep wounds and a lack of trust at an emotional and psychic level that makes it difficult to conceive. Sharing the yoga practices to reconnect the energetic flow from heart to womb, especially the inner form of the heart-womb river sacred greeting gesture (p.143) can help to heal such wounds. For more on fertility and its relation to healthy menstruation, see chapter ten.

Sexuality, PMS and menstrual pain

In relation to premenstrual syndrome, the positive flow and release of sexual energies can be of huge assistance in relieving the tensions and difficulties associated with intense emotions and physical challenges in the pre-menstruum. These premenstrual difficulties and menstrual challenges are greatly assisted by practising attentive cycle awareness (see chapter ten). Since a delightful side effect of practising such awareness is a heightened consciousness of the natural ebbs and flows of sexual feelings and responses through the cycle, then a respectful honouring of the peaks and troughs of woman's sexual desires can also provide a really effective support and encouragement for developing monthly cycle awareness. It's a positive feedback loop that can be happily entered at any point: paying attention to the rhythmic changes in our experiences of sexuality raises awareness of the monthly patterns of the menstrual cycle and vice versa. Awareness of our sexual rhythms and menstrual cycle patterns is mutually beneficial. One preventive measure for severe menstrual cramps is a positive experience of orgasmic release of the muscles of the uterus, and one perspective on premenstrual anger (in addition to the recognition that it is often simply a result of ignoring our body's signalled need for more rest) is that it is unresolved sexual tension. If more, better sex at other points in the cycle can help relieve PMS, then that is certainly a remedy worth exploring. The Deer exercise (pp.496–7) may also be helpful, especially for women coming off the Pill and looking to re-establish their own naturally occurring hormonal rhythms.
For guidance during and after menopause, see chapters fifteen and sixteen.

Breast health, the yoga of breast awareness and sexuality

At all stages of our lives, our relationship with our breasts nourishes and enhances our capacity for experiencing sexual pleasure. Sometimes the focus of attention in discussions of female sexuality is purely genital. But in fact, it is absolutely crucial to understand the primary significance of the breasts in relation to female sexual response. Contrary to many of the common assumptions about the singular importance of the clitoris, and patterns of sexual activity that emulate the usual goal-oriented 'excitement-arousal-orgasm' pattern of male sexual response, for many women, the deepest encounter with sexual pleasure needs to be focused on the breasts. There are many positive aspects to regular massage of the breasts, and frequent self-massage has the added advantage of helping a woman to be very familiar with the normal patterns of shift and change in her breast tissue (for example in tune with the menstrual cycle) in order to identify unusual growths and thus help to prevent breast cancer. For women who have had a breast removed, or otherwise surgically altered, the energetic flow of *prāṇa* to the breasts remains very powerful.

The yoga of breast awareness is fundamental to the experience of full spectrum female sexuality, because the fully awakened experience of the sensitivity and *prāṇa*-generating capacities of our breasts directly influences the degree of responsiveness and arousal in our vagina. The experiences of clitoral and vaginal orgasms are usually deeper and far more vivid when preceded and accompanied by attentive breast caressing. From a yogic perspective, it is not simply the external stimulation of the breasts that matters, but rather also a heightened internal awareness, a special kind of directed 'feeling into' the breasts from inside, that makes it possible to fully connect with the heights of pleasurable experience that breast arousal can bring. Clearly the most direct way to engage with this aspect of our sexuality in terms of yoga practice is the Deer exercise (pp.496–7), but all of the practices that encourage free movement of the arms and shoulders, thereby lifting and rhythmically moving the tissue around the breasts are helpful in this respect, e.g. Shoulder circling (p.506) the Seed-flower practice (pp.154–5) and the elegant circuits of the outer form of the Heart-river sacred greeting gesture, seated and standing (pp.144–5).

For the best discussion of the importance of respect, honour and love for breasts in relation to women's well-being, happiness and sexual satisfaction I recommend Diana Richardson's *Tantric Orgasm for Women* and Mukunda Stiles' *Tantric Yoga Secrets*. Both texts set out very beautifully the meditative approach to *tāntrik* encounters with human sensuality, and clearly convey the healing power of love in all dimensions of our being.

To support our energies in the early stages of a relationship

At any age, the experience of the emotional roller coaster of falling in love can be utterly overwhelming. Whilst this mental and emotional 'takeover' may be a delightful experience that we welcome and relish, it can also be a challenge to maintain balance and function in the rest of life. The drive for intimacy and intensity in sexual encounter can take over most of our waking thoughts, either because we are planning to maximise the opportunities we have for sexual encounter, or because, perhaps in later years, we are concerned about whether those encounters may cause us pain or frustration. For young women first encountering sexual intimacy, fears and anxieties about something so new and unknown can taint anticipation and experiences of sexual pleasure. Womb yoga provides many helpful practices to help maintain the heart-womb connection that enables us to fully encounter our sexuality as a manifestation of our capacity for love and nurture, and to welcome opportunities for sexual pleasure as an expression of our spirituality. Fundamentally, all of the womb greetings and honourings in chapters five and six bring us home to ourselves, so that we can positively embrace our sexuality. Especially in times when we are finding this experience to be overwhelming, then it is very helpful to do the Five dimensions of being practice (pp.183–7) and the *pūjā* to honour the elements with Sound and gesture *pūjā* (pp.189–99): both of these practices put our sexual experiences of intensity into a much broader philosophical and spiritual context.

This broader context provides a safe vessel to contain the intensity of sexual overwhelm and it can bring a deeper meaning to our understanding of these experiences. Barbara Marciniak gives an even broader, cosmic perspective: 'Sexual vibration has been your link with your cosmic identity, but this whole concept has been completely misunderstood and lost… Sexuality was left as a frequency for you to ride through the nervous system and connect with the higher mind by going out of the body… Your body has forgotten the cosmic orgasm of which it is capable because society has taught you for thousands of years that sexuality is bad... in order for you to be controlled and to keep you from seeking the freedom available through sexuality. Sexuality connects you with a frequency of ecstasy, which connects you back to your divine source and to information …the orgasmic experience brings about a healing and realignment of the physical body' (Marciniak: Chapter 21).

In times of celibacy

At any age, times of celibacy bring great challenges and immense rewards. Sometimes the celibate periods of our life are deliberately chosen, for example when we enter retreats, or spend time in religious or spiritual institutions where celibacy is one of the codes of conduct, and sometimes (for example as a result of exhaustion during early parenting) celibacy is not intentionally chosen, or may be an experience that we actively resent. At all of these times, yoga can help to support the experience of abstinence from sexual encounter by awakening our awareness to the free flow of *śakti*. All of the womb greetings in chapters five and six are helpful practices to connect our own flows of energies to the wider world of *śakti*, and the standing heart-womb river sacred greeting gestures are especially valuable during these times (pp.143–6), whilst some of the sequences of flowing movements, especially being in the cycles (pp.517–21), can assist us in embracing the experience of celibacy as part of a series of encounters with different manifestations of sexual energy in our lives. Practising the complete series of poses to liberate energy (pp.497–510) can be a practical way to identify energy blockages and obstructions, and to help to clear these to render a more harmonious flow of energy. All of the poses to unblock the life force energy (pp.511–5) are also very practical means to keep the creative and sexual energies in circulation so that they are available to nurture and enrich our creative, family, social and professional encounters.

At times of healing from abusive relationships or experiences

During these times, it can be helpful to evoke the sense of protection and self-healing that can come through the placing of *yoni mudrā* (p.150) over the womb, and the use of the deep connection with the circle of flowing breath (pp.128–31). All of the practices to greet the womb with love (chapter five), but especially the seated heart-womb river meditation (pp.147–8) can serve to bring healing love into the womb. The *yoga nidrā* that invites entry to the healing temple of the *yoginīs* (pp.454–9) may also be a positive step towards healing, forgiveness and acceptance. Additionally the semi-supine practices that support uplift and re-energising of the pelvic organs (pp.483–8) offer opportunities for deep healing. Practising the complete series of poses to liberate energy (pp.497–510) can support multi-dimensional energy healing at the levels of the body, breath, emotions and spirit.

Sexuality, prolapse and vulvodynia

Pain and difficulty of any kind relating to the vulva and the pelvic organs impacts upon on our experience of sexuality. Vulval pain (vulvodynia) can have many complex causes, including hypertonic (too tight) pelvic muscles. Long-term patterns of gripping our pelvic muscles can cause pain during intercourse, and can adversely effect the healthy function of our pelvic organs, for example causing painful urination and interstitial cystitis. Learning to release the pelvic muscles may assist recovery, so the breath and *apāna* energy release of the menstrual *mūla bandha* (p.475) and the feminine, pulsing release of the *bandhas* can be valuable.

In postnatal years, and also during and after menopause, pelvic organ prolapse can change our experiences of sexuality, making certain kinds of sexual intimacy unpleasant because of vaginal sensitivity and 'descended' feelings in the pelvic organs. Sexual arousal and pleasure, particularly those forms of pleasure that are not 'friction sex' (that involves rhythmic thrusting in the vagina) can be important keys to healing and relief. The physiology of female sexual arousal is such that the entire cervix and womb are lifted up and away from the vaginal opening by engorgement of tissue with blood and by rhythmic muscle movement. Christine Kent, in *Saving the Whole Woman*, her book on pelvic organ prolapse, includes an entire chapter on sex. She warmly encourages women with prolapse to express their sexuality, and to see sexual arousal and orgasm as part of a programme of self-help to tone, reposition and provide support for the pelvic organs: 'Sex is one of the best activities to aid in this process.' Clearly, this is an encouraging attitude, but it is important to be aware that changes associated with the ageing process may make the experiences of conventional sex acts, such as penetration without sufficient arousal, painful and unpleasant. For further details, see the section on sexuality post-menopause (p.305).

Perimenopause and sexuality

In relation to perimenopausal difficulties, many of the same tensions and difficulties associated with PMS can surface, along with additional delights such as memory loss, vaginal dryness and decrease or loss of libido. Positive engagement with sexual energy is a great support during the time of uncertainty and (often) exhaustion. In particular, it may become especially important for women at this stage in life to eschew conventional 'friction sex', since hormonal changes affecting vaginal secretions can make already sensitive vaginal tissue hypersensitive because it is dryer and thinner. A focus on breast awareness and tender touch is the most valuable aspect of sexual activity in case of vaginal dryness, because it is the overflow of energy generated in the breasts that has the capacity to enliven, awaken and lubricate the vagina. Those practices recommended above in relation to breast-loving sexuality (p.302) are also invaluable. Uncertain menstrual cycles can also have an adverse impact upon our patterns of sexual desire: for example, if cycle awareness has been a major part of a woman's contraceptive strategies, erratic patterns of ovulation and menstruation can be unsettling, and concerns about unwanted pregnancy can suppress or eradicate sexual responsiveness. For natural choices that support menstrual cycle-based family planning during this time of change, but provide the contraceptive security to enable a freer engagement with sexual desires, see p.306.

Sexuality post-menopause

There is much negativity and secrecy around the sexual experiences of older women. Both the physical changes that affect the sex lives of women during and after menopause, and older women's changing attitudes to sexuality, are taboo subjects. Experiences of the thinning and drying of the vaginal walls are generally referred to as vaginal atrophy (VA) and the medical response to this experience is often insensitive, focusing on attempts to remedy the physical problems without any awareness of the deep and multi-dimensional emotional and spiritual responses that these changes can evoke. There is a mistaken perception that because there are physical challenges, such as pain on intercourse as a result of VA, that postmenopausal women have no interest in sensuality or sexual experiences. Certainly many menopausal women report lowering of libido, and dramatic changes in attitudes towards sexual relations with male partners. But when viewed in the context of a yoga perspective on sexual energies, these shifts can be understood to have deeper meaning: it is not about 'giving up' on sex, but rather that these changes may signal an opportunity to broaden understanding of the nature of sexual energy.

From the perspective of yoga, that acknowledges all energy as a single force with many expressions, sexual energy is just one manifestation of the great life force of *śakti*. With this understanding, later life can be a time where the skills, experience and heightened awareness developed over years of practice can mean that sexuality, with all its attendant health benefits, can continue to be a vibrant part of life for as long as a women chooses, in whatever way suits her best. An encounter with the living force of one's own *śakti* may take the form of a solitary meditation, the development of a creative project, or a tender connection with one's partner. This may also be a time to explore beyond conventional sex acts into slower, gentler and less goal-orientated experiences of sex. The yoga practices which best support this expansive experience of *śakti* include the five dimensions of being (pp.183–7), the *prāṇa śakti pūjā* (chapter six) and the *yoga nidrā* with self-anointing ritual (pp.451–2). Practising balancing breaths (pp.466–7) and pelvic locks and seals such as the Root lock (pp.474–5) and the Reclining uplifting lock (p.485) may also be helpful to identify, develop and, if desired, to redirect sexual energies.

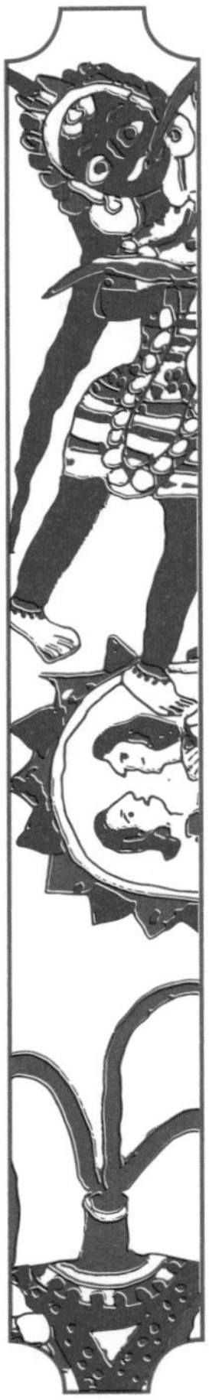

FEED THE WILD *YOGINĪ*

JUICE AND HONEY

During our menstruating years, if we're in tune with our cycles it is hard not to notice how juicy and desirous the *siddhi* of Kamalātmikā's capacity for sensual delight can be at the peak times in our cycles, perhaps at ovulation, or for some woman, just before menstruation. At these times, if the peak of our desire for sexual intercourse coincides with the peak of our fertility then we have some choices to make around contraception. If you're enjoying being in tune with your cycle then it's important to find reliable contraception that doesn't disrupt your own rhythms. This can be even more important as we come to the end of periods and our cycles become (more) erratic and unpredictable. At perimenopause, worries about unwanted conception can totally flatten an already perhaps fragile libido.

At these times, when a reliable form of contraception is needed, it can be delightful to discover that there exists such an item as a honey cap. Like a diaphragm, but a bit smaller, it's impregnanted with honey. You keep it in a pot of honey and pop it in your honey pot when you feel the need – up to four hours before intercourse, and then it stays in for four hours afterwards to ensure all the sperms, which hate honey, are well and truly dead. Using one of these little gems is like feeding the wild *yoginī* with juice and honey. See the listing below for Dr Dame Shirley Bond, who, as far as I am aware, is the only doctor in the UK who prescribes and fits these special treasures.

QUESTIONS AND REFLECTIONS

I invite you to explore your own experience of the relation between yoga and sexuality in your life by asking yourself some (or any, or all) of the following questions:

1. How do you describe the relation in your life between sex and spirit?
2. How has your experience of this relation between sex and spirit altered with different partners or different sexual encounters? Has this changed as you have grown up, and/or grown older?
3. How has your yoga / meditation practice influenced your experience of the relationship between sex and spirit?
4. What aspects of the relationship between sex and spirit do you feel that you would like to explore more fully? How would it be best to do this?

FURTHER READING AND RESEARCH

There are a lot of dodgy books out there about sex and women. The general tendency is to focus on sexual technique and to limit attention to the goal of a particular kind of orgasm. It can all become very fragmented and confusing, so that you end up with one book on female ejaculation and another on the clitoral orgasm and further separate manuals on the G-spot and *tāntrik* orgasm. None of this is very helpful when what you are after is a truly integrated and holistic approach to the cosmic wonders of sexual pleasure and loving union. So in all honesty, the only really truly reliable guides I can recommend on this topic are **Diana Richardson**'s *Tantric Orgasm for Women*, a beautifully spiritual and sensitive practical guide to the topic, and **Deborah Sundahl**'s radical work on female sexual experience and the G-spot, which is full of insight. In particular, her *Female Ejaculation and the G-Spot* is an inspiration. **Natalie Angier**'s *Woman: an Intimate Geography* gleefully sets out the science of 'liberation biology' with intelligent sassy cheek, and **Inga Muscio**'s super-radical *Cunt: a Declaration of Independence* places female genitalia and sexuality in the wider context of current cultural limitations. **Michaela Liedel**'s writings on *Yoni Massage* are also helpful, and **Sue Brayne**'s *Sex, Meaning and the Menopause* is a compulsively readable and generous guide to the experiences of decreasing libido and other aspects of female sexuality during and after menopause. For scientific explanations of why and how yoga makes us feel the way we do, the 'Divine Sex' chapter in **William Broad**'s *The Science of Yoga* makes fascinating reading. For a cogent summary of scientific research on the ill effects of menstrual suppression (through contraceptive pills, implants and injections) on libido and sexual response, **Susan Rako**'s *No More Periods?* is the business.

Other generally helpful, though not quite so woman-focused guides are books by **Mantak Chia**, **Rufus Camphausen**, **Nik Douglas** and **Penny Slinger**. For a genuine and heart-felt yogic perspective on love, sex and *tantra*, **Mukunda Stiles** *Tantric Yoga Secrets* is a gem, and his article on Śiva and Śakti in the anthology of fascinating essays in *Marriage of Sex and Spirit* is also worth reading.

Websites worth visiting in relation to the spiritual dimensions of female sexuality include the following recommended sites:

Deborah Sundahl's site is a superb source of information and support about female ejaculation and the G-spot: **www.isismedia.org**

Laura-Doe Harris's Yoniversity includes useful introductions to many aspects of women's sexual pleasure and self esteem, celebrating and educating on a variety of topics relating to pleasure, sexual health and well-being: **www.yoniversity.com.au**

Colette Nolan shares the cunt-loving adventures, workshops and artwork of the Lady Cunt Love: **www.cherishthecunt.com**

Jewels Wingfield's Living Love programme is an authentic and loving, holistic approach to women's sexuality and *tantra*: **www.jewelswingfield.com**

Diana Richardson's approach to neo-*tantra* and sexuality is set out on her site, which includes some interesting interviews with herself and her partner: **www.loveforcouples.com**

Sue Brayne's site offers many very useful links for information and support on sexuality during and after the menopause: **www.suebrayne.co.uk/links-for-sex-meaning-and-the-menopause**

Dame Dr Shirley Bond can be contacted via email: **drbond@bio-hormone-health.com**
or phone: 0207 467 8486. Her consulting rooms are at 10, Harley Street, London W1. There is also information about her work here:
www.bio-hormone-health.com/2010/02/02/dame-dr-shirley-bond
and a useful discussion amongst users of honey caps can be found here:
www.thewelltimedperiod.blogspot.co.uk/2007/05/honey-cap.html

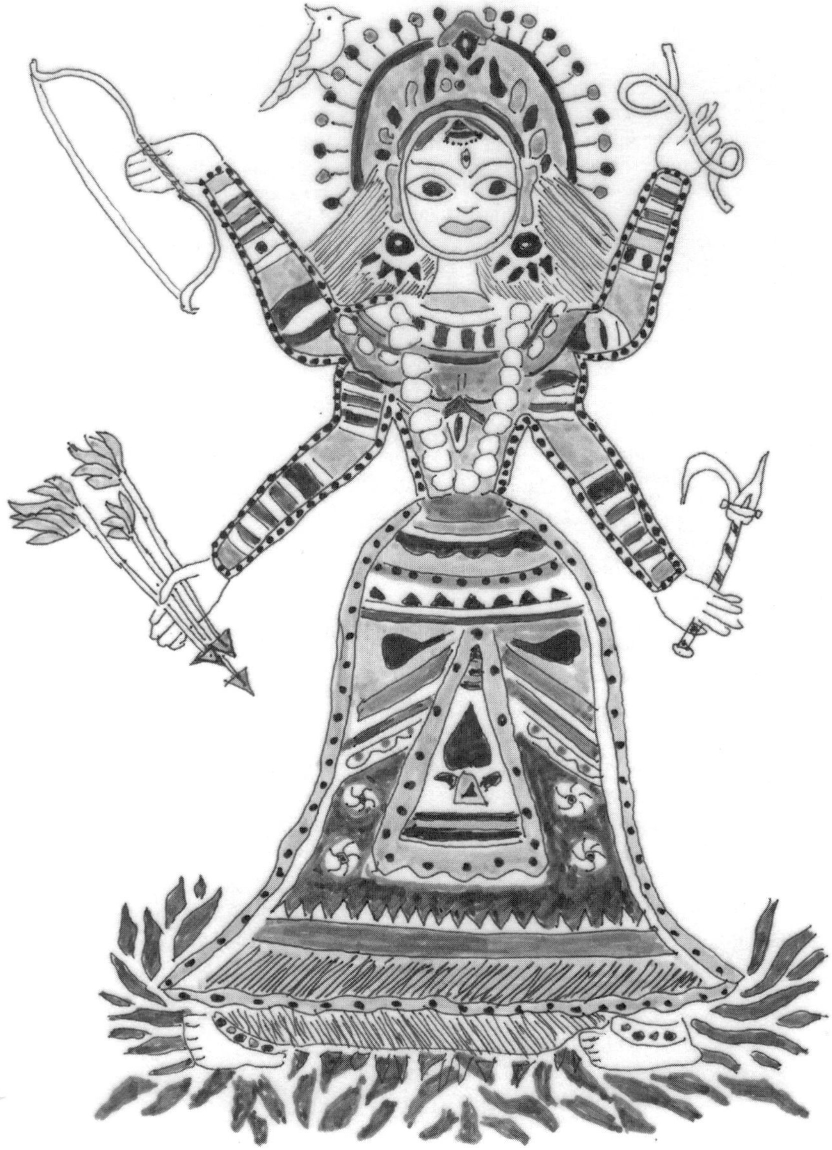

Mataṅgi embodies the power of creativity and visionary expression

CHAPTER TWELVE

Matańgi

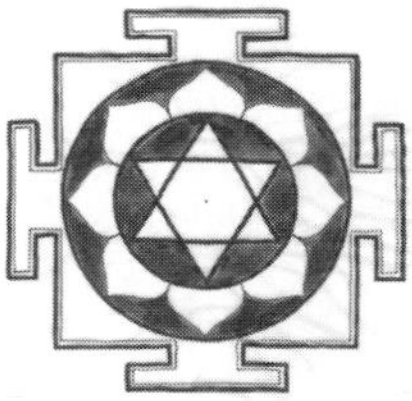

Manifesting the *śakti*: yoga and creative expression

> *Yoga and writing, I've found, both depend on a delicate balance between structure and freedom, will and surrender... through yoga, I cultivated the art of sensing what wanted to move – of trusting the subtle impulses that might be drowned out by my mind's ideas about the form a pose or a story should take. I trained myself to listen to the shouts and whispers of my body, and then took that listening into the dream space of my novel to hear what my characters had to say... Both yoga and writing can lead me into direct contact with the present. (Cushman, 2010)*

PREFATORY NOTE

The expression of creative power in a woman's life is simply another manifestation of the same *śakti* that enlivens our sexuality. Creativity and sexuality are two sides of the same coin. For a complete understanding of the relationship between freeing and manifesting this aspect of creative *śakti*, please read the following in the light of the preceding chapter on sexuality.

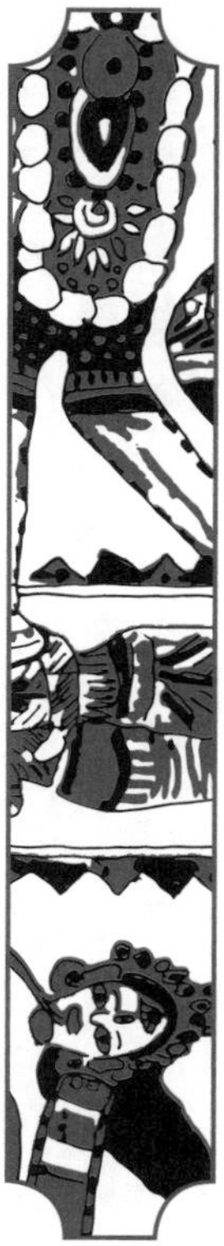

MAHĀVIDYĀ AND *SIDDHI*

WISDOM AND POWER

Matańgi is the outcaste or 'untouchable' poet who stands at the edges of conventional society. She is a visionary, wild and free from social constraints of any kind. She is associated here with manifesting the *śakti* (powerful energy) in creative expression. Her special *siddhi* is the capacity for abundant creativity and the expression of unique vision. To access this *siddhi* requires a consciously surrendered participation: for to create and manifest anything, be it a book or a dinner, a yoga festival or a vegetable garden, requires that we surrender entirely to the cyclical processes of creativity. Creativity may involve ecstatic outpourings that are joyous and free, but it always also involves spending time in uncertain places which are frightening and unknown, times when all there is to do is to wait (for the seeds to germinate, for the bread to rise, for the editor to get back with the comments on the manuscript). All these aspects of creativity are part of the process. Mataṅgi's great power is to be equally at home in all of these phases. Not only this, but her status as an outcaste gives her the power to inhabit the outer regions of consciousness where no-one else will go, to say outrageous and alarming things, to be vilified, despised and humiliated, and through it all to remain surrendered with a clear pure heart so that what needs to be manifested can find its way out.

The traditional form upon which to meditate on Mataṅgi is that of a beautiful goddess seated on a throne of jewels, playing a ruby-encrusted *vīna* (stringed instrument). She carries the same weapons of enticement and subjugation as the gorgeous Ṣoḍasī (Sundarī): the sugar-cane bow, the noose and hook, the arrows made from flowers. In comparison to the bloody choppers and deadly blades carried by Kālī and Chinnamastā, Mataṅgi's armoury is subtle, but no less powerful. For her deep and creative power can extend the boundaries of accepted thinking to reveal new perspectives. This *siddhi* can be dangerous to the stability of the conventional belief systems and norms of behaviour that rest on the boundaries of existing knowledge.

In specific relation to the creativity of women, Mataṅgi represents the power of women's creative voices to overturn or unsettle patriarchal patterns of accepted female behaviours and opinions. She pushes the boundaries and extends the limits of our horizons, so that when we manifest the power of our creative energies we can express what has previously been prohibited or reviled, and we can reveal what has been hidden and forgotten. Mataṅgi's position as an outcaste is an important aspect of her power because it places her outside of the normal social conventions. In her relation to creativity, especially speech and music, she is closely connected to the more well-known and better-behaved goddess Sarasvatī, but in her status as an outcaste she has a different power than Sarasvatī. 'Mataṅgi is the dark, mystic, ecstatic or wild form of Sarasvatī… Sarasvatī is often a goddess of only ordinary learning, art and culture. Mataṅgi rules over the extraordinary, which takes us beyond the boundaries of convention… she is that part of Sarasvatī that is allied with the transforming energies of Kālī' (Frawley 1994: 140).

These transformative energies are manifested through Mataṅgi in the form of her *siddhi* of creative expression, particularly of music and words, but also by extension, through healing, teaching and all other living forms of creative power. The name Mataṅgi can be translated or interpreted in various ways. The word *mata* in Sanskrit can mean a thought or opinion, so Mataṅgi implies the power of the goddess that has manifested as our thought processes or words. But *mata* also means wild or passionate, and so part of Mataṅgi's power derives from the quality of free abandon associated with ecstatic dance or inspired streams of words that are liberated when we surrender to let ourselves express the creative impulses we feel.

It is this quality of liberated power that gives Mataṅgi the clarity of vision to be like the little boy in the story of the emperor's new clothes who calls out that the emperor is naked, when everyone else in the crowd is too polite or too scared to say anything at all. But unlike the little boy, Mataṅgi knows the consequences of her revelation: she understands the power of saying what others fear to admit. She is fully aware of the position in which such observations place her and of her role as an object of fear and censure. So Mataṅgi's voice is brave, and terrifying to those who are constrained by fear to live their lives according to propriety and expectations. She rattles people, pokes holes in their comfortable boxes of convention, and embarrasses the cowed and silent by singing out loud and clear.

A crucial aspect of Mataṅgi's power is correct timing. To maximise the force of her power, the delivery of her observations and/or creative offerings needs to be perfectly timed and placed. In traditional village festivals in South India, a 'Mataṅgi' is a jokey but subversive and confrontational character whose role in village celebrations is to shove and push and insult village dignitaries, to belch and fart and gob at people for laughs, and generally to upset the status quo (Kinsley 1987: 207). The person who plays the 'Mataṅgi' in such festivals is a polluted, socially peripheral person, usually a woman of low caste. At all other times of the year such a person would be actively avoided, for simply to be seen to be close to her would be polluting.

For the duration of the festival, however, the saucy company of the 'Mataṅgi' is sought out as a blessing: to be shoved or poked by her is not just an amusement, but an auspicious sign, to be spat on or belched over by her is a welcome experience. It is all about timing: the role of the 'Mataṅgi' in such events is as an escape valve, a legitimate way for behaviours and opinions that are suppressed and devalued for the rest of the time to find their way out, and to be welcomed. The 'Mataṅgi' in these festivals plays a vital role in maintaining the health of social order, because she alone is permitted to upset the usual conventions. It's like turning over a stone to let the air in and the earwigs out:

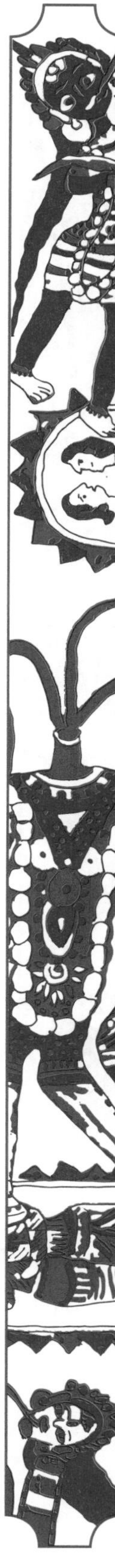

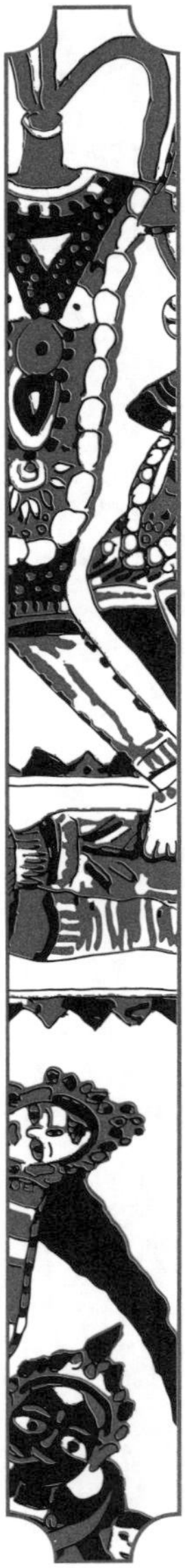

eventually everything crawls back the way it was before, but for a time, it's important to turn everything upside-down.

It is this aspect of timing that links Mataṅgi so directly to the preceding *Mahāvidyā*, Kamalātmikā. Because the creativity she manifests, just like the sexual energy liberated by Kamalātmikā, both utterly depend for their power upon correct timing. Just as there is no point in pressing a woman for sexual intercourse if she is too tired, or too premenstrual or otherwise at the wrong time of her particular cycle, so too there is no point in pushing for productivity in the reflective or evaluative phase of the creative cycle. Both *siddhis*—the capacity of sexual pleasure to lead us to experiences of cosmic loving connection, and the capacity of creativity to manifest with abundance – have their own particular cycles. Neither the natural flows of sexuality or creativity can be mapped by continuous linear progression. To receive the full power of either *siddhi* we need to respect the ebbs and flows of the cycles of their power. Mataṅgi and Kamalātmikā both teach us the importance of correct timing, and in relation to the dual creative and sexual powers of women, the timing is intimately linked to the phases of our menstrual cycles.

The visionary states that arise around menstruation can be living sources of Mataṅgi inspiration, and the upsurge in vitality and energy around ovulation, or around the pre-menstruum, can provide the power to realise these visions in the material world. Conscious recognition of the different capacities associated with these states can empower women to access deep and abundant creativity. In the section below I explore the changing phases of menstrual consciousness in relation to the spiritually transformative energies of Mataṅgi's creative power and her outcaste status. For in so far as the menstrual cycle has been reviled and dismissed, its status in our culture is very similar to that of the outcaste Mataṅgi: both have the potential to re-connect us to the forces of a wild and ecstatic creativity that expresses the long suppressed powers of the deep feminine.

LIMITATIONS: CULTURAL EXPECTATIONS

Sadly, many limits and constraints have been placed by our culture upon women's creativity. Traditionally almost every dimension of our capacity to create has been curtailed and controlled, with the possible exception of our capacity to birth and mind babies and to make homes and meals for our families and for the families of those who are richer and more powerful than us. Successive waves of feminist activism have brought welcome changes to this state of affairs, and certainly today having babies and cooking are no longer the only spheres of creativity in which women can be expressive. But this is a very recent shift.

Even in the traditionally acceptable spheres of women's creativity, the domestic realms of childbirth and homemaking, and even now, when you get right up to the top level of power-holding, our culture tends to hand even these womanly expressions of creativity back over to the men and to value their contributions more highly than those of women. For although women may birth babies and midwives may help them, it is the (usually, male) obstetricians who get paid ten times the rate of the midwives, and make the policies in the birthing units and labour wards. And although it is mostly women who are making homes and meals at the everyday, mundane level of getting food on the table every teatime and ensuring that the domestic environment is at least relatively non-toxic and that there is somewhere to sit down that is not covered in dirty laundry and Lego, most of the top paid TV celebrity chefs, restaurateurs and folks with their photos on the food packets tend to be men, and most of the wealthiest interior designers and retailers of home-making products, for example the CEOs of global homemaking powers like Ikea and Habitat, tend to be men. All this gives a clear message to women that although we may be creative in the domestic sphere, out there, where it really matters, and where the big money is to be made, it's a man's world, just like everything else, and so to compete with the guys you need to play the game their way or back out.

If this is the kind of message that we receive about areas of creative life where women have at least traditionally held some sense of limited power and authority, then it's way worse when we get out of the accepted avenues of female creative expression and begin to impinge on areas of creative life from which we have, until very recently, been excluded. When Virgina Woolf asked us in *A Room of One's Own* in 1929 to imagine the fate of Shakespeare's gifted sister (she ends up pregnant by a fellow actor and dies in ignominy before she even gets to write her first play), and when pioneering feminist art historians like Griselda Pollock and Germaine Greer kicked up a stink about the absence of the female Michelangelo or Leonardo, what these marvellously insightful women were doing was to shine their light into the dark corners of patriarchy, and show us just how and why it has been that women's creative endeavours have made such totally minimal impact on the unfolding of these aspects of human creativity. It's not that women weren't creative, it's just that we were a bit busy. For the past five thousand years we've been the ones wiping arseholes, cleaning up vomit, nursing sick children, minding babies, doing the cleaning or fixing dinner for some hungry tired man with dirty clothes that needed washing. Sorry we didn't quite get around to the final edit of the masterpiece, but that's how it was. God bless Jane Austen. And Frida Kahlo. At least they showed it wasn't because we didn't have the talent, we just had a lot of other stuff to do.

Certainly things have changed, and certainly now we have women artists and writers and musicians galore. We even have oodles of radical female pop stars and rock musicians, earning top dollar in areas of musical life that were until very recently utterly devoid of female presence. But still, in the context of five thousand years of patriarchal suppression of women's creative voices, these delightful developments occurred only recently. Proportionately, that's about yesterday afternoon.

And so for most of the rest of us right now, it's a bit of a struggle to believe that our own creative projects are worthwhile, or that we even have the skills and voices to realise them. The fact that most models of creativity are about the development of progressively greater brilliance on a relentlessly upward straight line of endless growth has also hampered us. Because most women are intimately, if not already consciously, working in circular patterns of creative processes that take time to unfold and may well still have to be fitted in around our other obligations.

So now some of us may be fortunate enough to have dishwashers and PhDs and support groups for women writers, and (ex-) husbands who might be willing to mind the children for us sometimes, just for a bit, on alternate weekends, now the field is a bit more open for women's creativity to unfold. What happens now? Now we've turned the stone over, we find the damp shady hiding place of all the reasons why we wouldn't really be able to express that powerful creative force that has been hiding with the earwigs in the dark all these thousands of years. This is what we hear:

> *'It's all been said before', 'I don't think anybody would really be very interested in what I have to say / sing / act / paint / make / dance', 'Well, I'm nearly finished of course, but I need more time to get it just right before I put it out there', 'No. I haven't finished yet. I've decided it's no good', 'In fact it's all crap and I don't know why I bothered to start in the first place. I've abandoned the project', 'Creative? Me? Not really', 'I suppose what I really lack is the confidence to make a proper start.'*

These and other forms of resistance to creativity that are especially popular amongst women, are sometimes identified as procrastination, worthlessness or lack of talent, but are all in fact aspects of the great cycle of the creative process. By recognising them as vital elements within a circle of shift and change, it becomes possible to embrace one's creativity, face one's inner critic with assuredness and crack on with the great task of filling the world's ears and eyes with the voices and creative outpourings of women who have the good fortune to be living right now, when the world really needs our voices loud and strong and clear. Almost every aspect of the challenge and difficulty of surrendering to the creative cycle can be met with a positive healing force through the great liberating power of yoga, so that the power of Mataṅgi may simply dissolve those limits that cultural constraints have placed upon women's creativity. In the next section I show you how to experience this particularly delicious form of freedom.

FREEDOMS: YOGA PERSPECTIVES, TECHNIQUES AND AWARENESS FOR BREATHING, MOVING AND BEING

The great freedom of yoga in relation to women's creativity is the gift of self-confidence. The first yoga book I wrote originally had the inspiring working title: *Yoga to Build Self-Esteem*. It was aimed directly at women, and used simple *haṭha* yoga to foster four qualities of strength, balance, flexibility and clarity. The book was in fact published under the title of *Feel Confident: Yoga for Living* (recently re-issued as part of *Yoga for a New You*). Twelve years ago when I wrote that book I believed, and I still feel now, that of all the positive things yoga could do for a woman, to foster her self-confidence and self-esteem was the biggest gift of all, because without this gift none of the others were ever going to see the light of day.

For women, the most important aspect of self-confidence is the confidence we have to trust our own inner knowing, to respect the wisdom of our bodies and to believe in ourselves that we are perfect just as we are. This is a yogic perspective on self-confidence. And there's an apparent paradox at work here, because this idea of building up self-confidence doesn't seem to sit too well with the ultimate aim of yoga, which is, after all, the dissolution of the limited sense of ourselves as identified with the 'I' that is Ego in order to return to the experience of undifferentiated oneness that is our true nature. But this is only an apparent paradox. Women still need self-confidence big time because it's simply not possible to even think about working to dissolve the Ego if your sense of self is so damaged and undermined by sexism that you believe yourself to be worthless to start with just because you are female. So self-confidence, from a feminist perspective, is a positive yogic attribute that fosters creativity and this section deals with ways to grow it well.

In particular, and in direct relation to the powers of creativity, it is truly confidence-building for us to recognise and honour the cycles of our lives and our bodies, in particular the menstrual cycle. These natural cycles offer great support for the unfolding of creativity. If we have confidence that we can trust what our bodies teach us, and that we do not have to mask over or run away from the changing shifts and moods and altered states of consciousness and awareness that these cycles are showing us, then we come into powerful alignment with the unfolding forces of creativity around and within us, and gain the sense of profound self-esteem that is a firm foundation for any creative act.

Because yoga and *tantra* give us tools to focus our attention within, they offer truly helpful support for learning to listen to the inner guide and to respect its voice. For menstruating women, the most important inner voice of all is the voice of the menstrual cycle; in postmenopausal years, it is the ebb and flow of the inner guide that connects us to the cyclical wisdom of life on earth through our connection with the phases of the moon, or other natural manifestations of change and shift, for example the rapid developmental shifts of our grandchildren, the unfolding waves of creative wisdoms, the deaths of our friends, or the seasonal shifts in our garden. Chapter ten provided general guidance on how to incorporate this yoga of menstrual cycle awareness into everyday life. The following reflections consider aspects of menstrual cycle awareness that are of direct benefit in relation to the support of creative processes. The two cycles are connected.

The first great awareness to develop is how the menstrual cycle herself provides a clear map for the creative process. Not just for women, but for all creative humans. 'I could teach this stuff to men!' quips Alexandra Pope with a cackle as she lays out the template for understanding the creative process in relation to the menstrual cycle on a recent women's leadership apprenticeship. Many of the insights that I offer here in relation to the yoga of cycle awareness and the support of creativity have been inspired by Alexandra's phenomenal depth of understanding of this work.

In particular, her perception of how every creative process finds its mother template in the qualities of experience that accompany the four phases of the menstrual cycle is of central importance to the whole of this section.

The four different seasonal qualities that unfold in the menstrual cycle – the springtime of the pre-ovulatory phase, the high summer of ovulation, the autumnal week/s of the pre-menstruum and the wintertime of menstruation itself – all provide a deeply practical way to understand and work with the cycles of creativity. Of course, the menstrual seasons usually unfold across something like twenty-eight days, and some creative projects might take twenty-eight years to complete their cycle. But the process remains the same, regardless of the nature of the project or the length of time it can take to complete. For example, my first and third books took less than four months from first commission to delivery of manuscripts, and *Mother's Breath* expanded to fill almost six months of writing, whereas *Yoni Śakti* took over three years. Big projects involving more people take longer to grow and mature, as I have seen with the on-going annual Santosa Yoga Camp project that has been developing over nine years.

These different creative processes all unfolded according to the same seasonal pattern of cyclical growth, expansion, harvest and internal focus that are played out each month in the menstrual cycle. In fact, in relation to the growth of the book you are reading now, the different qualities of the menstrual cycle became evident in the tones of voice that emerged from writing during different phases of the menstrual cycle. In the interests of sharing the benefits of cyclical awareness as a support for creative process, it is worth being transparent about the evolution of these voices. If you have read this far, you have probably already noticed that there are a number of different 'modes of address' in *Yoni Śakti*. Each voice emerged during a particular phase of the menstrual cycle. For example, the visionary fairy stories and parables of the yogic tower and the nine-gated city manifested themselves during the menstrual period, when inner vision was very clear. It was as if they arrived from nowhere and asked to be written down. There was nothing else to do.

The more critical arguments and the work around women's oppressions and disempowerments past and present flowed strong and clear during the pre-menstrual period, when my inner critic is in her full power as a terrifying form of feminist Darth Vader, breathing heavily and quite prepared to take on the forces of the universe single-handedly.

More poetic and lyrical descriptions of the womb yoga practices communicated themselves to me most clearly at times of ovulation, when I truly experienced that the process of sharing these practices was an act of spiritual generosity of which I was only capable because I had so abundantly received great teachings from so many wonderful teachers: I find it easy to share and smile during the summertime of my ovulation, and writing up the instructions for those practices is a form of sharing.

A wobbly point for me in my cycle is the early springtime of pre-ovulation when I am not quite ready to run full-pelt out into the blazing future abundance of summer, smiling and giving it all way, but am keen to protect the tender new growth of ideas from unexpected frost. At these points, some of the more radical ideas and writings took shape, in particular the deep engagements with the forms and qualities of the *Mahāvidyās* were developed in this tentative fashion, and edited later.

To read this account of the cyclical evolution of the different elements of *Yoni Śakti* through the writing voices manifested by the different qualities of the menstrual cycle makes it all sound tidy and coherent. But in fact, the creative process is rarely tidy, and I found myself in some very great messes along the way. This is a usual part of the creative process, so in the interests of exploring how the yoga of cycle awareness can provide support, it's worth setting out in some detail:

> *For the truth is, that as writer who's been turning out prose for publication all my adult life, when I came to review the first (incomplete) draft of the book I was seriously alarmed by what I read. Every editorial sensitivity I had ever developed through my journalistic and academic work screamed out in horror: 'EEK! This is nonsense. Start again!' Then it dropped the exclamation marks and got picky: 'You see, there is no single consistent mode of address here. This is a total mish-mash. It's uneven in tone. There is no reliable passive voice of guidance. It's too personal, then it's too strident. It's too academic, then it's too cheeky. It's got airy fairy visions and cosmic philosophical observations and anatomy and practical stuff and poems and REALLY RUDE WORDS all in one chapter, and that's just the introduction… It's just a mess. This isn't how books are supposed to be. You know that. Come on, you're a pro – you can see a total re-write when it's staring you in the face.'*
>
> *I struggled with this critique for a few months, experiencing it most intensely just before the bleed times of my cycle, when I considered either abandoning the whole project right now or re-writing the whole book with a single even-handed tone of address.*
>
> *It took me several more months to discover that neither of these courses of action would be the right thing to do. By the time I got around to the visionary part of the menstrual cycle once again, I could hear another voice. (Between you and me, I think it was probably Mataṅgi, who had silenced the super picky editorial critic by farting in his face and thwacking him off balance with her gorgeous hips). This voice told me that part of the value of this work is for it not to be like the other books. It said that 'Part of its message is to demonstrate how honouring different parts of the menstrual cycle is in itself a creative act, a means to access all sorts of different perspectives. This is a more feminine way to write, it's transparent and open and inclusive. A re-write would just kill it. Leave it how it is.' By the time I came around to the pre-menstruum again the critic had calmed down: 'OK, OK. But it's too long. It could do with an edit.' This time I listened.*

And so, the menstrual cycle as a map for the navigation of the creative process not only provided clear guidance and access to visionary material at certain times, it served to inspire confidence in the processes of my own creativity. Awareness of the menstrual cycle during the process of writing became a form of yoga in itself, a powerful technique for guiding awareness within to access the tools to manifest the *śakti*, the power of the creative work in progress. As a *yoginī* with very positive experiences around the connections between yoga and creativity, I understood this form of cycle awareness to be of great value for any woman involved in creative projects. My positive experiences with the yoga of cycle awareness in relation to creativity has given me a fresh perspective from which to view some of the other creative projects with which I have been involved in my capacity as a yoga practitioner and teacher. These two yogas – the forms of *haṭha* and *tantra* yoga practices that promote spaciousness and ease, and the form of menstrual cycle awareness that unfolds naturally (if not always consciously) in the lives of menstruating women – has helped me see how a positive relationship between yoga and creativity can truly empower women to manifest their *śakti*, to embody the creative *siddhi* of Mataṅgi.

For example, during my twenty-six years in London, I spent a lot of time with artists, writers and other creative people, and was always happy to offer support and assistance to creative women who were nurturing their projects through the practice of yoga. This willingness put me in some interesting situations in which to support the creative *śakti* of women. One of my favourite opportunities to serve this manifestation of Mataṅgi's *siddhi* came to me when I worked as a yoga teacher for an innovative Indian dance company, *Angika*, during the development and rehearsal periods for a number of dance pieces.

The artistic directors were looking for a yoga teacher to offer morning sessions for the company as a part of the rehearsal process. They were preparing a new work for a major international contemporary dance competition and had a feeling yoga would help them do it better. Whilst they had practised yoga before, they did not feel quite confident to design their own daily practice, and so they held an audition for a number of different teachers, inviting each of us to share the kind of practice we felt might be of support for the dancers in their creative work. To cut a long story short, I shared a number of different yoga practices from the nascent womb yoga programme that combined the athleticism of some *haṭha* yoga *vinyāsa* work with a *tāntrik* integration of *mudrā*, breath and sound and meditation. The 'audition' session also included a *yoga nidrā* of great spaciousness intended to support the creative process of working on a new dance piece. This combination was specifically designed to offer both the physical preparation to support and enliven the dancers during the long rehearsal period and the level of deep creative nurture to facilitate the growth of the dance work as it neared completion, for in terms of the creative cycle, the company had reached the height of summer and were preparing to harvest the fruits of their work in the form of performance.

The effects of this approach to yoga practice matched pretty exactly what *Angika* were looking for, and so over the years I had the good fortune to continue to work with the dancers and choreographers of the company during the rehearsal periods for a range of different dance pieces. I was often called in to support the later 'summer' or 'autumnal' phases of the project, and it was deeply rewarding work. The range of practices varied according to the nature of the dances. In particular, we discovered that the devotional quality of the dance piece *Bhakti* was well supported by the quality of spaciousness and receptivity created in the morning yoga practices, and that the combination of *mantra* and movement (similar to the sequences described in chapter seven) was very nourishing to the work of preparation for this piece. It was fascinating as a yoga practitioner and teacher to see very directly how the experiences of yoga informed the creative processes. One of the great delights of this period of my work as a yoga teacher was the opportunity to attend a special performance of *Bhakti* that was held in the Raphael cartoon room of the Victoria and Albert Museum as part of a festival of Indian culture. The piece was staged in the centre of the room, with the audience around the sides, and the quality of rapt, devotional focus which the dancers brought to the piece was exceptional, and so entrancing that even our two younger sons (aged three and five) sat in attentive stillness for the duration of the entire performance, much to the astonishment of the dancers and the rest of the audience. I like to think that the yoga practice that nourished the rehearsal and development of this piece was a helpful foundation also for the focused quality of its performance, a demonstration of the power of yoga as a support for creativity in action.

Other creative projects through which I witnessed at first hand the support and inspiration of yoga practice included some of the early work of Lucy Gunning and Clare Calvert. Both of these artists were regular yoga practitioners at the South London yoga venues where I was teaching and practising throughout the 1990s. For both of these women, the experience of practising yoga itself became an inspirational creative force that provided material for a number of projects.

> *One evening after our usual yoga class in a tenants' hall on a council estate in Camberwell, Lucy organised for a team of* yoginīs *who were proficient in headstand to accompany her to the building where she had her studio, in order to take some slides for her latest project. She promised us food afterwards, and it seemed like a bit of a laugh, so we all dutifully cycled up the Walworth Road on our bikes and stood on our heads in a cold hall for what seemed like ages as Lucy took photos of our feet nearly touching the ceiling. The inspiration for the idea had come from a previous video installation Lucy had made of herself doing headstand, simply called* Headstand *(1995). The piece was screened upside-down so that her head was by the ceiling and her feet hovering off the floor. And the idea for that piece had, in turn, come from from a mistaken insertion of a slide at a presentation she had made at Goldsmith's College in London: 'I showed many images and when summing up I had wanted to show a slide of myself doing a headstand – but it had been loaded in the wrong way up, which as it happened was more appropriate.'*

For Lucy, her practice of yoga, and her adaptive capacity to respond positively to surprising mistakes, had quite literally given her ideas. It had become part of her creative process. Not long after this little adventure, another yoga colleague who taught at a neighbouring South London venue requested for more *yoginīs* to work with her on an installation for her final show to complete her masters degree in Fine Art. This was not just a case of standing on our heads for our supper. It was a collaborative development of a repetitive sequence of movements that required regular attendance at rehearsals and a promise to show up for the duration of the exhibition to perform the piece.

> *Clare was clear about what was involved, and she was absolutely committed to the idea that yoga practice was part of the creative process of manifesting the movement sequences for the installation. It was yoga practice that had given her the ideas in the first place, and yoga practice that had given her the courage to develop the project, even though clearly some of the tutors at the college were more than a little sceptical. Everyone involved got free yoga classes with Clare for the duration of the rehearsal period. That was motivation enough for me, and, evidently also for the other half dozen* yoginīs *who showed up at the warehouse where we practised. To begin with, the movement sequences were based directly on certain* haṭha *yoga* vinyāsas, *and we were enjoying showing off complicated transitional shifts from headstands and forearm balances down into upward- and downward-facing dogs.*
>
> *As the creative process unfolded, and Clare moved the piece away from the exuberant liveliness of its 'springtime' birth to a stable and sustainable form that could be 'harvested' in performance, the more extravagant sequences were dropped and we ended up with a minimalist series of bounces, jumps and stretches that began and ended with each woman in corpse pose on her mat.*
>
> *For the performance of the piece, entitled* Still, *we were all dressed in identical blue outfits, and we ran through the sequence of repetitive movements continuously. We had the same starting time and the same routine, but because of the difference of each woman's breath we gradually came out of synch. Initial, unified and imposed order became seemingly chaotic due to everyone's different patterns, so that the whole room was full of what appeared to be random movements. It was pretty weird to watch. As unsuspecting show-goers wandered in we could see they were alarmed by the vision of an apparently comatose set of young women suddenly leaping up and down and periodically dropping as if dead to our mats before starting up again the whole cycle of jumps and bounces.*
>
> *It took people a while to discover, if they stayed long enough, that there was in fact a carefully orchestrated repetitive pattern to the apparently random motions. The effect of the piece was unsettling but hypnotic. The sceptical tutors saw the profound philosophical import of the piece, or at least that's how it seemed to us, because Clare graduated no problem after the show. She said she couldn't have handled the pressure without her yoga practice to sustain her.*

In all the stories above, there was already a positive experience of yoga practice that enabled the dancers, choreographers, artists and filmmakers to see exactly how yoga could support the development of their various creative projects, and to use yoga practice to sustain the various stages of the cycle through to the next phase of the process. Each of them, in her own special way, had found out that yoga was a positive help in the manifestation of *śakti* in the form of their dance, photography, or installation. Although each made use of yoga practice in a different way appropriate to the nature of her work, my understanding of how yoga helped all of these creative women is that, in fact, it basically offered the same thing to everyone. Yoga helps us to manifest our creativity because when we experience the effects of practising yoga, we know for certain that it links us to the fundamental source of creative energy in the universe: the life force itself. Yoga means union, and it works to connect us to the life force energy, the great *prāṇa śakti*, and that is what powers our creative projects. It is a direct line to the Source.

But the success of these creative women in integrating yoga practice into the support of their creative projects did not lie in any philosophical or intellectual understanding of why yoga might be of help – it actually lay deep in an *experience* of yoga that meant they simply knew from their feelings of practising yoga that it would be of help in their creative projects at every phase of development. It was experiential, not analytical understanding that motivated them. This is an important distinction. Because if we come at it this from an analytical angle, for example by thinking that we *should do* yoga because it might be a helpful thing to support our creativity, then it doesn't work so well.

For example, a well-known television actress who lived close to us in South London, made a sensible analytical decision that yoga would be helpful to her to manage stress and tension in order to prepare more effectively for her new role. So she contacted my husband for some one-to-one yoga sessions. At an intellectual level her decision to practise yoga seemed well founded – she had heard it helped you to relax, and she was so tense that this was affecting her creative capacity, and so she thought if she practised yoga this would help her work better.

The trouble was, because she had not actually encountered the experience of what it really felt like to do yoga, there was no experiential motivation for her to practise, or even to show up for classes. The idea that yoga would help was not enough to actually enable her to make time to do it. And so my husband would arrive at her home for the yoga session only to discover that the actress had been called away on an urgent performance issue, and had left an envelope with a cheque inside it taped to the front door. This was a fairly trusting thing to do in our neighbourhood. But this didn't happen once, it happened week after week.

At first there would be amusing little notes expressing her regret that she had to miss the yoga session again, but later the notes turned into longer, funnier and deeply apologetic explanations of exactly why she was so busy with her work that she couldn't practise the yoga that she knew would help her with her work. With the hilarious notes there were always cheques to pay for the missed yoga sessions. It was as if this highly creative and deeply stressed woman was writing to herself to justify why she couldn't take the time she needed to relax, and that she needed to make out the cheques so at some level she felt she was in fact paying for the time she really had wanted to be practising the yoga.

Every week for several months, my husband returned with a note and a cheque and a big smile, until he decided to call it a day. It was high comedy while it lasted, and I always hoped that this rather peripheral encounter with not doing yoga at least supported our neighbour's creative process as an actress.

From the perspective of cycle awareness, it was clear that this particular creative woman either had no reliable sense of where she was in the creative process of her working life as a whole, because if she had, then she would have known at the outset that now was not the time to be practising yoga. Or, perhaps if she had over-ridden the tremendous drive of her current creative state of super-busy-ness to find time for the yoga, then its practice might well have given her a deeper insight into the rhythm and nature of the creative process as it was unfolding through her work and life. That insight could have given her the motivation she needed to balance the two. Maybe she took up yoga later. Maybe she's still paying for classes she can't attend.

In this kind of scenario, it is only an *experiential* encounter with yoga that will actually provide the motivation to make yoga part of the creative cycle. We need to actually feel how the practice of yoga can nourish the creative process. Until that happens, the energy of the creative process itself can seem more powerful than anything that yoga could offer it, and so it becomes hard to resist the lure of the project in order to stop for long enough to do any yoga practice. My experience as a writer has shown me that when a person is deeply in the flow of the productive parts of the creative cycle, that it can seem completely nuts to stop to do anything, to brush your hair or take a pee or eat, let alone to pause and do some yoga. But over the years, and over the unfolding of various creative projects, I have experienced at first hand how vital yoga practice is to the sustained continuance of creative life.

It is all very well to go hell for leather on a few projects when you are young, but if what you need to manifest is a whole lot of work over an entire lifetime, then some kind of sustaining and nurturing practice is necessary. Otherwise important things like health can fall apart and then nothing at all will be manifested. And so this is why *yoga nidrā* practice has been a central part of the process of writing *Yoni Śakti*. This is not just because it is a book about yoga. Although the continuing practice of the *āsana* and *prāṇāyāma* described in chapters four to seven and in part three was helpful and necessary to ensure that the instructions given were accurate, it has been the practice of *yoga nidrā* that deeply sustained creative energies through what has been a very long writing period, punctuated by periods where work on the book needed to stop to make space for other vital activities. Especially in this kind of stop-start creative process, that is often the most common way for creative women who also have family and work responsibilities to honour, *yoga nidrā* can become a crucial receptacle for the creative project in times when work needs to stop temporarily. For example, it is possible to use *yoga nidrā* as a way to hold and nurture the creative project, a sort of 'back burner' where the creative process can continue whilst other work is attended to. *Yoga nidrā* can also be used as a problem solver when a project gets stuck: for example when a certain metaphor or form of language is eluding the conscious creative mind, it can be revealed to the writer in a state of *yoga nidrā*. *Yoga nidrā* can also be used as a way to re-enter certain dream states or scenarios in order to discover further guidance about the progress of a project. These are just some of the ways in which I have made use of *yoga nidrā* as a writer. The practical details of how to utilise this form of yoga for these purposes are described in detail in the next section.

YOGA PRACTICES

The following selection of yoga practices is recommended for nourishment and support of the creative process. Remedies for specific problems relating to creativity are offered in the next section.

Opening the lotus to *prāṇa śakti* (pp.136–9). When practised with the opening *mudrā* at every *cakra* this practice not only creates a powerful symbolic gesture of receptivity, but also establishes a hypnotic and settling rhythm to synchronise breath and hands. It is an ideal starting invocation for any creative act. Work upwards from the base *cakra* all the way up to the top of the head and then come back down to become open and balanced.

Being in the cycles (pp.517–21) This is a fabulously effective movement and sound sequence for reconnecting our flow to the cycles of life. It is a useful practice at any stage of life, but has special resonance for the creative process because it helps us to embody a very real experience of our own creative processes as part of the greater cosmic pattern of constant change and shift. Done early in the morning, barefoot in the dew, is best but at any time of day in any place this practice really enlivens and reconnects.

Honouring the power of the womb (pp.153–4) for the purposes of awakening and nourishing creativity from the primal energy of the womb, this can be practised from lying, sitting or standing, in synchronisation with the breath. The practice relates to the powers of the energetic centre of the womb, and not the organ herself, and so it can be practised with good effect in the absence of the womb.

***Bhrāmarī* series of humming breaths** (pp.469–70). Primordial sound vibrations represent the original source of the creative powers from which the whole universe was created, so this humming sound aligns the practitioner's energies with the powers of cosmic creativity. It's also calming and induces happy feelings. A positive remedy when feeling stuck, tired or uninspired.

Yoga nidrā (chapter eighteen) *Yoga nidrā* is of inestimable value in the support of creativity. There a number of different ways to make use of the states of *yoga nidrā* for different purposes relating to creativity:

1. To nourish the deep pulse of creative energies in a general sense through archetypal imagery. Use the basic *yoga nidrā* protocol and when you arrive at the visualisation section of the practice, invite the images to be of many flowers, all in bud and about to bloom. Visualise each bud bursting into flower in turn.
2. To get unstuck in a creative project. Use the basic *yoga nidrā* protocol, but when you arrive at the visualisation section, connect with the energies of the last portion of the creative project at the point where you left off, and invite the next stage to unfold.
3. To seek inspiration for a new project. Create a special *saṁkalpa* (yogic intention) relating to the project and ask for it to unfold in the appropriate manner at this time. Repeat the *saṁkalpa* at the beginning and the end of the practice. If the wording or feeling of the *saṁkalpa* is not readily available, then use the state of *yoga nidrā* to access what is right for you now, by simply resting in a receptive state of welcome to whatever the most appropriate *saṁkalpa* may be. Be patient.

YOGIC REMEDIES AND RESPONSES

As I set out in the 'limitations' section above, there are an impressive number of ways that women's creativity can be obstructed. You may recognise some of these critical or obstructive voices from experiences with your own creative processes. They seem to get around. Most women I have spoken to think it's 'only me' who hears them but in fact they are speaking to everyone at once, like a kind of undercover patriarchal ventriloquist. Below, I offer specific yogic remedies to help get us unstuck and to encourage the creative juices to flow (again).

Not believing in the existence of your own creativity: 'Creative? Me? Not really', 'I suppose what I really lack is the confidence to make a proper start.' One of the best ways to deal with this voice is to integrate calming and empowering yoga practices with tiny practical tasks to get your project off the ground. For example, use a balancing *vinyāsa* sequence that integrates consciousness and energy, such as the Fierce goddess / Lord of the dance sequence (pp.539–40), or the Palm tree *vinyāsa* (p.532), or a calming *bhrāmarī* breath (pp.469–70) to clear your mind and liven up your energy. And then immediately following the practice, do one small thing to advance the project, for example write one sentence of the email you need to send to your collaborator to follow through on your last meeting, or write three different possibilities for the project title. Alternating tiny tasks with your chosen yoga practice can inch you forward without even noticing it.

Being scared to start because you think it has already been done before and your voice has nothing to say: 'It's all been said before', 'I don't think anybody would really be very interested in what I have to say / sing / act / paint / make /

dance'. Bridge *vinyāsa* (pp.155–8) is a helpful antidote to this feeling because it creates an embodied sense of how the same supportive and creative energies work for each of us. There is no need to fetishise the value of one's own unique voice, for this can paralyse any creative impulse. Rather, simply experience how it is natural that when the creative energies flow through a particular woman, they take on her voice. All we need to do is to make space to create the conditions for this to happen.

Being stuck and/or finding excuses not to do it: 'I'll just trim my toenails / have another piece of toast / put a load of washing in / take the dog for a walk / clear up the kids' breakfast mess / go to the pub/organic veggie café / allotment / beach / or surf the internet for stuff to buy …' you say to yourself, and then give yourself a hard time for not getting on with the next vital stage of your project. Relax. Nothing is wrong with any of these things. What matters is timing, and if the creative process has reached a point in the cycle where there is nothing to be done it probably is better to head off to the allotment or get the laundry sorted than it is to sit staring at a laptop or a piano or that corner of the canvas you've been picking over for the past four hours, because if you have reached a part of the cycle where pause is required, then nothing much of any use is going to happen.

Yoga practice can teach us to respect the moment of pause in the creative processes, but to be fully aware of the difference between actually being stuck (in which case getting unstuck is a good idea) and being in a place of necessary pause and not doing. I have discovered that if there is any confusion between these two experiences then the best practice is the complete sequence for the liberation of energy (pp.497–510) with *ujjāyī* breath (pp.134–5), which effectively unsticks the *prāṇa* in every dimension of our being, and alternate nostril breathing or triangle breathing of some description (pp.464–5) which is a powerful re-balancer that helps us to discern the difference between genuine stuckness and temporary natural pauses. These practices serve to unstick us if we are stuck and to free up energy and focus to continue without further procrastination (well perhaps just one more cuppa).

Being scared to stop 'Well, I'm nearly finished, but I need more time to get it just right before I put it out there.' This can come from fear of critical response to the work, either your own or someone else's (see below), but may also be about wishing to perpetuate a certain part of the creative cycle indefinitely. Not stopping means you can continue doing it for ever – because if you stop then it will be finished, and if it's finished then it will have to be perfect – and then you will have to put it out into the world and if it's finished but it's not perfect then it's better not to finish at all, and so it's better not to stop and to continue with it forever so you never have to finish or make it perfect and you can stay in the creative zone for ever and never leave.

This one is also about timing. Developing an intimate relation with a breath practice such as the Circle of flowing breath (pp.128–31) or the Balancing breath (pp.466–7) is helpful here, because through it we encounter directly the need to shift, alter and respond to cycles as they flow. We feel how unsustainable it is to seek to remain in one part of the cycle continuously, and it becomes easier to apply this understanding to the balance of our lives and our creative work.

Thinking everything is rubbish: 'No. I haven't finished yet. I've decided it's no good', 'In fact it's all crap and I don't know why I bothered to start in the first place. I've abandoned the project'. Yoga is helpful here to bring a sense of proportion and respect to the manifestation of creative power as a cyclical process. This voice is often a sign of a particular place in the cycle where tiredness and despondency has set in. This can be the time to put the novel away in a drawer for a week or a month or more and to re-view it later. The best yoga approach is to enter the 'giving it up' experience by practising restorative yoga poses, especially those that foster a direct experience of surrender (e.g. Surrender and worship p.555). Use *ujjāyī* breath to enable you to completely let go into the pose. Take the time that you need to rest, perhaps even practising *yoga nidrā* whilst you are there. Before returning to review what you have done, change your perspective on life with an inverted pose (pp.488–91).

Dealing with the outer critics: Fostering a connection with Mataṅgi's *siddhi* is useful here. She connects us with the courage and conviction to stand firm and follow through with the particular aspect of creative expression that is right for us now. When we meditate on her power we gain the wisdom to discern that what others have to say about our particular creative project is not necessarily relevant or important. *Kapālabhāti* (p.516) is a helpful practice to create space, clarity and the possibility for discernment.

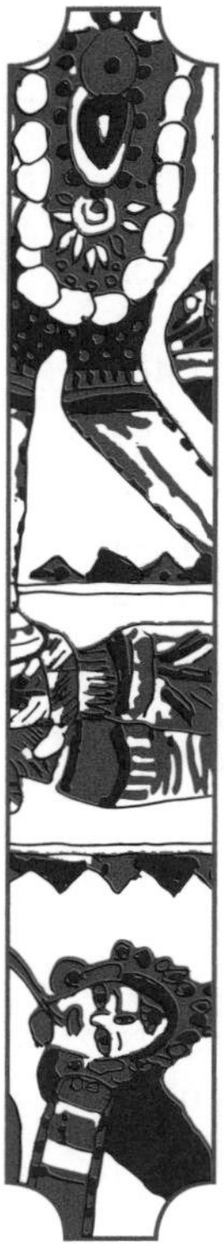

FEED THE WILD *YOGINĪ*

LUCID DREAMING RITUAL

In the midst of a period of creative abundance, or even during a drought, make an offering to the wild *yoginī*: feed her your dreams. Either offer up newly arising dreams or ritually recover lost ideas or dreams. Enter the state of *yoga nidrā* (chapter eighteen) with an intention to revisit a certain dream scenario or idea. At the point of the visualisations, actually recreate the same conditions you experienced in that dream or around that idea. Use all the sensory awareness you can to recall and step back into the scenario with the intention of recovering or continuing the train of thought / quality of feeling, awareness etc.

When the new dream comes, or the old dream comes back, gather up its quality of feeling in the very best way you can (writing, drawing, baking, collage, song, dance…).

Then give it away. Know that it's not really yours anyway. Offer it up to the wild *yoginī* safe in the knowledge that giving it back to her, to the source of story, dream and all creative energies, is a powerful way to develop a deep connection with her, to ensure the future abundance of creative flow. It works.

QUESTIONS AND REFLECTIONS

I invite you to explore your own experience of the relationship between creativity and yoga in your life by asking yourself some (or any, or all) of the following questions:

1. How does creative energy manifest most naturally in my life? What is it that I do that provides an outlet for creative expression?
2. How does that activity help me to feel? What happens to my state of mind and levels of vitality if I don't do it?
3. Could there be some creative activity that I wish I was doing, or wish that I had not stopped doing? If that is not in my life right now, could that provide a creative outlet?
4. How is creative energy flowing in my life right now? Draw comparisons with other periods and other times to get some clarity about what's needful right now.
5. If I am menstrual cycling, how do the phases of my cycle relate to my patterns of creative activity? (If you are not already tracking your cycle, experiment for a month or two by noting how moods and patterns of feeling may resonate with / obstruct / support your creative activities).

FURTHER READING AND RESEARCH

For an interesting account of a real-life 'Mataṅgi' at play in a village festival in South India, see **David Kinsley** (1987: 207). Gripping accounts of the curative powers of liberated *śakti* as embodied by female Tibetan shamanic healers are included in **Laura Amazzone**'s *Goddess Durgā and Sacred Female Power.* As a *tour de force* on the creative powers of menstrual visioning as creative guidance, **Alexandra Pope**'s *Wild Genie* is unsurpassed. In *Red Moon*, **Miranda Grey** offers a fascinating account of the relationship between her menstrual cycle and her creative powers as a writer and illustrator. For a helpful integration of creativity in the form of art therapy, and preparation for birth, **Pam England**'s *Birthing from Within* is invaluable. For an exploration of the scientific research into yoga as a support for creativity, read **William Broad**'s 'Muse' chapter in *The Science of Yoga*. As a source of inspiration and support I have also found that reading the published diaries of writers and artists is very helpful, so long as it doesn't become a replacement activity for the actual work of the project in hand.

Anne Cushman, US writer, *yoginī*, and author of *Enlightenment for Idiots*, has much of interest to say about yoga and creativity. Her site, including a long article on yoga and writing, is well worth a visit: **www.annecushman.com**

Lucy Gunning, artist and yoga practitioner: **www.tate.org.uk/art/artists/lucy-gunning-2644**

Linda Novick, artist, art teacher and yoga teacher, author of *Embodying Spiritual Discovery Through Yoga, Brush and Paint,* runs workshops on the relationship between painting and yoga: **www.kripalu.org/presenter/V0000634/linda_novick**

For an interesting article on yoga and creativity, I recommend: **www.yogachicago.com/jan10/neuroscience.shtml**

I warmly recommend Colette Nolan (aka Lady Cunt Love)'s poetry blog, which can be found here: **www.justcolette.wordpress.com**

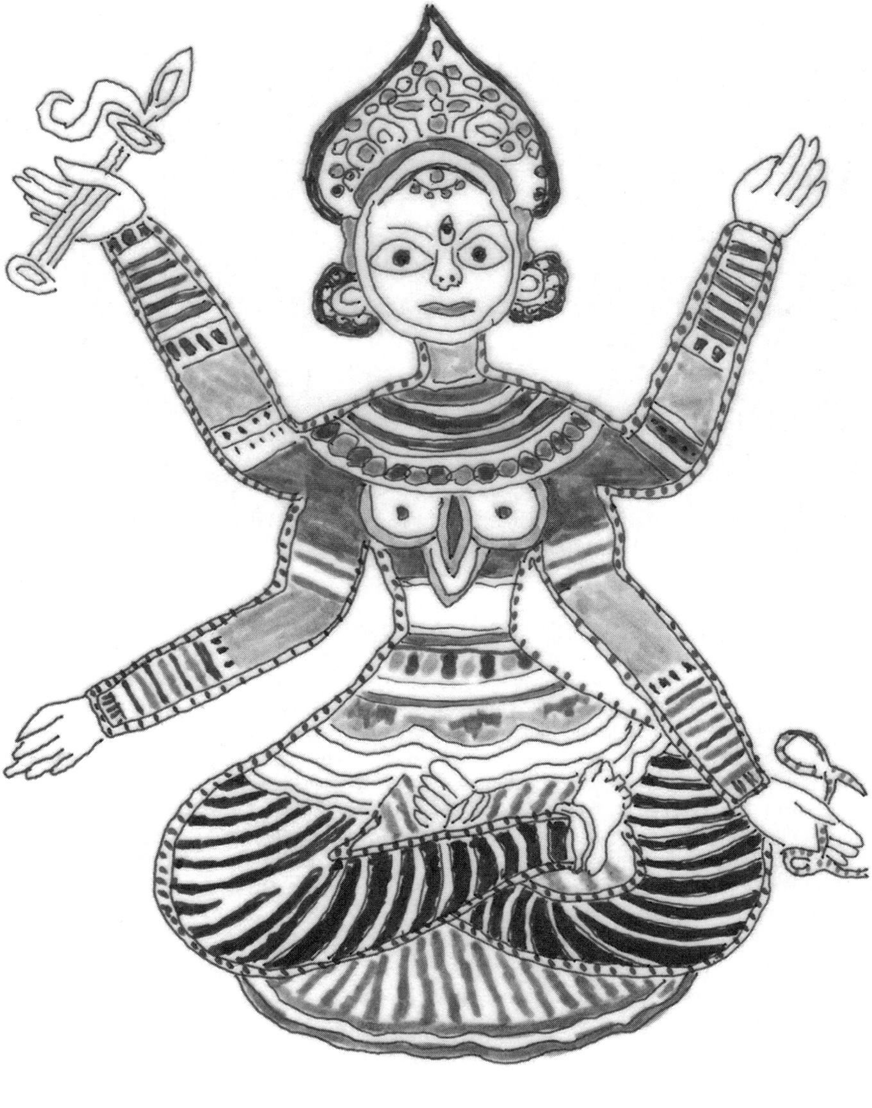

Bhuvaneśvarī holds the generous power of unconditional love, the most embodied experience of which can be during pregnancy, labour and birth

CHAPTER THIRTEEN

Bhuvaneśvarī

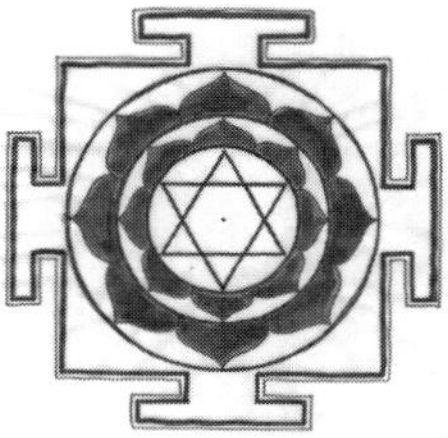

Nourishing the golden cosmic womb: yoga, pregnancy and birth

The goddess represents space. Space is the Mother and matrix in which all creatures come into being. She is the field in which all things grow. She is the receptive spirit who gives space to allow all things their place and function. She is the cosmic womb that gives birth to all the worlds. (Frawley: 1994: 96)

MAHĀVIDYĀ AND *SIDDHI*

WISDOM AND POWER

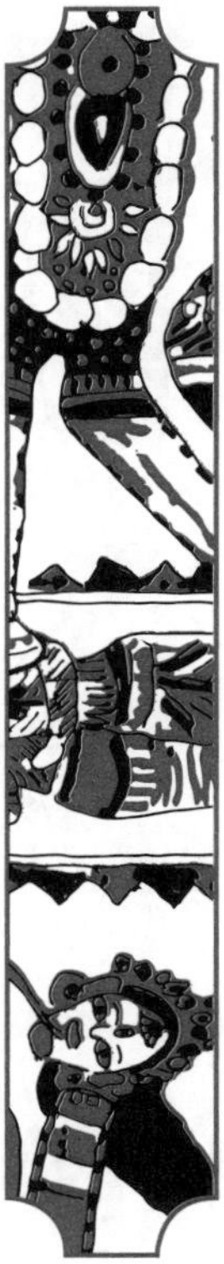

Bhuvaneśvarī, the goddess whose body is the whole universe, is also known as the divine mother of the universe. In the *Vedas* she is called Aditi, and in her creative acts she is the personification of mother nature. Bhuvaneśvarī holds the power of love and the creative aspect of space, and I have linked her here to the *siddhi* of conception, pregnancy and birth. This chapter is called 'nourishing the golden cosmic womb' in reference to the Vedic concept of the *hiraṇya garbha*, the great cosmic womb in which the whole of the universe is held.

The *siddhi* of Bhuvaneśvarī in relation to a women's life cycle is to empower the embodied experience of unconditional love. The experiences of conception, gestation and birth are remarkable events in a woman's life: they are simultaneously deeply visceral and intensely spiritual. *Mahāvidyā* Bhuvaneśvarī shares the wisdom and power of selfless generosity through the bodies of women as they conceive, gestate and birth babies. She is associated with the element of space, and she literally makes space inside the bodies and the hearts of mothers for babies to grow. Her power of selfless, spacious generosity is alive in women during pregnancy, whether they are prepared for it or not. For, in terms of the physiology of fetal growth and nourishment, to conceive a baby is to make space for creation within. As the

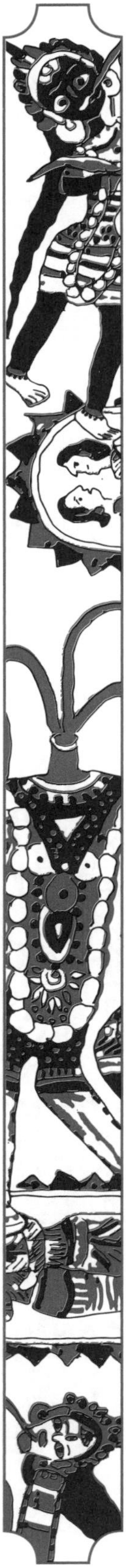

child grows, the pregnant body becomes a living manifestation of unconditional love in physical form: pregnant women breathe for two, sleep for two, and digest and eliminate for two. They also feel for two: they are twin-hearted. Everything about the experience of pregnancy manifests Bhuvaneśvarī's capacity to hold and expand space to accommodate living beings. The astonishing accommodations which women's physical and emotional bodies make to the growing presence and birth of another being are vivid, microcosmic testimonies to the power of Bhuvaneśvarī's boundless capacity for holding the cosmic space that nurtures and sustains all life.

At a philosophical level, the experiences of conception and pregnancy have the potential to open our consciousness to a truly vivid understanding of our physical self as a microcosm: of the experience of the forces of all the elements in the macrocosm at play within our own being. If that has not become truly apparent by the time labour begins, then the force of nature that is the power of birth offers a further, more direct encounter with the experience of elemental forces pulsing through our flesh and blood. A women in labour is like a tornado or a hurricane, or a great storm raging at sea. Her very breath and body are alive with the power of birth itself: 'Don't expect a lady to be reasonable when she is having a baby' (Gaskin: 348).

These direct experiences of the creative energies of the great mother's power are astonishing enough, but in many ways pregnancy and birth are merely a preparation for the profound *sādhanā* (spiritual practice) of mothering which follows, during which time the great *siddhi* of Bhuvaneśvarī's spacious capacity for love grows and matures as we negotiate the sometimes shocking and challenging demands of mothering. Mothers realise (sooner or later) that in order to mother well, a mother's love needs to be spacious as well as generous. As children grow and their needs change, then the deep *siddhi* of Bhuvaneśvarī teaches that a truly deep love is a love that gives a child freedom and space. As the mother of the universe, Bhuvaneśvarī is present in all space, for it is her ability to hold and expand space that creates a nurturing home (the world as her womb) for all beings.

Literally, Bhuvaneśvarī means the ruler (*īśvarī*) of the realm of beings (*bhuvana*). Her body is the universe itself, and everything in the universe, including all beings, are simply ornaments to decorate her form. There is a place for every living thing, and all have their own space within the loving embrace of the universal mother. Her traditional meditational form is very like the gorgeous Ṣoḍasī (Sundarī). Four arms hold a noose and a goad, and offer the gestures that grant wishes and banish fear.

She too is the colour of dawn light, and wears the crescent moon on her head. She too sits on a regal couch supported by five forms of Śiva, maintaining her own space of absolute serenity and peace, whilst directing and observing the actions of all beings.

One aspect of Bhuvaneśvarī's *siddhi* of spaciousness is the capacity to witness and hold the space in which everything unfolds. By the creation of spaciousness she invites generosity and the expansion of love – by giving it away. This aspect of her wisdom is especially resonant in the experiences of birthing and mothering, where the arrival of subsequent children is accompanied by an expansion of the capacity to love, and the often astonishing discovery that the intensity of love that can be felt for the first child readily expands and grows to include other siblings.

For those women who are not mothers, then the nurturing spaciousness of Bhuvaneśvarī relates very directly to the capacity to pour loving and nourishing energy into 'babies' of the mind and heart, such as businesses, creative projects and any form of work in the world that requires the holding space of nurture and attentive love in order to grow and thrive. For many women, the mothering energy of Bhuvaneśvarī's *siddhi* of deep love and generous spacious holding manifests in a life of caring and nurturing other beings.

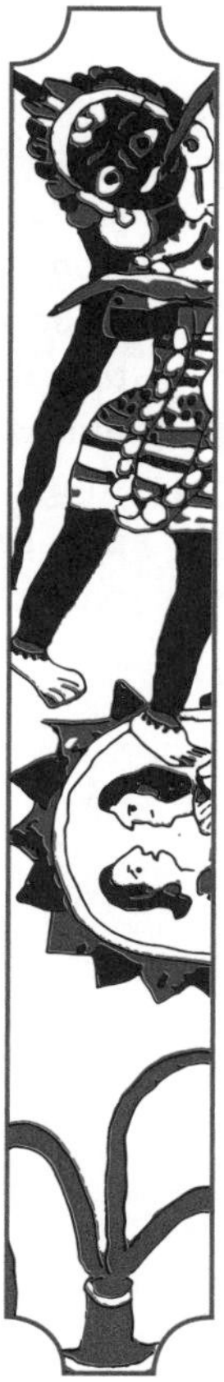

LIMITATIONS: CULTURAL EXPECTATIONS

> *... by the early 1900s ... the fast development of industrialised childbirth became visible ... the primary phenomenon was the increased control of the birth process by doctors ... Concentration in large hospitals is not the only characteristic of industrialised childbirth. There is also a striking tendency towards standardisation. 'Routine' and 'protocols' are key words in modern obstetrics ... In the age of industrialised childbirth the mother has nothing to do. She is a 'patient'. (Odent 2002: 24–29)*

In comparison to the spacious generosity that is the essence of Bhuvaneśvarī's immense power, many mothers in our culture experience a profound lack of time and space. The multitude of tasks and responsibilities that accompany motherhood fill women's space and time to the degree that they have not a single un-scheduled minute in their hectic days. Life for many working mothers becomes an exhausting marathon that has us literally running between workplace and childminders, from school to nursery, from late nights to early mornings, grabbing sandwiches and snacks to eat *en route* and dashing frantically from one overdue pick-up or late appointment to the next, whilst trying to fit in the shopping, cooking and laundry between work deadlines and last minute prep for whatever significant school event about which we may have almost forgotten (again).

This experience of a combined lack of available time and an intense pressure to get 'everything done' can begin during pregnancy, when the current pattern is for women to remain at work for as long as possible prior to the birth of our babies. The tendency is to save up whatever maternity leave is available in order to maximise the time with the baby before having to find a nursery space and return to work. Often, time is so scarce and the pressures are so intense, that mothers-to-be find ourselves struggling through late pregnancy and entering labour in a state of stressed exhaustion, having only recently handed over our workload, and packed in a few birth preparation sessions before the contractions start.

> *Jenny was a successful lawyer in a major London firm, working towards a partnership, up to her neck in cases and expecting her first baby. She routinely worked very late nights and was permanently exhausted. She planned to give herself a couple of days' rest before the due date she had been given for the arrival of her baby, but in the event she went into labour a week earlier than she expected and felt she had no time to ready herself: 'I remember falling into bed after working really late one evening, and thinking to myself "I'll never be able to labour in this state". When I woke up early in the morning with contractions starting I was still shattered. The whole labour was a disaster for me because I was tired to start with. I just couldn't cope.'*
>
> *Other women find that the pressures of work and family push them to the very edges of what their energy permits: 'I fall asleep every night at seven-thirty when I put my toddler to bed,' explained an exhausted teacher, thirty weeks pregnant with her second child. She was working part-time and taking care of her three-year-old daughter on her 'days off': the combination was wearing her out.*

In such circumstances, it is no accident that pregnancy yoga has become one of the forms of yoga whose popularity has increased most rapidly over recent years. Having taught yoga to pregnant women for the past eighteen years, I can testify to its astonishingly healing effect. When women who are scheduled to within an inch of their lives actually make space to attend even a single pregnancy yoga class each week they receive a remarkable range of benefits, from the obvious physical experiences of being able to move and breathe more freely, to a profound healing sense of deep rest and ease. The spaciousness and comfort of pregnancy yoga classes can support women's understanding of pregnancy as a multi-dimensional preparation for motherhood: for women who have never practised yoga before, yoga in pregnancy can open the door to a spiritual perspective on bodily experience that is really helpful during pregnancy. For women who already have a well-established yoga practice, then the opportunity to adapt and adjust their yoga practice during pregnancy can show how the essence of yoga is not tied to outward forms and familiar systems of practice, but resides rather in the experiences of connection that yoga facilitates.

For all pregnant women, especially those who are expecting their first babies, labour and birth can be anticipated with great fear. It is this fear that paralyzes women to the degree that we become willing to accept any kind of medical assistance or pain relief, often regardless of how these interventions may in fact be inimical to the natural and healthy unfoldment of labour and birth. The development of what Michel Odent describes as 'industrialised childbirth' has grown alongside this profound fear. A great disempowerment of women occurs when we become so afraid of this natural occurrence that we seek to avoid the experience of it completely rather than to discover that we have within our own selves an immense capacity to engage with its power.

FREEDOMS: YOGA PERSPECTIVES, TECHNIQUES AND AWARENESS FOR BREATHING, MOVING AND BEING

> *Practising yoga during pregnancy is one way to heal the split between soul and spirit found in our culture. Prenatal yoga sexualizes spirituality and spiritualizes fertility. It is the tantric practice of mothers. Once the babies come planetside, our yoga practice shifts into karma yoga beyond belief. We become servants to our babies and our path is* bhakti *yoga, the practice of devotion. Giving conscious birth is woman's vision quest, par excellence. It is ultimate* sādhana, *spiritual practice – which requires purity in strength, flexibility, health, concentration, surrender, and faith. (Baker 2001: xii)*

In a culture where birth is widely feared and the experience of pregnancy is largely medicalised and managed, pregnancy yoga has a vital role to play in awakening women's understanding of embodied spirituality. The souls coming to life on earth reside first within the wombs of the women who carry them, and the female *siddhis* of pregnancy and birth make these everyday miracles possible. The tides of blood and hormones which sustain these remarkable experiences operate under the direct influence of the moon. Ask any midwife when the labour wards are likely to be full to overflowing and she will point to the great tidal moments of full and new moons. The onset of labour, like the patterns of the menstrual cycle, can manifest the lunar rhythms at work in women's bodies. Yoga in pregnancy brings conscious awareness to the rhythmic changes at work in the physical body of the pregnant woman.

> *When asked to describe what really characterises the essence of the experience of early pregnancy, a yoga teacher in the eighteenth week of her pregnancy with her first baby waxed lyrical: 'It's the sensory vividness of the whole thing – I feel like I've never seen the world properly before. Now I'm pregnant every sense seems heightened: I notice the grass and the sky and the living energy of the trees and the birds – everything smells powerfully alive and I feel part of it all like never before. It's like how you feel just after you finish a really good yoga practice, but all the time!'*

From a yogic perspective, the practice of conscious breath, movement and meditations during pregnancy and birth are powerful means to re-connect the consciousness of pregnant women with elemental rhythms. Practising yoga when we are pregnant helps us to learn to respect and honour the immense forces of breath and growth at work in our own bodies, and to feel how to use yoga to allow these forces to flow healthily without obstruction or restraint. This is a powerful antidote to the medicalised, fearful attitudes to birth that are so prevalent in our culture. To do yoga during pregnancy is a very potent and precious experience because it has the potential to assist the woman not only to adapt and accommodate with grace and acceptance to the changes that occur during pregnancy, but also to make use of the powerful yogic consciousness of breath and movement during labour and birth. The experiences encountered during the practice of yoga for pregnancy can directly empower a woman to birth her baby in the spirit of conscious surrender to the forces of nature that are at work during the labour and birth. This is of world-changing significance, because the more souls who can enter the world through the bodies and on the breath of consciously surrendered, connected women, the more people there will be in the world who are empowered to arrive fully conscious and awakened to the life of the spirit.

Yoga for pregnancy is an immensely powerful transformative force in the world because it harnesses two of the most powerful female *siddhis* (pregnancy and birth) to the clarity of yoga consciousness. For many women who encounter yoga for the first time during pregnancy, there arises a permanently expanded consciousness of the healing power of yoga. It is often a time of 'embodiment', a time when women who have lived all their lives on their wits and in their intellects finally realise that: 'Giving birth is something a woman does with her body, not in her head.' (Pam England).

> *During her first pregnancy, Harriet discovered that yoga opened her awareness to a whole new way of life. A barrister who previously had been utterly focused on her very successful career and the material benefits it brought, Harriet started her pregnancy yoga classes determined that the best thing for her would be to 'Get it out and get it over with': if she couldn't book in for an elective caesarean then she wanted an epidural as early she could so that she had no experience of the labour pain. She saw yoga as a way to keep her fit and mobile so she could carry on regardless. She planned to work right up to the labour, to book a place in a nursery for the baby as soon as she could and to get back to work fast. 'I told them at work I'd be available for email enquiries right up until I went into labour and then immediately after the birth. I don't want to be wasting any time' announced Harriet at the first yoga session she attended when she was thirteen weeks pregnant. The other women in the class looked a bit shocked.*
>
> *Over the weeks, as Harriet settled more into the relaxing effects of the practices of pregnancy yoga, she began to review her plans.*

She started to move and breathe in ways that helped her to trust her own body. By twenty weeks along she began to feel that perhaps, after all, she and her baby would get off to the best start if she laboured as naturally as she could. She investigated the effects of epidural anaesthesia. She didn't like what she discovered. She felt deeply relaxed after her yoga sessions. Harriet made friends with a neighbour who was expecting about the same time as her and planning a home birth. They travelled to and from the pregnancy yoga classes together and they got talking. By the time Harriet was thirty weeks pregnant she was seriously considering a home birth.

In the end, much to her own surprise, Harriet opted for an independent midwife, had a very positive experience of homebirth and fell so deeply in love with her baby son and her new role as a mother that she couldn't face going back to work. She told the office she was not available for email consultations, and she started to see life differently: 'It was definitely something to do with the yoga,' she explained as she turned up for a repeat dose of pregnancy yoga when she found herself expecting her second baby. 'Everything about who I thought I was and what I thought mattered in life somehow shifted. The yoga helped me find my trust in myself as a woman, supported me through a phenomenal experience of birth, and now my whole life has changed.'

Harriet gave up being a barrister and retrained as a photographer. She specialises in photographing pregnant women and young families: 'I want for my work to capture the magical time of being pregnant and having young babies – it's a time in life when everything is open to review. Yoga helped me make the most of it. I'm a changed woman. I love life and I love yoga!'

For Harriet, her pregnancy yoga class was her first encounter with yoga. But for those women who have practised yoga before pregnancy, the experience of adapting and adjusting their practice through pregnancy and beyond can expand their previous concepts of yoga to include a more holistic and profound understanding of its transformative essence that reaches far beyond attachment to familiar forms or systems of yoga postures. I have lost count now of the numbers of yoga teachers and yoga practitioners who tell me that it was the experience of being pregnant that actually helped them to understand the real meaning of yoga.

Alex, for example, arrived at the integrated mother and baby yoga teacher training with a burning desire to share the great joy which yoga had brought to her during her pregnancy and during her son's babyhood: 'I thought I knew my body. I was a dancer. And I thought I knew all about yoga. I was a yoga teacher. But then I got pregnant and I realised I had to start all over again. I didn't really know anything, not from the inside. All the other yoga I had done before

I got pregnant was just about the outside stuff. Being pregnant and doing yoga really changed my understanding of what the point of it was. It opened my heart. It showed me the real transformations come from the inside.'

One of the great benefits of pregnancy yoga is that it can awaken women to their own capacity to labour well, and to encounter birth as an opportunity for a profound spiritual initiation. The breath, movement and meditation practices that are encountered in pregnancy yoga can provide a hugely supportive foundation for women to enter into labour and birth with a sense that they can trust an instinctual and embodied response to these great challenges. Of all the practices that empower women to experience conscious surrender, it is the practice of *prāṇāyāma* during pregnancy and birth that brings this home most completely. Practising yoga during pregnancy helps women to learn to follow the breath and to be guided by the deep blood wisdom of the body. This experience enables women to face the challenge of birth by letting the breath help us to make a conscious surrender to the great forces which are working through the body: it is a generous and spacious surrender, to 'get out of the way' of birth. This is the yoga of birth, the great *siddhi* of Bhuvaneśvarī. It is beautifully expressed by Karen, who gave birth to her daughter after attending pregnancy yoga classes from as soon as she knew she was pregnant:

What I learnt in those classes was totally invaluable. I learnt to breathe and to move, of course, and to be confident that I could birth my baby, but more than that, I learnt that I had a connection to my baby, and to my own inner guide. I trusted that inner guide when I went into labour and I breathed my way through the whole extraordinary experience. I feel it was a huge blessing, it was a rite of passage. Yoga helped me appreciate that.

Yoga practised during pregnancy helps to carry women through the challenging experiences of birth, not because it protects us from the pain, but because it makes it possible to find a deep strength and trust that help us to encounter that pain as a process, and to take each moment of the labour as it comes, without expectation that it will be anything other than what it is. This is a profound freedom. Every birth is different, and every woman is different, so even for the same mother approaching birth for each child reveals different ways in which yoga empowers us to be free to face to the special nature of each contraction with courage and trust.

All of my three children were born in our yoga space in Brixton Hill, South London, and I breathed through each labour with a very similar set of yoga techniques – ujjāyī *(pp.134–5) and Golden thread breath (p.462) in a Peaks and valleys sequence (p.463) – but at each birth these breaths revealed to me a fresh aspect of freedom. As a woman in her early thirties, giving birth to my first son, I encountered the freedom of realising that my labour did not match up to anything I had read about: after forty-eight hours in early labour,*

I spent six hours in a state of deep yogic meditation, breathing my Golden thread breath into the centre of a yantra *before moving into an effortless second stage labour that lasted barely twenty minutes before my son arrived with his hand on his head, like a silent philosopher pondering the meaning of life. He didn't cry.*

And so, two-and-a-half years later when I was in labour on my second son, I thought I knew what was what. I felt I was ready to birth him after a few hours of labour. But when contractions went into a state of suspended animation that nothing seemed to shift, it was the same yoga breath that carried me through the relatively easy birth of a loudly yelling baby, followed by a post-partum haemorrhage that sank me deep into an extended postnatal recovery period of anaemia and exhaustion, which lasted for over a year.

*By the time I came to birth my daughter when I was forty-two, I was pretty sure I knew what to expect: I was fitter and healthier than I had been on the second birth, but still utterly unprepared for an astonishingly long and drawn-out second stage labour that prompted all sorts of desperate measures to encourage my daughter to arrive. 'I've written a f*****g book about this' I panted, as I shoved and pushed down into my vagina with the next massive contraction. An hour later I was still shoving, and I was pissed off. 'In fact, I've written two f*****g books about this. I'm supposed to know what I'm doing. Why am I having to push? I have effortless second-stage labours.' But no matter how I bunny-hopped and swore, or sang raucously at the top of my voice, or sank my nails into my husband's arm, or breathed the great power of the breath right into my perineum, my daughter was simply not coming down. I kept breathing and singing, and in utter desperation I even turned a few cartwheels: 'Don't tell the ladies in the pregnancy yoga teacher training courses. This isn't very safe!' Maybe the cartwheels would have helped if I'd done a few more, but by that time I was out of juice.*

Eventually I just gave up. I admitted I had no clue what was going on, and I let the forces of birth take over. I just breathed and got out of the way. Bhuvaneśvarī gave me space and time. In the space between the breaths, what the great siddhi *of birth taught me was that some things cannot be rushed. And so it was not until I had given up on everything but my trust in the breath that my daughter chose her moment. When the time was right her arrival was indeed, at last, effortless.*

She was born singing. She sang out loud as her head was born, even before the rest of her body appeared. It was such an extraordinary experience that all I could do was breathe: the breath gave me a thread to follow, something to trust at a time when what was actually happening didn't seem quite possible. The midwives were so astonished that they went hunting through their textbooks that night and came back the following day to assure us that in the first place they had never seen anything like it, and in the second place it was impossible for a baby to sing before she breathed, but they had to believe it had happened because they had seen it with their own eyes.

Each of these three births was unique. Each birth on earth is unique, because every soul arriving has her own special way of getting here. Pregnancy yoga and yoga for birth is not about giving us a blueprint for doing birth the 'yoga way', it is about giving us the capacity to trust that our breath and our bodies will enable us to meet with an open heart whatever birth experiences we and our babies encounter: openness and acceptance to adapt and accommodate is the 'yoga way'. Bhuvaneśvarī's *siddhi* is the power to know that we can let labour happen well if we open our hearts, our breath and our bodies to the forces that need space to move through us to birth our children. Yoga helps us to do this.

YOGA PRACTICES

The small selection of practices identified below form the core of the yoga that I have found to be of most value to women during pregnancy and birth. Following these basic recommendations are a list of common experiences during pregnancy and some simple yoga responses / remedies. Because I have written at length on these topics elsewhere (see Dinsmore-Tuli 2006 & 2008), I have kept things here brief.

Āsana practice can be based around these three fundamentally helpful practice groups:

The **Mermaid twist (sacro-iliac joint-stabilising practice)** (pp.514–15) provides support and gentle rhythmic movement for the pelvis that is of especial value during pregnancy, when the pelvic joints come under stress.

The **Full moon salute** (pp.522–6) is a spacious and feminine version of the sun salutation (*sūrya namaskār*) that is especially suitable during pregnancy and can be practised in a delicious and leisurely manner right through until the end of pregnancy.

The **Rising snake series** (p.543) is part of the full moon salute, but can be helpfully practised independently throughout pregnancy as a wonderful way to maintain vitality and mobility throughout the spine. It is easily adapted by bringing the knees wider and using support underneath the buttocks and/or under the forearms to support the wrists.

In terms of resting positions, **Supported side-lying** (p.551) is a crucial pose that makes it possible to rest comfortably even at the very end of the pregnancy. It is also a valuable pose for breastfeeding.

Pregnancy (full womb) *mūla bandha* (p.475) provides a helpful expansion of the understanding of how to release the pelvic diaphragm and vaginal walls in preparation for second stage labour. This practice also prepares for an effective use of the Peaks and valleys breath (p.463, also used as Birthing breath).

Golden thread / *ujjāyī* peaks and valleys (pp.462–3) is the most helpful combination of breath to use as pain relief during labour and birth. Becoming familiar with this approach to breathing empowers you to make use of it however comes most naturally to you during labour, so that it ceases to be a 'learnt technique' and becomes instead your own inner resource.

***Bhrāmarī* (Tibetan version)** (pp.469–70) is perhaps the most calming breath practice to bring the attention and awareness within. It can be combined with postures or deep relaxation (for example the *yoga nidrā* below) to maximise its settling and calming effects. It also provides a very beautiful sonic massage for the unborn child, who will recognise these sounds after birth so, in this way, *bhrāhmarī* becomes a valuable mothering tool for soothing fretful or sleepless infants.

Nourishing growth *yoga nidrā* (pp.446–8) is the most beautiful and profound practice to connect with the unborn child and the protective space of the womb. Ideally, listen to the recording daily (or to the pregnancy *yoga nidrās* on **www.yoganidranetwork.org**), and then the benefits accumulate: complete rest, deep healing, access to intuitive knowing and the wisdom of the womb herself.

YOGIC REMEDIES AND RESPONSES

Set out below are nine common experiences during pregnancy and birth, together with suggested yogic remedies / responses to be free from the suffering they may cause.

Anxiety: This is often a direct effect of over-exposure to medical information or other people's horror stories about pregnancy and birth, so part of the yogic remedy is to eschew impersonal external sources of information (in particular the internet) and direct attention towards the discovery of inner knowing, supported by people whose approach to life (especially pregnancy and birth) makes you feel happy and safe. Techniques to support the discovery of inner calm and intuitive knowing which serve as antidotes to anxiety are *ujjāyī* breath (p.134–5), Nourishing growth *yoga nidrā* (p.446–8), and the Heart / womb meditation (p.147). Lack of sleep can exacerbate anxiety during pregnancy, so see also the recommendations below for insomnia. If the roots of your anxiety are fear of labour and birth, then the most helpful approach is to become deeply familiar with those breath and movement patterns that can be used as effective pain relief, for example, Golden thread breath (p.462) and Peaks and valleys breath (p.463). Practising daily, especially in combination with *yoga nidrā*, can assist in reducing fear and relieving anxiety about birth.

Breech baby: The position of the baby can become a major source of concern in pregnancy. Babies have plenty of room to spin and turn until at least thirty-six weeks of pregnancy when they begin to run out of space, so efforts to alter the final resting position of the baby are not often necessary until later in pregnancy. Generally keeping active and frequently practicing all-fours poses (especially the Cat, p.502 and the Rising snake series, p.543) can help to prevent babies from coming to rest in the breech position. But if your baby does end up bum down, then there are some helpful yogic remedies that can be effective in encouraging the baby to shift position, especially if they are combined with acupuncture. Be aware that many acupuncturists who have expertise in this work recommend beginning acupuncture treatment for breech babies from thirty-four to thirty-six weeks.

In terms of *āsana* to shift a breech baby, the basic idea is to do practices that tip the baby out of the pelvis. But there is no point in these practices if the baby/ies is/are asleep because nothing much happens. It is better to wait until your baby is awake and kicking, then you have more chance that she will actually shift. Either tip the pelvis higher than the navel using the Cat pose (p.502) modified by dropping down onto the elbows, and sticking the tail up into the air so that you can wiggle the pelvis. Or modify the Bridge position (pp.155–8) by putting a couple of bolsters in underneath the sacrum and feeling how high up you can rest comfortably, still with your feet on the floor, and rest there. To be honest, these *āsanas* are of limited use if you do not combine, precede or follow the *āsana* with a *yoga nidrā* (pp.446–8) where you take time to communicate with the baby, visualising the baby in optimal fetal position and explaining to the baby how important it is to come out head first. This is the most crucial practice of all, especially when the baby is awake.

Carpal tunnel syndrome: A number of women experience pain and restricted movement in the hand and fingers during pregnancy as a result of compression of the carpal nerve. This can mean that many yoga *āsanas* where weight is carried down through the wrists, for example the Cat pose, are uncomfortable or impossible. The easiest way to remedy the situation is to provide support for the elbows, wrists and forearms, so that the forearms are at a ninety-degree angle to the upper arm, for example by placing a stack (usually three is sufficient) of yoga blocks under each elbow so that the forearms and wrists can rest and no weight comes through the wrist joints. This means that all poses where weight is usually directed through the wrists become accessible. In terms of reducing the pain associated with this condition then the Golden thread breath (p.462) can be useful, and, some modified versions of wrist rotations in *pavanmuktāsana* (p.504) can be helpful, although in acute cases even these should be avoided because they can exacerbate the pain.

Haemorrhoids (piles): So many women experience discomfort as a result of haemorrhoids in pregnancy and the postnatal period, that it is useful to know the yogic remedy, which can be helpfully combined with whatever topical pain relief works best for the woman. *Ashvini mudrā* (the anal squeeze pp.476–7), especially when practised with the pelvis lifted higher than the navel and the weight resting on the elbows and forearms, provides a rhythmic squeeze and release to the anus. This optimises circulation to the area and can boost healing, whilst the inverted posture can relieve unpleasant sensations of pressure and pain.

High / low blood pressure: Changes in blood pressure are very common during pregnancy. The dance between increased blood volume and changes in the capacity of the cardiovascular system to transport the additional blood around the body can result in increased or decreased blood pressure depending on the constitution of the individual woman. Supported side lying poses (p.551) and deep relaxation such as *yoga nidrā* (pp.446–8) are very helpful in managing either experience. *Ujjāyī* breath (pp.134–5) is useful to lower raised blood pressure, and a steady even full breath pattern (pp.131–2) is helpful in either case. In postures where hands are raised above the head it is important not to maintain this position for long, but to move rhythmically through it: women with lower blood pressure will tend to faint if the hands are held up above the head for any length of time, whereas women with high blood pressure will raise it further by sustaining this pose.

Insomnia: so many of the challenges in adapting to pregnancy are exacerbated by lack of sleep. Attentive propping in restorative poses such as Side-lying pose (p.551) can help you to go to sleep easily and to remain comfortably asleep through the night. Calming breath patterns such as the Circle of flowing breath (p.128–31) and Humming breath (p.469–70) are invaluable in inducing sleep. *Yoga nidrā* (chapter eighteen) is also immensely helpful to catch up on lost sleep and to assist in getting to sleep, or to practise during wakeful hours to ensure you can face the day rested.

Lower back pain: because there is so much adjustment to the curves of the spine during pregnancy, lower back pain is a frequent experience. All the pelvic movements and snake undulations in standing positions (pp.168–72) can provide helpful relief from discomfort, whilst the Mermaid twist is also a boon (pp.514–5). Regular practice of all-fours poses, especially the Rising snake, provide a good preventive programme, and the Wall as teacher sequence (pp.546–9) is a useful way to correct any awkward postural developments. Be aware that much of the support necessary to keep the back pain-free comes from the arches of the feet, so regular practice of all the foot arch supporting techniques described in the awakening of the feet and hands section (p.472) are very helpful.

Oedema: Swollen joints, e.g. ankles, feet, wrists, can feel very tender and uncomfortable. The best approach to relieve these sensations is to practise the full series of poses to liberate energy (pp.497–510), especially those that relate to the effected joints because they improve circulation, including drainage of excess fluid from the joints. Complete breathing patterns can also be helpful (pp.131–2) as prevention and management, and sometimes inversions, such as those described in the pelvic organ support section (pp.488–91), are also useful.

Pelvic girdle pain: this can occur in any one or more of the three joints of the pelvis, and can range from being mildly annoying to extremely debilitating. It is exacerbated by activities that bring uneven weight into the pelvis, e.g standing on one leg, walking with long strides, cycling, or getting into a car by swinging in one leg at a time. The best remedy is to bring the sense of even balance that comes through good yogic standing posture (pp.494–5) into everyday activities, for example, by taking shorter steps when walking, and using upper body strength when rolling over in bed or sitting up. All the practices which use the wall as a teacher are helpful (pp.546–9), and building positive strength and support through the arches of the feet (pp.472–3) is also useful. Developing healthy pelvic and abdominal muscles is an excellent means to support the pelvic joints.

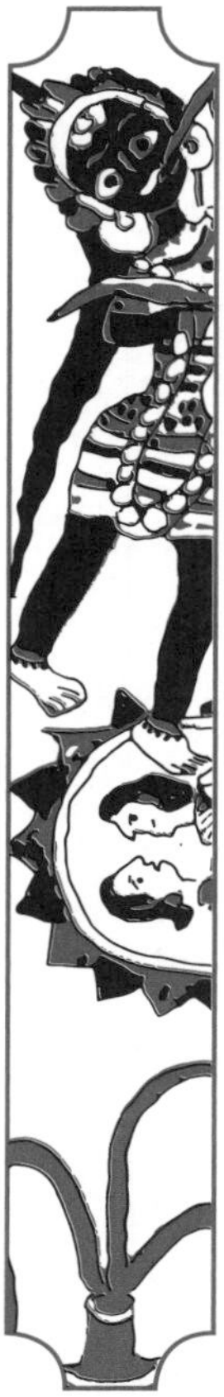

FEED THE WILD *YOGINĪ*

ON THE LAP OF THE COSMIC MOTHER

Pregnancy can be experienced as if we are opening our body to house and nurture the guest of the unborn child: every cell of our body is literally in service to the growth and well-being of the child. This can be very tiring. The energies of the *Mahāvidyā* Bhuvaneśvarī are kept very busy.

What a gift to be able to offer back the precious experience of rest. This is a radical act. Let yourself be like the little baby within the womb. Spare no expense, get extra cushions, take extra time and get yourself set up in the most super-delicious In the golden cosmic womb restorative pose (pp.552–3), or indeed whichever of the restorative poses you most enjoy (see chapter twenty-five). Give yourself an hour off. If you are minding small people, get others in to help. This is important. When your body is being the golden cosmic womb, you need to rest in the lap of the cosmic mother. Feed the wild *yoginī* with your renewed energy and vitality, recover your good humour, get some sleep, or do a *yoga nidrā* (chapter eighteen). Enjoy your ritual. If you feed her the fabulously rare delicacy of deep rest, then she will feed you. For certain.

QUESTIONS AND REFLECTIONS

I invite you to explore your own experience of the relationship between yoga, pregnancy, labour and birth in your life by asking yourself some (or any, or all) of the following questions:

1. What are you hoping to gain from practising yoga during pregnancy? Is your top priority the ability to move more easily, keeping / staying fit, getting in tune with your baby, preparing for change, having an easier birth? Be clear about what you think you want, and then re-visit this question again when you have had a chance to experience what yoga can bring you during pregnancy.
2. How do you feel after yoga class / practice? Are you more rested, calmer or more anxious, more physically comfortable, more tired / energised? Explore how these feelings feed into what it is that you want yoga to do for you, e.g.: if the class helps you feel more rested, how could you bring those practices into your daily life? Or what is it about the pregnancy yoga class / practice that helps me feel more comfortable? Perhaps you could do with some more pillows / bolsters at home to help get that

feeling when you settle down at night? If the class / practice is making you feel anxious or tired, then it might be worth exploring other teachers in your area, or considering another approach.

3 What do you most value from practising yoga during your pregnancy? Is it the emotional or physical experiences that are most important? Do you prefer to be still or to be moving? Do you mostly value yoga for pregnancy because of the time it gives you to connect with your baby, or just the precious feeling of having some time to yourself? Reflect on the possibility, especially if this is your first baby, that your answers will give you a sense of how to help yourself to be supported in your mothering. For example, if you most value time alone and quiet breathing, it may be important to re-connect with those practices once the baby is born (for hints on how to do this, see chapter fourteen).

4 What is it about birth that most concerns you? Consider how yoga may help you to address these concerns. For example, it may be helpful to develop familiarity with breath that relieves pain (p.462), or that assists in the birth of your baby (p.463). It can also be liberating to connect with the wider awareness of birth as a rite of passage and an initiation into spiritual power. Exploring the spiritual perspectives one brings to life as a whole is a starting point for engaging with this aspect of birth.

FURTHER READING AND RESEARCH

For a comprehensive guide to yoga breath practices during pregnancy, labour and birth see *Mother's Breath* and its accompanying audio recordings, on CD and downloadable from **www.wombyoga.org** and **www.yoganidranetwork.org**.

Clarity and safety are the hallmark of all the posture and breathing instructions in *Teach Yourself Yoga for Pregnancy and Birth*, which I wrote whilst I was pregnant with my daughter. It also has a useful chapter on using yoga during labour to promote a deep connection with natural and instinctive ways of moving and breathing that reduce anxiety and relieve pain. Available from **www.yogamatters.com**

The triple DVD *Mother Nurture Yoga* offers an accessible audio-visual guide to yoga during pregnancy and birth in the form of hour-long sessions with students at different stages of pregnancy. Shorter classes for relaxation and easeful movement during pregnancy are available online from the resources section of **www.wombyoga.org**

Other very valuable resources to support the experiences of pregnancy and birth are **Pam England**'s *Birthing from Within*, **Wendy Teasdill**'s *Yoga for Pregnancy* and **Françoise Freedman**'s *Yoga for Pregnancy, Birth and Beyond*. For teachers trained in these methods visit **www.birthlight.co.uk**, **www.birthingfromwithin.com** and **www.teasdill.com**

Janet Balaskas, the pioneer of Active Birth in the UK, has produced an impressive range of resources to empower and support active labour, and her material is accessible through **www.activebirthcentre.com**. An expanded network of teachers rooted in the principles of yoga for the empowerment of pregnant and birthing women can also be contacted through **www.yogabirth.org**

Sofya Ansari, an āyurvedic practitioner and yoga teacher specialising in yoga for pregnancy and women's health has produced a particularly sensitive and delicious audio CD of practices, that also includes a 32-page pamphlet of useful tips and instructions. Details of her work and the CD are available at **www.sofya.org.uk**

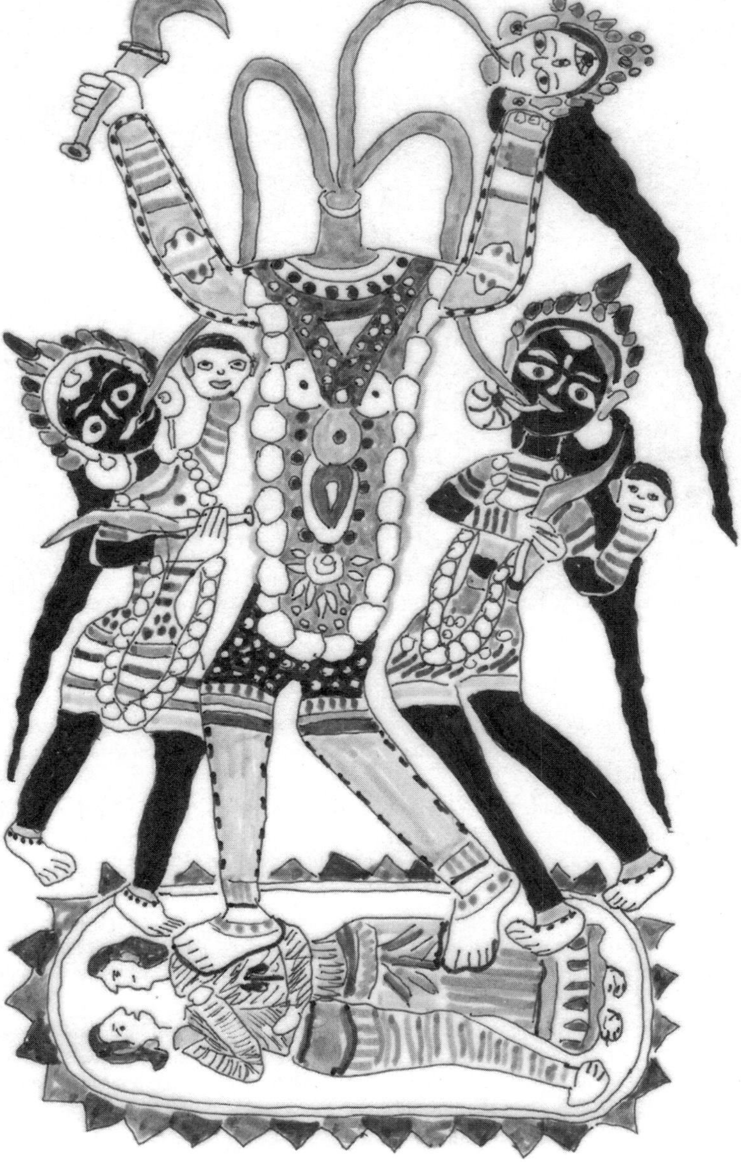

Chinnamastā holds the power of transformation at the precise moment of change, as manifested through the selfless sacrifice that can characterise postnatal recovery

CHAPTER FOURTEEN

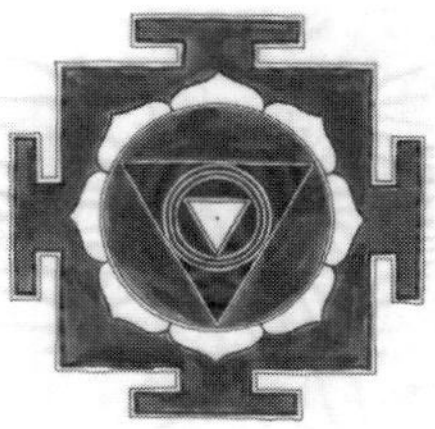

Chinnamastā

Thanksgiving, grieving and healing: yoga and postnatal recovery

> *Mothers live in a universe that has not been accurately described. The right words have not been coined. Using habitual vocabulary sends us straight down the same old, much-trodden footpaths. But there are other areas to which these footpaths do not lead. There are whole stretches of motherhood that no one has explored ... Mothers complain about their physical isolation, but surely a more fundamental isolation is about not being understood. That kind of isolation arises when a person finds it difficult to communicate an important experience to other people ... It's hard to find the words to communicate what "looking after my baby" really means. (Stadlen 2004)*

MAHĀVIDYĀ AND *SIDDHI*

WISDOM AND POWER

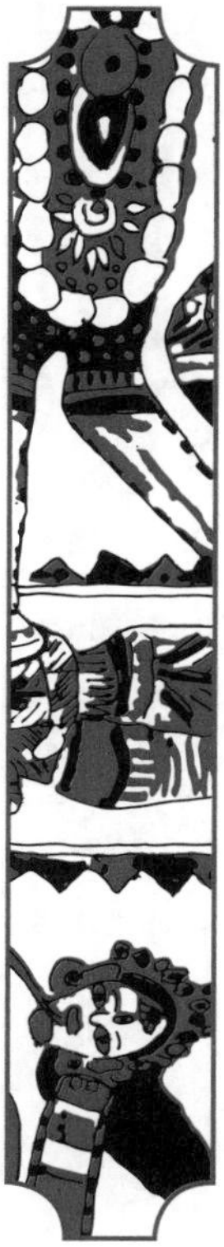

Chinnamastā, the goddess who represents consciousness beyond the mind, is perhaps the most terrifying of all the *Mahāvidyās*. Her name literally means 'she whose head is severed'. Her other name is Prachaṇḍa Caṇḍikā, the fiercest form of Kālī (Candī). She is usually placed as the sixth *Mahāvidyā*, coming in between Bhairavī the warrior goddess and Dhūmavatī the widow, but I have placed her in specific relation to the experiences of postnatal recovery, of thanksgiving and/or healing.

I link Chinnamastā to the female *siddhi* of transformation through postnatal recovery because the great power of Chinnamastā is her capacity to bring about a total and irreversible shift of consciousness, and the postnatal times in a woman's life demand complete transformation of every aspect of awareness. Chinnamastā represents the change-energy of Kālī when it is utterly focused at the moment of shift. The quality of her power is like lightning; a rapid illuminatory force that is both dangerous and utterly liberating because it breaks open the limitations of who we think we are. The time after birth carries precisely this charge of intensity. All previous notions of self-identity are immediately rendered null and void. Postnatal recovery of any kind (including after miscarriage, stillbirth and abortion, as well as after a live birth) is by its very nature a period of dramatic change in a woman's life. It is a time when we are forced to face loss and grief: we grieve for the death of the woman we were before we gave birth; for the passing of other potentials and possibilities; sometimes also for the death of the baby we have carried, and always, for every woman, the ending of a certain stage of our lives – the end of pregnancy, the end, especially after the first birth, of a certain innocence, and the end of illusion.

This time can often also be intimately linked to the experiences of nourishment and lactation. In relation to Chinnamastā, the intense and often dramatic transition from the pregnant to the postnatal state and the creation of a woman as a giver of nourishment are profoundly connected. For Chinnamastā is the self-decapitated goddess whose own blood feeds her devotees and herself. The startling image of her depicts the moment of change: in one of her hands she holds her own freshly severed head, whilst in the other she still brandishes the bloody sword with which she has beheaded herself. The blood that gushes from her neck flows in three red fountains into the hungry open mouths of her two devotees and herself. She and her devotees stand with their feet upon the bodies of a copulating couple. All three wear garlands of human skulls.

The usual interpretations of this image of Chinnamastā identify her severed head as a yogic metaphor for the death of the ego and liberation of consciousness from the limited identification with the body as self. There are a number of other severed heads to be found amongst the *Mahāvidyās*: Kālī holds a head that drips with blood and is also adorned with garlands of skulls; Bhairavī's breasts are smeared with blood from the severed heads that hang like a rosary around her neck; and Dhūmavatī also wears a garland of human skulls. But it is only Chinnamastā who severs her own head, and only Chinnamastā who feeds her devotees with her own blood. This image is clearly a graphic communication of the forces of transformation that bring about the shift of consciousness that disconnects us from ego-identification.

But in relation to this period of change in a woman's life, the image does not simply resonate at a general philosophical level. For a postnatal woman, the experience of transformation is direct, bloody and embodied. Whatever kind of birth a woman experiences, the transition from being pregnant to being a mother is an immense and rapid transformation at every dimension of being from the visceral to the spiritual. At a physical level the body changes overnight from a living embodiment of ripe fullness into an empty and often damaged and exhausted shell. Even after the most positive birth experience, the postnatal body can be left bleeding, leaking and broken. The shift in hormone levels is like falling off a cliff, or going cold-turkey from class-A drugs. From the astonishing experience of peak levels of pregnancy and birth hormones (the feel-good progesterone, oestrogen and endorphins that facilitate the super-human endeavours of late pregnancy and labour, and the massive adrenalin kick that actually births the baby), a postnatal woman encounters a dramatic hormonal drop accompanied by a chaotic vortex of shifting patterns of endocrine activity.

It is not fanciful to see in the self-decapitated form of Chinnamastā a powerful visual metaphor for the transformations which women encounter after birth: both are shocking and effect permanent shifts of consciousness. Overnight, the woman can change from being the blooming focus of everyone's attention and love, the 'pregnant queen' whose every whim is met, into a shattered shadow of a servant, whose well-being is only of interest in so far as she is the giver of nourishment and comfort to the baby who now becomes the absolute focus of attention. Evidently, the upside of all this is the profound experience of absolute love that can accompany the arrival of the child, but this maternal feeling does not always come straight away, and the physical encounters with exhaustion and hormonal chaos are immediate and powerful presences. For women who miscarry, or whose babies die before or soon after birth, then the physical and emotional challenges of postnatal recovery are not tempered by joy at the birth of the child. Grief replaces thanksgiving. The especially intense challenges of these aspects of postnatal recovery are explored in the next section.

Clearly, there are many approaches to postnatal care that place as much emphasis upon the well-being of the mother as the baby. However, it is not infrequent in western industrialised cultures, where postnatal care is woefully underfunded and undervalued, for a women to experience postnatal recovery as a time of neglect and dismay, as she struggles to negotiate the changed balance of focus in her life. High rates of postnatal depression, which affects ten to fifteen percent of all mothers worldwide and three in every ten new mothers in the UK, indicates a cultural difficulty with managing this change. The difficulty is deeply embedded in both our attitudes to motherhood and our capacity to embrace the changes that are part of the natural unfolding of cyclical wisdom.

Chinnamastā not only beheads herself. Part of her power is her capacity to provide nourishment for her devotees (and herself) from the streams of blood that flow from her own headless body. The complete surrender of the ego that is depicted by the decapitation makes it possible for her to do this: it is because she has no head that the streams of blood can flow from her body to feed into the open mouths of the devotees.

In relation to postnatal experiences that include lactation, this image carries quite a charge. I read it like this: in so far as a woman completely engages with the transformation of awareness that birth and motherhood invite, thus far is she able to engage fully with the role of her own body as the provider of nourishment for her child. For example, the many hours of intimate connection with a newborn that are necessary to establish and maintain milk supply to keep that baby well-fed initially requires the almost total surrender of whatever activities a woman may previously have used to identify herself. It is not that it is impossible to 'go back to normal' immediately and still take on the role of the mother as nourisher for a small baby. It is rather that by avoiding the all-encompassing nature of this role we are likely to miss the opportunity to engage with the fundamental power of the postnatal change. Resistance to the total (temporary) surrender of the activities by which we previously identified ourselves prevents a full encounter with the extreme energies of transformative power that Chinnamastā represents. For women who are able to embrace the experiences of the postnatal period as an opportunity for deep change and growth, the outcome can be astonishing. Sometimes women don't even recognise themselves in the mothers they become after birth: 'I was surprised I even had the same name' says one of the mothers in Naomi Stadlen's vivid account of *What Mothers Do* (2004).

The capacity to embrace the profoundly transformative experiences of postnatal recovery is not something that women can manage all alone. The image of Chinnamastā shows her flanked on either side by two kneeling female devotees. These handmaidens support her even as they drink her blood – they witness and affirm her experience. To be present at the moment of her transformation provides spiritual nourishment for the devotees who give Chinnamastā the practical support she requires to undergo transformation. This aspect of the necessity of support and witness that surrounds Chinnamastā is an important element of her resonance for the postnatal period, which I explore in detail in the following section.

Equally significant in relation to the experiences of postnatal recovery is the fact that Chinnamastā stands upon the bodies of a copulating couple. At a symbolic level, Chinnamastā is seen to be quashing the distracting energies of sensuality. The usual interpretation of this image is that the delusions of limited pleasure which copulation brings is nothing but dirt beneath the feet of the goddess who has the capacity to reveal ultimate reality through a profound change in consciousness.

At a very literal level, in relation to the postnatal period, the placing of the copulating couple beneath the feet of the goddess indicates where sex fits into the life of a postnatal woman. It is often at the very bottom of the list of her priorities. If you have just decapitated yourself, then your attention is unlikely to be upon what lies beneath your feet. In this way, Chinnamastā depicts a massive change—a different set of priorities. Because she has willingly transformed herself by the removal of her head, and has shifted her attentions to her role as provider of nourishment, her stance on top of the copulating couple indicates pretty clearly that now may not be the time for sex, or at least not in the way it had previously been experienced. The postnatal time can be a time for great tenderness between the parents of a new baby, but it may not be a good time to return to old habitual patterns of sexual relations, in particular the 'friction sex' acts that are mostly about responding in a limited and conventional manner to the arising of male desire for ejaculation.

Alterations in a woman's libido are a well understood aspect of the effects of lactation, and many lactating women experience such intense intimacy in the experience of breastfeeding that previously familiar patterns of sexual intimacy with their partners may well need to shift to accommodate these changes. This is simply one dimension of the free expression of energy (in its sexual form) that is likely to be changed by the 'Chinnamastā experience' of the postnatal period, and it can present an opportunity to expand consciousness of the nature of sexuality.

In the following section I explore in more detail the cultural expectations around new motherhood, and encounters with pregnancy loss, in relation to the stresses and challenges that can be experienced at this transformative time. The shocking image of Chinnamastā provides a reliable reference to make spiritual sense of these experiences because she gives the wisdom necessary to engage with the power of total transformation.

LIMITATIONS: CULTURAL EXPECTATIONS

The subtitle of this chapter is 'Thanksgiving and/or grieving and healing'. All three are equally important aspects of the postnatal recovery period. The difficulties often encountered by postnatal women in our culture stem directly from the fact that our culture tends to focus on the thanksgiving element of the postnatal period and to give no attention to women's deep need for grieving and healing at this time. The dominant message received by women after they have had a baby is to 'get back to normal' as swiftly as possible. Celebrities stroll smilingly out of hospitals with their newborns in their arms, wearing size eight jeans; top businesswomen and politicians work flat out until the first contractions and then are back at their desks within the week; even yoga teachers leap (literally) back into full teaching schedules, demonstrating fast-paced flows and advanced postures just weeks after giving birth. The message is clear: 'Get over it, get on with it, act like nothing has happened.'

There are many reasons why this is the dominant message, and none of them respects the realities of women's experiences at this time. In the first place, there is a huge pressure for women to return to work after the birth of their babies: family funds can precariously depend on two incomes, and/or a woman's commitment to the development of her career in the competitive environments of business or law, for example, can push her back to work for fear that she may lose her job or miss out on promotion. It is not legal, but far from unusual for women to lose their jobs simply because they are pregnant, or have become mothers. Provisions for paid maternity leave have certainly improved in recent years, but for most working mothers, the reality is that they need to get back to their jobs as soon as they can to protect their earnings and/or their professional status.

This 'back to normal' pressure manifests in many other ways and they are all deeply damaging to the bodies and psyches of postnatal women because they deny women the time they need to grieve and heal after childbirth.

> *Only a few days after the birth of her baby, one of our pregnancy yoga students was transported to hospital in an ambulance after collapsing to the floor whilst out shopping in the west end of London: she'd utterly mis-read the signs of her own fragility and forced herself up and out. 'I felt really lonely cooped up at home. I couldn't stand it for another minute'. Another local woman at the same early point after birth had fainted at the checkout of her local Tesco's: 'I just needed to connect with another human being, even the lady on till', and another found herself stranded in the park, unable to move: 'I didn't realise that I couldn't walk this far, but I really needed to get out of the house. Then I got stuck on the bench and couldn't stand up to go home.'*

All of these women's unfortunate experiences were motivated in the first place by a profound state of isolation. Being isolated and alone drove them to disregard the realities of their own need for a reasonable time of healing and rest. They only went out of the house far too early in their recovery because they were desperate for some company or food. It's simply crazy to expect that a single adult human without any other support would find it anything other than impossible to be the sole carer for a newborn baby, or babies, day in and day out. It takes more than one person to do this job well. And the woman who is expected to do the job single-handed is often in need of deep rest and healing. She requires a network of extended social and practical support for her own recovery and to keep the household running. Most of the hundreds of postnatal women I taught in London did not have any kind of family or neighbourly support. They were on their own, often many thousands of miles from home, just mother and baby all day long. No wonder these women started doing crazy stuff. I'm surprised that the floors of retail establishments across town aren't daily littered with the exhausted bodies of postnatal mothers. The fact that most of us manage to wait till we get home from the shops before we collapse is testimony to the astonishing resilience of women. That we are collapsing all alone back at home indicates the deeply isolated lives of many postnatal women in our culture.

When I worked as a volunteer breastfeeding counsellor for the Lambeth branch of the National Childbirth Trust (NCT), experiences of total isolation were the most common reasons why women telephoned in desperation to talk about why they couldn't breastfeed. When I listened for long enough what I heard was that the breastfeeding problems were just a tiny part of the whole sorry puzzle. Often, these women were actually just tired, hungry, lonely and very confused. If they had partners or husbands, they would have left early for work, and the women, exhausted and often injured after birth, would focus their entire attentions on their baby and simply forget, or be unable to feed themselves. I started bringing loaves of bread and jars of honey along with me on home visits, and every time I discovered that a woman had not eaten since breakfast, I would feed her first and listen to the energy and vitality beginning to pour slowly back into her voice after the third round of bread and honey. It usually took at least three rounds. The confusion and sadness and isolation of these women who called for help with breastfeeding problems had most often been exacerbated by the basic practical difficulties of actually getting enough food inside them: so I held the baby while they got a cup of tea, and then, with at least some basic support to get a little food inside them, they had the energy to start looking at things differently.

I am simplifying the issue of course. But isolation and neglect of postnatal women really cannot be helping our postnatal depression figures to decrease. There's even a new and fast developing genre of literature chronicling the descent into depression of new mothers, because if there's no-one around to talk to about it, then writing it all down is the next best thing, so long as you can stand the fact of doing it amongst the heaps of unwashed dishes in 'Hell's Kitchen'. That's how Rachel Cusk, whose *A Life's Work* is one of the most literary of this postnatal depression genre, describes the state of domestic chaos during the depths of her postnatal collapse.

When a woman is undergoing one the greatest transformations of consciousness which life can bring us, she needs a bit of help. The image of Chinnamastā shows us this very powerfully: she's the only one among the wisdom goddesses who is seen to have active support, in the form of a pair of devoted handmaidens who kneel close to her feet. She may be feeding them both and herself from the fountains of blood that flow from the neck of her own decapitated body, but at least she's got company. And they are respectfully involved in her moment of transformation. They kneel attentively (and gratefully – because they look thirsty) at her feet to support her.

Looking at it from a mother's point of view, through the eyes of a woman who has spent a lot of her time cleaning up bodily fluids of one kind or another, it's a good job those devotees are there drinking all the blood up nicely, because otherwise it would be ending up on the floor, making a nasty mess, which Chinnamastā herself would need to clear up later, after the kids went to bed and just before she collapsed in anaemic exhaustion after her massive blood loss. Poor love. Been there, done that; so I can offer you a 'mum's eye' interpretation of Chinnamastā and her blood-drinking helpers that you won't find in the scholarly texts.

The devotees are important in more ways than one. Chinnamastā's handily placed handmaidens have a vital spiritual as well as a practical function. In the tradition of yoga, keeping good company is a special practice of yoga called *satsang*, which literally means the company of the truth, or the company of wise people. It's the same concept as that of the *sangha* in Buddhism: it is spiritual community. *Satsang* is crucial to the effective support of the transformation of consciousness. It makes the difference between being able to sustain changed priorities or new perspectives on life, and reverting to the habits and patterns that existed before the spiritual transformation took place. Many wisdom traditions value this aspect of spiritual life. It's one of the reasons why Christians go to churches, Jews go to synagogues and Muslims go to mosques. When you value a particular perspective on spiritual life, then it's important to have this perspective supported by others who share it. The communities of people that form in response to this spiritual necessity also provide practical support for each other in times of need, for example the birth of a new human. The support of aunties, sisters and mothers, neighbours' grandmothers and a whole sisterhood of helpful local women is what a postnatal women needs to stop her from sliding, hungry and tired and lonely, into the deep pit of depression and domestic chaos that lies in the middle of Hell's Kitchen. This is the time of life when women really need the sisterhood.

But our culture's way of living means that these spiritual and practical support networks are rarely part of a postnatal women's life. There we all are, in our separate apartments and houses, each with its own washing machine and dishwasher and cable TV: utterly disconnected and totally miserable, talking to breastfeeding counsellors on the phone because we don't know any of our neighbours, or at least not well enough to ask them what they did when their nipples started to crack. Many new mothers experience extreme isolation because they are effectively living alone with no community at all except perhaps the network that was formed by work colleagues, from which of course they are temporarily exiled. Unless you know your line manager really well, they are probably not the person you'd call in the night when your milk won't let down or you feel too exhausted to pick up your screaming baby, or the mess in your house has got so bad you can't get out of your bedroom. Where are your blood-drinking handmaidens when you need them?

What do we have instead of the sisterhood of helpful local ladies who know their haemorrhoids from their blocked milk ducts, and who'll pop a nice casserole around to your doorstep when they see you're not up to cooking tonight? In place of these helpful folk, we now have a whole host of professional advisors. Many of these people make a living out of disempowering mothers. They (some of whom have never had a baby themselves) are the writers of books who tell women what to do to keep their babies happy. Their expert conviction that theirs is the right and only way to do this does a pretty marvellous job of helping women whose babies don't behave like the ones in the books to feel utterly despondent. There are websites and forums and text alerts to keep you updated about the latest developmental stage your baby should have reached. There are baby weighing clinics staffed by health visitors who tick the boxes in the health records of the babies to prove that they are still thriving, and who vilify those mothers who don't show up for the weekly weigh-ins because they feel they can tell without the box ticking that their baby is doing just fine.

There is a whole edifice of professional 'support' for growing babies in the way our culture approves, but absolutely nothing to empower mothers to trust their intuitions, to build their confidence in caring for their child their own way, nor to provide the practical and emotional encouragement they need to figure out what works for them and their baby. In the same way as women's creativity has been undermined by patriarchal oppressions and suppressions of women's innate creative spirit, so too has motherhood (which is of course, a deeply creative and intuitive adventure in figuring out what works for you and your child/ren) been cut off from the source of the sisterhood. There just ain't no blood-drinking handmaidens around when you need them, so, godammit, that means you've got to mop your own blood off the floor. Whilst feeding the baby.

For many *yoginīs*, the people they meet through their yoga classes and centres form powerfully important networks and communities of like-minded friends. It might be expected that such communities would offer a beautiful network of aware and concerned folk to support the transformations that come with life-changing experiences, such as having a baby, but this is not always the case. Many postnatal *yoginīs* find themselves and/or their babies excluded from the yogic *sangha*.

> *For example, Sarah was a long-term yoga student, and devotedly keen* yoginī, *who had been attending weekly classes regularly for many years. She signed up more than two years in advance for a yoga teacher-training course with her teacher, and in the interim before the course started she became pregnant with her second child. By the time the course was about to begin, her new baby was six weeks old and fully breastfed. With only a week to go before the first meeting of the teacher- training course, Sarah showed up at one of my integrated mother and baby yoga classes with her baby daughter. She wept as she took out a bottle of formula to feed the child during the final relaxation practice. 'I'm not really happy about this', she said as the disgruntled baby refused the bottle for the fourth time, crying. 'The breastfeeeding was going so well.' I asked her why then she was giving up breast-feeding so soon. 'Because of the yoga teacher-training course', she explained. I was bewildered. What did a yoga teacher-training course*

have to do with breastfeeding her baby? 'It's a requirement of the course,' she said rather tearfully, as she struggled to get her unhappy baby to take the bottle, 'I'll lose my place if I'm breastfeeding. They say it's too difficult to accommodate.' Sarah shed a few more tears as she endeavoured to get her reluctant daughter to drink the formula, even as her breasts were engorged with milk. By the start of that yoga teacher-training course, Sarah had completely stopped breastfeeding. Her baby was barely eight weeks old. Neither the mother nor the baby were happy about the rapid weaning, but Sarah had been offered no acceptable alternative: either she stopped breastfeeding or the trainer gave her place on the teacher-training course to another student, and she would need to wait another three years for the next course to begin.

This situation was of course, completely avoidable. From my perspective, some fourteen years later, having trained many hundreds of yoga teachers and yoga therapists, many of whom were breastfeeding their babies, I can testify that babes in arms can be a positive asset in any yogic environment, including teacher-training courses. I have discovered that genuinely welcoming the presence of the infant encourages both a sweet kindness and compassion in the hearts of everyone in the group, and provides the opportunity to practise the heightened awareness of the yogic values of *ahimsa* (kindness) and *santosa* (happy acceptance). The baby is no trouble at all, in fact people hardly notice they are there. The postnatal mother can be naturally and very easily well supported by the students in yoga group, who, if given a positive model to follow by the teacher-trainer, are very likely to enjoy 'passing the baby', especially during breaks, to give the mother a chance to nourish herself whilst the baby is happily cuddled by her colleagues. 'Think of it like having a room full of aunties and uncles,' is my guidance to the mother of a child in a yoga teacher training class, 'Everyone is likely to want a cuddle at some point!'

This attitude of welcoming the child into the yoga environment was modelled to me both by Françoise Freedman, whose encouragement of postnatal mothers in the yoga context is exemplary, and also by Mukunda Stiles, who happily welcomed myself and my own baby daughter onto a number of retreats and training courses with the simple greeting: 'Children are always a blessing.' Their open-hearted approach is in contrast to the more traditional response of many yoga teachers, as I discovered when I brought my silently breastfeeding first son along to *satsang* in the months after his birth: 'If you want to come, come!' smiled an ageing Indian Swami as he greeted our yoga group, 'But if you want to come with children and babies, then stay at home!' He laughed, and so did the other *yogis*. My son and I never returned to that yoga centre, and instead sought out spiritual teachings from another visiting Swami attached to a different yoga organisation. By dint of great effort, we arrived at 7:30am one cold winter morning to a lecture on the *Bhagavad Gita*, and sat at the front of the hall. We were discreetly breastfeeding, with my son practically invisible beneath my sweater. The spiritual teaching began. After five minutes, the holy Swami suggested 'the baby might be more comfortable at the back of the hall'. We moved. Ten minutes later he suggested we might be better off outside. We left.

Such exclusion of postnatal women and their infants from yoga teachings is never very kind. But it is the norm in many traditional yoga schools, and perhaps it is all that can be expected from male monastics who perhaps find the presence of a breastfeeding woman uncomfortable or unusual. Sadly, though, these unkind and exclusive behaviours are not only the preserve of male Swamis: female Swamis can also demonstrate even more damaging responses to postnatal women. In fact, in the years prior to Sarah's experience of enforced weaning of her newborn baby, and my own exclusion from *satsangs* and teacher trainings, Caroline encountered a truly shocking attitude of exclusion that was deeply damaging. When she shared her experience, sixteen years later, it still caused her to weep.

Caroline was a dedicated yoga practitioner and teacher, and regularly attended yoga classes and community events such as kirtans *(devotional singing). She signed up for a further yoga teacher-training course, and shortly afterwards became pregnant. Caroline recalled that when given the news of her pregnancy, the teacher trainer said, 'Oh no! There's always someone who gets pregnant on this course'. "The trainer delivered the comment with an air of irritation that women become pregnant, that 'no good will come of this'" recalled Caroline, "But she let me start the course anyway."*

She was twenty weeks pregnant when she began the course, forty-two years old, and had a thirteen-year-old son. She attended all five sessions of the two-year course before her breech baby was born by emergency caesarean (she had prepared for a second homebirth). During those five months, the curriculum of the teacher-training course was strictly adhered to. Caroline observed "In my view, variations and contra-indications for pregnancy could have been woven into the class, and used as teaching points, along with the sacredness of this time in a woman's life, but it was treated as a nuisance."

She left hospital two days after the birth, and two days later, the father of the child committed suicide. Caroline developed an infection in her caesarean wound. She had not arranged additional help because she had envisaged the father being there, and both her parents were ill. She breastfed the baby.

Four weeks after the father's death, Caroline attended the yoga teacher-training with the quiet breastfeeding baby. She was motivated by her ardent desire to pursue her yogic studies with the community of which she was a part. She could not drive, because of the caesarean wound, and so walked to the yoga centre. She did not feel able to attend the second day, exhausted and grief-stricken. She asked someone at the yoga centre to drive her home, but they 'could not because they were preparing an Upaniṣads *lecture.' Four weeks later, she went again, assuming that a quiet newborn could be accommodated in the group, but asked in advance that she could bring friends and her mum in shifts to be at the yoga centre to hold the baby while she was in class. Her ill mother was put on a hard bench for two hours in the kitchen and not allowed in the empty sitting room, and so she asked to sit in the car where the seats were more comfortable.*

Caroline remembers holding the baby at lunchtimes on the yoga teacher-training course, 'Everyone else was helping themselves to lunch, and filling their plates, and there I was famished from breastfeeding, one-handed, holding the baby, trying to make her seem invisible, and struggling to get myself something to eat. No one tried to help in any way. It was awful.'

She stuck at it, and triumphantly completed her seventh weekend of the course. But her triumph was short-lived. She was hauled into the yoga room by the teacher-trainer, who said: 'No baby'. 'She didn't say, "I find it difficult to teach with the baby here", she didn't say, "I can see you have had a difficult time, how about resting and joining the course next year?" She simply said, "NO BABY". Crying, I said, "But I'm breastfeeding, and I have no-one to look after the baby." And she said "NO BABY". So I left the TTC.' Caroline also gave up practising yoga within this lineage.

The trainer's desire to maintain total control over every aspect of the training course made it impossible for her to welcome Caroline's pregnancy, and then made it impossible for her to consider welcoming her mother or the baby. To do so would have required kindness, compassion, and the admission that yoga is about accommodation and adaptation, not about the eradication of any obstacle to total control.

In contrast, a yoga centre where Caroline had been teaching for the last six years, when they heard what had happened, kindly sent some practitioners round to give her treatments, and when she went back to teaching ten weeks after her caesarean, they allowed her baby to accompany her. She went along to a Chi Gung class there, where she was welcomed with the baby by the male teacher. She relaxed a little, but then, when she turned up with the still quiet baby for a musical evening at the same yoga centre, while the teacher was singing 'Lean on Me' she was told she could not come in, in case the baby made a noise. Caroline had attended classes at the Active Birth Centre, and when she went there postnatally and explained her financial situation, Janet Balaskas welcomed her for free, for as long as she wished. But it was too far to go and finally she had no choice but to stop going out with the baby and stay at home with her grief. In the end she gave in and sent her baby, aged seven months, to a childminder.

The behaviour of those in the yoga centres which excluded Caroline and her baby, and led Sarah unhappily to the enforced weaning of her eight-week-old baby, calls into question their definitions of yoga, and what kind of teacher-training they were offering. It demonstrates a deep lack of awareness of the kind of support and understanding needed by postnatal women, and shows how damaging it can be when yoga communities exclude postnatal women at this vulnerable time. Even if the women were well-rooted in those communities before they gave birth, they can feel abandoned and adrift once the babies arrive.

If the birth of the baby comes unexpectedly early, or the child is very sick, then the need for postnatal support intensifies. Women with premature infants, or babies who need intense medical care after birth can experience a very difficult postnatal recovery period. They fall into a kind of purgatory – they have given birth, but they cannot bring their babies home. Instead of the kind of deep nurturing, healing and rest that is required for effective recovery in the postnatal period, mothers of sick and premature babies are often caught up in a very demanding scenario that gives them no opportunity for self-nurture at all. They may be camping out in the hospital, or travelling daily in and out of the special care baby units, perhaps pumping milk to feed the baby through tubes because their sucking reflex has not yet developed to enable them to breastfeed. They may well be worried sick that the baby will not survive. In this kind of postnatal period, it can be impossible to put the necessary energy into healing. External support is crucial to sustain these mothers.

During our time in London, we spent two years working with the parent support officer at King's College Hospital to offer weekly sessions of healing and restful yoga for families whose newborns were sick or dying. The relaxation and breathing practices were very helpful in terms of giving these very stressed and worried people a little space to rest. But the most potent aspect of the class was the opportunity it gave for the women to share their experiences, and to know that there were other mothers who knew what it was like to encounter all of the physical and emotional challenges of having just given birth with the additional suffering of profound anxiety about the welfare of the child. There was no funding for this class because the available (limited) resources were all poured into caring for the babies. This economic pattern of diverting all resources towards the newborns reflects our culture's inability to recognise that postnatal recovery is an experience that requires support. It is not that there needs to be less funding for the care of the babies, but rather that meeting the needs of their postnatal mothers is, in the long term, a positive investment in the future health and well-being of the child.

And if women who have given birth to live babies, sick or well, full-term or premature, need more emotional and practical support than our culture will admit, then women whose babies are stillborn, or who miscarry, need even higher levels of support. The isolation of new mothers with live babies to care for is a happy cocktail party in comparison to the lonely sorrows of postnatal women whose babies are dead. This kind of isolation goes deeper, for miscarriage and stillbirth are experiences of which women rarely speak. The difficult experiences of postnatal mothers with new babies may be well hidden under a veneer of happy cooing over their gorgeous infants. But the experiences of women whose postnatal recovery is a time not of thanksgiving but of deep grieving have been rendered so invisible as to have become apparently forgotten or ignored by the general community. The women who encounter these experiences are often treated as pariahs by other mothers.

One of the bravest women I ever met was Heather, whose twin baby daughters died shortly after birth. Heather was a yoga teacher, and she chose to attend the postnatal recovery and baby yoga training course because she believed that her own experiences of postnatal recovery after stillbirth would provide a valuable perspective for the other teachers on the course. During the training she conceived another baby, and her delicate dance between grief and hope was played out in the context of a course that trained teachers to run healing yoga classes for postnatal women and their new babies.

'It's not all fluffy bunnies,' observed Heather as she gave a presentation to the training group about stillbirth. 'The worst thing about when my baby daughters died was how people avoided me. It was like having some kind of horrible contagious disease. Family wouldn't come near, and some neighbours would literally cross the road when they saw me because they just didn't know what to say.' Her sense of isolation had been so extreme that it made it even more difficult to bear the grief: 'If there's one thing I can share from this experience that would help make a difference to women in the same position, it's to make contact with her. Look her in the eye, tell her that you are sorry to hear of her loss, and that you can't possibly imagine how sad she feels. But let her know that you are there for her, that she does not need to grieve alone.'

Heather's experience of the death of her daughters occurred when her son was a toddler. She lived in a small town, and because of her son, she was already connected into the small world of playgroups and nursery. Her loss was widely known, and the lack of connection from the members of her community made the death of her daughters even harder to bear. For women living in a big city, the knowledge of their loss may be shared only with close family. In either place, the loneliness can be very painful. For Heather, one of her motivations to train as a postnatal yoga teacher was to be able to provide appropriate support through yoga movement, breath and relaxation, for all postnatal women, including those who had lost their babies at or before full-term pregnancy; she felt that the community created through yoga and benefits of the practices might be able to help counteract the deep loneliness which she knew from experience such new mothers experienced.

For women who miscarry in early pregnancy, the grief and isolation is of a different quality. To many people looking in at a miscarriage from the outside, it is as if nothing has happened. This means that early pregnancy loss can be an especially difficult postnatal experience. Lara Owen's description of her own experience vividly conveys the nature of the suffering:

'... when I became pregnant... I still had an attitude of neglect towards my body when its needs interfered with my work. I remember being extremely hungry but putting other things before eating. I miscarried, and the grief that I felt in my body for the lost baby and the frustration of a pregnancy cut short awakened me to my body and its essential femaleness in a shocking way...

This was an experience that set me apart from the world of men, and the intellect, in a stark and thorough way. I had no conscious resources within me to deal with the feelings that overwhelmed me. I was full of loss for a being that had at most been six weeks old. It didn't make any sense. But I could feel my body grieving in a powerful way. I cried endlessly, and was depressed throughout the rest of what would have been the pregnancy… I was lost in an unexpected sea of hormonal anguish… Being a woman was taking me into regions of feeling that were vast and uncontrollable. Why had no one prepared me for this? Why didn't anyone talk about the fact that a woman's physiology had such a powerful effect on her mental and emotional state? Was I some kind of aberration, or was this another of the facets of female experience consigned to the secret compartment of life?'

Lara Owen's grief, like that of many women who encounter pregnancy loss, is compounded by the hidden nature of the loss: because it is out of sight in the 'secret compartment of life', women who experience it are isolated from each other. Not only is there an experience of emotional grief that is rarely acknowledged by the wider culture, but at a physical level, women are dealing with bleeding and exhaustion, and with rapidly shifting hormones that may, depending on the length of the pregnancy, also result in lactation. Coping with all of these physical changes at a time of deep grief that may not be acknowledged by those around her is an enormous challenge. Only when one of her acupuncture clients spoke to her about her own experiences of miscarriage, did Lara herself begin to feel the healing significance of a circle of female support for the intense encounters with the female *siddhis*. The other woman tells her about her three pregnancy losses:

'… every time I felt the most terrible grief. No one who hasn't been through it understands the pain of it.' (Owen: 42–3)

Lara's sense of loss does not lessen because her client reveals her own sadness, but the fact that she knows another woman understands how she feels is a source of strength to her. There is a deep relief in knowing that other women have experienced the same losses, and a comfort in hearing others speak about what is so often unspoken. The sharing is healing. The support of other women who have been through these experiences is not just comforting, but necessary to ensure positive recovery.

The deep need for the presence of other women at moments of transformation and change encountered through the female *siddhis* is graphically depicted in the image of Chinnamastā (p.344): at the moment that she beheads herself, Chinnamastā's handmaidens are present to witness her transformation. The witnesses acknowledge the depths of the moment of change: so too, the experience of postnatal transformation is so intense that it demands full support. The key to healing at all dimensions of being after pregnancy loss or stillbirth is to acknowledge these periods in a woman's life as times for the grieving that is a natural part of postnatal recovery. It is important to remember that women whose babies have died have also given birth. Healing after any kind of birth is a serious business that takes time.

The same is also true in relation to the experience of abortion. But whereas the experiences of stillbirth and miscarriage, or the birth of a very premature or sick baby are generally shocking surprises, the process of deciding whether or not to terminate a pregnancy requires conscious decision. In some ways this may make the process of healing after the experience easier, but in other ways the fact of having chosen to abort may make healing more difficult. It all depends on the circumstances surrounding the conception. Some women arrive at the decision to abort rapidly, and describe their deep and uncomplicated relief at having terminated an unwanted pregnancy, like Caitlin Moran, who observes:

> *'... not even for a second do I think I should have this baby. I have no dilemma, no terrible decision to make... when friends come round with their new babies, I am hugely, hugely grateful that I had the option not to do this again.'*

Other women are deeply troubled and saddened by the choice they have had to make. Either way, the physical experience of terminating a pregnancy requires a time of healing and adjustment. Even though the woman's body may not have been pregnant for longer than a few weeks, she still needs to shift from the pregnant to the postnatal state, and this process is not always easy. Having a supportive circle of understanding women can change this process from an isolating ordeal to a time of change that includes the possibility of spiritual growth. The wider significance of these *śakti* circles of support and sharing is explored in chapter twenty-eight.

Whatever the nature of the birth experience, effective postnatal recovery requires patience, support and time. And genuine postnatal recovery is healing *from the inside out*. Crucial attention to inner healing in the early postnatal period is overlooked in our culture because it does not bring immediately visible results. Most often, the emphasis is on looking great, on having firm abs and buttocks, and toned arms and a well made-up face under a snappy haircut; but truly, what is the point of looking great in a bikini if you wee yourself every time you laugh? At this point so often in a woman's life, the true heart of our recovery is neglected. The experiences of women during the postnatal period reveal the sad limitations of patriarchal culture with regard to women: what is important is the visible, the external, the peripheral and superficial. The deep treasures lie neglected and unknown. Yes, if we neglect our own deep healing and buy into this limited vision of what it is to be a woman at this time in their lives, we might get nice tight abs and toned upper arms, but, more likely sooner than later, the bottom will literally fall out of our world. We'll be wincing every time we walk, weeing every time we sneeze, and we'll be back at the hospital eighteen months later in our high heels, checking in for prolapse surgery. This is not a fanciful imagining. In the crazy world of London yummy mummies, where the way a woman looks can be valued above and beyond any concern about her own level of deep recovery, it is commonplace:

> *'I see it all the time,' confided a postnatal yoga teacher about the women in her well-heeled community in South West London: 'they sign up with a personal trainer and are up there in the gym working their abdominals and obsessed with losing baby fat. They look great on the outside, but they've never really healed. It just makes*

everything worse. Half of them are back in the hospital for prolapse within a couple of years. They'd rather do that than admit that they need help to heal. It's sad because it's avoidable.'

Almost everyone in this culture has forgotten that postnatal women need to heal from the inside out, and that they need help and support from other women to do this. Thankfully, there are small pockets of resistance where these ideas are thriving, and women are slowly, authentically and completely healing from the inside out. These pockets of resistance are called postnatal recovery and baby yoga classes.

FREEDOMS: YOGA PERSPECTIVES, TECHNIQUES AND AWARENESS FOR BREATHING, MOVING AND BEING

I have discovered over the years that postnatal recovery and baby yoga classes are special *satsangs* that create perfect environments to nurture the important community-building element of the postnatal experience. There is a qualitative difference between the experience of those groups of mothers who come together to practice yoga with their babies, and the same women, getting together for an NCT coffee morning and a bit of a chat. Practising yoga together is a powerful balm for the soul. Whilst local baby and toddler groups can helpfully create communities of like-minded mothers who can support each other, the yogic perspective of groups like postnatal yoga and baby yoga groups offer an additional opportunity for physical healing and a spiritual perspective that is important to women's deeper well-being. One of my first postnatal recovery yoga classes created such a beautifully spirited connection between the women and the babies, that they continued coming to class together for nearly four years (the session morphed from postnatal recovery and baby yoga into mum and toddler yoga). The bond between these women was so strong that some of them supported each other when they moved out of London together, and more than a decade later they all still keep in contact.

One of the most beautiful aspects of classes that provide a welcoming environment in which mothers and babies can practise yoga together is the opportunity which it provides for postnatal women to welcome and honour their infant.

Kim returned to the postnatal yoga class in Bristol with her six-week-old daughter after spending a fortnight visiting the child in the local hospital's intensive care baby unit where she had been placed for observations after respiratory and digestive problems that occurred immediately after birth. Kim described after the first session how the class gave her a special chance to begin to acknowledge the arrival of her baby: 'You know this is the first time since she arrived that I have actually been able to really connect with her. I have been worried sick, and not able to even let myself relax and enjoy her.' As they cuddled up together in a Side-lying restorative yoga pose for the Sonic massage (pp.467–9), Kim and her daughter visibly settled. 'It's because we are here and being so nurtured. I can finally really welcome her. It feels like she has come home.'

Kim had attended the pregnancy yoga classes right up until her due date, and had especially enjoyed the breathing and sound practices. She immediately saw when she brought her tiny baby to the postnatal recovery and baby yoga class that the baby clearly recognised the rhythms and sounds of the practices. 'Look! You can see in her eyes, and how she's breathing – she remembers it. It's calming her down'.

What Kim observed is a common occurrence in these classes, and indeed when any mother continues to practise the yoga she did during pregnancy. The effect of hearing familiar sounds and feeling familiar movements after birth is clearly comforting to the infants. It is as if babies are reminded of their time in the womb. These techniques thus become very helpful mothering tools to sooth and calm agitated infants. Postnatal yoga, especially when it is a partial continuation of practices done during pregnancy, creates a genuine, positive connection between mother and child. It also offers powerful means for postnatal healing in mothers, and can be a great support during the establishment of breastfeeding.

Mel, one of the Greek yoga teachers attending a pregnancy yoga training course in Athens, testified with passion to the power of ujjāyī *breath as the tool that supported her during some serious challenges with breastfeeding: 'I wanted to train to share this with other women,' she said, 'because I know at first hand how it can help. When my son was one week old, I was in this awful situation, where it seemed as if I couldn't produce enough milk to feed him, and I was in huge pain trying to breastfeed. All my doctors, and family and friends were pushing for me to just give him formula, which I really did not want to do. I was being pressured on all sides, and was really upset by the threats and horror stories I was hearing – "your son will die of malnutrition" they were saying to me because he had lost weight, and we had been in hospital with jaundice and everything had got out of synch.*

I was crying with pain when I fed him, and my mother was waiting in the background, ready to give him a bottle. I was really desperate. The only thing that got me through was the breath. I held him all night and all day, and just kept breathing with ujjāyī, *which I had used during pregnancy and birth. It really calmed him down. But the main thing was it kept me together even when I thought I was going to fall apart. I kept my focus on my breath, and I believed I could do it, and the breath kept me going – after a couple of days with just resting and breathing and being close to my son I knew something had to change. I reached the point when I thought, if I haven't got this happening by the end of today I will give up. But the breath helped me stay with it, and the pain went away, and the milk began to flow. And I was able to feed him even though everyone said I couldn't. It was like a miracle. I fed him for nearly a year in the end, and I loved every feed. I couldn't have done it without the* ujjāyī *breath.'*

YOGA PRACTICES

The ***ujjāyī* breath** (pp.134–5) which Mel described as a 'miracle' of support can be combined with the **Golden thread exhalation** (p.133) and rhythmic pulsing lifts to create a profoundly **Healing breath** (p.482) that can not only help to restore muscle tone to the pelvic muscles, but also bring conscious awareness into the vagina and womb. This awareness helps a woman to understand where she is in the process of postnatal recovery, and to respect her own limits.

Semi-supine rest with chair (p.550) is probably one of the most helpful restorative poses a woman can do postnatally: it helps to release the lower back from tension, encourages a flow of energy and awareness in the pelvis and takes the pressure off feet, ankle and knee joints that can often be painful at this time. It's the perfect way to take rest when the baby is having a nap. Even if practised only for a few minutes it can totally revitalise a tired mother. One of the students at the weekly class in Stroud routinely arrived late because of multiple family obligations, and the only pose she ever got to do was this one. I wondered why she bothered coming at all. 'It's worth getting here just for this,' she said, 'I feel completely renewed.'

Of all the practices I have shared over fifteen years of teaching mother and baby yoga classes, the **Sonic massage** (pp.467–9) is the one integrated practice that I share in every single class, because it always brings joy and comfort to the mothers and their babies. It uses the mother's healing breath to carry her voice directly into the baby's body, reminding the child of the sonic landscape of the womb even as the mother rejuvenates and nourishes herself with sound and breath.

Kneeling salutations (p.542) is a very accessible and energising sequence that moves the spine through a gentle but revitalising range of movement (side bends and twists, and backwards and forwards), whilst keeping the mother close to the ground so that the baby can see her clearly and easily. It is ideal for the early months of postnatal recovery, before the baby is able to crawl. The **Postnatal sun salute** (pp.533–5) offers helpful modifications to the usual sun salute, safely encouraging postural readjustment to counteract the shoulder hunching that accompanies infant feeding and carrying. It gradually but effectively builds strength and support through the lower back, abdomen and pelvic walls.

All of the semi-supine practices to support **pelvic health and recovery** (pp.483–8) are very helpful during the postnatal recovery period. In addition the **inversions** (pp.488–91) give profound relief from the low, 'dragging' feeling many women experience in the pelvis. Whilst the semi-supine practices are suitable from the first days after birth, it is important to wait until after bleeding has stopped before doing the inversions.

The ***yoga nidrā*** for thanksgiving and grieving (pp.448–9) is a powerful healing process for postnatal recovery. It creates the space and time to grieve for what has been lost and left behind in your life so that you can fully embrace your present situation. This is a crucial component of postnatal recovery that is often overlooked.

YOGIC REMEDIES AND RESPONSES

The most important thing to know about yoga for postnatal recovery is that for it to really work, to bring long-term healing, it needs to be slow and steady. I have observed many *yoginīs* leaping back into a dynamic practice of *āsana* after the birth of their children, desperate to get the 'vitality kick' that fast *āsana* practice can sometimes bring. They are tired, and they believe that working hard and fast in a yoga class will rejuvenate them. But this is not what happens. The postnatal body is fragile and leaky, literally and energetically. Dynamic practice at this time tends to deplete women. Think of it like this: if you go to collect water in a leaky bucket, then no matter how much you put in, most of it will end up pouring out of the holes in the bottom of the bucket. This image of the leaky bucket was shared by Mukunda Stiles during the structural yoga therapy training, as a general metaphor for the importance of sorting out pelvic and abdominal tone in all yogic practice, but is particularly pertinent to postnatal yoga.

Deep healing to fix the holes in the bucket is the prerequisite for more energising practice. When women practise too fast or too hard it actually retards postnatal recovery: it's one step forwards and three steps back. I have seen women who were super-fit yoga teachers before they gave birth flinging themselves back into hectic teaching and practice schedules in the weeks and months after birth, only to damage their pelvic ligaments so profoundly that they are practically unable to walk for years, and I have watched women retire weeping and exhausted from their old *aṣṭaṅga vinyāsa* classes as they discover too late that their body is simply not ready for this practice, and they have caused injuries to their joints, or they have begun bleeding again from the healing site of the placental attachment.

None of this suffering is necessary, because there are loads of practices in yoga that actively support deep postnatal healing. To get any positive healing benefit from yoga at this time it is necessary first to *nurture* the mother, and then to proceed to *stabilise* her pelvis and whole musculoskeletal structure by doing practices that bring sustainable strength. Last of all, once she feels nurtured and stable, then, and only then, will practices intended to *revitalise* actually have the desired effect. This nurture – stabilise – revitalise sequencing is the structure for the postnatal yoga remedies for some common postnatal experiences set out below.

Exhaustion: This is the organising principle of the postnatal period. Yoga for postnatal recovery is yoga for exhausted and sleep-deprived women. Even if the babies are in fact sleeping well at night, there is inevitably a deep exhaustion that persists after pregnancy and birth and can often be difficult to address because the demands on a mother's time are so intense. Those practices that most directly support a woman's energy levels at this time are *yoga nidrā* (pp.448–9), semi-supine practices to support pelvic health (pp.483–8) and the complete series for the liberation of energy (pp.497–510). The revitalising effects of all these practices are intensified by combining them with the Healing breath (p.482).

Grief for pregnancy loss and healing after miscarriage or abortion: Because emotional and physical tiredness can exacerbate the feelings of hopelessness and sadness at these times, the practices recommended above for exhaustion are of great value. In addition, all of the yoga greetings that bring love into the womb in chapter five are comforting and healing. Of particular importance after such losses is the *yoga nidrā* practice (pp.448–9) that gives you an opportunity to bid a proper farewell to the woman you were before this experience. This is a vital part of the grieving process. To nourish the body after a miscarriage, it is important to rest, but it is also helpful to introduce gentle movements, especially those that revitalise the pelvic muscles and the lower back, because these build a strong foundation for regaining strength and confidence. All the Standing womb pilgrimages (pp.170–2), Snake circles the womb (pp.168–9) and the Spirals and snakes from all-fours (p.541) are useful in this respect, and also the Healing breath with *mūla bandha* (p.482) (but only after bleeding has finished). Depending on circumstances, the main aim for a woman after the loss of a baby may be to re-conceive as quickly as possible, or to give thanks that the pregnancy did not result in a live birth, and to resolve to avoid future conceptions. In either case, the deep healing practices of the Healing breath (p.482) and *pūrṇa pavanmuktāsana* (pp.497–510) are a good place to start. In the case of wanting to re-conceive, then it is helpful to move on to receptive practices such as the Seed–flower pose (pp.154–5) and *śakti bandhas* (pp.164–8).

> *For example, Sita came for her first yoga therapy session four days after a miscarriage following a conception that had been assisted by taking the fertility drug Clomid. She was determined to heal and re-conceive as rapidly as she could. Sita practised the Womb greetings (pp.143 and pp.147–8) and Seed-flower pose (pp.154–5) with* ujjāyī *breath (pp.134–5) and the New beginnings* yoga nidrā *(p.442). Within two cycles, and without the use of Clomid, she was ovulating naturally and had conceived again, this time carrying her baby to fullterm. She effectively used the yoga practices of healing after miscarriage to lead directly into another pregnancy, and, two years later, is pregnant with a second baby. For her, the healing after miscarriage was welcomed as an entry point into further conceptions.*

At the opposite end of the spectrum, Angela, who already had three boys, conceived a fourth child and miscarried at sixteen weeks.

> *At forty-four, she experienced this fourth pregnancy and miscarriage as a shocking encounter with the reality of her physical age and her incapacity to summon up the resources she knew were necessary for mothering a fourth child, so she grieved for the loss of the baby, but welcomed the healing process as a way to nourish herself and to recognise that in fact, the loss was for the best: 'I really thought I wanted the fourth child,' she said, 'it was my secret dream. But when I actually felt how exhausted and wiped out the pregnancy made me feel, I knew in my heart I just couldn't do it. It was simply too much for me at this age. The miscarriage was really a blessing, and now I can heal, and recover and know clearly that my family is complete.'*

Angela used the Healing breath (p.482), Deeply restorative poses (pp.546–55) and *yoga nidrā* (pp.448–9) to rebuild her energies. It took three months, but in the end she felt her body re-balanced and she was able to grieve fully, recover and heal well.

Whereas for Angela and Sita, the ending of their pregnancies was not planned, for Sam, her third abortion was a carefully considered decision. As a film-maker in her early thirties, she had conceived a child with a colleague whilst on a research trip for a documentary film project. She felt instantly that neither she nor the father of the child were ready to be parents, and that for many personal and professional reasons, pregnancy and birth at this time in her life would be absolutely wrong for her. When she returned to the UK she arranged to terminate the pregnancy.

> *At the time she knew this was a completely appropriate decision and she recovered rapidly: 'I was totally relieved. I did the right thing. Realistically, it was the only thing I could do.' Ten years later, following a miscarriage, Sam sought yoga therapy to support recovery with a view to conceiving a child through IVF. 'I met the love of my life,' she explained, 'I knew that I wanted to have babies with him, and then I began to realise how difficult that might be. Even though I consider myself to be 'super-fertile' and have conceived very easily in the past – hence the need for the three abortions – we had problems with conceiving together, and so we went for IVF.'*

Sam conceived easily but then miscarried. Her decision to come for yoga therapy was in many ways a sign that she was at the end of the line: she was forty-five and beginning to face up to the fact that she might never conceive again. At this point, she looked back at her previous decisions to abort from a different perspective.

> *'I know that I made the right decisions for me in my life as it was then. I know that I had the capacity to conceive children then. And now that has changed. It's just how it is.' For Sam, the most useful aspect of yoga therapy was the space and skills it gave her to be kind to herself, not to judge the decisions she had made in the past with hindsight, to embrace everything that was positive in her life and to adjust her expectations to include the possibility that she might well not conceive. She learnt* ujjāyī *breath and a simple form of* yoga nidrā *that invited her to discover her own* saṁkalpa *or guiding affirmation. Instantly she recognised how helpful these practices were, saying: 'I can just know how useful this will be for me. I can feel this breath helps me to let go, and be in the here and now. I feel its power to help me get through this.'*

Whilst breath, movement and relaxation practices can offer very practical support for the adjustments needed to recover from abortion or miscarriage, the broader philosophical perspectives of yoga can provide an even deeper level of support. To promote psychic and emotional healing after pregnancy loss and abortion it can be very helpful to view the experiences from the point of view that sees acceptance and adaptation as positive responses to grief. For example, a gifted midwife who contributes to the pregnancy and postnatal yoga training courses, and has worked all over the world delivering babies and supporting women's health, views miscarriage and pregnancy loss as a positive opportunity to admire the womb's capacity to encourage a deep preparation for motherhood.

> *'It's like when you are expecting a special guest,' she explains, 'you take extra care with the cleaning, and make the room really beautiful and fresh. That's what happens after miscarriage – it's as if the womb is making herself ready for the arrival of the special guest. Sometimes those few weeks of a pregnancy that end in miscarriage are really a preparation to be totally ready when the baby who is going to come into your life arrives.'*

I have found this perspective to be of great help to many women recovering from miscarriage and hoping to conceive again soon. Personally I also found great solace in another perspective that was offered to me by a yoga teacher friend who had spent a lot of time in Tibet, and who explained her understanding of the Tibetan Buddhist belief that babies who don't make it to birth are the incarnations of souls who do not actually need a full human birth, they simply need time in a human womb to resolve some past karmas, and then they are free to move on.

> *'Perhaps they are people who died suddenly or accidentally, and they have some unresolved karma that doesn't require a whole lifetime,' she explained to me when I was recovering after my second miscarriage. 'All it needs is a few weeks' gestation in the soul of a willing human mother. These babies have a special karmic bond with the woman whose body provides this opportunity for healing their karmas. That's why we feel sad when we lose them, but we have offered a service to them that they truly appreciate.'*

After a stillbirth, when a mother has had a whole pregnancy to develop a special bond with the child, the feeling of sadness at their parting can be even greater, so in such cases it can be very healing for the mother to recognise that the child she has grown has already thanked her for her special service:

> *'Think of it like this,' explained a healer to my friend in Ireland who was grieving after the stillbirth of her second daughter, 'one day you will be able to say thank you to this soul: for she gave you a precious gift. You may not feel like this now, because you do not understand the nature of the gift that she has brought, but in time you will be able to appreciate how her presence and her death have changed you.'*

Such spiritual perspectives on the experiences of grief after an unexpected pregnancy loss or stillbirth may also be very valuable to women healing after a planned abortion, whether that was recently or farther in the past. In Sam's case, for example, when she was adjusting to the realisation that she might not conceive another child, having a broader philosophical picture that included the three babies she had conceived and aborted made it easier to come to terms with the decisions she had made in her life. At these times, it can be extremely supportive to practise the 'thanksgiving and grieving' *yoga nidrā* practice (pp.448–9) that gives us the opportunity to offer kindness and support to the woman we were at the time of previous decisions to terminate pregnancies. Above all it is crucial to understand that the feelings we experience after abortions are signs that we are passing through a time of postnatal recovery: this is an initiation into the *siddhi* and power of Chinnamastā, a moment of deep transformation. Postnatal recovery certainly requires physical and emotional support and nourishment to enable us to heal well, whatever the circumstances that have brought the pregnancy to an end.

Being 'out of cycle': no menstrual cycles during breastfeeding (lactational amenorrhoea): After giving birth, some women's periods return within the space of a few weeks. For breastfeeding mothers, the range of time it takes for the menstrual cycle to return varies enormously, from a couple of months to a couple of years. Within this spectrum every woman finds her own rhythm and response, and the length of time without periods is related to all sorts of factors, including general health, diet, proportion of body fat, the amounts of breast milk being made and rest that is being taken. Many postnatal women welcome the 'period without periods', and other women find it very disturbing to be 'out of cycle' for months or years on end, especially if they are very connected to the experience of cyclical wisdom which their cycle brings.

> *My colleague Sjanie, co-founder of Women's Quest, struggled with this experience of being out of cycle while she breastfed her first daughter because she missed the sense of 'home-coming' when she arrived at menstruation each month; without it she felt lost. Certainly, many women experience a welcome sense of being 'back to normal' with the first period after birth, especially if there has been a long gap. My first period of lactational amenorrhoea lasted for two years, and there was only one cycle between the birth of my eldest son and his brother two and a half years later (whom I then breastfed for a further two and half years). So over four years I experienced only one menstrual cycle. I conceived my daughter one cycle after a miscarriage, and breastfed her for three years, creating a further span of over four years with only one cycle. During these years, whilst I was relieved not to be menstruating because my body had a lot of other things to do, including dealing with an intestinal parasite that caused me to lose a third of my body weight, and recovering from a post-partum haemorrhage after the birth of my second son. But when my bleed finally returned I experienced a sense of elation and relief, especially because, at the age of forty-four, I had wondered if I would ever menstruate again.*

Whether the period of lactational amenorrhoea is long or short, such experiences of being 'on pause' or 'out of cycle' are part and parcel of a postnatal experience that is often characterised by a deep disruption of many other important cycles in life, most significantly the disruption of regular sleep patterns, and the departure from weekly patterns of working hours, so at a profound level the postnatal woman can feel as if everything in life is chaotic and random. This kind of chaos is hard to cope with for anyone, but is especially difficult if you are tired and confused, for example because you don't understand why your baby is crying so much. Being 'out of cycle' postnatally evokes intense but often hidden emotions at either end of the spectrum, from missing the period, to wishing it would never come back.

Whichever end of the spectrum you are at, it can be a challenge to find a 'holding rhythm' to life during this chaotic time, and so it is very helpful to use yoga to heighten an awareness of the other naturally occurring cycles in life, for example connecting to the *svara* of the breath in the nostrils (p.466), honouring lunar cycles, and creating patterns of activity in daily life that bring a sense of order into the postnatal chaos. For example, setting aside a time for a daily nap, or even better, a daily *yoga nidrā* (pp.448–9) at about the same time each day can be very nourishing. Yoga practices that emphasise steady rhythm and synchronisation of breath, movement and awareness, especially *pūrṇa pavanmuktāsana* (pp.497–510) are also reassuring and revitalising.

Mastititis: Prevention of mastitis is better than cure. The awful flu-like symptoms and intense pain that this inflammation of the breast brings are so nasty that women who have experienced it will often say they would rather be in labour than have mastitis. Whilst there are remedies to ease the pain, for example, placing chilled cabbage leaves inside the bra, combing the breast, bathing the breast with hot and cold water, taking the homeopathic remedy phytolacca, or massaging the breasts in the bath, there is sometimes also a need for antibiotics. The best yoga support for healthy breast tissue and to prevent mastitis is to ensure, in the first place, that you have plenty of rest when you are breastfeeding, because getting tired and depleted can predispose you towards mastitis. Restorative yoga poses that enable you to feed the baby at the same time, e.g. side-lying (p.551) are ideal. Shoulder circling (p.506) and all practices from *pūrṇa pavanmuktāsana* that give space and movement around the armpits help to keep the breast tissue well-drained and healthy.

If you suspect you may have mastitis, get straight into bed, drink plenty of water and feed your baby. Use the pain-relieving breath practices (p.463). Consult your doctor and also get the support of an experienced breastfeeding counsellor. Act fast to hasten recovery because full-blown mastitis is so nasty that it is absolutely to be avoided if at all possible.

Haemorrhoids (piles): One of the most frequent comments I hear from postnatal women is 'Why did nobody tell me about how painful piles are?' Experiencing pain from distended blood vessels around the anus is a postnatal experience that causes many women deep distress. The classic yoga remedy is to stand on your head and do *ashvini mudrā* (pp.476–7), but since headstand is not an accessible or safe posture immediately after giving birth (there is not sufficient abdominal strength to support inversion of the spine, and inversions are not a wise idea when you are bleeding), a modified version is sensible. Simply take a basic all-fours position, perhaps with the elbows on the floor if the wrists are troubled, and lower the head and shoulders so that you can raise the bum. In this partial inversion, practise rhythmic *ashvini mudrā* (pp.476–7) with *ujjāyī* breath (pp.134–5). Drawing the anus in and out in this way can improve circulation and help to relieve pain and heal the piles. It is also helpful to use pain-relieving breaths (p.463) when pooing, and to sit with your bum in a bucket of warm water as the poo comes out so that it doesn't hurt so much. Plenty of fluids and a high-fibre diet are important to ensure the poos are regular and not hard, because getting constipated and straining will intensify the pain of the piles.

Pelvic organs and muscle problems including incontinence and prolapse: There are often problems with the pelvic muscles and organs after birth (sometimes during pregnancy). Healing is best achieved through a holistic programme that brings awareness of positive pelvic angle to provide optimum support, together with practices to tone and promote the healthy capacity for release in these muscles. Little and often, always working with the breath is the best way. Once bleeding after birth has stopped, then all of the practices to support the pelvic organs are really helpful (chapter twenty-one), and paying attention to postural adjustment is vital (p.481) because the angle at which the pelvis is held has a big impact upon the support available for the pelvic organs. Integrating these practices with those that raise the arms (e.g. Palm tree *vinyāsa* p.532) and that encourage a full yogic breath (pp.131–2) promote positive pelvic organ health and general vitality.

Depression: The most helpful yoga practices during postnatal depression are those that nourish the mother whilst promoting a positive bond with the baby: Sonic massage (pp.467–9) does both simultaneously. Kneeling salutations (p.542) with the baby in front are best practised with lots of clapping and clicking and sounded exhales, for example vibrating the lips loosely to make 'horse lips' on a noisy exhale, or humming and singing when moving close to the baby. Moving from Cat to Sphinx (p.535) with kisses on the exhalation can build a light and positive connection with the baby, and seeing how much all of this amuses the babies can be a delightful and cheering experience for even the most deeply depressed mother. It can also be nourishing to use the Wall-supported standing poses (pp.546–9) with the baby positioned underneath the mother, keeping eye contact and letting there be freely sounded exhalation to entertain the baby as the mother explores some energising standing stretches that are not as depleting as unsupported standing poses. Resting together with the baby in a Supported restorative pose (p.551) doing Healing breath (p.482) can relieve the exhaustion that underlies some of the desperate feelings that lead to depression postnatally. But above all it is the healing of being in community with other mothers, the yoga *satsang* (p.352) that can be the most profound yogic remedy for this experience.

Abdominal weakness, 'split rectus' and lower back pain: Abdominal weakness is a natural effect of having been pregnant for nine months. In the case of caesarean birth, the healing of the scar brings a clear focus of attention to the need to go gently with the abdominal muscles, but this caution is also helpful for women who give birth vaginally. Working with the Healing breath (p.482) is an effective way to strengthen gently from the inside out, using the pelvic muscles in tandem with the movement of the abdominal wall. The Circle of flowing breath and the Full yogic breath in chapter four are also very helpful to bring energy and tone back to the abdominal muscles. All the Heart-womb river practices in chapter five are effective to revitalise the subtle energy flows in the abdomen, and bring a loving touch along the front of the belly.

As the muscle tone improves, the semi-supine work to support the pelvis can also be utilised (pp.483–6), as can the Kneeling salutes (p.542) and the Postnatal sun salutation (pp.533–5). Gentle and very slow twists (p.159) can also be positive encouragements for the two bundles of the rectus muscles to move back closer together, but only if they are done with great attention to completely engage the breath and the pelvic muscles simultaneously with the abdominal muscles. Engaging oblique abdominal muscles without proper attention to their effect on the whole abdominal wall can pull the rectus muscles further apart.

Healing *from the inside out* slowly and steadily is what works best postnally. It is very important not to isolate the healing of the abdomen from the rest of the body, especially from the pelvic muscles and the lower back. Developing strength and tone in the rectus without integrating the pelvic muscles and awareness of pelvic angle can provoke or exacerbate prolapse.

> *For example, Nina, a tiny and vital New Zealander who had three children in quick succession in her mid-thirties, developed a split in her rectus muscles during third pregnancy. After the birth she assiduously worked with a personal trainer to build strength in that part of her abdomen. 'It worked,' she said 'only in so far as I got great strong abs that stood out nice and clear. The trouble was, they were nice and strong on either side of the gap. The gap between them didn't disappear, it was just fixed there. The stronger the muscles got, the clearer the gap seemed, and now it's permanent.' The other side effect of focusing attention on building abdominal strength in isolation was that, the more strength work Nina did on her belly, the less secure her pelvic organs felt. "Eventually, I could sense that every time I contracted my abdominal wall I could feel my pelvic organs descending. It was horrible. Everything I had been doing to help myself recover was actually making things worse: I ended up with great abs to show off a massive gap, and a constant dragging feeling in my pelvic floor.'*

With yoga healing that seeks to nurture and stablise first, this kind of thing doesn't happen, because the woman learns to lift and engage her pelvic muscles whilst she is contracting the abdominal muscles, and to hold her pelvis at the optimal angle to provide effortless postural support for the pelvic organs, and so they are not 'pushed' down. This is real healing, from the *inside* out, not just on the surface.

Aching knees, wrists and other joints: One of the most common complaints in postnatal yoga classes is knee pain. Wrists, ankles and feet can also be aching and painful, but the knees can really cause trouble. This is partly because the postnatal hormonal picture, especially during breastfeeding when there are high levels of oxytocin and prolactin in the body, can create a general ache in all the joints that is exacerbated by exhaustion. But this is only part of the problem. The deepening curves of the spine, which develop during pregnancy so that it's possible not to fall flat on your face at full term, tend to alter the angle at which the pelvis is held relative to the spine. This angle is maintained partly by the action of the quadriceps, and so it is referred to as the 'Q' angle. After pregnancy and birth, this angle re-adjusts, and the process of readjustment, which can take months, brings quite a lot of strain down through the knees and ankles as they re-adjust to the different weight loadings in relation to the changing angles.

What all this means is that usually the knees themselves are fine, but they are taking the rap for the adjustment of the pelvis. So working against the wall (pp.546–9) with bent knees can help to support the readjustment and lessen the pains in the knees, and paying attention to the fluid motion of the spine in the Snake circles the womb pose (pp.168–9) is a positive way to encourage a happy angle that does not trouble the knees. *Pūrṇa pavanamuktasana* (p.497–510) can strengthen those muscles above and below the knees that provide support during this time of readjustment, and restorative poses that elevate the knees and ankles (p.550) can also help.

If wrist pain is troubling, pay especial attention to the way you use your wrist when holding and feeding the baby, and in all-fours poses, rest the elbows and forearms on the ground instead of the palms of the hands, or use a stack of foam blocks to support the forearms.

Being postnatal and pregnant at the same time: This particular combination of challenges in the cycles of women's lives is becoming increasingly common as women leave having babies until later in life and then go on to have two or three in quick succession. The general medical opinion about the optimum time to conceive after a birth is a minimum of two years, whilst traditional Chinese medicine recommends a gap of five years as the optimal spacing. But very often women re-conceive before the previous baby is a year old, and 'Irish twins' (when two siblings are born within the same twelve-month period) are not uncommon. Whether or not the newly pregnant mother is still breastfeeding the previous infant, the experience of growing another baby so swiftly after birth places intense demands on every dimension of a woman's being. The crucial yogic component to support this experience is to take as much high-quality rest as possible. Restorative yoga poses (chapter twenty-five) preferably in combination with *ujjāyī* breath (pp.134–5) and *yoga nidrā* (chapter eighteen) are the most helpful things to do. Full and free breathing, and gentle revitalising practices such as *pavanmuktāsana* (pp.497–510) are the best option. It is also very helpful to develop a relaxation practice, for example using *bhrāmarī* whilst lying down (pp.469–7) that can be enjoyed together with the older sibling, so that they feel included in the process and do not become resentful of the unborn child who seems to be taking their mother away from them.

FEED THE WILD *YOGINĪ*

RADICAL RITUAL RECYCLING 1: DRINK YOUR OWN BREAST MILK

Breast milk is a homegrown energy boost. It is packed full of fabulous nutrients, which is why it is so good for babies, and why breastfeeding mothers need to eat and rest plenty: for food, rest and love are the raw materials of breast milk.

When I was pumping breast milk during a weekend course two hundred miles away from my youngest son, there was no way to get the milk back to him to drink. He was nine months old and I had to pump off my milk to avoid breast engorgement. At the end of the first day, I found myself poised over the sink with a flask of milk in my hand, wondering what to do. It seemed an awful waste of resources to pour it away. I am a keen recycler. And so I decided to make a ritual offering of the milk back to the divine mother, to honour all the effort that had gone into its creation. Gesturing with humility from my own heart, I offered my milk back to myself, by pouring it over my porridge, and savouring a highly nutritious breakfast. It was tasty.

See this act as a practical form of radical ritual re-cycling, marvel at the astonishing *siddhi* of lactation, and feel the great power of Chinnamastā to feed herself and her devotees. Even if you can't quite do the literal thing, then just thinking about this does a good job of shifting our perspectives on breastmilk: it helps us to appreciate breastmilk as a valuable resource, not only in nutritional terms, but in terms of the massive investment of energy that it represents. From an ecological perspective alone, it makes sense to perceive breastmilk as a precious natural resource worthy of attentive recycling. I'm not proposing that you neck gallons of the stuff, I'm just suggesting that next time you spill a few drops, have a taste. It's pretty amazing. And if you don't want it, and the baby's had enough, then the cat wouldn't say no.

RADICAL RITUAL RECYCLING 2: GIVE THE PLACENTA BACK TO THE EARTH

If you can shift your awareness to perceive breastmilk as a valuable natural resource, and view menstrual blood as the world's best plant food (p.269), then it's not such a leap of faith to regard the placenta as a truly precious item. After all, menstrual blood is the product of a twenty-eight-day cycle, and

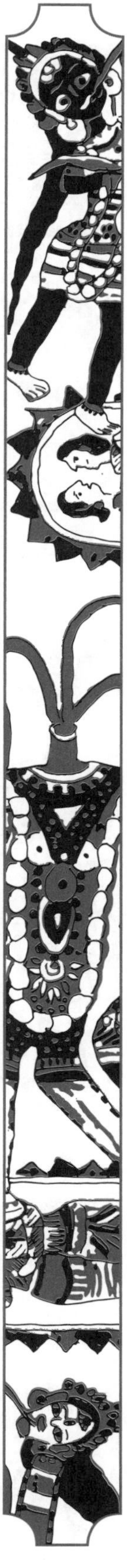

breastmilk is on an even faster turnaround, but the placenta, she takes nine months to develop, and is thus a far more significant investment of energy and resources. Such a complex, beautiful and life-sustaining organ merits respect.

In its most intense form, this respect for the placenta can take the form of a 'lotus birth', where the placenta remains attached to the child until the umbilical cord naturally comes away and the baby and the placenta part company very gently indeed. But there are other ways to demonstrate respect for the placenta, and to honour the remarkable energies that have taken nine months to grow this astonishing life-support system. Appropriately reverent treatment of the placenta after the baby is born is not simply a form of ritual recycling, but can also be a healing act of closure on the experiences of pregnancy and birth.

Burying the placenta in the earth is a powerful way to feed the wild *yoginī*. It's not something you need to do straight away. A placenta freezes very well. Wait until you feel ready to give energy to the ritual of recycling, and then dig (or ask someone else to dig) a nice deep hole and place the placenta underneath the roots of a young tree, or other plant, to nourish new life and to let the earth feel the arrival of the child who has no further need of the placenta. The act is a ritual offering of something your body has created to sustain the future creativity of the earth. I've always found this to be a deeply satisfying closure on pregnancy, even if it usually took me over a year (in my daughter's case, four years) to get around to doing it. The three placentas of my three children have fed the roots respectively of a very productive apple tree, fig tree and a hawthorn. Eating the fruits, and admiring the blossoms of these trees nourishes my sense of connection with seasonal cycles.

A more direct experience of recycling the placenta comes to women who consume their placentas, either as a cooked food or as a specially prepared medicine. But the experience of eating the fruits of the trees that are nourished by the placenta seems to this wild *yoginī* to carry a similar energetic effect, even if the nutritional benefits are perhaps not so impressive.

And if it wasn't possible or practical for you to obtain your placenta, then the same powerful effects of the literal act of ritual recycling can be obtained through a meditative virtual burial, or the planting of a special tree or bulbs. All of these gestures invite surrender to the reality of the cycles of experience: a vivid encounter with our direct connection with earth and the nourishment of life on the planet. This form of ritual recycling feeds the wild *yoginī* in many different dimensions of her being.

QUESTIONS AND REFLECTIONS

I invite you to explore your own (current or previous) experience of postnatal recovery and how it may be supported by yoga by asking yourself some (or any, or all) of the following questions:

1. How much rest (not sleep, but rest) did I get after the birth? What yoga practices helped me to feel rested?
2. What did I miss most about my 'ordinary' yoga practice after birth? Did I find any way to recover that precious aspect of yoga practice during the postnatal time?
3. What aspects of my life before birth do I miss most? Have I grieved for their loss? Do I need time to say a proper goodbye to the woman I was before this baby arrived?
4. Were there any yoga practices I did during the postnatal period that actually made me feel worse?
5. Were there any yoga practices I did during the postnatal period that made me feel better?
6. What yoga practices worked for me to do together with my baby?
7. What yoga practices worked better for me to do alone?
8. What elements of the power and wisdom of Chinnamastā have I experienced in this time of postnatal recovery? E.g. what are the deepest changes have I noticed, what support do I have, how am I nourishing myself now?

FURTHER READING AND RESEARCH

The Politics of Breastfeeding: When Breasts are Bad for Business, is **Gabrielle Palmer**'s classic exposé of the impact of big business on breastfeeding. It helps us to see this *siddhi* as a truly precious natural resource and breastfeeding as a radical force for change. **Sally Placksin**'s *Mothering the New Mother* provides a wealth of information and helpful tips for the community support of postnatal recovery, and **Jill Rohmer**'s *Postnatal Healing* is a goldmine of practical suggestions that actually work. A*fter the Baby's Birth... A Woman's Way to Wellness* by **Robin Lim** is also warmly recommended, as is her exploration of the placenta in postnatal healing, *Placenta: the forgotten Chakra*. **Dr Lesley Regan**'s book *Miscarriage: What every woman needs to know* is a reassuring overview of current medical thinking and case studies.

Rachel Cusk's *A Life's Work* is an illuminating and depressing classic in the 'my tales of postnatal depression' genre. Her grim experiences contrast with the more poetic Californian perspectives of **Francesca Lia Block**'s *Guarding the Moon*.

There are helpful healing tips for effective postnatal recovery in **Emma Cannon**'s *You and Your Bump*, and a very useful chapter on yoga for postnatal recovery in my own book, *Teach Yourself Yoga for Pregnancy and Birth*. For inspiration on yoga practice with your baby, see *Yoga Baby* by **DeAnsin Goodson Parker** and *Yoga for Mother and Baby* by **Françoise Freedman**.

Stillbirth and neonatal death charity, SANDS provides excellent support, community and information for those recovering from stillbirth: **www.uk-sands.org**

The Miscarriage Association offers support and useful information through its website, and operates a telephone helpline during office hours (01924 200 799). **www.miscarriageassociation.org.uk**

The UK charity 4children campaigns nationally to raise awareness of postnatal depression, and their 'Give me strength' project seeks to provide better support for mothers with postnatal depression. They also provide local links and good information on postnatal depression and family crisis: **www.4children.org.uk**

Another useful source of information and support for postnatal depression is **www.pni.org.uk**

The National Childbirth Trust runs postnatal discussion groups and other local events around the country that offer opportunities to connect with other new mothers in your area: **www.nct.org.uk**

TAMBA provides support for the families and carers of twins, triplets and higher-multiple births: **www.tamba.org.uk**

The following organisations all offer breastfeeding support by telephone and in person:

National Childbirth Trust: **www.nct.org.uk/parenting/breastfeeding-common-concerns-and-questions**

La Leche League: **www.laleche.org.uk**

Association of Breastfeeding Mothers: **www.abm.me.uk**

To locate teachers for postnatal recovery and baby yoga classes, see the listings at **www.wombyoga.org**, **www.yogaseva.org** and **www.birthlight.co.uk**. Yoga birth teachers (**www.yogabirth.org)** also provide some postnatal classes, as do those trained by the Active Birth Centre (**www.activebirthcentre.com**).

For a sweetly integrated mother and baby yoga class that includes postnatal recovery yoga for the mother and fun for the baby, the Sitaram *Mother Nurture* DVD is a helpful resource. It is available from **www.sitaram.org** and **www.yogamatters.com**. Other valuable DVDs demonstrating postnatal yoga include those produced by **Tara Lee** and **Wendy Teasdill**.

CHAPTER FIFTEEN

Bagalāmukhī

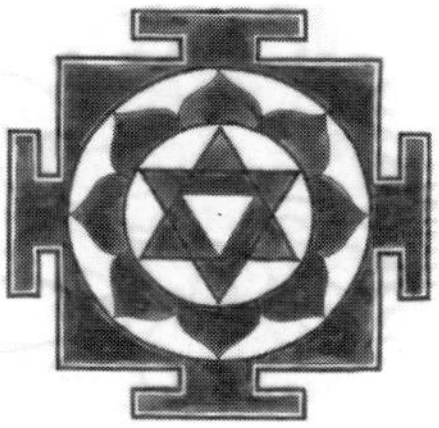

Stepping into the unknown: yoga and perimenopause

> *Menopause can be a disconcerting experience. Just when you think you have your act together… just when you have finally reached a comfortable level of poise and self-confidence, menopause causes you to sit up and take nothing for granted.*
> *(Janine O'Leary Cobb, in Taylor and Sumrall 1991: 26)*

PREFATORY NOTE ON PERIMENOPAUSE AND MENOPAUSE

The term 'peri' simply means 'around the edge'; it's at the root of the word 'perimeter'. Perimenopause is the time leading up to the edge of menopause. It is characterised by changes in the menstrual cycle and many other aspects of women's experience. Perimenopause does not have a clear start, like the first period, or the conception of a baby; and it only comes to an end when the menopause itself can be understood to have fully arrived. It is a lead-up to menopause, and it can last for many years. The time of onset is variable: in the same way that menarche can arrive any time between the ages of nine and seventeen, so too perimenopause can arrive at different times. Most often it begins around forty-five, but sometimes much earlier, and usually it has ended by the mid-fifties, but sometimes it may extend past sixty.

Menopause is the permanent end of menstrual cycles. The time of perimenopause and menopause are times of especial uncertainty in a woman's life, because they are experiences whose beginnings and ends can only be identified in retrospect. Only once it is over, and we know that our periods actually have stopped completely, can we tell absolutely for certain that we have been in menopause at all, and that it has ended. From a medical perspective, menopause ends with the one year anniversary of the last period but, in women's lived experience, things are not often so clear-cut.

This chapter addresses the issues that are raised by the experience of stepping into and living through the unknown. It covers the time from when changes first appear in a woman's cycle until she knows for certain, following a year without menstruation, that her periods have ceased. Although there are women who do experience a return of menstruation following a whole year without periods, it is most usual for twelve months without menstruation to be a clear sign that perimenopause has finished, and that this particular period of 'unknowing' has been completed.

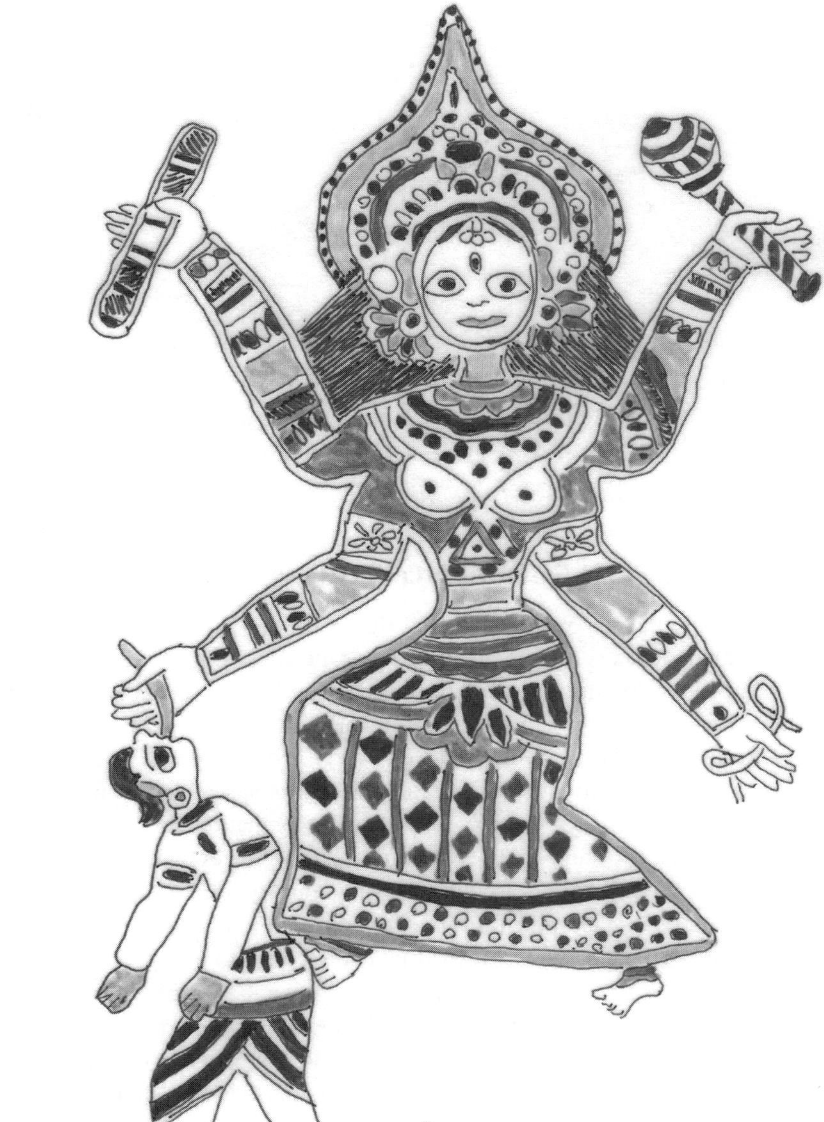

Bagalāmukhī manifests the turning-inward of consciousness that can occur during perimenopause

MAHĀVIDYĀ AND *SIDDHI*

WISDOM AND POWER

The *Mahāvidyā* presiding over this uncertain and challenging time of life is known as Bagalāmukhī, the 'paralyser'. She is associated in this chapter with the sometimes paralysing experience of stepping into the unknown as a woman encounters perimenopause. Bagalāmukhī literally means the face (*mukha*) that catches you like a noose (from the Bengali *bagalā*), and so she can be understood at one level to be the kind of beauty that is literally stunning. At the level of the deepening wisdom of midlife, the power of the 'paralyser' is to cause us to stop, to look back and review who we are and where we have come from, so that we may more clearly evaluate where it is that we would like to be heading in the future.

Perimenopause is often a time of confusion and sometimes anger or dismay, when the forward dash of younger years and the outward focus of mothering or minding businesses and professional or creative projects may reach an impasse. At the level of our bodies, this is often a time when we notice changes or pauses in the menstrual cycle, or become aware of the signs of incipient ageing and the effects of having lived in our bodies for forty-five years or so. All of these signs direct us to turn our attention inwards, to stop the outward activities, at least temporarily, to enter into stillness and reconsider everything we think we know: to 'grow or die'. It is a time when regrets and anger about things we have not done, or energies we may have misplaced in activities we no longer value, need to be faced.

The person whom Bagalāmukhī paralyses at this stage in life is ourselves. David Frawley puts it perfectly when he observes that 'The truth is we have forgotten ourselves and are hypnotised by the allure of external objects and identities. Bagalāmukhī breaks this eternal hypnosis through the greater hypnotic power of spiritual knowledge that causes us to lose interest in the idea of an external reality' (Frawley 1994: 133).

What this means at this point in our lives is a growing sense that it is imperative to follow the promptings of the inner guide. Women who experience the power of Bagalāmukhī can become transfixed by the unfolding of an inner wisdom that ultimately provides direction. For those women who embody the wisdom of Bagalāmukhī, the allure of outward focus, in particular the focus on outward trappings of youthful glamour, begin to lose their attraction. A deeper magic is at work, and we may become enchanted by the emerging sense of a profound calling, a way to be in the world that truly honours our power.

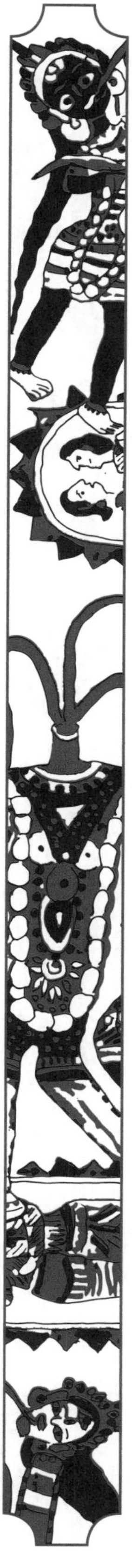

In this sense, Bagalāmukhī is directly expressive of the powers of the 'great enchantress' or 'Maga', the sorceress, who represents a fourth aspect of women's life experience that comes after the 'Mother' and before the 'Crone' in Celtic images of the goddess. This time of holding the powers of enchantment is not about bewitching others, but about being deeply drawn into the magical and empowering discovery of our own true nature, as the earlier, more outwardly directed roles of 'Maiden' and 'Mother' fall away.

Bagalāmukhī's great *siddhi* is the capacity to transfix and disarm us: to halt us in our habitual patterns of thought and belief. This is the quintessential experience of perimenopause: everything begins to stop, and we question deeply how we are to live in the chaos caused by the falling away of habitual patterns and rhythms. We are caught firmly by her, and she renders us speechless to stop the usual flow of our thoughts. Ultimately, Bagalāmukhī gives us the gift of clear speech, for she is associated with the power of speech in so far as it expresses the ultimate truth. Once the initial shock of our encounter with Bagalāmukhī is processed, we gain the perspective of middle age on the activities of our youth. Then we are empowered to pronounce on them, to voice the truth of how we now really feel about all of these things that have passed. There can be a stunning quality to the pronouncements of middle age, a sense that the words we speak carry the weight of experience and the clarity of regret or knowing that only comes through years of reflection. If we have never really stopped to think about what we have been doing all this time, then this time of life can come as a bit of a shock: it literally can paralyse us.

In specific relation to the menstrual cycle and the changes that can begin to occur at perimenopause, the harvest we begin to reap is the harvest of attitudes and experiences that we have brought to all of our monthly cycles over the previous thirty years or more. If we have spent our lives ignoring or demeaning the experiences of the menstrual cycle, if we have endeavoured never to speak about them or to pretend that the cyclical peaks and troughs of monthly moon cycles have not been a significant part of our lives, then now is the time when decades of suppressed experiences are likely to resurface. For some women, there is a graceful, gradual tailing off of menstrual experiences as hormonal levels begin to shift, but for others there is a dramatic set of alarming changes.

Although, when the pelvis is angled optimally, the effects of forty-five years of gravity should have nothing but the positive effect of creating intra-abdominal pressure to support our pelvic organs effectively, often our posture has not been helping our pelvic organs, especially if we've been walking and standing in high heels, or tucking our tailbones under to make our bums look smaller. When we've experienced decades of these forms of postural self-abuse, then the effects of forty-five years of gravity on the pelvic organs in a poorly positioned pelvis can combine with a changed hormonal environment to manifest as prolapses and pelvic organ shifts.

The effects of forty-five years of suppression of menstrual visions and revelations can erupt with such power as to stop us in our tracks, wondering 'where did that come from? We can speak with such vehemence and power that we and others are shocked. These voices, the voices of the middle aged women whose decades of experiences are beginning to bubble up and are wanting to be heard, can be a treasure trove of wisdom and guidance. The perspectives of women at this stage in life are often clear and direct, having gained through experience the broader vision that empowers us to leave aside distractions and confusions, and to arrive at a clear sense of what really matters, and the confidence to voice it.

The force of that voice, and its ability to speak ultimate truths that are not always welcome or comfortable, has the capacity to silence others. Bagalāmukhī's voice is a direct line to wisdom and power. She has no respect for false mental constructions or vanities. This voice of spiritual wisdom often only begins to become audible once women get over forty-five. But in our culture, this time of life is often feared and denigrated as a time when the power of youth and beauty is beginning to fade and women become crabby, irritable and marginalised.

In the domestic arena, women of this age who gave birth when they were over thirty are often co-existing with teenaged children who are undergoing their own powerful transformative shifts. The relationship between adolescence and perimenopause is intimate and inverted; an empathic understanding of the experiences of adolescence can be helpful to those women who experience the menopause as 'puberty backwards'. For those perimenopausal women sharing domestic space with pubescent offspring, it is not uncommon for the combination of these two different life stages to bring family life to a total standstill, as wild arguments or profoundly uncomfortable silences erupt.

The capacity for powerful argument is one of the key characteristics of Bagalāmukhī. The traditional form of Bagalāmukhī depicts her facing her armed opponent, with one hand around his tongue, holding tight, and the other hand wielding a mace

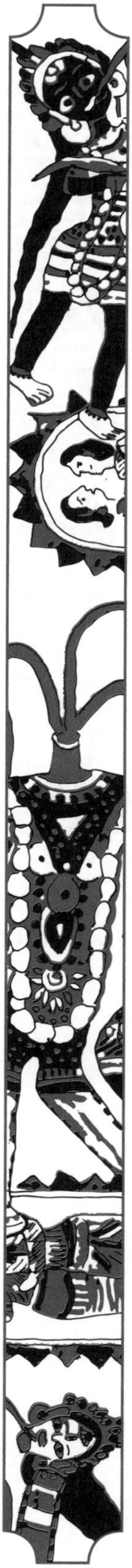

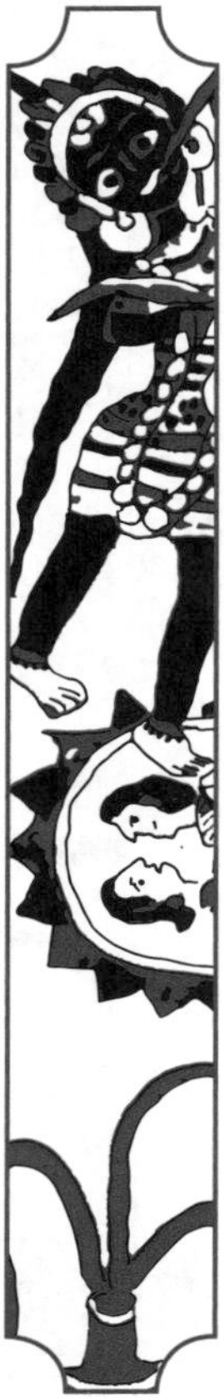

with which she hits him on the head with such force that he drops his weapon. The image is a powerful depiction of her capacity to stop all argument: not only does she literally render the opponent speechless by immobilising his tongue, but she puts a stop to his capacity to think by striking his skull with her mace.

Because she is seen to be grasping her assailant's tongue, the purifying power that she holds is related to the capacity to cleanse and transform through changes in speech pattern and content. For example (and this resonates particularly with midlife changes in perspectives and values) Bagalāmukhī eradicates pointless gossip and chatter. When her wisdom is at work to literally hold our tongues, then the power of speech is in service to the ultimate truth. *Prāṇa* can then be re-directed to the development of true wisdom and understanding to make sense of the challenges of midlife and beyond.

Bagalāmukhī gives the capacity for us to see the opposite quality in everything, and this is a mark of the clarity of thinking that can come at midlife: to perceive the light which can illuminate the darkness of struggle or sorrow, and to taste the true freedom which comes as the options and choices of youthful opportunity begin to close down. For a woman at midlife, Bagalāmukhī is the immense power of clarity and understanding that arises out of confusion. She recalibrates our priorities, and she brings the words to articulate this deep knowing.

LIMITATIONS: CULTURAL EXPECTATIONS

> *The fifty-year-old woman has no option but to register the great change that is taking place within her, but at the same time she is forced to keep this upheaval a secret. The shame that she felt at the beginning of her periods is as nothing compared to the long-drawn-out embarrassment occasioned by their gradual stop-go ending; no woman would step into a shop or an office or a party and announce in ringing tones that she expected special consideration because she was struggling through menopause. (Greer 1992: 390)*

In contrast to the immensely transformative powers of Bagalāmukhī and the understanding that she brings us of perimenopause as a positive, expansive opportunity for self-evaluation and reflection, perimenopause in our culture is demeaned, belittled and hidden. Cultural and social pressures and expectations around perimenopause are profoundly limiting. At a time in our lives when women prepare to step into the unknown inner territory of perimenopause, the judgements of the outer world begin to systematically devalue and disempower us. This is a toxic combination.

Inside we are confused and possibly alarmed, whilst outside we are expected to keep up appearances for fear we lose our usual roles. Our current cultural climate does not nourish the perimenopausal woman, neither does it support us in the inner work we need to do to find our way through the times of challenge and change at this time of life. At the level of deep nurture and support, our society has practically nothing of value for women as we enter the change. All that's on offer is stuff to buy to help us pretend it's not happening. Consumer culture is keen for us to invest our money in many means to remove or mask any evidence of change. Hair dye and anti-wrinkle cream are big business. Hairdressers make their livings out of eradicating the evidence of greying hair. They are clearly doing pretty well out of our fear of appearing to admit to change, because in many circles, even those where women in their late forties and fifties form the majority (for example certain parts of the yoga world), it is unusual to see women's hair greying naturally.

This may seem to be a small point, but it reveals a big truth. This truth is not about passing judgment on the millions of women who cannot bear to look in their mirrors and see their hair colour fading, it is about understanding the deep disrespect for older women that is at the heart of our culture. At the bottom of every purchase of every pack of hair dye, and prompting every effort to 'hide our roots' as the grey grows back, is a powerful fear that to be seen to be a woman over forty is to be seen as worthless. Such is the destructive power of our sexist culture's desire to deny women access to the deep freedom of just being ourselves, especially our older selves, just as we are, that many women clearly cannot even conscience the idea of visibly ageing. It is as if, out of fear of this deep disempowerment, we have all agreed to conspire to pretend that there is no change occurring. To deny this small aspect of change makes it harder to accept the profound changes that are occurring at a deeper level. And this utterly disconnects us from the possibility of recognising the inner shifts and empowerments that this stage of life can bring us.

One of the reasons why perimenopausal women feel obliged to act as if nothing has changed is because any mention of the shifts and signs that we are entering the change are met with derision, disgust or the desire to control. Instead of being recognised as a natural rite of passage, and a powerful and necessary initiatory process, the experiences of perimenopause are treated either as a joke or as a set of medical problems to be fixed. There is a long and appalling history to the medicalisation of menopause, well told in other places (see Foxcroft 2010 and Greer 1992). Perimenopausal women quite understandably keep our experiences largely to ourselves or attempt to hide the evidence of the changes because if we don't we're likely to be laughed at or medicated or perhaps lose our jobs.

Women who openly respond to the shifts of changes, the mood swings and energy troughs, the despair and hot flushes are often greeted (by husbands and doctors and line managers) with the response that if it is causing difficulty then the woman should just 'do something about it' for example by taking HRT. The logic of these responses is rooted in a belief that women's primary function is to provide discrete and efficient service to the world of men, and that if we are unable to do this, then we cause the men in that world serious problems, which need to be fixed. This logic extends out to those women who no longer engage in traditional activities of mothering or housewifery: if we play a role in the male worlds of corporate finance, or law, or academia, for example, then there are clear limits on the degree to which we can be permitted to disrupt these institutions, for example by honouring our menstrual cycles, or by taking time out to respond to menopausal experiences that may need periods of rest and self-care which the working environment simply does not allow. Germaine Greer writes acutely about the 'social invisibility' of menopause and points out that:

> *There is no rite of passage to surround the middle-aged woman with solemnity, no seclusion ordered for her, no special periods of rest. She cannot withdraw to a menopausal hut and sit and talk with other menopausal women. She simply has to tough it out and pretend that nothing is happening. (Greer 1992: 39)*

The trouble with this is that it makes it seem as if there are no women going through menopause: there are simply younger women, or those who appear younger than they are, and older women who have passed over the climacteric and are on the other side. The experiences of getting from one side to the other are neither valued nor discussed openly, and so this challenging time of life is largely an 'undescribed experience', a journey without any reliable signposts or maps. In this way the experience of the perimenopause has many similarities with the postnatal experience that also is overlooked, disrespected and largely hidden from view.

My intention in the next section is to tell the stories of those perimenopausal women whose experiences transcend the limits of our expectations of this time of life, so that they may help to provide reassurance, support and positive role models. The stories continue also in the next two chapters, where I consider the role of yoga in the lives of menopausal and postmenopausal women.

FREEDOMS: YOGA PERSPECTIVES, TECHNIQUES AND AWARENESS FOR BREATHING, MOVING AND BEING

> *Perimenopause, which coincides with the well-known midlife crisis, is a biologically and psychologically supported opportunity for total rebirth and rejuvenation of body, mind, and spirit, one that results from addressing and healing the unfinished business of the first half of our lives. That's why so many midlife women remember and then let go of childhood trauma at this time.*
> *(Christiane Northrup 2005: 30)*

The experiences of perimenopause are all about change. The intensity of the experiences can force us to let go of habits and ideas that have been central to our sense of who we are. This can be painful. The heart of a positive yogic response to the experience of perimenopause is to acknowledge the challenges this pain may bring, whilst we embrace the experience as a fabulous opportunity for re-evaluation, reflection and change at every level of being. It is helpful also to see the full circle of women's life experience at this time as a cyclic progression from bud, through flower, fruit and returning to the deep wisdom of the seed. In terms of attending to the needs of the perimenopausal time of life, it is especially valuable to recognise that the process of transformation from flower to seed is a powerful rite of passage that constitutes a life stage all of its own, a time of letting go and acceptance. This is the focus of the *yoga nidrā* ritual at the end of this chapter.

At the heart of yoga philosophy is the concept of *saṇtośa*, which means the happy acceptance of what is, as it is, and *ahimsa*, which is often translated literally as non-harming, but can also be understood as kindness. These two concepts from the philosophical bedrock of yoga take on a particular value during the perimenopausal years of our lives. To practise yoga with attention to this philosophical framework invites the opportunity to practise inner *saṇtośa* and *ahimsa*, in terms of offering kindly tenderness to oneself to help with the process of acceptance of change.

One of the most difficult aspects of the perimenopause to deal with is the experience of uncertainty, irregularity and lack of rhythm in terms of monthly cycles at a physical level, but mental and emotional life generally. This is where yoga has a deep and powerfully healing role to play: promoting acceptance of change in preparation for a safe journey through the passage to power that is the menopause. It is also important to acknowledge the powerful influence which culture and environment have upon our expectations of this point in our lives, and to see positive roles for menopausal and postmenopausal women in our families and wider social networks, which I explore in the next chapters.

The yoga practice of *satsang* has huge importance during perimenopause, and the support, sharing and wisdom of older women is absolutely crucial to the positive experience of perimenopause. Happily, opportunities for hearing menopausal stories and sharing experiences are increasing. This is partly due to a natural demographic shift (more women are living longer after menopause and have more chance to share their experiences) and partly due to a change in cultural attitudes towards menopause. In terms of demographics, it is clear that there is a 'critical mass' of women coming through to menopause now who have experiences of conscious menstruation, and possibly also of the conscious initiations of birth and breastfeeding. As these women pass through menopause, there will be on the planet an astonishingly large number of the kinds of humans who could never before have existed: few of our grandmothers got to do 'conscious menopause', many of them didn't live long enough to have many years after the menopause, and hardly any of them would ever have even spoken about their experiences of menstruation and menopause.

The influence of younger women upon their elders is not to be underestimated: in the same way as women who have consciously engaged with their menopause can share experiences with younger women to provide support and inspiration, so too the shifts in attitude towards menstruation can positively impact on peri- and postmenopausal women.

> *My mother, who began menstruating at the age of ten and continued with regular cycles until she was sixty-two, was afforded no opportunities to speak about menstruation as a young woman growing up Catholic in Dublin in the nineteen-fifties, but as a postmenopausal woman she has attended three Womb Wisdom retreats and enjoyed*

the experience of the group work and visualisation exercises facilitated by Alexandra Pope. In the presence of menstruating and perimenopausal women who are both conscious and openly sharing about these experiences, there is an opportunity to heal the previously unacknowledged wounds and griefs caused by shame, guilt and secrecy around menstruation and menopause. 'You girls are so lucky to have this work,' she announced each year, 'in my day, nobody spoke of these things. It was all a curse.' Other women working in the field of menstrual awareness report the astonished new freedoms and intimacies experienced by their grandmothers: 'She's ninety-eight, and when I first told her about the workshops for menstrual health she was totally delighted. She told me she had never before, not even once in her life, had a single conversation with anyone about her periods.'

Eighty years of silence is a long time. When the silence is broken, there is great healing and support to be had, not just from speaking the truth of one's own experience, but also from hearing other women's stories. In an environment of a supportive womb-friendly yoga class or retreat, women have the opportunity to acknowledge with sensitivity the coming to the end of their menstrual periods. These acknowledgments allow the release of grief and regret which no doubt shapes our experiences of perimenopause. Speaking and hearing stories of menstrual life and its conclusion is powerful medicine. Perimenopausal women in particular are hungry to hear the experiences of women who have 'gone through it'. The most moving part of the well-woman yoga therapy course is often a section of the training that involves listening to the passage to power of a postmenopausal *yoginī*. Many of the women attending the training are in their thirties and forties, and they are keen to hear 'good news from the other side' to counteract the relentless negative portrayals of perimenopausal trials.

One such positive story that has been shared in this course is yoga teacher Frances Lewis's remarkable account of the ritual release of her old self, and her conscious embrace of freedom postmenopausally. Her experiences are described in the next chapter, and Frances has been generous enough to share them with women on the womb yoga training course over the past four years. The reception her story receives is inevitably tearful. All the perimenopausal women in the room weep with relief: 'We never get to hear these stories. Thank you so much for sharing your experience. I don't feel so frightened now about what is starting to happen to me.'

On another training course, Colette, a vibrant yoga teacher in her mid-fifties, held the circle of thirty younger women spellbound as she described her own experiences during the perimenopause and how yoga had helped her to hold down her day job as a bank cashier in the face of what she described as 'mind-wipe'. 'I would be counting out money, or cashing up, or about to complete a transaction for a client and then all of a sudden I would forget everything completely. I would be totally and completely unable to think. I couldn't concentrate or focus. And if it wasn't 'mind wipe' then it would be wild mood swings or I'd be drenched in sweat from a burning hot flush. I had to go and change in the toilets. I was really worried that I'd lose my job.'

The intensity of the experiences she described were common, but what was unusual about Colette's delivery was that instead of a litany of complaints and horror stories, she was able to share strategies that had helped her cope with her experiences and find freedom in her own attitudes to what was happening to her:

' I couldn't have survived without my yoga. It kept me sane.' The programme of yoga that Colette developed to support herself through the change was a combination of management and prevention. In addition to attending a regular weekly yoga class Colette had her own practice to use during the day at work to help handle symptoms, for example Cooling breaths (pp.470–1) to reduce temperature, ujjāyī *breath (pp.134–5) to assist concentration, combined with breath counting in small batches to hold focus. She also used breath-balancing practices to maintain equilibrium. In terms of prevention, Colette found that more vigorous practices at weekends including sun salutations and backward-bending practices, and some inversions would all help her burn off excess heat and create a state of balance and calm that could carry her through the week.*

But above and beyond the practical assistance that the yoga practice of posture and breathwork brought her, it was the regular practice of yoga nidrā *(chapter eighteen) and meditation each evening before bed, which really provided the deep sense of calm that carried Colette through perimenopause with a sense of graceful acceptance and openness: 'The* yoga nidrā *brought me home to myself each night,' she explained, 'and so I could touch base, rebalance, and treat the whole thing as a pretty amazing adventure. What a trip!'*

The experiences of *yoginīs* like Frances and Colette are precious to hear. Yoga sessions that include opportunities for such sharing can make a big difference to our experience of perimenopause. Women are thirsty for this.

At a recent womb yoga for menopause workshop in Cork city, attended by perimenopausal and postmenopausal woman, the aspect of the session that most women prized the highest was the sense of deep relief that came from making even a little time to hear each other's experiences. 'It was worth coming just to hear you all speak!' enthused one yoginī *in her mid-forties, 'I had been feeling so alone. My mothers and older sisters just call menopause 'the thing'. They refuse to talk to me about what's happening. I thought*

I was going mad. After this sharing I feel reassured that I am not on my own in this. I feel miles better already.'

At one level, the *satsang* or sharing may reveal emotional and spiritual concerns, but at another, equally useful level, it can be about pooling helpful practical strategies to cope with the challenges of this time.

> *The top two menopausal tips from a postmenopausal yoga therapist of my acquaintance included a recipe for 'menopause cake' that included plenty of nourishing seeds and fruits, and her fulsome testimonial to the best quality, highest thread count, pure organic Egyptian cotton bedsheets 'because you sweat less in them. And if you do get a flush, then they really soak the night sweats up way better than anything else. If you're sweating every night then these things really matter.'*

Another perimenopasual *yoginī* put me on the track of natural progesterone cream, because her experiences with even the most minute doses of the stuff had helped reverse hair loss and make more manageable for her the intense rages that were consuming her during her perimenopausal pre-menstruums:

> *'No-one else is going to tell you this: it only works if you are cycle aware,' she explained 'because you use the cream for three weeks of the cycle, from the week at the end of your bleed through to the first day of your period. I only use a fraction of the recommended dose, so it lasts for ages and it's like a ritual of self-anointing. You mustn't put it in the same place each day, so I follow a pattern that moves the placement of the cream around my body on the twenty-one days of each month that I use it. It's a literal kind of* yoga nidrā*, and it's really helped me.'*

Sharing tips like this is valuable, especially if we have information that is not so readily available from our regular healthcare providers. Because of the widespread promotion of standard forms of HRT, most family doctors tend not to give out information about the subtle dance of self-titration and responsive dose-reduction that a woman can negotiate with bio-identical hormone cream, because they are simply not familiar with this option for hormonal support during perimenopause. To share strategies that empower us to respond sensitively and with awareness to the changes that we experience is a great service we can do for our sisters.

Sharing and letting go are important ways to access the healing power of yoga, but of course there are many other ways in which yoga may be of support during the perimenopause, as the following section demonstrates. Deep nurture and sharp awareness are the keys to utilising the tools of yoga to help ride hormonal fluctuations, and offer relief and support during times of challenge. This selection of yoga practices are all techniques and approaches which work to dignify and honour the depths of challenge at this time whilst offering support for the practical difficulties which may arise.

Yoga to support pelvic organ shift and unstable foundations: Many perimenopausal women experience the feeling of our pelvic organs descending, dragging or shifting from their previously accustomed places. This can manifest as a distinct sense of the organs literally dropping, for example the uterus prolapsing into the cervix, or the bladder into the uterus. These experiences can be very mild or they can be intense: when we have these sensations at this stage of life we can usually relate them directly to long-standing postural stress, and/or to earlier experiences of labour, birth and the postnatal period. Sometimes the sense of pelvic organ descent has already arisen during pregnancy. Often these earlier experiences are overlaid or exacerbated by continuing postural habits or health issues, for example the occupational stresses of work habits that place the body in an unhelpful posture for many hours daily (e.g. driving seats that tilt the pelvis backwards, standing in high heels or shoes that constrict the feet and limit their capacity to support a healthful pelvic tilt, or computer work stations that don't permit free rocking and moving of the pelvis), or temporary but intense stressors such as periods of strong coughing and sneezing.

There are many factors that may bring about the sensations of pelvic organ shift, and very many different degrees and varieties of pelvic organ prolapse that can be considered to be 'serious enough' to warrant surgical intervention. Women in their forties and fifties who consult orthodox medical care givers for advice on dealing with the sensations of pelvic organ shift are frequently alarmed by the rapidity with which our doctors will offer surgical solutions, including minor 'repairs' and full hysterectomies. Depending upon the severity of the sensations and the degree to which they are compromising daily activities, it can be a great comfort to discover that there is a range of yoga-based techniques and practices that can help to manage these sensations without surgical intervention. Women often express absolute relief that by taking the time to explore how these practices can help them, they can honour their own deeply held belief that these sensations can really be alleviated by appropriate rest, subtle posture adjustment and breathwork.

For the posture adjustment and breathwork to be effective really depends on taking the time to explore how each technique affects the organs of the pelvis and the feelings in the pelvic muscles. It is not something that offers an immediate rapid fix, but then, the problems generally did not occur overnight.

In energetic terms, what these experiences are about is a powerful sense of losing our life's foundations: the earth and water elements are no longer securely contained within us, we may wee when we cough, fart when we run, or have the feeling that our insides are heading outside. These sensations can be alarming. One of the most helpful aspects of any yoga theraputic work to manage and alleviate the sensations of prolapse is exploring the development of our current experiences with a caring yoga therapist: someone who will listen attentively and provide the assistance (often in the form of questions and enquiries) to help us unravel the tangled set of factors which may have led to pelvic organ shift in the first place. There is a healing empowerment in this process of self-discovery.

At a first therapeutic encounter with a women experiencing these problems, I ask a lot of open questions, and discover through the women's answers that they do, when they give themselves the time to explore the situation, actually already really know what has led to the current situation. The women generally also have a powerful intuitive sense of the sort of thing that will help them to manage the sensations. This self-awareness has often been dormant, or in the interests of 'getting on with things' and leading busy lives, may well have been strategically ignored for decades.

> *When talking to mothers of teenage and young adult children, those women frequently will recall very specifically the times during their labours when the initial damage was done: 'I can even see the words 'PUSH' on the hospital doors as they wheeled me through on the gurney, and I remember thinking at the time, I just shouldn't be pushing right now, even if that's what they are telling me to do, because this baby is just not ready to be born. I just know that is what started this problem off,' recalled one fifty-one-year-old yoga teacher of the birth of her third child. Or, 'There was always loads of fuss and worry about the state of my cervix during my first pregnancy,' recollects another yoga practitioner whose uterus had prolapsed into her cervix in her late forties, 'And I knew myself then that birth was going to really stress that part of me because of the history of cervical surgeries I'd had in my twenties.' Or again, 'I knew at the time of the birth I'd done some damage,' reflected a woman whose twins were seventeen years old by the time she really had the time and space to address the gradual feeling of descent in her pelvic organs, 'but there just never seemed to be a moment to do anything about it. And now it's really got much worse.'*

It seems that these earlier experiences can cause problems during perimenopause partly because the changing hormonal patterns during this time can reduce the supportive, 'uplifting' effects of oestrogen, and partly because of the cumulative effect of unhelpful postural habits. Additional stressors, such as respiratory problems that cause extended periods of fierce coughing can also be present. It is truly helpful for women to explore the benefits of postural change and free movement of the pelvis to re-energise this area of the body. It is also valuable to gain experiential understanding of exactly how the yogic approach to full-body breathing, that includes the activation of the feet and legs and hands, can all assist in providing a sense of uplift and support for the pelvic organs.

The practices described in chapter twenty-one assist a woman to explore and encounter the effects of holistic breath, movement and positive posture in relation to her pelvic muscles and the angle of her pelvis to help her manage the sensations of pelvic organ shift in daily life.

YOGA PRACTICES

Balancing breath (pp.466–7). This breath practice, especially when preceded or followed by **Triangle breath (psychic *nāḍī shodana*)** (pp.464–5) is a remarkably calming and settling practice that produces a sense of balance and quiet. Psychic *nāḍī shodana* (alternate nostril breathing) alone is invisible and portable, so can helpfully be done undetected anywhere.

Moon phase salute (pp.527–31). This sequence in honour of the moon is a beautiful way to connect through rhythmic movement and breath to the phases of the moon. When practised with conscious awareness of the current phase and position of the moon, it can provide a helpful means to maintain embodied contact with these rhythmic patterns at a time when the cycles of the inner moon may become erratic or confusing.

Wall sequence (pp.546–9). At a practical level, these practices are helpful means to create postural awareness that may relieve certain experiences of joint pain (especially in the feet, shoulders, neck and lower back). They are also a good way to do effective and revitalising standing poses that are not too tiring because they use the support of the wall. At a symbolic level, using the wall in this way creates a real sense of having something solid to rely upon when everything else in life may be feeling rather wobbly.

Golden thread breath (p.462). Although originally designed for use in labour as a pain reliever, this breath practice is also effective at calming intense mood swings. It's soporific, so may be used to assist in dropping back to sleep or at least calming anxiety during wakeful nights.

Śīthalī and sitkarī prāṇāyāma (pp.470–1). These are highly effective breaths to lower body temperature.

YOGIC REMEDIES AND RESPONSES

Anger: Many perimenopausal women encounter alarming levels of anger during this time, and can discover untapped depths of rage and resentment surfacing, often very rapidly and unexpectedly. Being with not knowing *yoga nidrā* (pp.450–1) is a deeply effective way to develop some distance and objectivity in relation to these experiences, and to promote levels of deep rest that act as a preventive for mood swings, which worsen under conditions of stress and exhaustion. Golden thread breath (p.462) is a positive resource to encourage release and rebalancing if anger has surfaced.

Depression: Often related to the experiences of unexpressed anger or fear, there are so many different manifestations of depression that it is difficult to offer a single set of remedies to suit all women. In general it can be extremely helpful to use gentle flowing movements such as Being in the cycles (pp.517–21), or *śakti bandhas* (pp.511–5) to get 'unstuck' and move through depressive experiences. Paired work such as the Spiritual warrior dance can also be useful, as can the flowing sequences such as the Sun and Moon salutations and the Palm tree *vinyāsa* (chapter twenty-three).

Exhaustion: Being exhausted exacerbates all the other experiences of perimenopause. Regular practice of 'awakening to *prāṇa śakti*' (chapter four) maximises the awareness and amount of available *prāṇa*. Deep relaxation such as *yoga nidrā* (pp.450–1) especially when practised in restorative poses such as the Golden cosmic womb (pp.552–3) or Super deluxe *savasana* (p.550) builds energy and promotes rest.

Erratic periods / bleeding: Many women suffer for years with almost constant bleedings, or are utterly confused and bewildered by erratic and surprising start-stop bleeds. The best help yoga can offer is to maximise opportunities to rest and recover energy (see Exhaustion above), and to promote a sense of rhythm and pattern in life by establishing regularity (little and often is best) of practice to create some sense of order at a chaotic time. During bleeds, avoid inversions and pumping breaths and only practise the menstrual variation of *mūla bandha* (p.475). The practices for the menstrual part of the cycle in the menstrual *mālā* (pp.560–3) are helpful to manage any pain or cramping that may accompany bleeding.

Forgetfulness / absent-mindedness and confusion: Any practice that promotes the direction of focus into a single point of awareness is helpful in managing perimenopausal mind-wipe. For example, balancing breathing practices (pp.466–7) both require and promote mental focus, whilst Triangle breathing in alternate nostrils trains mental attention (pp.464–5). The complete series of poses to liberate energy (p.497–510), especially when done with the focus on attentive counting of repetitions, is also a useful mind training, as is *yoga nidrā* (pp.450–1), particularly if done in the morning when you are more likely to stay awake and follow the instructions with detailed attention.

Hair loss: Practices that promote hormonal balance and reduce stress provide the best yogic response to hair loss. In particular, *yoga nidrā* (pp.450–1), Alternate nostril breathing (pp.464–5), *pūrṇa pavanamuktāsana* (p.497–510), Deep restorative poses (p.546–54) and Supported inversions (pp.488–91) are especially valuable. Massage of the scalp with a good āyurvedic medicated oil, and the use of a wooden comb may also be helpful.

Hot flushes and night sweats: The Cooling breaths (pp.470–1) are the first port of call for management of dramatic shifts in temperature. In terms of prevention, there are two basic yogic approaches, the first is to make time for more deeply restful practices (see Exhaustion recommendations above) and the second is to discover which of the more flowing and vigorous sequences (chapter twenty-three) work best to 'burn off' excess heat so as to lessen the intensity of hot flushes. A combination of these two approaches can work well, but discovering which approach suits you best depends on getting to know your own constitution, and for help with this it is may be worth consulting āyurvedic and/or homeopathic practitioners.

Vaginal dryness: Practices to balance hormones and reduce stress (see Hair loss, above) may improve this symptom. The Deer exercise (pp.496–7) can also heighten awareness of and sensitivity to signs of arousal in the breasts, and this is a powerful way to promote the ready flow of juices in the vagina.

FEED THE WILD *YOGINĪ*

SELF-ANOINTING FOR ACCEPTANCE

Part of the huge challenge of the perimenopause is noticing the early signs of ageing: our silver hairs and wrinkled eyes, our shrinking breasts or whiskery chins all bring us messages that whisper to us of the future. We may not be enjoying what we hear. We can get some nasty habits as we watch things change, and the hardest habit to kick is the habitual self-deprecating, 'Look, I'm starting to get old!' that can become an almost constant voicing of critical disatisfaction with what is happening to our physical vehicle.

It's a burden we can do without, so why not ditch it now? Get yourself some of the most delicious rose otto oil, the fragrance of which is the essence of femininity. Prepare for *yoga nidrā* (pp.450–1) by literally anointing each of the parts that are named. Set aside a long time to engage with the practice of *nyāsa* (rotation of consciousness), and before you lie still to do the practice, anoint yourself with the fragrant oil.

Once you have anointed yourself, let the fragrance of the rose carry the focus of your mental attention to each part of the body in turn, mentally anointing each place with the rose fragrance and with a loving mental caress.

Move the awareness first to the crown of the head, the third eye centre, between the eyebrows, the soft space between the collarbones, the top of the right shoulder, right elbow, right wrist, the tip of the right-hand thumb, and then the tip of each finger in turn: index finger, middle finger, ring finger, little finger. Bring the awareness and the rose fragrance back to the inside of the right wrist, the inside of the right elbow, the right shoulder, and then back to the soft space between the two collarbones. Then over to the top of the left shoulder, left elbow, left wrist, the tip of the left-hand thumb, and then the tip of each finger in turn: index finger, middle finger, ring finger, little finger.

Bring the awareness and the rose fragrance back to the inside of the left wrist, the inside of the left elbow, the left shoulder, and then back to the soft space between the two collarbones. Invite the awareness to bring the rose fragrance gently down to the middle of the breastbone, the left breast, the right breast, and back to the middle of the breastbone. Allow the attention to descend to anoint the belly at the navel, and down to the pubic bones, and then on down to bring the awareness gently to the right hip, knee and ankle, and onto the tips in turn of the big toe, second toe, third toe, fourth toe and fifth toe. And back up inside

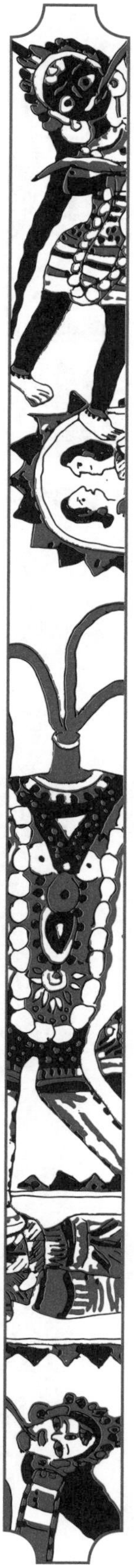

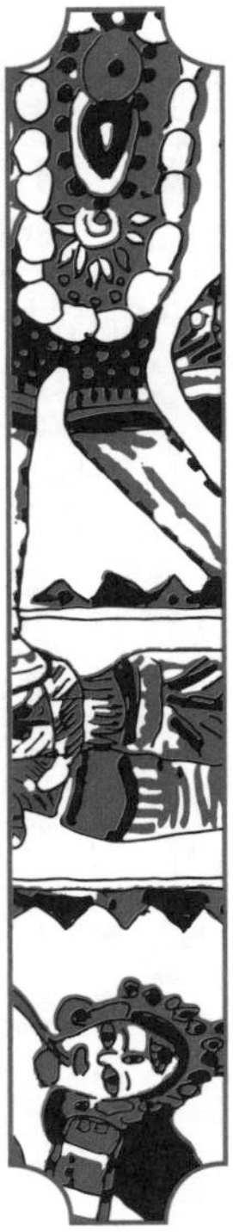

the right ankle, knee and hip. Return the awareness to the pubic bones, and then on down to bring the awareness gently to the left hip, knee and ankle, and onto the tips in turn of the big toe, second toe, third toe, fourth toe and fifth toe. And back up inside the left ankle, knee and hip. Lift the awareness back over to caress the pubic bones, and lift it again to anoint the belly with the fragrance of the rose oil.

Finally bring the awareness home gently to caress and anoint the place of the heart, in the centre of the breastbone. (Now continue with the remainder of the Seed at the heart of the fruit *yoga nidrā* practice described on pp.450–1).

Feed the wild *yoginī* with the rich food of deep self-love and acceptance. Nourish your heart, nourish her heart and feel by such nourishment that you are strengthened and protected as you step onwards into the unknown.

QUESTIONS AND REFLECTIONS

I invite you to explore your own (current or previous) experience of perimenopause and how it may be supported by yoga by asking yourself some (or any, or all) of the following questions:

1. What might you be able to do to build healthy rhythms into your daily life? For example, if you have the choice to determine eating and resting habits, then might it be possible to opt for regular times to eat and a fairly similar pattern of sleeping and waking times?
2. If you have a daily practice of yoga, when do you usually do it? Is it possible to make it the same time each day? Building rhythmic patterns into daily life sustains and nourishes every dimension of our being. Rhythm and regularity (not fixed rigidity, but healthy rhythmic patterns) create a helpful framework within which it is possible to adapt and respond to change more effectively.
3. The inevitable uncontrollable disruptions and powerful changes we can experience at this stage of life are better sustained when we have a sense of steadiness underneath. What makes you feel steady and secure? What can you do to deepen your connection with this steadiness?

4 What is your relationship to uncertainty? How comfortable are you with being in a space of not knowing and/or confusion? It can be helpful to explore this at a small scale, by reflecting on how you may have responded in yoga classes, for example, to the introduction of a new practice, or when you have needed to adapt to surprising changes, such as the last-minute arrival of an unexpected new teacher, or a departure from the usual contents of a familiar class.

5 What might you be able to do to nourish your capacity for spontaneous and adaptive response to change and disturbance? For example, on a micro-level, it may be useful to invite opportunities for new learning and challenge into your experience of being a yoga student by choosing once or twice to shift to a different teacher or time than usual, or to explore an unfamiliar practice with the support of written or audio-visual instruction. Are there other areas of life that might sustain a few small adventures into conscious engagement with beneficial change, for example diet or sleep patterns?

FURTHER READING AND RESEARCH

As a great support for the experience of *satsang*, I warmly recommend **Suza Francina**'s *Yoga and the Wisdom of Menopause: A Guide to Physical, Emotional and Spiritual Health at Midlife and Beyond*. It offers an inspiring combination of true life stories from yoga women, and sound advice from an Iyengar yoga perspective. Especially helpful are the sections on yoga and perimenopausal bleeding, osteoporosis and the emotional experience of menopause.

Bonnie Horrigan's edited collection of inspiring feminist stories about menopause, *Red Moon Passage*, offers a range of perspectives from women whose lives are dedicated to the unfolding of spiritual understandings, including **Clarissa Pinkola Estes** and **Barbara G. Walker**. This is the only book on menopause recommended to me by **Alexandra Pope**, because she feels it gets to the heart of the menopausal journey as a quest for deep wisdom. It's gripping.

San Francisco medical doctor and women's health expert, **Susan M. Lark** has written a range of practical handbooks on women's health. Her *Menopause Self Help Book* describes many natural methods of responding to the experiences of menopause, offering useful self-evaluation tools and sensible guidelines on diet, exercise and self-care including herbs and massage.

For an informative read on the subject of menopause I recommend **Louise Foxcroft**'s *Hot Flushes, Cold Science: A History of the Modern Menopause* in which she presents an utterly compelling account of the medicalisation and cultural construction of what we understand to be the menopausal experience. Her perspective is a helpful antidote to the prevailing notion that menopause is always a problem which needs fixing. **Germaine Greer**'s *The Change* does an equally brilliant job of this, but from a more literary perspective.

For information about bio-identical hormones and natural remedies for osteopaenia and osteoporosis, see the work of *Dame Shirley Bond*: **www.bio-hormone-health.com/2010/02/02/dame-dr-shirley-bond**

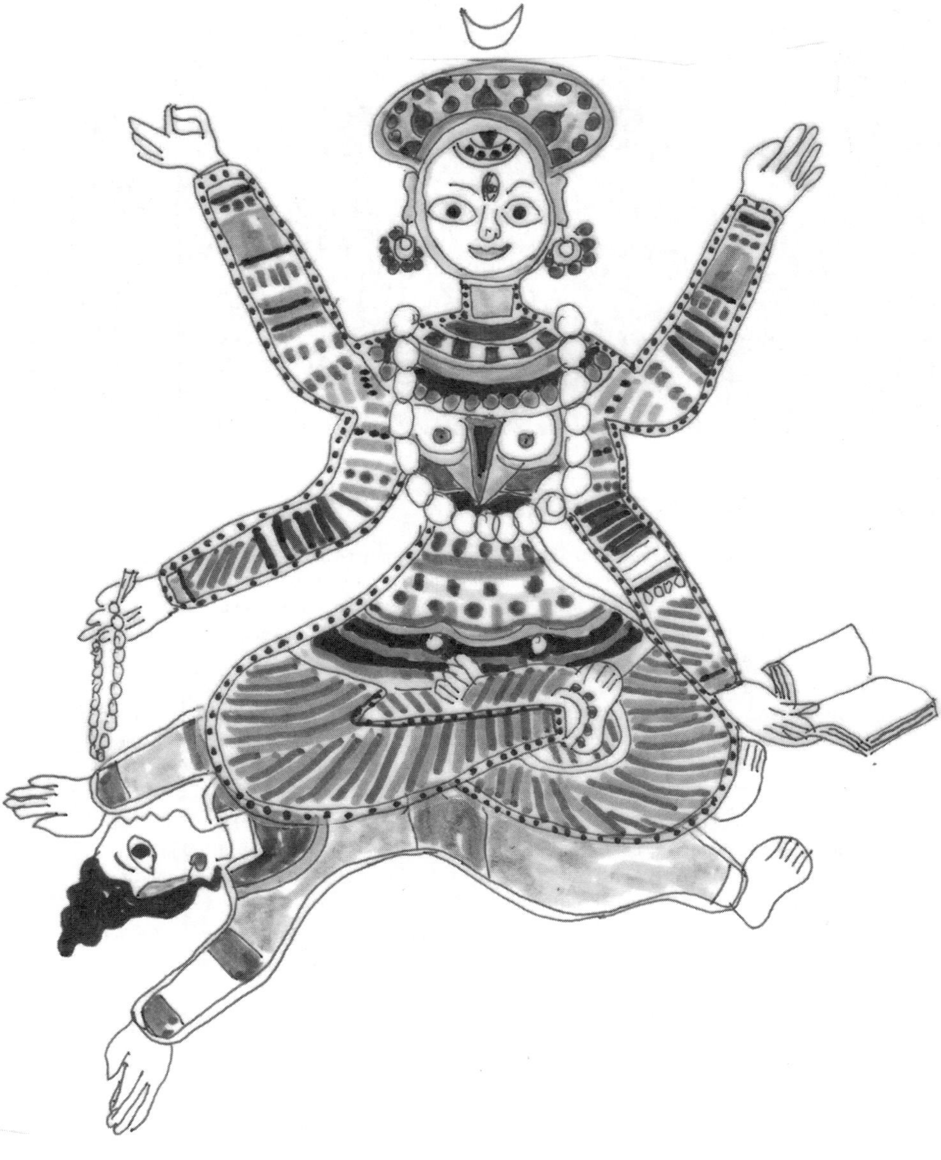

Bhairavī emanates the fierce clarity and fearlessness that may arise during menopause

CHAPTER SIXTEEN

Bhairavī

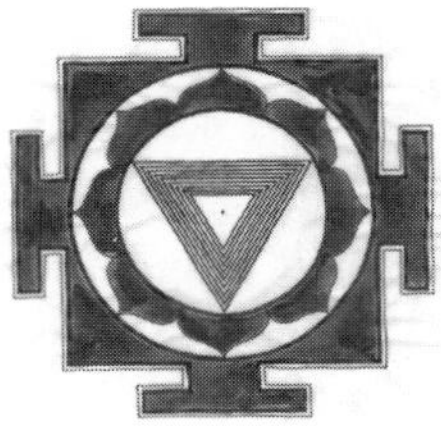

Embracing our power: yoga and menopause

I realised that I and others in our culture were being methodically starved of substance, that something was awry in some of the "wisdom" of our culture, that it did not have our best interests at heart, that it saw those who are "menopausal" as somehow less. It is not so, we are instead more. Much, much more. (Clarissa Pinkola Estes, in Horrigan, (ed.) 1997)

We should never judge how any woman experiences menopause. Each woman is just trying her best to make peace with herself. (Alexandra Pope, lecture on Spirituality of Menstruation and Menopause, May 2012)

MAHĀVIDYĀ* AND *SIDDHI

WISDOM AND POWER

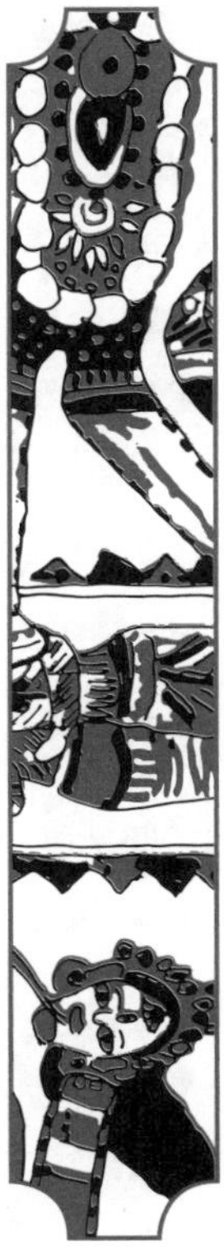

Bhairavī, whose name means 'the terrifying fierce one', is a warrior goddess associated closely with Kālī, and I have invited her to stand guardian over the chapter on menopause. This time of life is often defined simply as the point when menstrual periods have permanently ceased. Although 'the menopause' is often understood to be an initiatory experience that marks a specific turning point in a woman's life, for the purposes of this book I have chosen to extend our understanding of the limits of its influence into the fourteen years following the last period. It is these years that are the focus of this chapter.

Clarissa Pinkola Estes identifies this as a very special time in a woman's life, with the ages from forty-nine until fifty-six being the 'age of the underworld', a time of deep re-evaluation and fear-facing during which a woman learns 'the words and rites' of the powerful initiation that enables her to enter the 'age

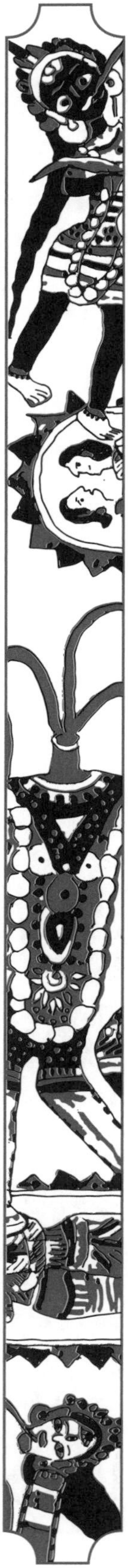

of choice'. The age of choice extends from the ages of fifty-six to sixty-three, and the 'choice' refers to the freedom to 'choose one's world and the work yet to be done' (Estes). This special time is often one of deep challenge and great rewards, which is why I have placed the goddess Bhairavī as its fierce guardian.

Bhairavī is a terrifying form of the goddess, whose breath is the word of fire, of truth. In particular, Bhairavī is a powerful manifestation of woman's wrath, especially the fierce anger of a mother in the face of any threat to her child. She is the power of light and fire, the strength of focused discipline, and the triumphant goddess as she returns from the defeat of her enemies of ignorance and fear. The *yantra* of Bhairavī distils this impressive and frightening form of feminine energy into a graphic essence that can be used for meditative purposes.

I have worked closely with the graphic essence of Bhairavī for many years, and she has been a powerful presence and impetus in the communication of yoga teachings relating to mothering and birth. As the fiery aspect of the power of the word, Bhairavī provided the impulse to communicate the teachings in my second book, *Mother's Breath*. *Mother's Breath* was literally Bhairavī's breath, and it was her energy that presented the breath and awareness practices held by the framework of the *Mahāvidyā*'s deep knowledge. There were over three hundred images of Bhairavī in that book: the cover carried the colourful geometric form containing nine concentric triangles, and the *yantra* also appeared as a graphic thread on every page of the book. In *Mother's Breath* I called upon Bhairavī's presence to link the practices I described into the unbroken stream of knowledge represented by the ten wisdom goddesses. For me at that time, Bhairavī was a powerhouse of wisdom and energy. When people asked me how on earth I managed to find the time to write such a book when I had two little boys (my youngest son was four), two jobs and a household to run, I simply used to answer that I got up very early and listened to what Bhairavī wanted to say and then I wrote it all down. The graphic presence of a host of Bhairavī *yantras* on every page of the book was a vivid gesture of thanksgiving to the source of the wisdom shared in that book.

I put so many of Bhairavī's images into *Mother's Breath* because I felt at the time that in the context of pregnancy, birthing and mothering, the power of Bhairavī was a very positive and empowering aspect of feminine energy to acknowledge, accept and channel. Looking back now, from the vantage point of middle age, I can sense that what I was calling upon as I wrote *Mother's Breath* was the protective power of a very fierce goddess whose energies in fact resonate far more deeply with the qualities and experiences of women at menopause. These older and often wiser women have the capacity to lend their power to the mothering years, to provide support and context for the women who are giving birth and minding babies. But in fact the essence of Bhairavī's wisdom is more closely related to the time of life after the cessation of menstrual cycles, when steadiness and clarity give women the perspective and understanding to become fierce guardians, not only of their own children, but of all life. This is peri-crone, or enchantress energy at its fiercest and wildest, putting wisdom and power in the service of those vulnerable beings who need it most. In her writing on the power of crone energy, Jean Shinoda Bolen (2003) has identified the protective and nurturing energies of older women as a world-changing force: activism powered by empathy. The fierceness of Bhairavī as a warrior goddess carries this same charge. The wisdom of Bhairavī is fierce because it challenges us to stand up for what we know is important. The process of menopause brings us face to face with who we really think we are, and what matters to us, our true 'calling'. The postmenopausal experience may involve standing in defence of the choice we have made to answer our calling.

Bhairavī is the feminine form of the word Bhairava. It has two key meanings: the state of consciousness preceding the ultimate union with universal consciousness, and a name for a terrifying manifestation of Śiva that causes annihilation. Bhairavī is related to the Sanskrit verb *rāvayati*, which means to 'howl' or 'wail', and this can be understood as the expression of the grief of the individual soul at the separation from universal consciousness. This is the root of Bhairavī's fierceness. It is as if, having felt the pain of separation from the universal soul, she knows the nature of real suffering, and is fiercely empowered to distinguish between what matters and what doesn't at the level of ultimate reality. This fierce clarity resonates with the deep self-knowing and self-acceptance that comes after the passage through menopause. Women at this time in life are 'on the other side' of the cyclical patterns of shifting moods and awareness that come during the menstruating years, and have come through the uncertainty of perimenopause.

A part of ourselves dies when our childbearing years end, and we are freer because of this. Because menopausal women are now beyond bearing any (more) of our own children, we are more directly connected with the source of life itself. We have a closeness and reverence for light and life because our reproductive capacity has died: our power to give life in the limited

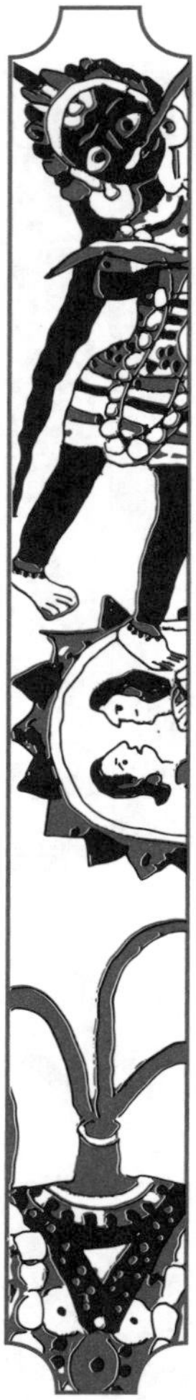

physical sense of being pregnant and giving birth is replaced by a broader connection and reverence for life in a wider sense. And so Bhairavī's powerful ability to protect the vulnerable child – like the anger of a mother roused in the defence of her child – is in fact the wisdom of Bhairavī in the form of the older woman, whose protective power extends to defend the whole of life.

This expanded consciousness is possible at this time of life because by this stage a woman has literally passed through the perimenopausal fires: *kuṇḍalinī* rising in the experiences of hot flushes and/or hot tempers. Her very physical being has changed to the degree that the energy of Bhairavī glows within her: 'She represents transforming heat or radiance, Tejas, which is the primal power or Divine energy. This we experience as a frightening thing because it burns away and destroys all the limitations and illusions of egocentric existence' (Frawley 1994: 104). The powerful clarity and energy of women who are past the menopause is greatly feared and suppressed by patriarchy. The transformations which Bhairavī represents are literally enacted through the changed behaviours and priorities of postmenopausal women, who have been down into the underworld of re-evaluation and self-scrutiny and whose life experience and understanding can lead them to become radicalised activists and powerful *yoginīs* at this time:

> *When we come up out of the underworld after one of our undertakings there, we may appear unchanged outwardly, but inwardly we have reclaimed a vast and womanly wildness. On the surface we are still friendly, but beneath the skin, we are most definitely no longer tame.*
> *(Pinkola Estes: 455)*

LIMITATIONS: CULTURAL EXPECTATIONS

The cultural pressures and expectations around menopause are immense and generally very negative. To say 'she's menopausal' is usually used to demean or humiliate a woman, or possibly to excuse some behaviour that is judged unfeminine or unsuitable for a woman of a certain age. To be recognised as 'menopausal' is often to be the butt of many jokes about the perceived ugliness and unattractiveness of the female body at this time of life. To be honest the prejudice against menopausal women in our culture is so dreadful and so deeply engrained that sometimes the best thing to do is laugh about it, as the following story shows.

For several years I had the honour of sharing the teaching on the well woman yoga therapy module with retired anatomist and busy yoga therapist Ruth Gilmore, about whom you can read more in the next section. Our remit was to cover all aspects of women's health in relation to yoga therapy. Ruth taught the anatomy and physiology. When she reached the topic of menopause in her opening lecture on women's life cycles, Ruth reduced thirty *yoginīs* to paroxysms of uncontrollable laughter by thus describing a medical textbook slide depicting a menopausal woman:

> *'What a tale of woe have we here! I mean, will you just look at this miserable woman: droopy boobs, saggy tummy – her hair is falling out, her uterus is prolapsed, her vagina is dried up and she's growing a beard. Oh yes, and it says she is depressed. I'm not surprised. Her kids have left home, her husband's probably gone off with a younger woman, she's spent her life looking after these people and now she feels as if life is utterly pointless. She's probably also experiencing deep despair, rage and anxiety too. She's in a sorry state, I can see. Who wouldn't be?'*

When the laughter died down and everyone had a chance to examine the image Ruth was describing we saw that it was all true: the woman indeed was experiencing every one of these miseries all at once. What a terrible prospect. Not only is she experiencing all the challenges of an ageing body, but her psyche is in total meltdown because she's failing to match up to all the criteria by which she used to be valued as a woman.

This is the frightening image of menopausal experience that is most current, and it is this image that makes menopausal women either invisible to popular culture, or objects of ridicule. If popular ideas and widespread media images are one's only source of information on the topic, then there is evidently not one single positive experience that can be expected during and after menopause. Such is our culture's obsessive equation of woman's value with youth and sexual availability that any woman who does not display signs of fertility is considered to be worthless. This idea is explored more fully in the next section, but it is sufficient to observe here that menopause is widely regarded as an experience to be feared, postponed, or avoided if at all possible.

Most of the popular discussions about women's 'age of choice' are really about limitation and avoidance. The only real choice on offer is often how long to stay on hormone therapy (HT, previously known as hormone replacement therapy or HRT). The prevailing cultural belief is that somehow, if we can pretend menopause has never happened, then we can carry on as usual, and if we're lucky we'll die young and beautiful before any one notices we've got old. This kind of patho-adolescent, mid-life arrested development is a profound denial of our right to wisdom and power. It's a dead end street, and to allow ourselves to be driven down it is deeply damaging to every aspect of our being.

> *As Joan shared her experiences with the other women attending a womb yoga workshop in the north of England, she wept with fearful anger and sadness: 'I started taking HT in my early forties,' she explained, 'because I was frightened. Both my mother and sister had early menopauses, and*

I was noticing symptoms in myself that I did not like. I was worried the same would happen to me. I'd been on it for eight years when I started to be frightened that it wasn't good for my health. But when I stopped taking it, things got even more terrifying. All the symptoms came straight back again, but worse. So I went back on HT. I just couldn't face what was happening to me. And now I'm really scared. I worry that I should stop taking it, but I don't want that experience again. It was like falling off a cliff.'

What Joan had discovered was that the shift into 'act three' of life is inevitable, and that putting it off for as long as possible just made the transition experience worse: faster, and more intense. Of course, there are women who find helpful ways to use HT, or its more delicate cousins, bio-identical hormones and natural progesterone cream, and to integrate these hormonally supportive strategies into a more gradual and graceful arrival at the postmenopausal place. Everyone discovers menopause has to happen, but the pressure to deny the reality of our ageing process and to imprison ourselves in a cage of outgrown behaviours and experiences is so intense that it can be hard to escape. Thankfully, the practice of yoga provides many keys to free us from this particularly uncomfortable cage.

FREEDOMS: YOGA PERSPECTIVES, TECHNIQUES AND AWARENESS FOR BREATHING, MOVING AND BEING

Metaphorically, the three phases of the moon – waxing, full and waning – the three phases of the ancient goddess – maiden, mother, crone – and the three biological markers of menarche, menstruation and menopause divide women's lives into a three-act play. This is Act 3. The curtain will come down at the end of it. In Act 3, you may pick up on threads of meaning from earlier phases of your life and find yourself absorbed in something new. There are completions and endings; doors close and others open. Whatever the particulars, what makes life juicy is being deeply involved in life. (Bolen 90)

This is the time in life when a woman finally is asked to accept herself for who she really is: to give birth to herself as herself. (Alexandra Pope, Women's Leadership Apprenticeship, Spirituality Module, May 2012)

Part of the freedom that the practice of yoga brings to us as women is the capacity to accept ourselves. At the start of the third act of life, self-acceptance is the key to being able to 'pick up the threads' of earlier life experiences and welcome them into the weave of menopausal life, or to shift our attentions to new aspects of life. The positive stories I have to tell are about women whose yoga practice empowers them to embark on this new phase of life by picking up, sometimes in a surprising manner, the threads which may have been present or even perhaps unrecognised in their earlier years. These experiences give women opportunities to truly embrace their own deep sense of self as it emerges.

Perhaps the world's most famous postmenopausal *yoginī* was the Florentine yoga teacher Vanda Scaravelli. She did not begin practising yoga until she was forty-seven, only started teaching when she was sixty, and then went on, through her own uniquely passionate engagement with the liberatory powers of yoga practice, and through the work of a devoted band of less than a dozen main students, to become one of the world's most influential yoga teachers. Speaking about her own evolution as a *yoginī* after menopause, Scaravelli has said,

> *'We say flowers blossom in the spring, and certainly that is true,*
> *but also sometimes in the autumn there are flowers blooming.*
> *It was like that for me. I could feel myself re-awakening.'*

For Scaravelli, the practice of yoga brought deep freedom. With this awakening to her freedom came a fierce and generous courage, a Bhairavī-like capacity to share the treasure she had discovered with her students. To watch archive footage of Scaravelli in her yoga practice, or to read the memoirs of her students as they warmly recall her fearless desire to share what she knew, is to perceive the presence of a deep wisdom that comes only through self-acceptance.

Sometimes yoga supports a woman to let go of old practices and habits that no longer suit her newly postmenopausal way of being and to make new choices that resonate with this new phase of life.

> *Yoga teacher Frances marked her journey towards Bhairavī consciousness with two rituals that brought depth of meaning to her experience. After six months with no periods, and at a time in her life marked by bereavement and loss (both her parents had died, her children had left home and she had let go of her previous work patterns), Frances asked friends to help her shave off all her long hair. The ritual was designed to assist in the grieving process that Frances felt she needed. As a side effect, she was delighted to discover that she looked absolutely stunning with a crop, and has kept her hair short for many more years.*
>
> *Frances's second special menopausal ritual was conducted a year and a day after the end of her last period, to celebrate her transition into the postmenopausal state: she stepped across a sacred stream to signal that she had completed her passage into the postmenopausal world. 'I wore a red dress as I approached the stream' she recalls, 'to symbolise my menstruating years. I took off the dress and stepped naked through the water to the other side. When I got out, I was free to choose to wear a dress of any colour I liked. I chose gold. For me that was an expression of my choice to "go for gold" in every aspect of my life at this time.' Having previously practised strong, fast* vinyāsa *yoga, Frances found that she was now drawn to a quieter and more meditative practice. She spent much time resting, practising* yoga nidrā, *and realising her dreams of living in simple abundance, by moving to a cabin in the woods:*

'My daughters had left home, my parents were dead, and I had allowed my investments in previous patterns of work to fall away. I felt that once I had crossed the menopause I was free to create a way of life that genuinely supported my well-being.'

For Frances, the insights she had gained through the practice of yoga gave her tools to honour her newly-born postmenopausal self. She had positive experiences of managing deep exhaustion and uterine prolapse through a restorative and intuitive yoga practice that gave her the time and space she needed to heal and spontaneously revitalise. She now shares what she learnt through her own postmenopausal experiences with other women, and has collaborated with two other teachers to establish a new yoga centre in Swindon that offers yoga, massage and other tools for holistic healing. The choices that women can make at this time can often lead them into a different relationship with the yoga they had practised earlier in their lives.

Whereas Frances discovered that what truly supported her needs as a postmenopausal woman was a slower restorative yoga practice, Janet and Sarah both found that stronger and more vigorous practice was helpful. Sarah discovered that a regular practice of hot yoga helped her to minimise the intense and uncomfortable experiences of night sweats and hot flushes, whereas Janet discovered that regular practice of the primary series of *aṣṭaṅga vinyāsa yoga* provided the healing movement that relieved intense pain from spinal problems that had intensified postmenopause. (More details on the use of yoga to minimise perimenopausal symptoms are provided in the previous chapter). Both women had previously practised more gentle forms of yoga, but postmenopause had picked up on nascent interests in other approaches when they discovered that they suited them better.

This process of picking up the threads of previous interests and a deepening connection to one's deepest sense of self sometimes manifests as big changes in terms of career and work patterns as postmenopausal life unfolds. For women who have had children, this can seem to be a natural unfolding that is related to the experience of the empty nest – and it is often described in the wider culture as a looking for something to 'occupy oneself' and one's energies once the children have left home. To see it this way is to miss the point that vivid clarity of purpose and re-direction is often equally present in mothers and in women who have not brought up children, as the following two stories reveal. I've already described my colleague Ruth Gilmore's amusement about general attitudes towards postmenopausal women, and her own trajectory as a menopausal women has been inspirational. When I first encountered Ruth she had only relatively recently shifted from being a practitioner of yoga to training as a yoga teacher and yoga therapist.

Combining her previous experiences as an anatomist at Queen's University Belfast with her love of sharing yoga, Ruth had become involved in an experimental project to offer anatomy and physiology teaching on a yoga therapy training course in London. She'd teamed up with her own yoga teacher trainer and the pair of them would fly over from Belfast to London to run sessions that were fizzing with excitement and the desire to share valuable knowledge. As a student on that training course I could feel the passion that was driving Ruth: a lifetime's experience of teaching medical students was being poured into the service of educating yoga therapists. In the 'age of choice' Ruth had clearly responded to her opportunity to 'choose one's world and the work yet to be done'. She had clearly found a way to redirect her vast professional knowledge into a new path: she reviewed everything she knew, reframed and simplified it for yoga therapists, and then delivered the information with palpable delight. She'd found a new audience of people who were utterly receptive to what she had to share, and what she had to share was coming directly out of her own unique perspective as anatomist turned yoga teacher / therapist.

Ruth's postmenopausal shift of interest and her willingness to follow a new line of work is a shining example of the creative embracing of our power, of Bhairavī's wisdom in action. Having let go of her previous life as a university professor, and followed the calling of the deep self whom she had rediscovered through her yoga practice, Ruth stepped into a whole new life.

Her combined skills as a retired university anatomist, a yoga therapist and a wickedly humorous raconteuse means that her lectures are always pertinent and never dull. Her passion is palpable and her teaching is accessible. So, flying back and forth from Ulster to the UK for many years, Ruth's contributions and involvement in yoga therapy training increased, and her distinctively humorous and direct style became widely acknowledged and respected.

Everything useful I have ever learnt about human anatomy and the relationship between yoga therapy and medical conditions I have learnt from Ruth Gilmore. But I am only one of thousands of her students. For once she had established her reputation on the yoga therapy training, many other courses began to request Ruth's input. Eventually she and her husband moved to London, she dropped most of her weekly yoga classes and concentrated on training for yoga teachers and therapists. She became the country's most in-demand lecturer for yoga teachers and therapists. 'This is what I have to offer. It's what I know only I can do in this particular way at this time, and so I wanted to give it my full attention and energy' she told me when I asked for guidance about the balance of my own work as a yoga teacher and trainer.

Ruth's clarity of understanding about her unique gift and how best to nurture and share it is refreshing, and carries all the weight of knowledge and understanding that comes when a postmenopausal woman completely embraces her power. By honouring her own special combinations of experiences and utilising the abundant energies which were liberated from the care and nurture of her children once they left home, Ruth found a new interest and outlet for her energies that was hugely beneficial to many people in the yoga world. Fifteen years on, and now a delighted grandmother, Ruth is poised to take the next step and to begin to retire from a full programme of yoga teacher-training initiatives that has resulted in re-designing the entire anatomy component of one of the country's most widely followed yoga teacher-training syllabi, and the creation of a fully integrated diploma course training in yoga therapy that attracts students from all over the world. She's also written two yoga therapy books based on her long-running series of popular articles in a yoga magazine that are widely consulted by many UK yoga teachers as a reference for reliable information on medical conditions.

Ruth's shift of energies is a classic manifestation of postmenopausal re-evaluation and redirection. The story pans out in different ways across all of our lives. In all corners of the yoga world, the effects of women consciously welcoming the opportunities offered at the 'age of choice' are inspiring. We can optimise our capacity to 'choose one's world and the work yet to be done' at this time in our lives. In Ruth's case, the key elements in her capacity to choose were her commitment to the healing effects of her own yoga practice, which she wanted to share, and the feeling that her grown-up children no longer needed her focused attention.

In the case of Dr Sue Edgely (widely known by her spiritual name Bharati), this first element was present, but not the second: Bharati was a medical doctor and a psychiatrist who had also trained as a general practitioner. She was also a *bhakti yoginī* with a heartfelt devotion to the south Indian saint Ammaci, and a personal practice of devotional song. For all sorts of reasons her work within the orthodox medical establishment was becoming less satisfying. Bharati's professional focus shifted to providing more holistic support for mental health and well-being. Postmenopause, questions began to arise about exactly how Bharati wanted to be spending the rest of her life, and what use to make of her skills and experiences.

'A wise guide told me that I should "Start by using my voice"' Bharati told me, 'I thought that meant lecturing or counselling: something to do with my doctoring. But now of course I realise it's the bhakti *yoga – my 'voice' is my singing voice. That's the path. That's the right thing for me to be doing for the rest of my life.' It was Bharati's own spiritual practice, and her desire to share the benefits of* bhakti *yoga that guided her to know what choices to make: together with her musician husband who is also a* bhakti yogi, *Bharati began to share* kirtans *and* bhajans. *First she sang at home, then at yoga festivals, and then she began to organise events where such practices could be shared more widely. She has found her postmenopausal calling and has become well known in UK* bhakti *yoga circles for her warmth of voice and her openness of heart.*

It takes courage to follow this kind of calling, and this courage is the hallmark of Bhairavī energy.

YOGA PRACTICES

The following yoga practices support women in developing the courage to practise self-kindness and self-acceptance. They also help to foster the states of mind and heart that enable us to make the most of the opportunities for self-evaluation and choice offered in this period of life.

All of the **womb greetings** in chapter five, in particular those done from supine and semi-supine positions can encourage a continuing sense of self-nurture and connection to the presence of the womb. At this time of life, whether or not the organ of the womb is still present, the experience may well be of a connection beyond the physical presence (or absence) of the uterus, to the experience of the world-womb or the sense of being held in the golden cosmic womb (*hiraṇya garbha*): at this stage these greetings can serve to connect our awareness outwards into the world and the service we may offer.

Supta uḍḍīyāna bandha (p.485) and **Womb elevation sequence** (pp.155–8). These practices can be a helpful support for the experience of living with prolapsed or otherwise shifted pelvic organs. They can help to maintain tone in the abdominal wall and pelvic diaphragm, and provide a revitalising lift of energies that can be very refreshing.

Agnisāra kriyā (pp.515–6) has a similar uplifting and revitalising effect to the previous practices.

Feminine strength: spiritual warrior (pp.536–8) is a positive sequence to refine and connect with the fierce energies of this time of life. It is beautiful to practice this alone, to tap into one's own experience of how to direct this fierceness, but is also supportive and fun to practise in a pair with another woman. This experience helps us to become aware that this fierce energy is present in our sisters too.

Inversion sequences (pp.488–91). Being upside down changes our perspective on life and revitalises us. These are both welcome experiences especially during our later years, when unless we respond sensitively to the ageing process it is easy to become fixed and limited in our views of the world. Some of the classical yogic means to be upside down can either be uncomfortable or unsuitable during this stage of life, in particular if bones are weakened by osteoporosis. Depending on your existing familiarity with inverted postures, and your current state of health, you may or may not find it comfortable to continue to practise the standard approach to inversions. Gentle, supported inversions, however, are generally enjoyable for everyone at this time of life.

Opening the lotus to *prāṇa śakti* (pp.136–9): this practice has an especially beautiful resonance at this time of life. Bring to it an awareness of being open to sharing your own wisdom of experience with the world, even as you receive the energising vitality back into yourself. Either focus simply on being open-hearted by resting the practice at the breastbone, or move the gesture up and down the body, bringing awareness to each energy centre.

YOGIC REMEDIES AND RESPONSES

Breast cancer: Although breast cancer can affect women of all ages, I have gathered the information about yogic responses to this experience here. One of the most supportive and valuable approaches to managing experiences of breast cancer with yoga is to combine deep meditative and healing work in the Self-anointing ritual *yoga nidrā* (pp.451–2) and restorative yoga with gentle recuperative exercise. In particular the complete liberation of energy series (pp.497–510) is very helpful to encourage the healthy flow of *prāṇa* that encourages positive healing. The shoulder circling and shoulder rotations are especially pertinent at this time, so extra focus can be brought to the effects of these movements, for example by reducing their range of motion in cases of discomfort, or extending into the full circles as a means to encourage optimal lymph flow if larger movement is comfortable.

Remember that even though it is helpful to bring extra focus to these parts of the sequence, they have most potency when done as part of the full series. Resting In the golden cosmic womb (p.552) can be a very positive way to promote the receptive and welcoming attitude that encourages deep healing. For a very positive and encouraging account of a breast cancer survivor who combined orthodox western medical approaches with yoga, acupuncture, Chinese herbs and emotional freedom technique to create a truly holistic treatment, see Emma Cannon's introduction to her book *The Baby Making Bible*. See also the end of this chapter for contacts to yoga programmes specifically designed for women with breast cancer.

Hysterectomy and recovery after pelvic muscle and organ repairs: these surgeries may be encountered by women at any stage of life, but are most likely to occur in the years around and after menopause. If it occurs anytime before the natural onset of menopause, then the effects of a full hysterectomy that also includes the removal of the ovaries (and sometimes also, those hysterectomies that leave the ovaries behind) creates an immediate 'surgical menopause' that can be shocking in its intensity and rapidity. Self-nurture and care at this time is the essential ingredient of any yogic remedy.

The Seed at the heart of the fruit *yoga nidrā* (pp.451–2) may be helpful, and all the womb yoga breath practices in chapter four are very sustaining and nourishing. The practices to greet and honour the womb (chapters five and six) may be helpfully used at this time for two purposes. In the first place they invite powerful healing *prāṇa* into the belly to promote optimal post-operative recovery, and in the second place they offer an opportunity to acknowledge both the absence of the organ/s of womb and/or ovaries, and the continuing presence of those energies of nurture and creativity and cyclical wisdom which are associated not with the absent organs, but with the energetic space of the *yonisthāna*. The practices can help us to recognise that the qualities associated with the functions of the organ of the womb are in fact fully present even in the womb's absence. This awareness can make it easier to give thanks to the womb for all she has done, and to move forward into life without a womb, and with the freedom to embrace new perspectives that are genuinely supported by the continuing experience of the *yonisthāna*'s energy of nurture and creativity.

Because yoga helps us to understand that we have five bodies, not just one (see pp.181–2), yogic practice enables us to connect with the continuing presence in the energy body of all of the qualities associated with the functions of the womb. Nurturing, creativity, and the capacity to gestate new ideas and projects are experiences that depend not upon the presence of the womb, but upon the healthy flow of *prāṇa* through our earth and water energy centres (see pp.141–2).

Osteoporosis: This condition can affect women of any age, but becomes much more prevalent after menopause, when bone density can decrease often very rapidly. Osteopaenic women (those on the borders of developing osteoporosis) are well advised to investigate dietary and lifestyle changes to prevent the development of osteoporosis. For full details about yoga to support osteoporosis, please see pp.423–4, and the references at the end of this chapter.

Living with pelvic organ prolapse: It is not unusual for some of the shifts in the placement of pelvic organs that may have become apparent during the perimenopause to settle into a long-term sensation of having 'dropped'. Sometimes the sensations may have gone relatively unnoticed, or just been something that was coped with earlier in life, but gains more significance and urgency later on. The full range of practices for yogic management of pelvic organ prolapse is described in chapters twenty and twenty-one. In particular, it is helpful to incorporate awareness of optimal standing, sitting and walking postures into everyday life. By integrating the beneficial effects of precisely the right angle of pelvic tilt, spinal curves and foot awareness into daily activities we can build on the sensations of uplift and support that come through these practices.

Continuing perimenopausal symptoms: Although the experiences of 'mind-wipe', hot flushes and night sweats, for example, are often focused around the years of transition into the menopause, for many women they can continue sporadically or frequently for many years. It can be extremely debilitating and exhausting for these intense sensations to continue for any length of time. The disruption to sleep is profoundly depleting, and the challenges of managing the experiences whilst going about daily life can be extremely tiring and upsetting.

In addition to the detailed, symptom by symptom suggestions presented in the previous chapter, the following yogic practices can be helpful: *yoga nidrā* (p.451–2) as a daily practice creates a cumulative credit of deep rest that nourishes every aspect of being, and on its own may well help relieve every single one of the symptoms of menopause. It is also a useful strategy for insomnia, and may be used in wakeful periods in the middle of the night or early in the morning. Balancing breath (pp.466–7) and all of the breath practices described in chapter four are very effective in the management of disturbed emotional states. Some woman find that using a series of flowing *āsana* sequences (chapter twenty-three) that warms the body is an effective way to minimise hot flushes, because they feel as if the heat is 'burnt off' by the yoga practices, but this is not always the case, so it is worth experimenting to discover if this approach works for you.

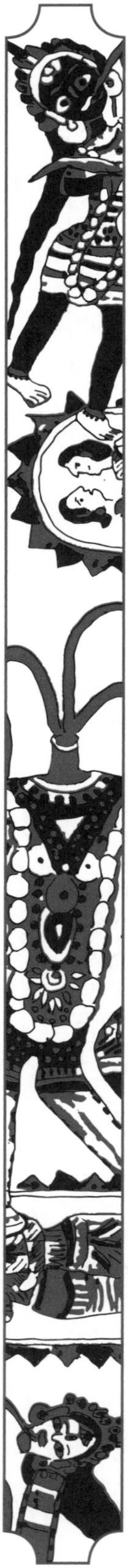

FEED THE WILD *YOGINĪ*

RADICAL RITUAL RECYCLING 3: DRINK YOUR OWN *AMAROLĪ*

Menopause is often described as a time when a woman 'gives birth to herself', when she comes face to face with herself, with her true nature. At a time when other roles we may have played in the past have possibly fallen away, at a time when perhaps we are making space in our lives to connect with what really fires us up, this is the time to get super-radical – to face our truth and live out who we really are, in and of ourselves, and not just in relation to services we may have always provided for others. Take this opportunity to clear out what's no longer necessary and to purify, simplify and focus your attentions on what really matters.

The practice of *amarolī* (p.478) is literally drinking our own urine. There are many profound changes in attitude and behaviour that come about as a result of even thinking about practising *amarolī*. Now is the time of life when many of those changes of attitude and behaviour may be very naturally unfolding: clearing a house, downsizing to a home with fewer bedrooms, passing on clothes that you never liked in the first place, pouring a lifetime of business administration skills into a local co-operative to support a venture that makes your heart sing. All of these acts are forms of 'recycling' – giving things back you have finished with, so that they can be used again in a different way.

You can make what you do in this sphere of change and simplification into an offering to the wild *yoginī*. Pass on to her your feeling of freedom as you unburden and rediscover yourself. The wild *yoginī* has a taste for genuine offerings of this nature. It doesn't necessarily have to be your own urine that you toast her with, but it could be. Whether at the literal or metaphorical level, make a conscious offering that testifies to your new state of freedom: the freedom to be yourself. Work with just the idea of *amarolī*, or the literal reality of quaffing a glass of your own special vintage. Drink to deep freedom. The wild *yoginī* wants us all to be free. She'll be celebrating with you. For sure.

QUESTIONS AND REFLECTIONS

I invite you to explore your own (current or previous) experience of menopause and how it may be supported by yoga by asking yourself some (or any, or all) of the following questions:

1. How did you experience, or how might you imagine, grieving for the end of your monthly bleeds? Would you / were you simply glad to see them go, or would there be / were there elements of sadness?
2. What other cyclical rhythms are part of your life? How aware are you of lunar phases and seasonal shifts? Does your yoga practice reflect/ honour such cycles?
3. Have you ever taken time to evaluate your life so far, for example through journaling or writing a thank-you letter to yourself? These practices are forms of yogic self-study and can be especially helpful in the preparation for this stage of life, or as a means to create space to help digest experiences at this time.
4. How many postmenopausal women in your life have told you their story of menopause? If the answer is not many, then would you be willing to ask them, and keen to listen? If so, this could be an effective way to experience *satsang*, to support this stage of life.

FURTHER READING AND RESEARCH

Julie Friedeberger's *A Visible Wound,* about her journey with breast cancer, is comforting and practical.

In a crowded field, *Yoga for Osteoporosis* by **Loren Fishman**, M.D. and **Ellen Saltonsall** takes the biscuit.

Jean Shaw Ruddock's *The Second Half of Our Lives* is an upbeat vision of a new approach to the social place and possibilities for postmenopausal women. A more subtle, gentle view is *The Warmth of Our Heart Prevents our Body from Rusting*, in which French psychologist **Marie de Hennezel** shares realistic but uplifting perspectives on the ageing process. **Christiane Northrup**'s *The Wisdom of Menopause* addresses not only the physical aspects of menopause, but also the shifts of attitude and understanding necessary to ensure a positive connection with our lives postmenopause.

Frances Lewis's positive experience of yoga and menopause can be read here: **www.franceslewis.co.uk**

For information and archive footage of **Vanda Scaravelli** practising yoga see **Ester Myer**'s site: **www.estheryoga.com/history/lesson-in-freedom**

Dr Sue Edgley's websites include information about her therapeutic work, and listings of events for devotional music and chanting : **www.drsueedgley.co.uk** and **www.bharatidinesh.co.uk**

For specialist yoga therapy developed to support women with breast cancer, visit: **www.yogaseeker.co.uk**, **www.breastcanceryoga.com**. **www.ucalgary.ca/healthandwellnesslab** is a Canadian programme that is beginning to train instructors in the UK, whilst the Penny Brohn centre in Bristol is a UK beacon for holistic responses to breast cancer, including yoga: **www.pennybrohncancercare.org**

For an overview of issues relating to hysterectomy, **www.hysterectomy-association.org.uk** is a useful site, and the '101 Handy Hints for a Happy Hysterectomy' is reassuring and sensible. Blogging Bhairavīs with sites worth a visit include: **www.mymenopauseblog.com**, **www.menopausegoddessblog.com**. For an overview of useful links: **www.menopausetheblog.com/2011/02/17/the-top-30-menopause-blogs**

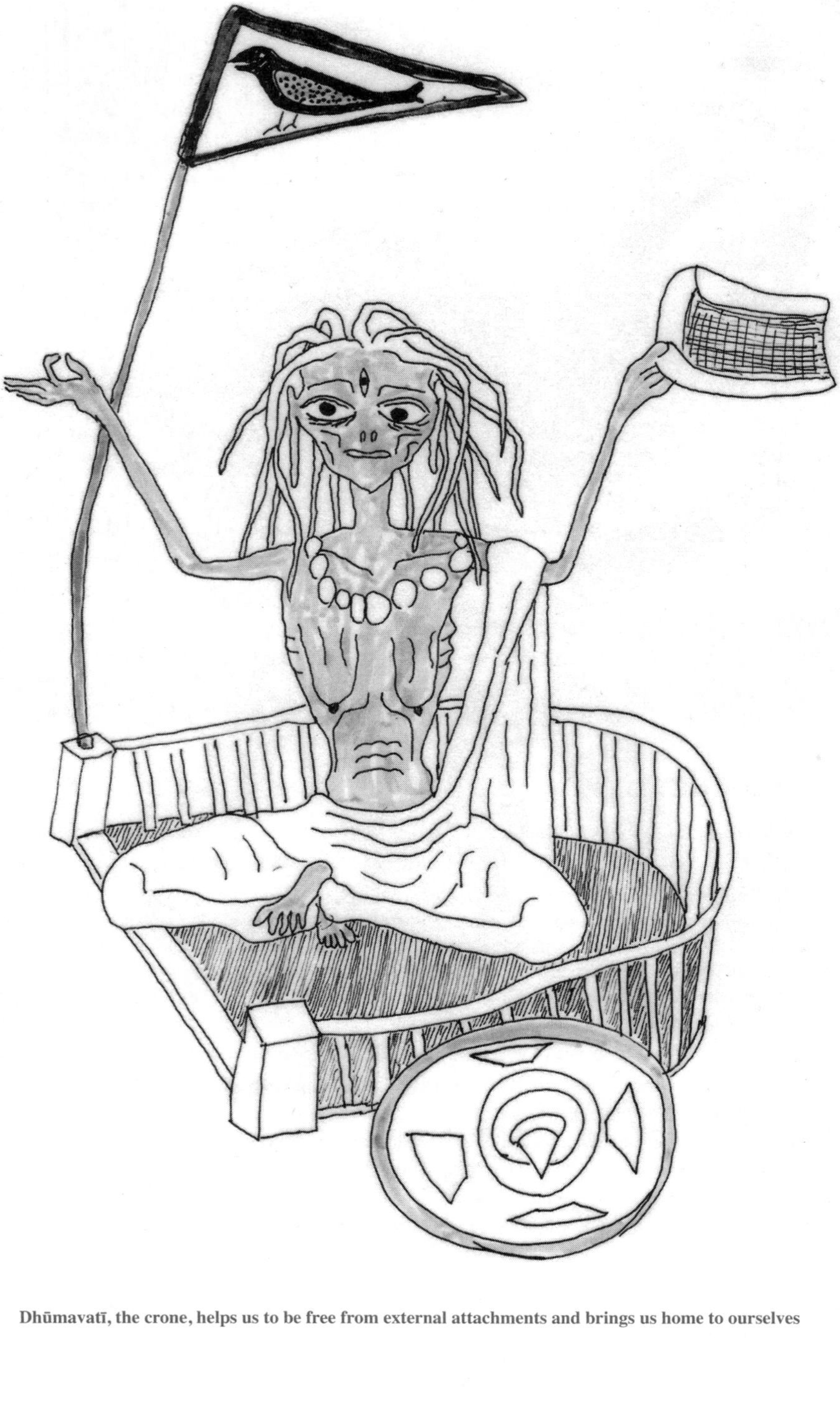

Dhūmavatī, the crone, helps us to be free from external attachments and brings us home to ourselves

CHAPTER SEVENTEEN

Dhūmavatī

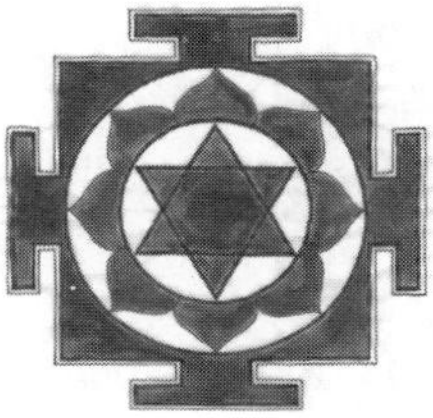

Living our wisdom: yoga and the crowning of a woman's life

> *... crone is not an acceptable mainstream word for women over fifty. Juicy crone however, struck a chord. The juxtaposition of these two words seemed both a contradiction in terms and a welcomed possibility; "dried up and old" were after all, the more usual adjectives attached to "crone." ... the juice that truly vitalizes us is unconditional love, which is the one source of energy that is never depleted; on the contrary, the more we give away, the more there is. (Shinoda Bolen 2003: 100)*

MAHĀVIDYĀ AND *SIDDHI*

WISDOM AND POWER

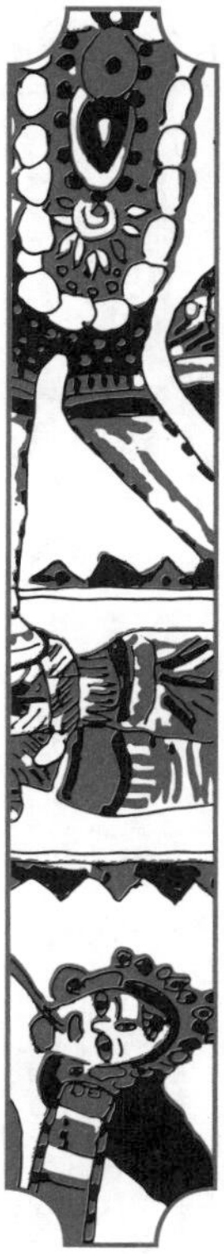

This chapter deals with the years from the end of the fourteenth year after menopause until the end of life, the time in which a woman lives her wisdom. Dhūmavatī [the widow] is the grandmother spirit whom I have placed as guardian over this precious time. She is the ancestral guide for all of the preceding *Mahāvidyās*, the oldest and wisest crone of them all.

Dhūma literally means 'smoke', and in comparison with the bright effulgence of the other nine *Mahāvidyās* who all radiate light, Dhūmavatī is the goddess made of dark smoke, the one who can obscure our view of the light with her clouds. At one level, her 'smoke' is the clouding of our vision and understanding of ultimate reality through the experiences of hardship and suffering. When we are caught up in the gloomy world of our own sorrow and regret, or we stumble through life in the darkness of loneliness, illness, poverty and humiliation, then it is as if we inhabit a smoky cloud where nothing can be seen clearly. Pain and disappointments of all dimensions can seem to block out the light and we lose our way home to ourselves.

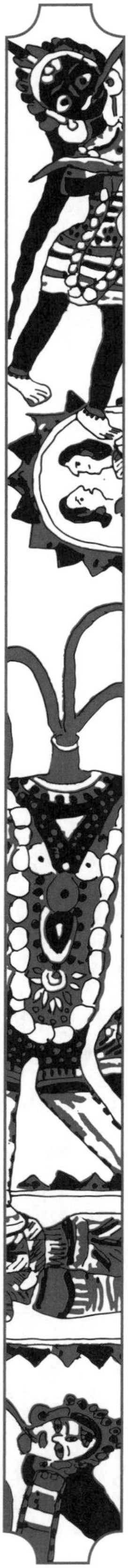

Having clouded our vision with the smoke of suffering, Dhūmavatī's great power is to show us that these experiences can in fact be welcomed as opportunities for spiritual growth and the expansion of wisdom. In this sense Dhūmavatī's wisdom brings a vital perspective to the experiences of the whole life cycle, and her power underpins the wisdoms of each of the other goddesses. This is why she is seen to be the ancestral guide for all of the *Mahāvidyās*. In relation to the years after menopause, Dhūmavatī's power is paradoxical: the nature of her smoky darkness brings us into the obscuring clouds of pain and difficulty that may accompany the ageing of the physical body, whilst her capacity to reveal the truth through suffering teaches great patience, tolerance, perseverance, understanding and forgiveness. These are the great powers of the crowning of our lives. When we learn what Dhūmavatī has to teach, our consciousness expands to see the light in the cloud, to gain detachment, perspective and the deep insight that comes from a capacity to see all angles of a situation and to appreciate the profound power of time as a healer.

Dhūmavatī is a widow and is depicted as a solitary figure, alone even among the other *Mahāvidyās*. In Indian philosophical terms, she represents the feminine principle of pure energy, without the consciousness of the masculine principle of Śiva to provide motivation and direction. She can also be understood as the power of negation, or the void, in the absence of light or positive charge. And so the great *siddhi* of Dhūmavatī is stuck, only existing as a potential force until such time as the sufferings that she brings awaken our own consciousness to provide a motivating directional focus to release her immense energy. In yoga *tantra*, goddesses are most usually understood to be one half of the pair Śiva / Śakti: consciousness and energy. So the solitary aspect of Dhūmavatī is very unusual and significant.

Whereas the rest of the *Mahāvidyās* are accompanied by other human forms, sometimes by assailants or devotees, and sometimes seated upon copulating or other prone figures, Dhūmavatī only has crows for company. There is even a black crow on the flag which waves atop the roof of the wheeled cart in which she sits alone. She is old and ugly and skeletally thin, always hungry and always thirsty. Half her teeth are missing, her wild hair is matted, and she wears dirty old rags and a rosary of human skulls. There is a sharp look in her wrinkly face and she is known as a troublemaker who is always starting pointless arguments and causing confusions and disagreements.

One of Dhūmavatī's hands is held in *cin mudrā*, the gesture of knowledge, whilst the other carries a threshing basket with which to sort chaff from grain. The basket signifies Dhūmavatī's power to teach us discrimination through suffering, to show us how to perceive what really matters in life. At the end of the threshing process, the chaff in Dhūmavatī's basket is discarded as unfit to eat. In the same way, our encounters with the sufferings that Dhūmavatī brings teach us how to discard thoughts and beliefs which are unfit to feed the life and growth of the spirit, and to recognise that even negative experiences can be an aid to spiritual awareness. Her *siddhi* is to give us the power to recognise this: the gift of vision that sees clearly even in the dark clouds with which she surrounds us.

Another perspective on Dhūmavatī defines her paradoxically as the 'wisdom of forgetting'. This aspect of her relates very directly to the understanding we gain towards the end of our lives as we review our many decades of accumulated human experience and choose to let go or forget those aspects of our lives that bind us to a limited understanding of who we really are.

Dhūmavatī as the wisdom of forgetting can be encountered as a special form of *yoga nidrā*, the yogic 'sleep' which is really an awakening, because it brings us back to the pre-creation experience of pure bliss, a time before our consciousness became identified with names and forms and distractions and illusions. As the power of *yoga nidrā*, Dhūmavatī has the capacity to help us dis-identify with all that is extraneous and irrelevant, and to connect instead with the truth of ultimate reality. The accumulated experiences of a lifetime bring us to the possibility of acquiring the discriminative power to choose to forgive and forget those experiences and people that distract us from the pure state of being. Dhūmavatī teaches us to let things go.

Dhūmavatī is Kālī as an old woman, she is time that has passed. Her *siddhi* gives us the wisdom to recognise transience and impermanence as the only constants in life, and the power to live with our presence focused on what truly matters in a state of freedom from attachments.

LIMITATIONS: CULTURAL EXPECTATIONS

> *Yes. We're all dying. We're all crumbling into the void, one cell at a time ... But only women have to pretend it isn't happening. Fifty-something men wander around with their guts flopped over their waistbands and their faces looking like a busted tramp's mattress in an underpass ... Men age visibly every day – but women are supposed to stop the decline around thirty-seven, thirty-eight, and live out the next thirty or forty years in some magical bubble where their hair is still shiny and chestnut, their faces unlined, their lips puffy and their tits up on the first third of their ribcage. (Moran: 291)*

> *Patriarchal culture does not provide women with the necessary tools to prepare their Crone persona in advance, to make the transition without trauma. Neither does this culture provide the ageing woman with any sense of purpose or usefulness after she is no longer needed by dependent children. (Walker 1985: 37)*

The great wisdom and power held by Dhūmavatī in the form of older women is widely reviled and demeaned in our culture. To call any person 'an old woman' is to insult them. To comment that a woman is 'showing her age' is to humiliate her. To say that a woman 'looks like someone's granny' is to ridicule her appearance. Even the term 'crone', which I used positively in the previous chapter (following Jean Shinoda Bolen's and Clarissa Pinkola Estes' shining rehabilitations of the word), still carries an unpleasant charge for many, especially in the phrase 'dried up old crone' which is used to insult any older woman.

The cultural and social pressure around women and ageing is a poisonous brew: a mixture of deep disrespect and profound disempowerment. So insistent is our culture on setting women's value solely by our appearance of youthful fertility that there is simply no space or role for older women to occupy in public life. The public face of female presence, at least in the media, is under forty. Female newsreaders and TV presenters are retired (or relocated to radio) once they reach fifty, whereas their snowy-haired and craggy featured male colleagues continue to appear on screens for decades more. Older women in the public eye are generally expected somehow to remain young and glamorous forever, or to disappear from view once they can no longer manage the effort of appearing to be young. Those older women who remain active and present as actresses or entertainers do so only for as long as we can marvel at 'how good they look for their age'.

In private, the comments made by other women about the signs of an older woman's ageing process are often the cruellest of all: judgmental and spiteful comments are passed on every visible dimension of a woman's surrender to age, from her white hair and whiskers to her varicose veins and bunions. The implication of such comments ('She's really let herself go', 'That hairdo does her no favours', 'A woman her age should look after herself better') are that any evidence of ageing is a sign of defeat, and that a woman's true role once she gets over sixty is to stop the clock by becoming the ideal consumer of every potion and product that claims to help her to retain her youth and beauty forever. This demands considerable money, time and energies that are simply not available to most postmenopausal women. The judgmental comments passed by other women about the appearance of older women are mostly about how, in the absence of some seriously nasty disease that would understandably consume all her energies, she is somehow letting the side down if she doesn't make the necessary efforts to pretend that she is not ageing.

One of the resources available to wealthy older women in response to all of this is cosmetic surgery. Caitlin Moran, in her acerbic and hilarious exploration of *How to be a Woman*, observes acutely that the surgically lifted faces of the wives and partners of rich older men all bear the same expression, one of terror.

> *To be as privileged and safe as they are – but still to go through such painful, expensive procedures – gives the impression of a roomful of fear. Female fear. Adrenalin that [takes] them all the way to a surgeon, and a ward full of bandaged faces. (Moran: 288)*

Moran has a helpful standard test query to reveal whether an activity or attitude is anti-feminist: ask yourself simply 'Are the men doing this?' '... You can tell whether some misogynistic societal pressure is being exerted on women by calmly enquiring, "And are the men doing this, as well?" If they aren't chances are you're dealing with what we strident feminists refer to as "some total fucking bullshit."' (Moran: 289). Ask this question in relation to the phenomenon of plastic surgery and other means to remove evidence of ageing, and the answer is no the men are not doing this. Not usually. Men are not queuing up to get their faces lifted, and their wrinkles botoxed. They are ageing, visibly, proudly and with additional power and kudos accruing with every additional silver hair. They are not, usually, endeavouring to appear to be boys. Old men have roles to play and power to wield. Old women have long since had these powers stolen from them. The disempowerment and humiliation of older women is one of the most long-standing and unchallenged effects of patriarchy. As a result, ageing women are often engaged in an indecorous struggle to deny their experience and to act as if we were still young.

FREEDOMS: YOGA PERSPECTIVES, TECHNIQUES AND AWARENESS FOR BREATHING, MOVING AND BEING

In contrast to the doom, gloom and disempowerment of cultural expectations and responses to older women, the yoga perspective can help us to appreciate that these are indeed the years of living our wisdom. One of the great freedoms of living and working in the yoga world is the honour it can pay to older *yoginīs* and *yogis*. All of my most inspirational teachers have been women over sixty, and now that most of these teachers are well into their seventies, it has been a great source of strength and encouragement to observe how the profundity of their teaching has matured and deepened as they have aged.

Clarissa Pinkola Estes helpfully describes this time of life in a number of attractive and intriguing ways, including the 'age of becoming watchwoman' from sixty-three to seventy, during which time a woman has the opportunity to 'recast all she has learned'. Estes also describes the experience of 're-youthanization', the paradox of fully meeting the realities of ageing with a youthful spirit of acceptance and trust, which one sees clearly evident in the lives of the many elderly *yoginīs* whose stories fill this chapter. Observing and learning from their life stories can expand our ideas of what it is to live life after seventy fully as a crone. Moving into the 'age of the mist beings', as Estes describes the age of seventy-seven onwards is an evocative idea that connects our last decades with the living presence of the spirit, whilst the bright examples of those women who demonstrate successful ageing in an extreme form by living, as my paternal grandmother did, until the age of one hundred and four, show how the closing decades of our lives may well be filled with a rare and beautiful energy that is generated by connecting an elderly but freely zestful vitality with a clarity of perspective and understanding. Estes identifies a series of seven-year cycles that extend right through later life up until the age of one hundred and five, and perceptively observes that :

> *'... as a woman transits through these cycles, her layers of defence, protection, density become more and more sheer until her very soul begins to shine through. We can sense and see the movement of the soul within the body-psyche in an astonishing way as we grow older and older.' (Estes 1993: 448)*

The value of yoga for older women is not that it helps us to look young again, but that it gives us the tools and attitudes we need to align our focus with the growing presence of our soul life, ensuring that the energy and power we have can move freely to enable the full expression of our wisdom at this time. Yoga over seventy is not about sticking to the same practices we did in our twenties and thirties in the vain hope that we will appear to be as youthful as we were then, but rather it is about adapting and accommodating the practices we do to enhance our understanding of who we are now. When we encounter women who have discovered this then we come into the presence of powerful beings with much to teach us.

As a teenager, I had the great good fortune to have a part-time job in a village dressmaking workshop where a small team of skilled makers and designers created very gorgeous garments, and the occasional theatrical or special outfit. The lead designer's speciality was painted silk appliqué, and her most popular items were knitted and quilted mohair jackets with silk flowers. Most of those wealthy enough to afford these bespoke clothes tended to be older women, and as a sixteen-year-old I was so wrapped up in the world of youthful self-obsession that all these ladies tended to merge one into another. My job was to make silk buttons and bias cut loops, to stitch hems, brew coffee and sometimes (rather nerve-wrackingly) to cut out at speed half a dozen bridesmaids' dresses from great bolts of dupion silk. I was pretty delighted with myself and my job and I took very little notice of the customers. However, one day even I sat up from my sewing and took notice of a most remarkable customer who was quite unlike any of the others.

> *She was called Olive, and she was a yoga teacher. In rural Buckinghamshire in the mid 1980s this was rare and exotic.*

Olive was a special being in many ways. Unlike all the other women who frequented our shop with thick make-up and expensive hairdos, dyed and permed and coiffed, Olive had straight grey hair screwed up tight into a chignon on the top of her head, and her face was scrubbed clear of any makeup except for bright red lips and a pair of startling black eyebrows. She was tall to start with, but she stood up so straight that everything about her looked elegant and graceful. She dressed in stretchy black flared trousers and skinny tops and black leather boots and the jackets we made for her had luscious scarlet poppies embroidered extravagantly right across the back.

I was impressed by all of this, but what was even more remarkable was what happened to everyone whenever Olive entered the shop. She was like a sunny day. She smiled and chatted and cackled and thoroughly enjoyed every moment of the process of getting her jackets made. Other customers grumbled about the fitting process, and found picky complaints to make about the stitching or the buttons or the colours of the painted silk, but not Olive. She knew exactly what she wanted, and she took ages at the start choosing the yarn and the colour and the styles (and the buttons), but once that was all clear, she had a joyous bubbling spirit that took huge delight in everything. It was contagious. We all looked forward to Olive's arrivals and revelled with her in just how gorgeous she looked in her lovely jackets. She couldn't thank us enough. 'Not bad for an old yoginī*!' she would trill as she struck a pose.*

Olive's joyous spirit and ready laugh was a testimony to her years of yoga practice and teaching. She taught several classes a week (there were not many yoga teachers to go around in those days) and she shared her great delight in the benefits of yoga with scores of devoted students who all loved Olive as much as we did.

As a hypercritical adolescent, evaluating the models I was being offered by the older women around me, there was something about Olive that really lit me up. Although I wasn't able to put my finger on it at the time, I certainly felt that it would be pretty cool to be like Olive when I got old. She seemed so happy in herself. I understand now that she was a powerful manifestation of the liberated wisdom of Dhūmavatī, in that she had long since accepted the physical signs of her ageing and turned her attention elsewhere: she wore her grey top knot with elegance and pride, and instead of fixating on the loss of youthful beauty, had devoted her energies to the cultivation of a vibrant inner life that brought her great joy and abundant vitality to do the work she still chose to do.

Olive was the first yoga teacher I ever met in person (I didn't count Richard Hittelman because I'd only ever seen him on the telly, in *Yoga for Health* in 1969), and she showed me how a deep pulse of vital energy could be nurtured into old age through the life-long practice of yoga. As I widened my yogic horizons I began to see that there were many other ageing *yoginīs* like Olive, women who moved through their seventies with grace, power and levels of energy and enthusiasm that would be remarkable in women half their ages.

> *When seventy-four-year-old Angela Farmer leads a yoga workshop, she overflows with quietly joyful exuberance that is quite contagious. It is because of her own way of being at ease in her body that she is able to share her delight in the freedom of movement and openness of heart that have been gifted to her through her lifetime practice of yoga. She moves gently and elegantly, and she smiles often. She graciously welcomes students from all over the world to the retreat space she runs with her husband Victor in Eftalou, on the Greek island of Lesbos, and the rest of the year she maintains an international schedule of teaching that brings her across Europe and into the US and the Far East.*
>
> *Her vitality and energy are sustained by yoga, and she is quite clearly practising what she preaches. Angela's yogic trajectory led her to move away from her roots in Iyengar yoga to explore her own fluid practice style. Her contemporary, Gurmukh Kaur Khalsa, who has spent over forty years spreading the message of* Kuṇḍalinī *yoga, is still firmly rooted in the organisation established by her guru, Yogi Bhajan. Gurmukh's Los Angeles yoga centre is a thriving spiritual village powered by her own immense energies, and she has produced a wealth of teaching and training materials that share the techniques of* Kuṇḍalinī *yoga, especially in relation to pregnancy and postnatal recovery. At seventy years of age, she is still happily on the road, and like Angela Farmer, divides her time between welcoming students to her own yoga space, and teaching workshops all over the world. Her motivation to share is powered by her own living experience of the benefits of yoga practice.*

But in the world of the Dhūmavatī *yoginīs*, these impressive women in their seventies are at the youthful end of the spectrum. Angela and Gurmukh are twenty years younger than the woman who currently holds the Guinness record as the oldest yoga teacher in the world.

> *Tao Porchon-Lynch is ninety-four, and still teaching four weekly yoga classes in New York State and workshops all over the US. She's also a keen dancer and an active campaigner for world peace projects, including Yoga for Peace's initiatives in the Middle East. Tao began practising yoga in her twenties and studied with Indra Devi and B.K.S Iyengar in India. She has made innumerable trips back to India, bringing students with her on retreats and yoga trainings. Tao still travels in support of peace projects, for example, visiting Vietnam in 2012 as part of the World Karma Project.*
>
> *In video demonstrations of her teaching, she exudes a gentle but vital energy and a palpable sense of delight in both her students' and*

her own practice. In an interview about her recognition as the oldest yoga teacher on the planet, Tao affirms with a laugh, 'I'm going to teach yoga until I can't breathe any more and then it's going to carry me to the next planet… I love yoga! It brightens my day and it makes everybody smile.'

At every dimension of their being, these inspiring *yoginīs* are ageing with an authentic connection to the wisdom they have practised throughout their lives. Angela Farmer, Gurmukh, and Tao Porchon-Lynch have each devoted a lifetime of commitment to the practice of yoga that has placed them all now in a space where they are able to devote most of their abundant energies to the service of yoga. But for many older women, yoga is not a way of life, rather just a small but important part of their week. But even just by attending a regular class, the healing powers of yoga are evident as a great support for the well-being of women over seventy.

When I was teaching in London, two older women became regular students. Wealthy and conservative in many ways, they made a commitment to a Saturday morning yoga class because they could see for themselves that yoga worked. Sarah had been convinced of the healing power of yoga for many months before she brought along her friend Helen, who had been complaining of lower back pain. Initially she was sceptical. 'I am old' she warned me, as she filled in the registration form. 'And I have been around. I've tried everything. This pain doesn't seem to want to shift.' But she had cycled over to the class, given up her Saturday morning to be there, and she placed great faith in the positive testimony of her friend Sarah, so there was some hope that the yoga would be useful to her.

After twenty minutes of gentle work from a semi-supine position, breathing and moving the pelvis and the legs, Helen let out a very loud sigh. I was worried she might have hurt herself. 'It's gone!' she announced joyfully to the class, 'I am no longer in pain.' Delighted with herself, she became a regular student and continued to practise at home to maintain her newly discovered freedom from pain. What yoga did for Helen was to enable her to get on with doing the other things in life that really mattered to her: 'I'll be back Highland dancing next week,' she told her friend at the end of the first class.

For Sarah and Helen, who were both in their mid-seventies, their enthusiasm for yoga was sparked by the sense that its practice could help them to sustain the kinds of activities that made their lives worth living, like Highland dancing and cycling. For Sophie, who first encountered yoga on a post-retirement trip to India, yoga became important to her because it showed her ways to question the values of the life she had been living and to re-consider the focus for the rest of her life.

I first heard about Sophie from a friend who'd been assisting at the aṣram *where Sophie and her daughter went for a yoga holiday.*

'We only really went for a laugh' recalled Sophie later. But the experience of holistic yoga living and practising in the aṣram *for a month changed Sophie's perspective on her life. At the age of sixty-seven she trained as a yoga teacher herself, became actively involved in yoga workshops and classes in her community, and by the time I met her when she was seventy-one, she had signed up for an intensive residential retreat training in Vedic chant. Sophie's focus, clarity and open-heartedness are powerful testimony to the joyful nature of her encounter with yoga. Her good-humoured immersion in the power of Vedic chant showed me that a profound dedication to living yoga can be rooted very effectively in our later years.*

The willingness to let go of previous patterns of behaviours and values which no longer serve us, in order to make space and time for the pursuit of activities and attitudes which nurture the growth and radiance of our spirit, is the *siddhi* of Dhūmavatī. It brings great wisdom.

YOGA PRACTICES

The yoga practices recommended below are intended to support and sustain energy and strength in the years after seventy without causing injury or depletion. The womb yoga greetings and meditations presented in chapters five and six can be helpfully practised as techniques to honour the final stage of life's unfolding by honouring blood wisdom as a means to reconnect the physical body with the earth.

The womb yoga greetings, in particular **Opening the lotus to *prāṇa śakti*** (pp.136–9) can be done with tender attention to the effect of the practices as yoga to support the dignified and heart-felt experience of loss, grief and regret.

Pūrṇa pavanamuktāsana (pp.497–510). This remarkable sequence is an effective way to keep *prāṇa* flowing and to optimise range of movement, stability and strength. It is an ideal daily practice at any point in life, but has a particular value in later years because it is gentle and can be done even whilst lying in bed, for example during recovery from illness. The series in this book brings together three different approaches to this kind of practice: the original *pavanamuktāsana* series devised by Swami Satyananda; additional base positions and movement guidelines from Mukunda Stiles' joint-freeing series; and a number of strategic and therapeutic refinements from an inspiring yoga teacher in her seventies, who is so modest that she prefers to remain anonymous.

Palm tree *vinyāsa* with *yoni namaskār* (p.532). This sequence combines the gradual mobilisation of the spine with the flowing womb greetings from the opening chapters. It is revitalising without being depleting.

Supine twist (p.159) Resting in this open twist revitalises through repose: a passive twist is both energising and quietening, promoting a special, free and easy quality of rest. Twists are delightful to practise before *yoga nidrā*.

Shining skull *breath (kapālabhāti)* (p.516) This is a *kriyā*, a cleansing practice. It clarifies the thought processes, and is a valuable tool to lift energy and focus up into the head to establish a positive link with the realms of the spirit.

Circle of flowing breath (pp.128–31) The particular resonance of this practice with the later decades of our lives is the sense of cyclical wisdom and constant return that this breath brings. From the perspective of the third act of life, when many cycles of life have already unfolded, then simply observing the cycles of breath can be profound teaching.

Super deluxe five-star *savasana* (p.550): The basic corpse pose is not always a comfortable resting place for older bodies. This five-star version brings deep comfort and joy to aching bones by way of many props.

Heart-womb river meditation (pp.147–8): this is a valuable practice to maintain a sense of flow and renewal. At this stage of life it can be helpful to focus upon the renewal of compassion in the heart through the river of creativity and nurture from the womb, and to foster a sense of giving thanks and love down to the womb or the space of the absent womb for her lifetime's work.

Awareness in *yoga nidrā* and other meditative work: a helpful and nourishing focus for these practices can be on the experience of passing wisdom to future generations, for example with metaphors such as spreading the seed, growing the future crops, nourishing and giving back to the community. In the *yoginīs*' temple *yoga nidrā* (pp.454–9) is also a positive practice at this time.

YOGIC REMEDIES AND RESPONSES

Insomnia: *Yoga nidrā* (chapter eighteen) can be a helpful way to get to sleep, or a practice to re-introduce yourself to the sleeping state if you wake up in the night or early mornings. Womb breathing (p.153) can be a powerful sedative, a calming way to enter the sleep state. But from another perspective, it can be wise to embrace sleeplessness as an opportunity for meditative practice and, especially in the early morning hours, a way to devote more energy to the cultivation of the inner life.

Osteoporosis: Osteoporosis affects women (far more than men) of all ages, but is especially prevalent in later years. It is a condition in which the density of the bones begins to lessen, and eventually, the bones begin to crumble away. The good news is that it is detectable very early on and is reversible. The yogic and ayurvedic perspective on osteoporosis connects it to our root *cakra*, to the earth, and to our sense of being stable, supported, sheltered and safe. In *Women's Power to Heal through Inner Medicine*, Mother Maya Tiwari observes that:

> *Osteoporosis is a condition that literally relates to strength and support in the body and the sense of security in the mind. It occurs most frequently in women who have psychologically not come to terms with the absolute and personal reality of their own ageing, death, and dying. (225)*

This perspective on osteoporosis is unusual and helpful. Essentially, it enables us to understand the condition as being related to 'first *cakra*' (p.141) experiences of insecurity and confusion about our right to be safe and present in the world. We can see how the framework of bones that hold us up can crumble away if we doubt our own worth as we age and feel that we have no longer any right to belong in the structure of societal and familiar networks that hold our culture together. If older women have a sense of their own intrinsic value as they age (and this involves embracing the reality of the ageing process), goes this argument, then the internal structure of support is matched by the outer support of a culture which accords the ageing woman a sense of deep respect and value, and so bones stay strong. In addition to this philosophical reflection on the deep cultural roots of osteoporosis, Mother Maya presents in her work a number of rejuvenating āyurvedic tonics and medicines, and promotes very positively the idea that osteoporosis is in fact a reversible condition. Nutrition, food *sādhanā* and meditation are key to the ayurvedic response to the condition.

The possibility that osteoporosis is reversible and certainly preventable is also borne out by the inspiring work of Loren Fishman and Ellen Saltonsall, whose fabulous book *Yoga for Osteoporosis* sets out a full range of *āsana* to build bones. Osteopaenic (early signs of possible osteoporosis) and osteoporotic versions of all poses are included, and the emphasis is on weight-bearing poses to build strength:

> *'Yoga safely stresses bones without impact…with many poses that avoid moving joints altogether, yoga has been shown to strengthen bones without any evidence that it weakens joints. …'*

The positive effects of yoga for maintaining healthy bones is beginning to be well recognised by orthodox medicine in the UK. Whilst interviewing women's health specialist Dame Shirley Bond for this book, she affirmed that her Harley Street colleagues who specialise in treating osteoporosis are very familiar with yoga's beneficial impact on bone-building:

> *Whenever they do a DEXA scan [the scan which measure's bone density] they can tell that if the reading is high they are likely looking at a women who practises yoga, and so the first thing they ask when they get a good reading is: "Have you been doing your yoga?"' It's definitely a helpful practice.'*

Weight-bearing practices described in this book that are helpful in the management of osteoporosis include the paired balancing poses (p.539–40), the Spiritual warrior sequence (p.536–8) and Being in the cycles (pp.517–21). Work with the Cat pose variations (p.502) and the Wall as teacher sequence (pp.546–9) can also be useful. Inversions (pp.488–91) may also be of value, but can be dangerous in cases where the osteoporosis is advanced. It is not within the scope of this section to offer fully detailed yoga therapeutic programmes for reversing osteoporosis (for guidance on that please see the references), but it is helpful to know that, in most mild cases, a full programme of weight-bearing *āsana*, combined with a healthy diet and plenty of sunshine, is a positive way to reverse osteoporosis, and that regular checks on bone density can be useful to monitor progress.

Arthritis: When the inflammatory condition of rheumatoid arthritis is relatively mild, and movement is not causing acute pain, then the limitation of joint movement can be helpfully relieved by the practice of *pūrṇa pavanamuktāsana* (p.497–510). At times when the inflammation is acute, then the practice of *yoga nidrā* (chapter eighteen) and the pain-relieving *prāṇāyāmas* (pp.462–3) are the best course of yoga therapy. The same programme may also be helpful for osteoarthritis.

Recovery after heart attack: Restorative poses, in particular In the golden cosmic womb (pp.552–3) are valuable at this time, and Out of the smoke *yoga nidrā* (p.453) can be of huge benefit in terms of creating space for reflection and understanding of what changes may be needed to support future health. The full *pavanmuktāsana* series (pp.497–510) is a helpful way to maintain mobility and strength during any period of rest and recuperation.

Pelvic organ prolapse / dysfunction: For full details on the use of yoga to manage pelvic organ prolapse, please see the practices in chapters twenty and twenty-one, especially the uplifted vaginal locks (pp.474–6) and the semi-supine and inverted practices (pp.483-91). In terms of living long term with the effects of prolapse, then all of the pelvic movements and womb greetings described in chapters five and six, especially Snake circles the womb (p.168), and Standing womb pilgrimages (p.170), can help to adjust habitual posture to provide optimal support. It can also be very helpful to explore the perspectives offered by Christine Kent, whose *Prolapse First Aid for Elders* is a valuable resource specifically created for the support of older women living with pelvic organ prolapse.

FEED THE WILD *YOGINĪ*

ENCOUNTER YOUR OWN DEATH

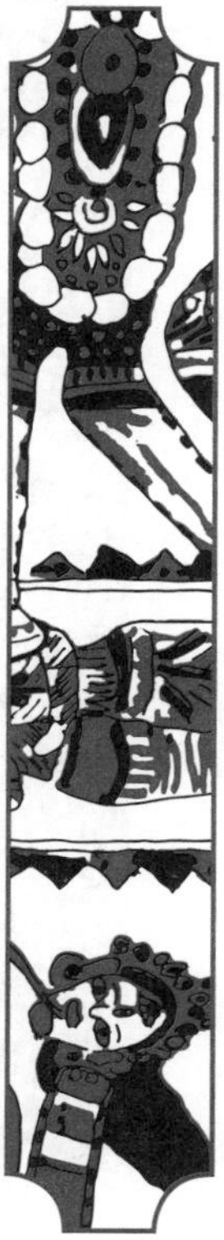

In the yogic tradition, there is an understanding that it is only the most enlightened of beings who know in advance the nature and time of their own deaths. Reports from those close to Paramahamsa Satyananda Saraswati, who died in 2009, describe how he prepared for the moment of his death by taking his *mālā* and sitting for meditation. 'I'm going now, don't try to stop me,' he advised his disciple Swami Satyasangananda. And then he sat meditating as he took his last breath. Such a passing is the sign of a highly evolved soul, and it serves as an inspiration to use our yoga practice as a preparation for our own departure.

When asked to recommend yoga practices for the older woman, Menaka Desikachar, senior Vedic chant teacher of the Krishnamacharya Healing Yoga Foundation, and herself in her seventies, said with a big smile, 'The end of life should be preparation for final take-off. Definitely, no doubt, focus should be on final take-off.'

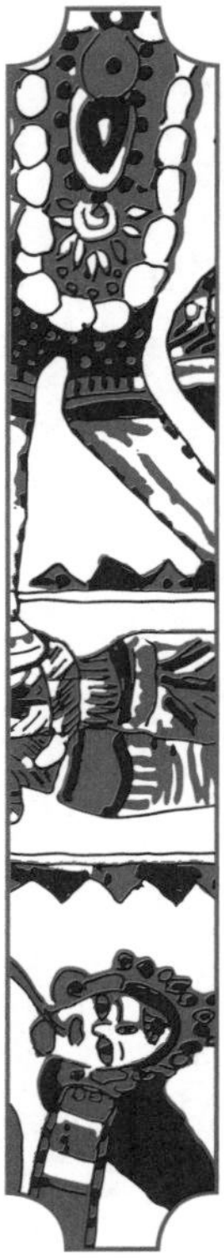

The practice of *yoga nidrā* gives us the opportunity to prepare for this 'take-off' as consciously as we are able. When next settling down to do *yoga nidrā*, imagine that you are laying down your bones for the last time. As you experience the heaviness, sense the dead heavy bones returning down to the earth, and as you experience lightness, sense the lifeless body going up in smoke, wafting high into the sky. Alternate between these two experiences and encounter the reality that, however vital and strong yoga practice may help our bodies to be, at some point we have to leave aside this physical vehicle. It makes sense to bring this awareness of being in 'death's anteroom' to consciousness and to get intimate with the fact of our mortality.

When you think about it, that's largely the point of all meditations anyway, and lying down as if dead for *yoga nidrā* is perhaps the most vivid way to encounter this awareness: 'The older woman knows the truth of the advice that the Duke gives Claudio in *Measure for Measure* … "be absolute for death; either death or life / Shall thereby be the sweeter."' (Greer 1991: 314).

QUESTIONS AND REFLECTIONS

To connect with the *siddhi* of Dhūmavatī is to become open to the experience of letting go, for forgiveness and forgetting in order to make more space for the expansion of our spirit.

1 Was there ever in your life a positive or inspiring role model for a woman over seventy? Who was she and how did she inspire you?

2 Was there ever in your life an older woman whose behaviour and attitudes alarmed or depressed you? Who was she, and what was it about her behaviour that you did not enjoy?

3 What are the qualities of older women that you most admire? And what are the aspects of older women that you most fear to embody yourself?

4 Have you met (in person, or by reputation) any old *yoginīs*? Who were they, and what elements of yoga did they practise?

5 What elements of your current yoga practice do you envision continuing into your life after seventy? What elements of your current yoga practice do you envision dropping out of your life after seventy? Are there new aspects of yoga practice that appeal to you as something that you would like to learn to practise after seventy?

6 If yoga is part of your working life (e.g. as a teacher or a trainer), what does your yoga retirement plan look like?

7 What elements of the power and wisdom of Dhūmavatī do you imagine (or experience) yourself embracing as you age?

FURTHER READING AND RESEARCH

Recent feminist scholarship has helpfully rehabilitated the word 'crone' and produced a number of very inspiring books that provide clarity of thinking around the relationship between women, ageing and power. I warmly recommend the writings of **Barbara G. Walker** on this topic, in particular her book *Crone*. **Jean Shinoda Bolen** also has a hotline to the great crone goddess, and all her reflections, especially those in *Crones Don't Whine: Concentrated Wisdom for Juicy Women* are pure gold. It goes without saying that **Christiane Northrup**'s opinions on the topic of later life are as valuable as those she has on all other aspects of womanhood, and she writes with attention to this time in *The Wisdom of Menopause*. The penultimate chapter of **Caitlin Moran**'s *How to be a Woman d*elivers a cracking rant on the craziness of surgical and other interventions to disguise the ageing process in women, and the last chapter of **Germaine Greer**'s *The Change* offers a beautiful literary-philosophical reflection on the growth of the life of the spirit in older women. **Jean Shaw Ruddock**'s *The Second Half of Our Lives* sets out an upbeat vision of older women as dynamos for positive social engagement and new business projects and *The Warmth of Our Heart Prevents our Body from Rusting* by **Marie de Henneze** shares a profound and uplifting perspective on menopause and after.

There's an engaging profile of **Jean Shaw Ruddock** from the Daily Telegraph: **www.telegraph.co.uk/health/women_shealth/9226756/The-Second-Half-of-Your-Life.html**

Websites that relate to this stage of life are less numerous than those dealing with younger women's issues. To be honest when searching for an internet presence for 'Old Women' what turned up were mostly dating agencies and scuzzy titillation about granny-sex. It was pretty disappointing. However, with diligence and wider enquiries I have uncovered a few sites worth visiting, and a lot of blogging crones.

Crone Magazine is available by subscription, but the freely accessible part of the site has many interesting articles celebrating the spirituality of older women: **www.cronemagazine.com**. For positive perspectives on women and ageing: **www.yoni.com/crone.shtml**

Perspective on crones in stories from the Celtic tradition are posted at: **www.suppressedhistories.net/secrethistory/crones.html**

Sensible information and guidance on the prevention and management of osteopaenia and osteoporosis through diet and lifestyle changes are available from **Dr Shirley Bond**: **www.bio-hormone-health.com/2012/01/05/10-key-facts-about-osteoporosis-and-osteopenia**

The National Osteoporosis Society has a helpline, and a wealth of valuable leaflets and good information on preserving bone density and living with osteoporosis: **www.nos.org.uk**

Angela Farmer and **Victor van Kooten**'s website lists their teaching schedule and outlines their approach to yoga: **www.angela-victor.com**

There are videos and messages from **Gurmukh Kaur Khalsa** on her website **www.goldenbridgeyoga.com**

To view a short interview with **Tao Porchon-Lynch**, the oldest yoga teacher in the world, visit: **www.bbc.co.uk/news/world-us-canada-18068548**. Tao Porchon-Lynch's own website: **www.taoporchon-lynch.com/**

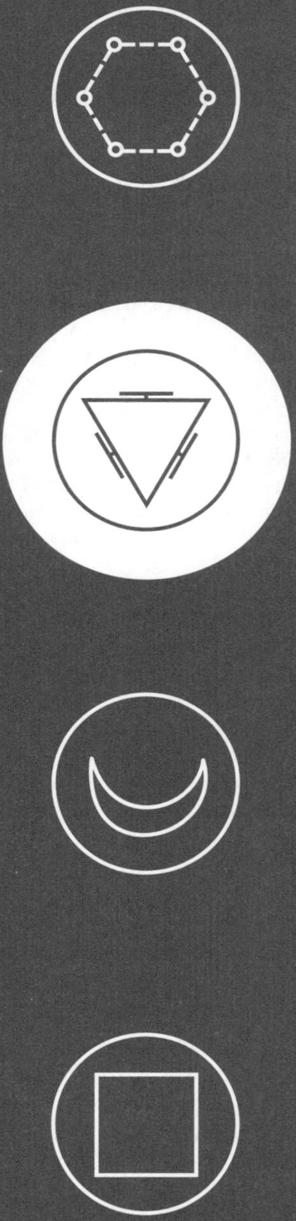

PART THREE

FURTHER PRACTICES OF WOMB YOGA

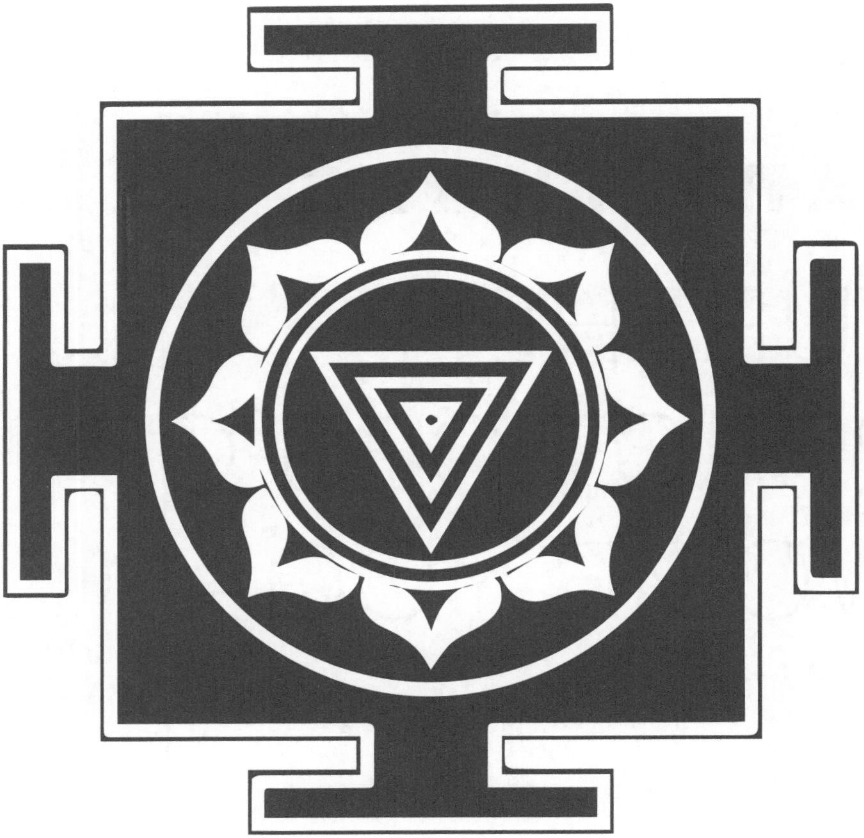

Please note that the techniques included in this part of the book are supplementary to those fundamental breath practices of womb yoga, the womb greetings and the energy invocations presented in chapters four to seven. In combination with the use of appropriate *yoga nidrā*, the practices presented here are nourishing and helpful to any woman at any time in her life. For practice suggestions that relate to a particular time in your life cycle, please consult the life cycle sections in the previous part of the book, where recommended practices are identified in terms of their relevance to certain life experiences.

The practices described in the chapters in this part of the book are organised in terms of the type and focus of the practice (e.g. all the breathing practices are grouped together, all the foundational [feet, pelvis and breast] practices are gathered together, and so are most of the pelvic health and awareness practices). The breath practices, and those specifically for the feet and the pelvis, are presented first since an understanding of these practices is crucial for everything that follows. The intention of this way of organising is to make it easier to find the practice for which you are looking.

For more detailed guidance on how to select specific practices for therapeutic use, please see the therapeutic index (pp.657–61). If you know the name of a particular practice and just want to find the instructions, then it is probably easier to search in the practice title index (pp.662–4). Suggested sequencing is offered in chapter twenty-six, where you will find suggestions for creating your own womb yoga programmes, for example to support menstrual health, or to connect with lunar cycles.

CHAPTER EIGHTEEN

Yoga nidrā: an inner ritual of healing and homecoming

Yoga nidrā literally means 'yoga sleep'. It is a special and effortless state of consciousness in which deep healing can occur. The healing that happens in *yoga nidrā* is multi-dimensional: it affects every level of our being, including our emotions and mental constructions. The physical body comes into a state of extremely deep rest, whilst the mind is guided through various activities intended to induce states of *yoga nidrā*. It is a remarkable experience, a practice that invites us into a state of awareness that is utterly free and profoundly nourishing. It is both a homecoming and a release, a settling into the deepest layers of our true state of freedom.

Richard Miller, the non-dual psychotherapist whose development of *yoga nidrā* in the US over the past thirty years has been very influential in ensuring global recognition of the power of this practice, calls it the meditative heart of yoga. Swami Satyananda, who first adapted and developed the practice to make it accessible for modern yogis, describes it as 'aware sleep'. However you chose to define *yoga nidrā*, it has an astonishing capacity to relieve mental and emotional tension, creating spaciousness to allow for authentic healing and transformation to occur.

Over the past forty or fifty years, *yoga nidrā* has become understood as 'set' form that we can 'receive' when it is delivered by a teacher. In fact, with experience and commitment, the state of *yoga nidrā* can be encouraged to arise naturally, and many original and creative manifestations of the form awaken within us. *Yoga nidrā* is alive in the sense that these states of being are accessible to every one of us. All we need to do is welcome in the guidance of the inner teacher. It is this approach to *yoga nidrā* that I take in my own practice and teaching, and it is through this approach that all the practices in this chapter evolved.

In relation to the stages of women's life cycles as set out in the previous section, I have over the past fifteen years developed a series of ten *yoga nidrā* practices to support women's health. Each practice resonates with particular issues and concerns at different times and stages in our lives, and draws from the insights offered by an understanding of female *siddhis* and the *Mahāvidyās* as described in the previous section. These practices are available for download at **www.yonishakti.co**. The best way to experience *yoga nidrā* is simply to lie down and listen to the track that resonates with you right now. Although the practices are presented as a chronological unfolding, each one relating to a particular chapter in the previous section (with the notable exception of practice four which presents sexuality and creativity in a single practice), this does not limit the application of any given practice to the specific life stage to which it refers. For example, the menarche *nidrā* may be just what you need to hear if you are just coming off the Pill and reconnecting to your menstrual cycle, and the pregnancy *nidrā* may work well to support the growth and development of a creative project that is beginning to feel as if it has a life of its own. There is much to work with here, so do allow time to explore the different practices and discover for yourself the power of *yoga nidrā*.

In the first instance, the Starry night pure *yoga nidrā* or the opening invocation at the start of the book (p.17–20) are good places to start because they offer the simplest *yoga nidrā*, without any particular visualisations or imagery. Each of the other practices offers a short image to evoke an inner ritual of healing and connection. Below I set out the structure and content of each practice as a way to convey the tone of each track in order that you can be guided in the choice of the tracks that suit you. Each track begins and ends with much the same format as the first one, but offers at the point marked * an opportunity to engage with the imagery of the inner ritual that is specific to that particular practice. The final practice 'In the *yoginīs*' temple' uses a different rotation of consciousness than the previous practices. Each track is about twenty-five minutes long, but the first one is only twenty minutes, and some of the other tracks are slightly longer or shorter than the average twenty-five-minute running time.

With all of the *nidrās*, before you start listening, it is important to create a secure and safe place where (ideally), you will not be interrupted for the duration of the practice. Turn off phones and computers before you start. Dim the lights, draw the curtains or wear an eye pillow. Rest on a mat on the floor or on a sofa or a bed: so long as you are warm and comfortable, that is the main thing.

LIST OF PRACTICES

Please visit **yonishakti.co/audio** to download or listen to these practices.

***Yoga nidrā* 4: In the wild garden, joyous freedom to flow**
Sexuality, creativity and juice (Kamalātmikā and Mataṅgi) (pp.445–6)

***Yoga nidrā* 5: Nourishing growth**
Nurturing the capacity to support new life (Bhuvaneśvarī) (pp.446–8)

***Yoga nidrā* 6: Thanksgiving and grieving**
Postnatal recovery, transformation and adaptation (Chinnamastā) (p.448–9)

***Yoga nidrā* 7: Being with not knowing**
Perimenopause and the inevitability of change; becoming the seed at the heart of the fruit (Bagalamukhi) (pp.450–1)

***Yoga nidrā* 8: Self-anointing ritual**
Embracing power, menopause and the confidence to speak one's own truth; empowered by nature to be your true self (Bhairavī) (pp.451–2)

***Yoga nidrā* 9: Out of the smoke**
Touching the power close to the bone (Dhūmavatī) (p.453)

***Yoga nidrā* 10: In the *yoginīs'* temple**
Resting and healing to live in wisdom and power (Full constellation of *yoginīs*) (pp.454–9)

SCRIPTS FOR *YOGA NIDRĀ* PRACTICES

Please note that these scripts are provided for reference and self-exploration only, for example, you may enjoy reading the scripts before or after you listen to the audio recordings. They are intended to deepen your experience of the recorded yoga nidrā *tracks. Never just read out a script to a person or group of persons, because this will send all your energy into the paper, depleting your listeners of vitality. To experience* yoga nidrā *it is best either to have the practice 'running' in your head, or to listen to a living practice, delivered for you by an experienced teacher who is responsive and attentive to your needs, and not simply reading out a script. In the absence of such a person, then listening to a recording is the next best thing. The following practices are offered as audio recordings on* **www.yonishakti.co**. *To access downloads and for listings of further* yoga nidrā *teachers worldwide, please see* **www.yoganidranetwork.org**

NB If you are over 30 weeks' pregnant, when resting to practise yoga nidrā *you are advised to lie on your left side, supporting your head and right knee with cushions and bolsters.*

YOGA NIDRĀ 1: STARRY NIGHT PURE *YOGA NIDRĀ*

THE FUNDAMENTAL PRACTICE OF AWARENESS (KĀLĪ)

Welcome to the practice of *yoga nidrā*. Welcome home. The first part of the practice is to get comfortable. Lie down on your back (or side, if you are pregnant, or if you prefer this to lying on your back). Take time to arrange your body so that you feel that you are well supported. Place cushions and pillows under your head and wherever else suits you so that you can feel absolutely at ease. Having support underneath the knees can really help to let the lower back settle well. Bear in mind that body temperature may drop during the practice, so if you feel the need, cover yourself with a blanket, or put on socks or a sweater to keep warm.

When you feel you are able to rest comfortably, settle into your chosen position and allow the body to become still, knowing that there is no need for any further physical movement during this practice. Experience the state of zero desire for movement. If that state is not present, then make whatever adjustments are necessary so that you feel super comfortable. The ideal state for the physical body during *yoga nidrā* is zero desire for movement. If the desire to move does arise during the practice, simply watch it. It will probably go away and you can remain still. If the desire to move returns then that may be a signal that you do actually need to move, so do so with awareness, and with the intention to regain comfort and stillness, returning to the state of zero desire for movement.

Now become aware very precisely of the position in which you are lying. Know the shape and the posture of the body; know the shape and arrangement of the room. Feel the points of contact between the side or the back of the body and the floor.

Be aware now of the gentle rhythm of the natural breath. Feel the breath coming in and the breath going out. If the breath moves freely and easily through the nostrils, breathe that way. If it is more comfortable to exhale through the mouth, then do that. Let whichever is the most comfortable and easy way of breathing arise naturally.

Allow the outgoing breath to release the weight of the body down into the support of the earth beneath. With every exhalation now, consciously transfer the weight of the body, down through

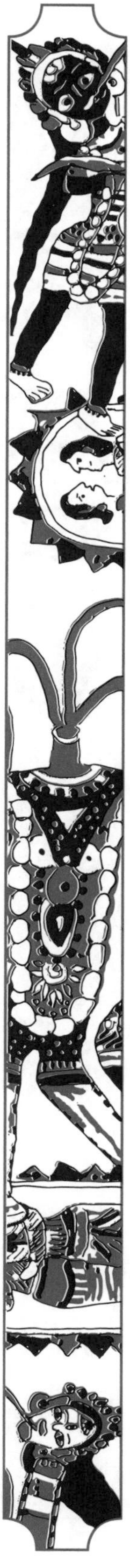

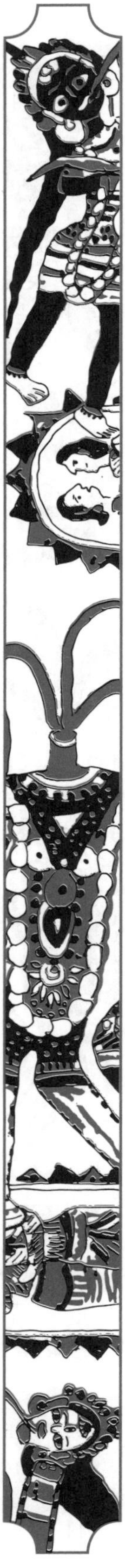

its points of contact with the floor, into the support of the floor beneath. Every exhalation is a letting-go, as if you could give away the whole weight of the body. Be with the gentle rhythm of the natural, easy breath. Allow the body to settle deeper into stillness with every outgoing breath. You are in the lap of the mother earth, let her carry your weight.

Now take a moment to observe the stillness and quietness of the body.

As the body comes into a state of deepening stillness, allow for the breath to become more spacious and free. Listen to the sound of the breath. Hear all the other sounds that are audible right now. Now let the focus rest with the intimate sound of the breath coming in and going out, the sound closest to you.

Feel the stillness of the body and the spaciousness of the breath. Know that your practice of *yoga nidrā* is held safely in a place of protection and security. Know that the boundaries of the practice are secure, and that as you enter into the state of consciousness which is *yoga nidrā*, you are held safely within this protected space. Invite now the mind to follow the example of the body and the breath, to become stiller and quieter. Invite the mind to create a single form of consciousness: Allow that form of awareness simply to be: 'I am practising *yoga nidrā*. I am practising *yoga nidrā*. I am practising *yoga nidrā*.' Let that be the form of consciousness for the rest of the practice of *yoga nidrā*.

And now allow the focus of the mind to accompany the breath.

On the next exhalation, breathe down as if the breath could enter into the space of the heart. Feel as if the heart herself is breathing. Evoke there in the heart a feeling of thankfulness, a sense of gladness simply for the opportunity to practise *yoga nidrā*. Feel this gladness as a gentle warmth that radiates from the heart. Breathe into this warmth and be thankful for the opportunity to practise *yoga nidrā*. As the mind enters the heart, hear the breath of the heart as if it were the voice of the heart's own wisdom. Listening to the breath of the heart, there are two ways to be with it. You can repeat your own *saṁkalpa*. If you have your own positive affirmation, a heart's prayer or resolve, then allow for the words of this affirmation to be repeated over three times, in the present tense as if it has already happened.

Alternatively, simply rest in receptive relationship to the heart's guidance. Be open now to whatever wisdom may come through to you on the breath of the heart. Welcome it. Know that the heart's prayer, or resolution, the *saṁkalpa* or the guidance of the heart is now like a seed that has been planted in the fertile soil of gladness and thankfulness. It is surely already growing and thriving, manifesting in your life.

And now take the attention back to the physical body, and prepare to guide the mind around the body, as if the light of the mind's attention comes to shine on each part of the body in turn. Whilst the mind travels freely, following the instructions, the physical body remains motionless, and takes deep rest.

Allow for the light of the mind's attention to take the form of bright little stars. As consciousness travels to each part of the body that is named, place a star on that part of the body, leaving it to twinkle there. It is as if the whole body begins as a dark night sky, and as the mind travels around it, bringing bright starlight to each part, the body is illuminated like a great constellation of stars in the sky.

Bring the awareness to the tip of the tongue and shine a bright star at that point. Then place twinkling stars on the floor of the mouth, the roof of the mouth, the upper teeth and gums, the lower teeth and gums, the inside of the right cheek, the inside of the left cheek. Move the awareness to the inner part of the right ear, and shine bright stars all the way through and around the ear, right through to the outer part of the right ear, the lobe of the ear, the shell of the right ear, the whole of the right ear. Move the awareness to the inner part of the left ear, and shine bright stars all the way through and around the ear, through to the outer part of the left ear, the lobe of the left ear, the shell of the left ear, the whole of the left ear. Feel both ears, twinkling with the starlight of conscious awareness.

Then shine a bright star on the back of the head, in the place between the two ears. Shine a bright star on the back of the top of the head, and have a star twinkling on the very top of the head: a bright star on the crown of the head. Then place a twinkling star at the right temple, left temple, and the forehead. A star on the right eye, and one on the left eye; stars at the right eyebrow, left eyebrow, eyebrow centre, the right cheek, left cheek, the nose. Shine a bright star on the right nostril, left nostril. Let there be a star at the bridge of the nose and a star at the tip of the nose. Move the awareness down to shine a star on the upper lip, lower lip, the chin, and all along the jaw line.

Be aware of the whole head, feel the whole head: twinkling with tiny stars, the light of conscious awareness. Move the awareness to the neck and the throat. Shine a star on the right collarbone, on the left collarbone, and one twinkling in the place between the two collarbones.

Then move the awareness to shine stars on the right shoulder and armpit; the right upper arm, elbow and forearm; right wrist, back of the right hand and palm of the right hand. Take the awareness to the right-hand thumb and shine a little star there, and one each twinkling on the index finger, middle finger, ring finger and little finger. Be aware of the whole of the right hand, twinkling with the starlight of conscious awareness.

Now carry the attention back up the right arm and across, over to the left side.

Shine stars on the left shoulder and armpit; the left upper arm, elbow and forearm; left wrist, back of the left hand and palm of the left hand. Take the awareness to the left-hand thumb and shine a little star there, and one each twinkling on the second finger, middle finger, ring finger, and little finger. Be aware of the whole of the left hand, twinkling with the starlight of conscious awareness.

Now carry the awareness to the centre of the chest. Place little stars twinkling now along the length of the breastbone, into the right side and ribs, left side and ribs. Shine a star in the middle of the right shoulder blade and the left shoulder blade, and a star twinkling in the space between the two shoulder blades. Stars in the back of the waist, and the right side of the waist, left side of the waist. Stars twinkling in the lower back, and on the right side of the pelvis and the left side of the pelvis. A star shining in the right buttock, and the left buttock. A bright star at the navel, and a star at the pubic bones.

Now take the attention to the right groin, and shine stars there, and on the top of the right thigh and back of the right thigh. A star twinkles at the kneecap, and in the back of the knee, calf, shin, ankle, heel. Shine stars along the sole of the right foot, the top of the right foot. Five little stars are twinkling, one each on the right big toe, second toe, third toe, fourth toe, fifth toe. The whole of the right foot and leg are twinkling with the starlight of conscious awareness.

Now take the attention to the left groin, and shine stars there, and on the top of the left thigh, back of the left thigh. A star twinkles at the kneecap, and in the back of the knee, calf, shin, ankle, heel. Shine stars along the sole of the left foot, the top of the left foot. Five little stars are twinkling, one each on the left big toe, second toe, third toe, fourth toe, fifth toe. The whole of the left foot and leg are twinkling with the starlight of conscious awareness.

Be aware now of the whole body, be aware of the whole body. Be aware of the stars twinkling now along the whole of the right side: foot and leg, arm and hand, the whole of the right side, twinkling with the light of conscious awareness. Be aware of the stars twinkling now along the whole of the left side: foot and leg, arm and hand, the whole of the left side. Both sides together.

Bring the light of the mind's attention to shine now inside the body, up into the womb or the womb space. Let the light here shine in the form of a little moon, a moon inside you.

See the light of the inner moon shining. See all the little stars twinkling now in the constellation of the whole body. Bring the light of the mental awareness to the whole of the right arm and hand. And now take the awareness to the whole of the left arm and hand. Now be aware of both arms and hands together. And now take the awareness to the whole of the right leg and foot. And now take the awareness to the whole of the left leg and foot. And now be aware of both legs and feet together. Be aware now of both arms and both legs together. See the starlight twinkling through the whole of the right side, the whole of the left side, both sides together. Be aware of starlight twinkling in the whole of the head, and the moonlight shining in the pelvis.

And now be aware of the whole body, like a constellation of tiny stars shining. Be aware of the whole of the body, like the night sky, twinkling with the lights of conscious awareness.

Feel the whole of the physical body resting on the floor. Remain alert and attentive to the practice; 'I am practising *yoga nidrā*'. Let that be the form of awareness. And now as the breath goes out, experience a sensation of extreme heaviness. Feel that the physical body is so heavy that the bones might settle right down into the earth, so heavy, so heavy. And as the breath comes in, experience a sensation of lightness, as if the body was so light that it might even float up, like a puff of smoke, moving up into the sky, so light, almost weightless.

As the breath moves, alternate between these two sensations: heaviness on the exhalation and lightness on the inhalation. Exhaling heavy, inhaling light. At a certain point now, stop alternating between the two extreme sensations, and invite both to be held simultaneously in the witness consciousness: be aware of heavy and light at the same time, together. And now let go of this practice, and simply become aware of the natural weight, shape and form of the physical body as it rests on the floor.

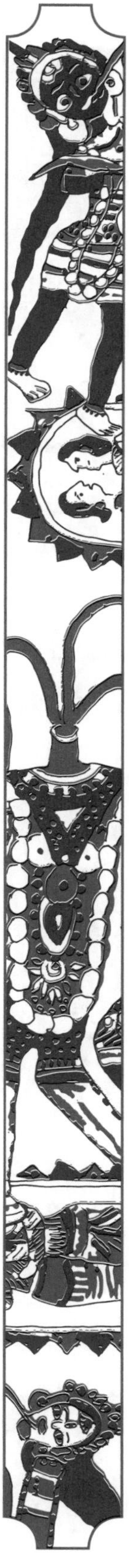

Feel the whole of the physical body resting on the floor. And now as the breath goes out, allow for the light of the mind's attention to focus entirely on a single point in the centre of the heart, like a little point of light is there. On the exhale, gather the attention further and further inwards to rest at this single point of focus, a tiny point of light in the centre of the heart. And as the breath comes in, experience a sensation of expansion, as if that tiny point of light were radiating outwards through the whole body and beyond. On the inhale, carry the light out into a expanding field of spacious awareness, radiating from the heart.

As the breath moves, alternate between these two experiences: inward gathering and focus on the exhalation and outward expansion and radiance on the inhalation. Exhaling into the single point in the heart, and inhaling outwards to expand the light. At a certain point now, stop alternating between these two extremes, and invite both to be held simultaneously in the witness consciousness: be aware of the single point and expanded awareness at the same time, together. And now let go of this practice, and simply become aware of the natural boundaries, shape and form of the physical body as it rests on the floor.

And then just notice the body breathing. Be aware of the breath entering and leaving. It is as if the body is being breathed. There is no effort involved. The breath is simply coming in and going out, as if the body and the breath were very old friends, and the breath simply lets itself in and out of the body with no formality, it just comes and goes. Be aware of the body being breathed. Let the focus of the mind's attention rest with each breath. Count these breaths, starting with the next exhale: let that be number nine, and then count on down to zero. If the count goes astray, it doesn't matter. Simply begin counting again. The point of the counting is to keep the mind attentive to each breath.

And now leave off the counting. *(* This is the place to insert any of the visualisations from the other sections if desired).*

Now direct the whole of the focus of mental attention back into the space of the heart on the next exhale. Hear the heart's breath and know that it carries the voice of the heart's guidance. Listen now to the guidance of the heart's wisdom or hear the words of your own *saṁkalpa*, your positive affirmation or resolve. Hear it repeated over three times, in the present tense as if it has already happened. Nurture the seed of the resolution that you planted at the beginning of the practice. Know that the *saṁkalpa* grows and flourishes now in your life. Feel how it is actually to inhabit the reality of this resolution. Experience the feeling of embodying the reality of the heart's guidance, of living the *saṁkalpa*. Now.

Remind yourself of the form of awareness that has been present throughout the practice: 'I have been practising *yoga nidrā*, I have been practising *yoga nidrā*, I have been practising *yoga nidrā*.' Know also that the practice of *yoga nidrā* has been held safely around you in a place of protection and security. Know that the protective nurturing that has held the boundaries of this practice of *yoga nidrā* continues to surround and protect you as you come towards the end of this practice of *yoga nidrā*. Be aware that the protection and the blessings of the practice of *yoga nidrā* come now out with you into your everyday life.

Once again direct the attention to the rise and fall of the natural breath. Allow the breaths to become a little deeper, a little noisier, so that you can hear the sound of your own breath entering and leaving your body. Listen to the sound of your own breath. Feel your body moving with each inhalation and exhalation. Sense now that each inhalation is a waking breath, bringing vitality and strength to the body. With each inhalation, feel the body returning to a waking state, full of energy and life. Be aware now that the body is refreshed, the mind is wide awake. Begin to make tiny movements. Touch the tip of each of your fingers in turn with the tip of the thumb. Stretch out the fingers and wriggle them. Wriggle the toes. Turn the wrists and the ankles. Stretch and release through the muscles of the arms. Stretch and release through the muscles of the legs. Turn your head gently and slowly to either side. Bring your head back to centre and take a long comfortable stretch through the whole body in whichever way pleases you most. Then roll over to the side and pause, resting and getting ready to sit up. Wide awake. Wide awake. Wide awake. The practice of *yoga nidrā* is now complete.

When you feel ready, slowly ease yourself into a sitting position, and open your eyes. *Hari Om Tat Sat*.

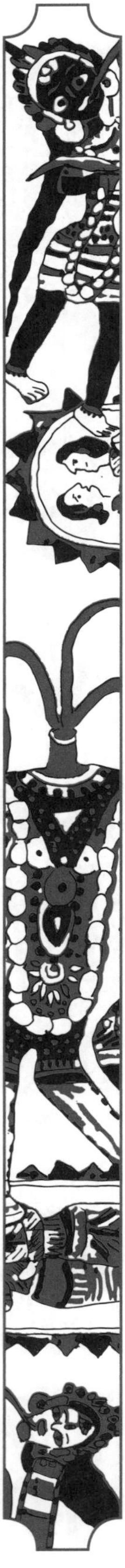

YOGA NIDRĀ 2: NEW BEGINNINGS

MENARCHE, INNOCENCE, TRUST AND POWER (ṢOḌASĪ)

*At the point marked * in the first* yoga nidrā *(p.440), the following visualisation may be used:*

Look into the space in front of the closed eyes. This is the mind-sky. Right now it is night. See into a darkness so deep that it seems to extend for ever. The inner gaze rests quiet because this darkness is so profound that there is nothing to be seen – until a tiny point of red in the distance draws your gaze. The point becomes a sliver, and the rosy light brightens. It grows. More red light emerges from the darkness. Its radiance fills the whole sky. A new day is dawning. You behold the arrival of the morning with wonder and delight.

The point of light grows and slides higher into the mind-sky, spreading a warm and gentle glow right across the mind-sky. It shines on your hands. You hold the tips of the fingers together and the two palms facing inwards, gently cupped around something very precious and new. The tender presence within your hands is radiant with the pink dawning light.

Expectantly, you look into your hands, and slowly open the palms. In the cup of your two hands lies a magical red rosebud. The morning light shines upon it. Soft warmth emanates from its centre. Almost imperceptibly the closely furled petals begin to uncurl. You sit to honour this miracle of awakening in your hands. The rosebud is beginning to flower in the dawn. Time moves differently now.

You gaze into the opening bud with a tender wonder and warmth. As the scene fades from view, this feeling of wonder settles softly into your heart, and you sense the opening energies of new beginnings within.

*Now return to complete the remainder of the practice that follows from point * (p.440).*

YOGA NIDRĀ 3: CYCLICAL WISDOM UNFOLDING

MENSTRUATION, CYCLES AND SEASONAL TURNINGS (TĀRĀ)

*At the point marked * in the first* yoga nidrā *(p.440), the following visualisation may be used:*

NB Your own experiences of the qualities of feeling associated with each of the menstrual seasons may not be fully reflected in this suggested sensory visualisation. If the suggested experiences do not resonate with you, then edit or create your own seasonal encounters in the cycle of the womb world.

Look into the space in front of the closed eyes. Exhale and bring the focus of your attention down to the space of the womb: *yonisthāna*. Breathe your inner gaze down inside the womb and find yourself at the heart of a warm red space. See yourself lying there, inside your own womb, comfortable and perfectly at home.

As you lay there in your womb, feel her to be an entire world in herself. Feel a soft breeze blowing across your skin and look up to see the branches of a beautiful tree above you. You are lying beneath a great womb tree, and her roots reach deep down into the earth. She is growing in the very centre of the wombworld.

You can see blue sky bright behind her branches and it is spring. Tiny baby leaves are curled up tight on the branches and as the sun shines they begin to unfurl. The quality of feeling is fresh and expectant, as if the air itself is full of the possibilities of new beginnings. You feel excitement and wonder at all the newness around you. A sudden little shower of raindrops falls, and the water kisses your face with a gentle, sweet tenderness. More tiny droplets of rain now fall to the ground as the leaves open out in the warming air.

It is high summer in the womb world. The tree is decked in the finery of full green leaves and beginning to be heavy with fruit. Beneath the tree, the heat of the season warms you deep inside and you feel full of life, overflowing with love and ready to give. You stand to stretch and move with a conscious delight, suffused by the power of simply being so vibrantly alive, strong and full of abundant energy. You watch the branches of the tree bending under the weight of the ripening fruit. Everything feels abundant and all is possible.

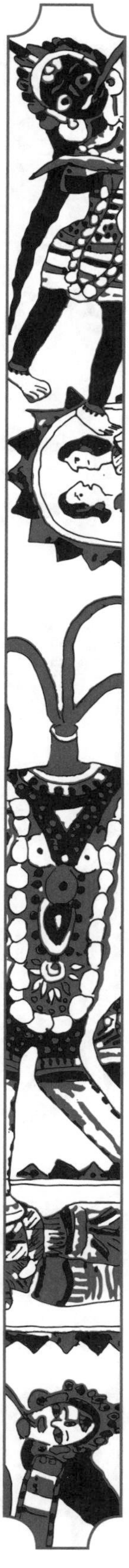

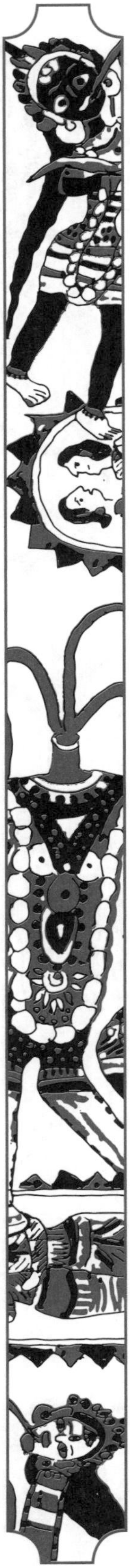

It is autumn, and the fruits on the tree are ready for harvest. In the magical womb world, the fruits harvest themselves, rolling softly to the ground. The leaves in the tree begin to change colour, curling into fiery twists of orange and red. The wind grows cooler and leaves begin to fall to the ground. You begin to feel the need to tidy and sweep: after the growing seasons, it feels as though the garden needs tending, and you begin clearing the fruits and fallen leaves that have accumulated, sorting and reflecting, preparing for the resting time of the coming cold.

It is winter in your womb world, and you are sheltered warm inside by roaring fire. There is nothing to be done. You respond to the need to rest deeply. In this state of stillness you experience a state of gracious peace, as if you had been washed out to float on a river of blood. With a visionary clarity you enter deep inside your own awareness, and experience a powerful energy of descent. The blood tide inside is pulling you home to yourself. The womb world is cleansed by the red river flow, as if it were washing through you. When the last wave passes, you feel quietly renewed and revisioned. In your hand you hold a golden chalice that contains blood: your flow. You walk to the great tree in the heart of the womb world. Kneeling reverently, you pour the blood down into her roots, to nourish future growth.

The blood is received back into the earth, and you sense the beginning of a slight shift in your energies and interests as the seasons in the womb world begin to turn. You greet the coming cycle with the deep wisdom of a woman who respects the special qualities of each season, and responds to the changes each brings as it turns in the womb world of your inner life.

*Now return to complete the remainder of the practice that follows from point * (p.440).*

YOGA NIDRĀ 4: IN THE WILD GARDEN, JOYOUS FREEDOM TO FLOW

SEXUALITY, CREATIVITY AND JUICE (KAMALĀTMIKĀ AND MATAṄGI)

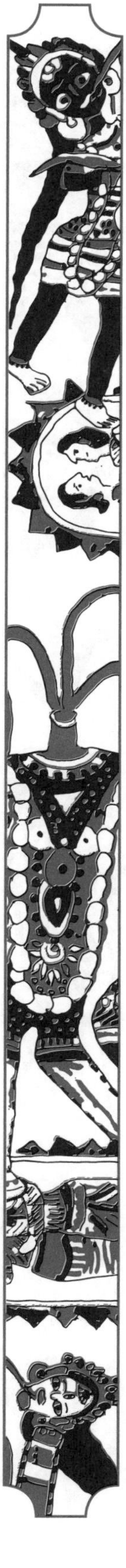

*At the point marked * in the first* yoga nidrā *(p.440), the following visualisation may be used:*

Look into the space in front of the closed eyes. Exhale the focus of awareness far out into the mind's sky. And then, from the magical perspective of your internal heavenly heights, look back to see yourself lying here, practising *yoga nidrā*. See your body from the outside, looking down from above. See yourself. Then let the awareness shift so you can look up from beneath your body, seeing it from underneath. See yourself. Then shift the perspective so you are poised by your feet, and look up through your body from the soles of your feet. See yourself. Take a look at yourself from the right side. See yourself. And take a look at yourself from the left side. See yourself. And then, seated close by the crown of the head, look down at yourself as if you could see through from the crown of the head all the way down to the soles of the feet. See yourself.

Return to the viewpoint that you had at the start: looking down from on high. And see now that this body is resting in the most luscious and abundant garden. It seems to have no limits. There are flowers and fruits and birds and gorgeous plants and trees. The colours are extraordinarily vivid. The garden smells fresh, wild and spicy. There is the sound of running water and beautiful birdsong. Everything is warm and enticing: the ripe fruits on the trees are dripping with juice, the blooms of the flowers are so bright they seem to be on fire, and every plant and creature in the garden is overflowing with life and energy. Even the light is alive here. As you watch yourself lying there, the outward shape and form of the physical body becomes transparent and translucent. Everything that is outside in the garden is inside this body. The body contains the abundance of the garden. You watch and know: I am the garden. I feel it within me, vivid and alive and utterly entrancing. Stay in the garden as long as you like.

And when you are ready to leave the garden, exhaling now, the focus of mental attention comes to rest back in the space of your heart. The breath grows deeper and louder. As you begin

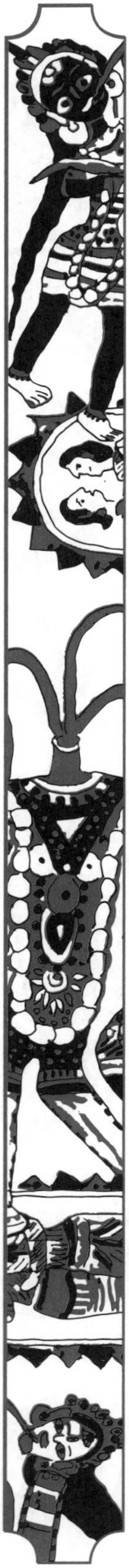

to reconnect your perceptions to the world within your physical body, the breath of the heart is whispering softly to you, 'How wild is your garden?' and every cell of your whole being sings out in response: 'I am the garden. I am the garden that is wild and free in its beauty. I am the garden that is abundantly juicy and creative.'

*Now return to complete the remainder of the practice that follows from point * (p.440).*

YOGA NIDRĀ 5: NOURISHING GROWTH

NURTURING THE CAPACITY TO SUPPORT NEW LIFE (BHUVANEŚVARĪ)

*At the point marked * in the first* yoga nidrā *(p.440), the following visualisation may be used:*

Now take the attention within. Be aware of the round, nurturing swell of the belly, and feel the thriving new life which is growing inside. With the clarity of the mind's eye, see the shape and form of your little baby resting within the womb. See the baby in an optimal fetal position, with his or her head down, their bottom pointing upwards into the top of the womb and their spine curved outwards into the curve of the mother's belly. See the curled body of the baby as he or she floats inside the safety of the womb, and guide the attention now around this tiny body. Know that as the attention moves to each part of the baby in turn, it is as if every part of the little body is being caressed. Allow the movement of mental attention around the baby's body to send a loving, gentle mother's touch to each part of the new being growing inside the womb.

Begin by sending the attention now to the baby's right hand where you see the thumb and four perfect little fingers. See the left-hand thumb and four perfect little fingers. See the baby's arms wrapped around their body, giving himself or herself a hug. Now carry the loving gaze of mental attention down to the baby's feet. See five perfect little toes on the right foot, and five perfect little toes on the left foot. See the baby with his or her knees bent, curled up inside the womb. Trace the loving awareness of the mind's attention to the baby's bottom, pointing upwards into the top of the womb, and let the attention stroke down from the buttocks to the base of the spine and all the way along the whole of the length of the baby's spine, curving out into the curve of the mother's belly, up to the back of the baby's neck. See the baby with the chin tucked in and the head well down, beautifully relaxed and optimally positioned for an easeful arrival in the world when his time is ready.

And last of all bring the attention to the baby's face. See the baby's face peaceful and smiling sweetly. There is a contented smile on the face of the unborn child. Seeing that smile makes you smile too. As you smile, the attention moves away from the image of the baby and back into your heart. As the image of the child fades from view, allow for the quality of feeling in that contented smile to remain in your heart. Feel the sweet and peaceful smile of the baby warming your heart. Take the attention to the breath. Know that the mother's breath is the link between mother and child. Feel the very gentle movements of the body that accompany every breath in and every breath out. Observe the subtle rhythm of the easy natural breath. Be aware now that this continuous rhythm is comforting the baby within the womb, as they gently rock to and fro, in time with every breath in and every breath out.

Be aware of breathing for two, of how the mother's breath is the baby's breath. Be aware now that every inhalation is a nourishing breath, bringing life-giving strength to the baby growing within the womb. Be aware now that every exhalation is a softening, releasing breath, allowing the baby to relax in readiness to receive the nourishment of each inhalation. Know that the very rhythm of this natural breath is the living assurance of the baby's nourishment and life within the warmth and safety of the womb.

Feel how the easy rhythm of the life-giving mother's breath forms a direct link with the well-being of the baby within the womb, a powerful link between mother and baby. Moment by moment, breath by breath, every inhalation and exhalation comforts the baby. The rhythm of the breath creates a gentle rhythm in the amniotic fluid, the ocean within the womb. Be aware that every part of the baby's body is bathed in the nourishing ocean of breath. Sense that the gentle rhythm of your breath is nourishing and comforting the baby. See now, in your mind's eye, that as the baby floats in a private ocean of warmth and love within the womb, so you too are completely supported by the gently lapping waters upon which you float effortlessly. Feel that these waters are moving in time with your own breath, cradling you and rocking you gently back and forth, just as your own breath rocks the baby within the womb. Be with the natural rhythm of your own easy breath, and know that both you and the baby are being comforted and nourished with every single breath in and every single breath out. Know that this rhythm is continuous and universal, the rhythm of life and growth.

*Now return to complete the remainder of the practice that follows from point * (p.440).*

YOGA NIDRĀ 6: THANKSGIVING AND GRIEVING

POSTNATAL RECOVERY, TRANSFORMATION AND ADAPTATION (CHINNAMASTĀ)

*At the point marked * in the first yoga nidrā (p.440), the following visualisation may be used:*

Look into the space now in front of the closed eyes. Looking into that space, as if you were looking down from above, see yourself lying here now practising *yoga nidrā*. As you look down at yourself resting, observe with kindness the woman you are now. See everything about you, how tired you are, and how you feel, what you are wearing and how you are lying. Shine upon yourself the full light of the attentive observation of the mind's eye. As you observe, let there be compassion in the mind's eye, to acknowledge who you are right now.

And see yourself now, as if watching a film playing backwards, making your way back through the hours that have preceded this moment. As you recollect the activities of the previous hours, then watch yourself moving backwards farther into your past. See the woman you were yesterday. Then see the woman you were last year. And then see with clarity the woman you were the year before that. Observe with kindness the woman you were then. Observe the woman you were before everything in your life changed. Carry your awareness back as far as you choose, pausing at each point in your life to acknowledge with kindness the woman you were at that time. Welcome her and greet her from the warmth of your heart. Let your mind's eye carry kindness to her.

And then, when you have carried your awareness back as far as you want to go, pause. Observe that woman you were then. Notice everything about her: what she wears, how she stands, what she does for fun. And know that woman is in the past. With warmth and compassion, turn to face her. As you prepare to say goodbye to her, she smiles and holds out to you a gift saying: 'Carry this with you. It is precious.' You receive the gift, and as you walk away you hold it close to your heart. See yourself walking into the future that is the present moment.

As you watch yourself walking towards the woman you are now, pause as often as you need. Greet the changes that have come to you, meet all the women you have been. Honour each one with the kindness of observation and understanding. Close to your heart through this journey, carry with you the precious gift you were given by the woman you once were.

Finally you arrive at the present moment and once again see yourself lying here, practising *yoga nidrā*. Gently approach yourself and place the gift from the past on your heart. It is a magical gift. The moment it arrives in the here and now, in the present moment, the outer package disappears. What remains is a powerful feeling in your heart, a sensation of warmth and tenderness, as your whole being is suffused with the potent essence of all that you loved most about who you once were. You feel spacious and free. Everything that truly matters about the essence of your true nature is here now. The gift from the woman that you once were is the gift of freedom to be who you are now. You inhabit the present moment completely, and give thanks for it with a consciousness of who you are able to be at this point in your life.

*Now return to complete the remainder of the practice that follows from point * (p.440).*

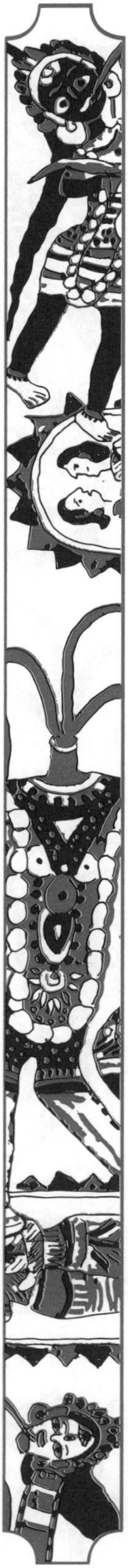

YOGA NIDRĀ 7: BEING WITH NOT KNOWING

PERIMENOPAUSE AND THE INEVITABILITY OF CHANGE; BECOMING THE SEED AT THE HEART OF THE FRUIT (BAGALĀMUKHĪ)

*At the point marked * in the first* yoga nidrā *(p.440), the following visualisation may be used:*

See your body resting in the shape of the Open flower pose (soles of feet together, knees out to the sides and supported over a bolster). Send consciousness into the womb.

Find that you literally are lying in the centre of a dark red soft place. It is fragrant. You are a tiny seed in the middle of a huge cosmic rose. It is huge, its scent is heavenly, and its petals are protecting you, as if you are lying in the centre of a circular palace whose walls are made from the living petals of the rose. The touch of the petals on your skin is soft like silk. Gently, as if blown away by a warm breeze, each petal of the rose separates from the stem, floats away on the breeze and disappears. Watch as slowly, one petal after another does this. It takes a long time before you realise what is happening because the rose is so luscious and with so many petals that the outer ones have long since gone before you become aware that they are falling away. See yourself like a tiny seed-child-woman resting with open eyes in the centre of this womb rose chamber, and become aware, as the outer petals fall away, that eventually they will all be gone and the red rose room will disappear.

The quality of feeling is perfectly serene, utterly beautiful and faintly curious. Watch the petals blow away and begin now to marvel at the beauty of each one. Give each one your full focus of attention as they detach from the central stem and float away.

Soon there are only a few remaining. And now the real beauty of the vision intensifies: become aware that a gorgeous golden light is bathing you – before it has been shining through the red petalled walls but now it is direct and strong. It shines on you as you rest in the centre of the rose room that is now an open platform totally bathed in this powerful light. As the last petal blows away, realise that you have magically become entirely naked, lying in open view in the golden light. It illuminates you and as it does so it awakens within you a radiant light that shines from within your heart.

Rest in the illumined nature of the menopausal woman – naked, clearly your own self, and radiant at the centre of the rose like the seed that remains to carry the essence of the flower itself when the rose has finished blooming. Let yourself receive the kindness of your gaze. Feel that you have become the seed in the heart of the flower: seeding vision and wisdom to grow the next generation. Have a sense of real connection to this powerful image – tender and very potent.

*Now return to complete the remainder of the practice that follows from point * (p.440).*

Complete the exit process for the practice of *yoga nidrā* and then carry the blessings and wisdom of the vision of yourself at the centre of the rose out into your daily life, where it continues to nourish and reassure your spirit.

YOGA NIDRĀ 8: SELF-ANOINTING RITUAL

EMBRACING POWER, MENOPAUSE AND THE CONFIDENCE TO SPEAK ONE'S OWN TRUTH; EMPOWERED BY NATURE TO BE YOUR TRUE SELF (BHAIRAVĪ)

*At the point marked * in the first* yoga nidrā *(p.440), the following visualisation may be used:*

Now bring the full attention into the space in front of the closed eyes. Look into that space where dreams appear at night and see yourself walking through a beautiful forest on a warm spring afternoon. Trees grow tall around you and the sunlight warms your face. You are carrying a small bag and a warm blanket. You arrive on the banks of a fast-flowing stream. You place the folded blanket on the soft bed of dry leaves and when you sit down on it you instantly feel absolutely comfortable and at peace. The folds of the blanket wrap around you, and you feel warm and protected. Across the stream, flowers are growing, blooms of blue and white and yellow. The only sound is the running water and the birds singing in the trees. It is a sacred peaceful space. It smells fresh and alive.

You open the bag you have been carrying and take out the precious objects within: the bag contains everything you need. There is a bright red cord, which you lay around you in the form of a circle, securing the boundaries of your circular space. There are flower

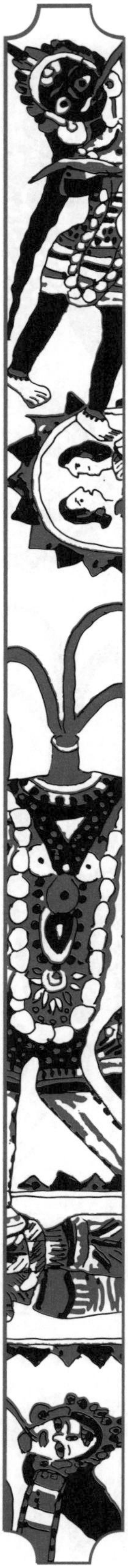

garlands which you lay on the earth in front of you, and there is a small red candle in a golden bowl whose sides are pierced with little heart-shaped cut-outs. When you light the candle with the matches that you find in the bag, the flame of the candle glows bright and its light shines out through the hearts in the sides of the bowl.

As you light your candle you feel that you have begun a ritual process of great beauty and power. The light shines on you. You sit comfortably on the warm blanket and hear the sound of the running water by your side. You take the flower garlands and place them around your neck, smelling the fresh smell of the blooms. Their fragrance is exquisite. You reach out your hand to touch your fingertips in the running water of the stream and lift them up to your head. Drops of water touch the crown of your head. You feel yourself anointed.

You are at one with the stream and the trees, flowers and creatures of the forest. The mother of the forest embraces you, the water from the stream anoints you and you hear the words from your heart: I feel myself anointed by the whole of nature, I honour my own power and wisdom. I am fully myself. I fully inhabit the world in my power. I am ready for this next phase of life: I am met and honoured.

Knowing that the ritual is complete, experience the quality of feeling that it creates. Savour the sense of peaceful welcome that the whole forest extends to you, and know that you are at home in the world: your own true self. You are free to be simply part of the living pulse of the planet: a woman who embraces her own power to live her truth. The ritual has affirmed this. Have a sense of real connection to this powerful image – tender and very potent.

*Now return to complete the remainder of the practice that follows from point * (p.440).*

YOGA NIDRĀ 9: OUT OF THE SMOKE

TOUCHING POWER CLOSE TO THE BONE (DHŪMAVATĪ)

*At the point marked * in the first* yoga nidrā *(p.440), the following visualisation may be used:*

Now bring the full attention into the space in front of the closed eyes. Look into that space where dreams appear at night and see a vast cloud of dark smoke. It is dark, thick and swirling. So big you cannot see the edges of the cloud. The smell and feel of the smoke in your nose is powerful and pungent. As you look deeper and deeper into the smoke, your eyes water. You blink and see glimpses of a figure in the darkest part of the cloud. She is an old woman. She sits in the middle of the darkest heart of the cloud, absolutely still.

She sits alone, really deeply depressed: cold, sick and tired, gnawed by hunger, parched by thirst, racked by pain, and experiencing the deepest levels of suffering and grief. She is you, in the depths of your deepest challenges.

In the midst of the smoke, the you that is she is sitting and waiting for it all to pass. She embodies everything there is to be learnt from suffering, loss and despair. This is a strong wisdom, born of experience of events which have shaped and scarred her. Old and alone, this crone you see in yourself is pared back to the very bone and close to death, but she is powerful. The you that is she calls upon the deepest inner resources simply to survive. And she still sits. She faces death and her wisdom is power.

The smoke clears, and light shines. The brightness illuminates the scene as it fades. The quality of feeling remains: a deep sense of inner resilience, a power that is close to the bone. This strong wisdom, this feeling of resilience and inner power, this feeling travels with you as the scene disappears.

*Now return to complete the remainder of the practice that follows from point * (p.440).*

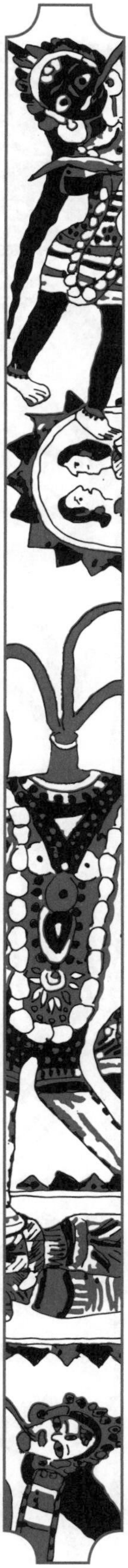

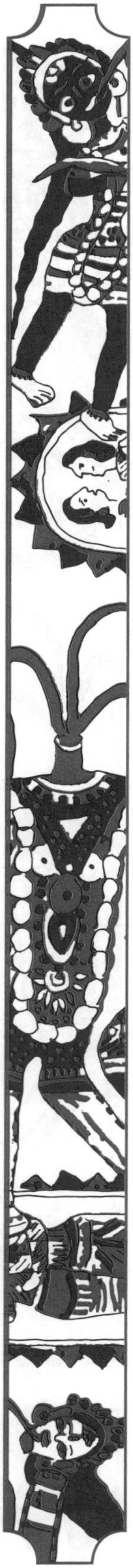

YOGA NIDRĀ 10: IN THE *YOGINĪS'* TEMPLE

RESTING AND HEALING TO LIVE IN WISDOM AND POWER: FULL CONSTELLATION OF *YOGINĪS*

Welcome to the practice of *yoga nidrā*. Welcome home. The first part of the practice is to get comfortable. Lie down on your back (or side, if you are pregnant, or if you prefer lying on your side). Take time to arrange your body so that you feel that you are well supported. Place cushions and pillows under your head and wherever else suits you so that you can feel absolutely at ease. Having support underneath the knees can really help to let the lower back settle well. Bear in mind that body temperature may drop during the practice, so if you feel the need, cover yourself with a blanket, or put on socks or a sweater to keep warm.

When you feel you are able to rest comfortably, settle into your chosen position and allow the body to become still, knowing that there is no need for any further physical movement during this practice. Experience the state of zero desire for movement. If that state is not present, then make whatever adjustments are necessary so that you feel super comfortable. The ideal state for the physical body during *yoga nidrā* is zero desire for movement. If the desire to move does arise during the practice, simply watch it. It will probably go away and you can remain still. If the desire to move returns then that may be a signal that you do actually need to move, so do so with awareness, and with the intention to regain comfort and stillness, returning to the state of zero desire for movement.

Now become aware very precisely of the position in which you are lying. Know the shape and the posture of the body; know the shape and arrangement of the room. Feel the points of contact between the side or the back of the body and the floor.

Be aware now of the gentle rhythm of the natural breath. Feel the breath coming in and the breath going out. If the breath moves freely and easily through the nostrils, breathe that way. If it is more comfortable to exhale through the mouth, then do that. Let whichever is the most comfortable and easy way of breathing arise naturally.

Allow the outgoing breath to release the weight of the body down into the support of the earth beneath. With every exhalation now, consciously transfer the weight of the body, down through its points of contact with the floor, into the support of the floor beneath. Every exhalation is a letting-go, as if you could give away the whole weight of the body. Be with the gentle rhythm of the natural, easy breath. Allow the body to settle deeper into stillness with every outgoing breath. You are in the lap of the mother earth, let her carry your weight.

Now take a moment to observe the stillness and quietness of the body.

As the body comes into a state of deepening stillness, allow the breath to become more spacious and free. Listen to the sound of the breath. Hear all the other sounds that are audible right now. Now let the focus rest with the intimate sound of the breath coming in and going out, the sound closest to you.

Feel the stillness of the body and the spaciousness of the breath. Know that your practice of *yoga nidrā* is held safely in a place of protection and security. Know that the boundaries of the practice are secure, and that as you enter into the state of consciousness which is *yoga nidrā*, you are held safely within this protected space. Invite now the mind to follow the example of the body and the breath to become stiller and quieter. Invite the mind to create a single form of consciousness: Allow that form of awareness simply to be: 'I am practising *yoga nidrā*. I am practising *yoga nidrā*. I am practising *yoga nidrā*.' Let that be the form of consciousness for the rest of the practice of *yoga nidrā*.

And now allow the focus of the mind to accompany the breath:

On the next exhalation, breathe down as if the breath could enter into the space of the heart. Feel as if the heart herself is breathing. Evoke there in the heart a feeling of thankfulness, a sense of gladness simply for the opportunity to practise *yoga nidrā*. Feel this gladness as a gentle warmth that radiates from the heart. Breath into this warmth and be thankful for the opportunity to practise *yoga nidrā*. As the mind enters the heart, hear the breath of the heart as if it were the voice of the heart's own wisdom. Listening to the breath of the heart, there are two ways to be with it. You can repeat your own *saṁkalpa*. If you have your own positive affirmation, a heart's prayer or resolve, then allow this affirmation to be repeated over three times, in the present tense as if it has already happened.

Alternatively, simply rest in receptive relationship to the heart's guidance. Be open now to whatever wisdom may come through to you on the breath of the heart. Welcome it. Know that the

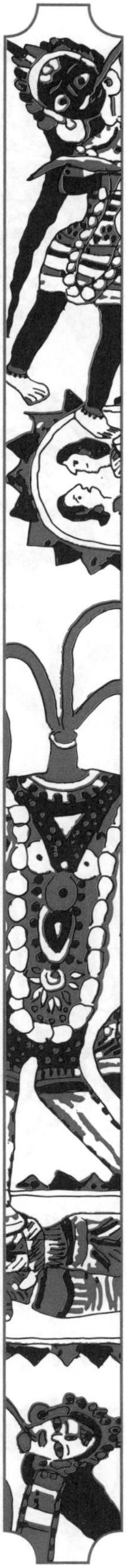

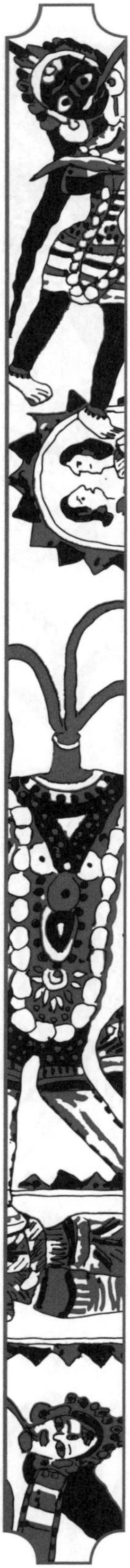

heart's prayer, or resolution, the *saṁkalpa* or the guidance of the heart, is now like a seed that has been planted in the fertile soil of gladness and thankfulness. It is surely already growing and thriving, manifesting in your life.

And now take the attention back to the physical body, and prepare to guide the mind around the body, as if the light of the mind's attention comes to shine on each part of the body in turn. Whilst the mind travels freely, following the instructions, the physical body remains motionless, and takes deep rest.

Allow for the light of the mind's attention to take the form of bright little stars. As consciousness travels to each part of the body that is named, place a star on that part of the body, leaving it to twinkle there. It is as if the whole body begins as a dark night sky, and as the mind travels around it, bringing bright starlight to each part, the body is illuminated like a great constellation of stars in the sky.

Place a bright star to shine at each of these points in turn:

crown of the head
eyebrow centre
throat
right shoulder
right elbow
right wrist
right thumb
index finger
middle finger
ring finger
little finger
inside right wrist
inside right elbow
inside right shoulder
throat
left shoulder
left elbow
left wrist
left thumb
index finger
middle finger
ring finger
little finger
inside left wrist
inside left elbow
front left shoulder
throat
centre of breastbone
left breast
centre of breastbone
right breast
centre of breastbone
navel
pubic bone
right hip bone
right knee
right ankle
right big toe
second toe
third toe
fourth toe
fifth toe
inside right ankle
inside right knee
inside right hip
pubic bone
left hip
left knee
left ankle
left big toe
second toe
third toe
fourth toe
fifth toe
inside left ankle
inside left knee
inside left hip
pubic bone
navel
centre of breastbo
throat
eyebrow centre
crown of the head

Be aware of the whole body.

Be aware now of the whole body, be aware of the whole body. Be aware of the stars twinkling now along the whole of the right side: foot and leg, arm and hand, the whole of the right side, twinkling with the light of conscious awareness. Be aware of the stars twinkling now along the whole of the left side: foot and leg, arm and hand, the whole of the left side. Bring the light of the mind's attention to shine now inside the body, up into the womb or the womb space. Let the light here shine in the form of a little moon, a moon inside you.

See the light of the inner moon shining. See all the little stars twinkling now in the constellation of the whole body.

Feel the whole of the physical body resting on the floor. Remain alert and attentive to the practice; 'I am practising *yoga nidrā*'. Let that be the form of awareness. And now as the breath goes out, experience a sensation of extreme heaviness. Feel that the physical body is so heavy that the bones might settle right down into the earth, so heavy, so heavy. And as the breath comes in, experience a sensation of lightness, as if the body was so light that it might even float up, like a puff of smoke, moving up into the sky, so light, almost weightless.

As the breath moves, alternate between these two sensations: heaviness on the exhalation and lightness on the inhalation. Exhaling heavy, inhaling light. At a certain point now, stop alternating between the two extreme sensations, and invite both to be held simultaneously in the witness consciousness: be aware of heavy and light at the same time, together. And now let go of this practice, and simply become aware of the natural weight, shape and form of the physical body as it rests on the floor.

Feel the whole of the physical body resting on the floor. And now as the breath goes out, allow for the light of the mind's attention to focus entirely on a single point in the centre of the heart, like a little point of light is shining there. On the exhale, gather the attention further and further inwards to rest at this single point of focus, a tiny point of light in the centre of the heart. And as the breath comes in, experience a sensation of expansion, as if that tiny point of light were radiating outwards through the whole body and beyond. On the inhale, carry the light out into a expanding field of spacious awareness, radiating from the heart.

As the breath moves, alternate between these two experiences: inward gathering and focus on the exhalation and outward

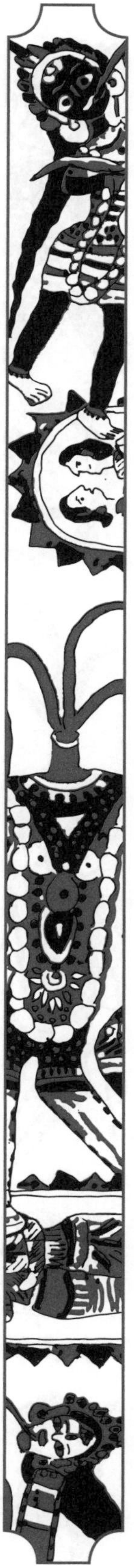

expansion and radiance on the inhalation. Exhaling into the single point in the heart, and inhaling outwards to expand the light. At a certain point now, stop alternating between these two extremes, and invite both to be held simultaneously in the witness consciousness: be aware of the single point and expanded awareness at the same time, together.

And now let go of this practice, and simply become aware of the natural boundaries, shape and form of the physical body as it rests on the floor.

And now just notice the body breathing. Be aware of the breath entering and leaving. It is as if the body is being breathed. There is no effort involved. The breath is simply coming in and going out, as if the body and the breath were very old friends, and the breath simply lets itself in and out of the body with no formality, it just comes and goes. Be aware of the body being breathed. Let the focus of the mind's attention rest with each breath. Count these breaths, starting with the next exhale: let that be number nine, and then count on down to zero. If the count goes astray, it doesn't matter. Simply begin counting again. The point of the counting is to keep the mind attentive to each breath.

And now leave off the counting.

Now bring the focus of attention to the space in front of the closed eyes, the space where the dreams appear at night. Looking into that space, there see a dark night sky, with stars twinkling. See a big silvery moon shining among the stars. And as if from the vantage point of that moon, look back down at the earth and see yourself lying here, practising *yoga nidrā*. And now, looking again, with such clarity of vision that everything on earth is visible in detail, see that you are in fact resting in a very special place, a place where you feel completely at home. Look down and see that you are resting on the warm earth on a balmy night in a beautiful circular stone temple. It is a healing temple, and you feel that you are completely at peace and relaxed in this place. It has no roof, and the light of the moon shines right down into the middle of the temple.

Set in the stone walls all around the circle are carved images of goddesses, and resting all around the temple are many other women. You are dreaming together, all of you women, at home in your beautiful temple. You are resting on the earth with your heads pointing into the centre of the temple and the moonlight is shining down on you, bathing you in its healing light. You are at home, at peace and in a place of deep healing and power. You are in the temple of the *yoginīs* and you are welcome there. You are one amongst many. You and the other women rest in your power in the temple under the twinkling stars in the moonlight.

As the moonlight grows brighter and clearer, the scene fades from view, so that all that remains to be seen is the light of the moon and the stars shining in the night sky. Deep in your heart there remains a potent quality of feeling: a sure sense of homecoming, a feeling of being healed and empowered. You know that feeling will remain with you to nourish you, and that you are always welcome to visit the healing temple of the *yoginīs*.

*Now return to complete the remainder of the practice that follows from point * (p.440).*

FURTHER READING AND RESOURCES

For a comprehensive and systematic support of your own experiences of *yoga nidrā*, the workbook *Total Yoga Nidrā* is invaluable. It provides helpful exercises and suggestions on how to get the most from *yoga nidrā*, including explicit guidance about developing your own creative responses to *yoga nidrā*, and strategies for accessing the deep well-spring of limitlessly abundant *nidrā* practices that support your own needs and interests. There is also a selection of complete scripts, and a fascinating survey of responses to the practice from long-term practitioners. It also sets out the practical, historical and philosophical background of the practice, and compares the frameworks of a number of different approaches to *yoga nidrā*. This workbook was originally developed as a resource for students on the Learn to Teach *Yoga Nidrā* course and will soon be available to a wider readership. It is the ideal companion to the practice and sharing of *yoga nidrā*. For details of the book, training courses and for free *yoga nidrā* downloads in a variety of languages, visit **www.yoganidranetwork.org**

There are many traditional *yoga nidrā* recordings available. Amongst the most reliable and effective are those created by experienced practitioners and teachers such as **Swami Pragyamurti Saraswati** in the UK:
www.syclondon.com/wp/swami-pragyamurti-saraswati
and available from **www.yogamatters.com**; and **Richard Miller** in the US: **www.irest.us** and at **www.soundstrue.com**

Rod Stryker's recordings are also helpful resources: **www.parayoga.com/**

Practising *yoga nidrā* is more beneficial than reading about it, but helpful books on the subject are **Swami Satyananda Saraswati**. 1984. *Yoga Nidrā* , Bihar School of Yoga, Munger, Bihar; and **Miller, Richard**. 2005, *Yoga Nidrā: The Meditative Heart of Yoga*, Sounds True, Colorado.

Useful articles that explore the effects of yoga nidrā include **Kelly McGonigal**, 'Inspired Intention: the nature of Saṁkalpa', in *Yoga International* (Winter 2010-11) pp.44–49. and **Swami Jnaneshwara Bharati**: 'Yogic Conscious Deep Sleep' available at **www.swamij.com/yoga-nidrā.htm.** These articles are available to download from **www.yoganidranetwork.org.**

CHAPTER NINETEEN

intimacy: mind and breath

MEDITATION: WELCOMING INNER SILENCE, CONNECTING WITH THE INNER TEACHER (*ANTAR MOUNA*)

The basis for this calming and nurturing breath and sensory awareness practice is a meditation from the *tantras* called inner silence (*antar mouna*). Usually it is taught very formally, as a sequential progression of directed awareness leading to deeper enquiry and mental focus. Below I offer a more fluid and informal approach that builds an evolving connection between the senses and the elements, and places the whole meditation in relation to the inner teacher of the heart.

1. Sit or lie comfortably. Slowly establish full yogic breath (pp.131–2) or *ujjāyī* (pp.134–5). If it feels right, close the eyes. If not, let them relax, cast down.
2. Rest the palms of both hands, one on top of the other, over the heart space in the centre of the chest. Palms flat and fingers relaxed. Breathe awareness down to direct focus of mental attention into that place. Breathe into the protective warmth and weight of the hands. Invite an experience of gladness into the heart. Be thankful for the people, creatures or circumstances that are making it possible for you to sit right now and do this practice. Breathe into that feeling as if the heart is breathing. Honour the presence of the inner teacher with the words (silent or voiced): *With great respect and love, I honour my heart, my inner teacher.*
3. Rest the hands down in the lap in *bhairavī mudrā* (hands palms up, back of the left hand supported by the palm of the right hand and two thumb tips touching), or in any of the other hand gestures that feels appropriate to you right now.
4. As breath comes in and out through the nose, be aware of the rhythmic cycle of breath. Allow this natural flow of breath to continue easily as you shift the focus of mental attention from one sense to the next.
5. First bring full attention to the sense of hearing. Exhale awareness into the sense of hearing and be aware of sounds around you. Notice sounds furthest away from you. Then notice sounds closest to you. Draw attention closer until you are just focusing on the sound of your own breath as it moves in and out. Listen to this intimate sound. Let each sound be heard. Give full attention to the sense of hearing.
6. Especially now listen to the sound of the breath as it comes in and out of the nostrils. Shift the focus of mental attention to the sense of smell.

7 Be aware of all the odours and aromas you can detect as the breath comes in. Give full attention to the sense of smell. Be connected to the qualities of earth: stable, nourishing, supportive.

8 Inhale awareness right up to the top of the inside of the nostrils, and then over into the back of the throat and into the mouth. Shift awareness into the mouth, and the sense of taste.

9 Exhale full awareness into the sense of taste. Become aware of different tastes experienced on the surface of the tongue. Notice which tastes seem most easily detectable right now, sweet, or sour, hot or salty, bitter or astringent, like vinegar? Give full attention to the sense of taste. Be connected to the qualities associated with the element of water: fluidity and creativity.

10 Run the tip of the tongue along the inside of the closed lips and be aware of the gentle touch of the upper lip on the lower lip. Shift the awareness up to the eyes and feel the same gentle touch between the upper and lower eyelids.

11 Feel the delicate skin on the eyelids and feel the eyelids resting against the eyes. Exhale awareness into the sense of sight. Rest with all interest at the relaxed eyes. What is there to be seen in front of them, colours or darkness, movement or stillness, patterns or random shapes? Whatever you see, just observe. Give your full attention to the sense of sight. Be connected to the qualities associated with the element of fire: warmth and illumination, the light by which we see.

12 Again bring attention to the skin on the eyelids and shift the awareness into the sense of touch. Notice the different temperatures and textures you can detect through the skin. Be aware of different temperatures of covered skin, compared to uncovered skin. Notice each touch sensation, its temperature, its texture.

13 Feel the air on the skin. Give full attention to the sense of touch. Be connected to the qualities associated with the element of air: openness and movement.

14 Especially now feel the air on the skin around the ears. Direct the focus of attention into the ears, feeling the air inside the ears. Be aware of the air carrying sound vibrations into the spaces inside the ears. Bring attention back to where you started, to the sense of hearing. Notice the intimate sound closest to you: the sound of your own breath. Gradually begin to move attention outwards from this sound, to become aware of sounds in the room around you, sounds outside of that room, sounds of the wider world. Be aware simultaneously of sounds closest and sounds furthest away. Give full attention to the sense of hearing. Be connected to the qualities associated with the element of space: the spaciousness through which the sound vibrations travel, the spaciousness within which all the other elements exist.

15 When you are fully aware of all the sounds, breathe a little deeper, take a yawn or two, and open your eyes. Honour the presence of the inner teacher with the words (silent or voiced):
With great respect and love, I honour my heart, my inner teacher.

BREATH DANCES (*PRĀṆĀYĀMA*)

NB These breathing practices are all built upon the foundations of the basic breath awareness techniques described in chapter four. Please be familiar with the foundations before proceeding to the practices below.

Golden thread breath

This is less a 'technique' than a way to become more aware of the power of the breath. It is the most valuable tool to promote relaxed acceptance, and focuses upon exhalation to ease the body into deep rest. The Golden thread works well in any position, but be aware that if you practise lying down you are likely to fall asleep. There is a fuller explanation of the breath on p.133, and a summary below.

1. Tune into a gentle pattern of effortless full yogic breath (pp.131–2).
2. Yawn several times to release jaw and throat.
3. Sigh loudly for three rounds of breath on the exhalation.
4. Open your mouth very wide and sigh out a very soft 'aaah' for the next three exhalations.
5. Let your lips be soft and breath out like a horse so the lips vibrate against each other.
6. Gradually let the space between the lips get smaller and smaller.
7. Let the lips be very soft. Allow there to be a small space between top teeth and bottom teeth, between top lip and bottom lip; just enough of a gap that you might imagine a piece of tissue paper held between. Find the size of gap that works for you.
8. Breathe in through nose using *ujjāyī* breath (pp.134–5) if that is comfortable.
9. Breathe out between slightly parted lips. Feel a fine cool breeze passing out between the lips.
10. Cheeks, lips and face are relaxed. There is no pursing the lips. They are soft.
11. Feel breath travelling in through the nose, and out through the mouth. Allow the breath to be so fine that it feels as if a fine golden thread is spinning out between the lips. It's a thin, golden thread, like embroidery yarn, smooth and silky, spinning out with every exhalation.
12. Allow each exhalation to lengthen, without forcing, but simply letting the out-breath increase in length, as the golden thread of breath spins out in front of you.
13. With each inhalation allow for the breath to go in through the nose and feel the breeze of exhalation travelling out between the lips, into the air in front of your closed eyes.

14 Let the end of the golden thread carry the mental attention farther and farther away with each exhalation.

The heart of this practice is softness. You are not pursing the lips, or making them tight as if to whistle. The lips are soft, and the breath is silent and gentle. The exhalation lengthens effortlessly: simply because the gap through which the breath passes is so tiny, it takes a long time for all the breath to exit. There is no sense of force; simply watch the breath lengthen, following it out into the space in front of you. It should feel entirely effortless, completely comfortable and soothing. If you are struggling to exhale because the gap is too small, simply widen the gap.

Any exhalation is an antidote to pain and tension. The Golden thread's extended exhalation makes this antidote more powerful. While staying within the comfortable limits of your own easy breath, the longer the exhalation, the more effective this breath is as a form of pain and anxiety management. The longer the exhalation, the farther out the mental attention travels, and the more the body can relax into a quiet, mind-free space of healing and ease. Exhalation is the antidote to pain.

Peaks and valleys breath (also used as Birthing breath)

This 'breathing journey' was initially developed for use during first-stage labour, but it is very valuable at many other times of life. It helps you shift between periods of intensity, pain or anxiety into restful spaces on the exhalation. The instructions are not intended as a set script, rather they show how to breathe to encourage an instinctive response to cope with pain and other challenges.

1 Close your eyes and begin with slow, even *ujjāyī* (pp.134–5).

2 Imagine you are about to experience intense pain or face a frightening situation. Use the Golden thread exhalation (p.462) to release any tension associated with your response. Inhale with *ujjāyī* and exhale with Golden thread.

3 Sense that the intensity of the fear or pain builds to a mountain peak or wave crest, with the most powerful sensations at the top, and the quietest place of rest in the valley, or in the still quiet trough between the waves.

4 At the start, in the valley, or in the still waters between the waves, the Golden thread exhalations can be long and smooth.

5 Let the exhaling breath lead you up the slopes and over the peaks, or up from the trough and towards the crest of the next wave.

6 Each time you get to the end of the exhalation, settle back down into your resting place, down in the valley, or in the still waters between the waves, where you are ready to take your next breath.

7 As the fear or pain builds in intensity, it may be difficult to exhale for long. Even so, each time allow the exhalation to lead you up the steeper slopes or up over the crest of the wave as the intensity increases.

8 It may be harder now to exhale back down to the resting place.

9. Use the exhale like a rope, to pull you up and over the peaks or the tops of the waves, to guide you through the intensity.
10. Once over the top, start moving down the other side – sensations may still be intense, and breaths may still be short, almost like panting at this stage, but focus on lengthening the exhale.
11. Know that the Golden thread breath is leading you down the mountain, or down into the trough between the waves.
12. Let exhalations grow longer as you return to the state of rest, sinking back down to the peaceful valley, or to the quiet space between the waves, the place where you find all your resources.
13. Down in that place of rest, let go of the Golden thread breath and return to effortless *ujjāyī* for exhales, its sound marking the end of this stage of the journey.

Triangle breaths and psychic alternate nostril breathing

These are hands-free versions of the classic yoga alternate nostril breathing practice, *nāḍī shodhana*. All these techniques return our state of mind to balance and calm, bringing focus and clarity. It is easiest to learn the triangle breaths lying in Corpse pose (p.550) but once you are familiar with them they can be used in any position.

First stage triangles

1. Close your eyes and breathe fully.
2. Sense the flow of breath in the nostrils, and imagine the shape of a triangle in the nose, so that the two nostrils form the base corners of a triangle and the point between the eyebrows is the top of the triangle.
3. Feel the inhalation moving up the two sides of the triangle to its tip, and the exhalation moving down from tip to base. Take three breaths like this.
4. Exhale the awareness down to the tips of the fingers, and imagine the shape of a larger triangle so that the two hands form the base corners of a triangle and the point between the eyebrows is the top of the triangle.
5. Sense the flow of breath along the arms, and feel the inhalation moving up the two sides of the triangle to its tip, and exhalation moving down from tip to base. Take three breaths like this.
6. Exhale the awareness down to the heels, and imagine the shape of an even larger triangle so that the two feet form the base corners of a triangle and the point between the eyebrows is the top of the triangle.
7. Sense the flow of breath along the sides of the body and down along the legs into the heels. Feel the inhalation moving up the two sides of the triangle to its tip, and the exhalation moving down from tip to base. Take three breaths like this.

Reverse the process, and bring the awareness back from the largest triangle, through the triangles that end at the hands and then back to the small triangle of awareness in the nose. Take three breaths in each triangle.

Second stage, alternating flow of breath in triangles

NB The instructions specify right and left, but once you are familiar with the practice, it is helpful to start on the dominant (more open) nostril at the time of practice.

1 Inhaling, direct the focus of mental attention into the left nostril, and follow the breath up to the top of the triangle at the point between the eyebrows.

2 Exhaling, direct the focus of mental attention from the top of the triangle to follow the breath down the right nostril and out at the base of the triangle.

3 Inhaling, direct the focus of mental attention into the base of the right nostril, and follow the flow of breath up to the top of the triangle.

4 Exhaling, direct the focus of mental attention from the top of the triangle to follow the breath down the left nostril, and out at the base of the triangle.

5 One complete round draws the inhalation up through the left nostril, exhalation out and down through the right nostril, the inhalation up through the right nostril and exhalation out and down through the left nostril.

6 Feel the triangle of breath in the nose, and imagine it flowing up and down each side.

7 Repeat five rounds and pause for a round of full yogic breath with awareness in both nostrils.

Once you have alternated the breath in the small triangle of the nose, do the same in the other two triangles that end at the hands and the feet. Reverse the process, and bring the awareness back to the nose triangle to finish.

Keep breath flowing in an easy rhythm, and allow awareness to move only at pace of breath. As an 'invisible' *prāṇāyāma* that no one else can see that you are doing, psychic alternate nostril breathing is handy to use in daily life: in crowded buses or trains, in cars, and during stressful moments at work or home. Awareness of the rhythm of the triangular flow of breath can help restore balance, equanimity and poise when you are under pressure.

Additional triangles of awareness can be brought to the following places using the same directional techniques described above:

1 Breasts down to pubis.

2 Breasts to third eye or crown of head.

3 Heels to pubis.

For a complete *yoga nidrā* practice that utilises these additional triangles, see the invocation at the start of the book, and **www.yonishakti.co**.

Balancing breath (*padadhirasana*)

The flow of breath in the right and left nostrils has a direct impact upon brain function. In yoga this flow of breath is called *svara* and it is naturally shifting from one nostril to the other, typically changing after about ninety minutes of flow. At any given point, the dominant nostril is the one through which the breath can be sensed to flow most easily. If the dominant nostril is the left, then the right hemisphere of the brain is most active, and vice versa. By becoming aware of the natural changes in the flow of breath we can become more sensitive to the natural range of activities and attitudes that are most suited to whichever nostril and thus, whichever hemisphere of the brain is dominant.

Pressure under the armpits has a direct influence on the flow of the breath in the nostrils. If pressure is applied under the right armpit, then breath in the left nostril tends to flow, and vice versa.

1 Sit in any comfortable balanced position. Have a straight spine, and let the shoulders drop away from the ears. Watch the breath as you breathe fully. Observe which nostril is dominant.

2 When the breath is rhythmic and even, cross your arms over your chest, tucking the fingers of the right hand under the left armpit and the fingers of the left hand under the right armpit. The thumbs are free, and rest on the front of the arm, pointing up towards the shoulder (1). Work the fingers deep up into the warmth of the armpits, and then let the elbows drop down. Alternatively, place the thumbs in the armpits and rest the fingers on the arms (2).

3 Close the eyes and focus the attention on the flow of breath in and out of the nostrils. Be aware of a triangular pattern, as the air flows into the nostrils and up the sides of the nose to the tip of the triangle at the point between the two eyebrows. Be aware of that same triangle as the breath flows out and down.

4 Watch the shifting balance of the breath in this triangle of the nose. When you want to release the pose remove the hands from under the armpits and rest the backs of the hands on the thighs. Observe the pattern of the flow of the breath in the nostrils. Note any changes that may have occurred.

1
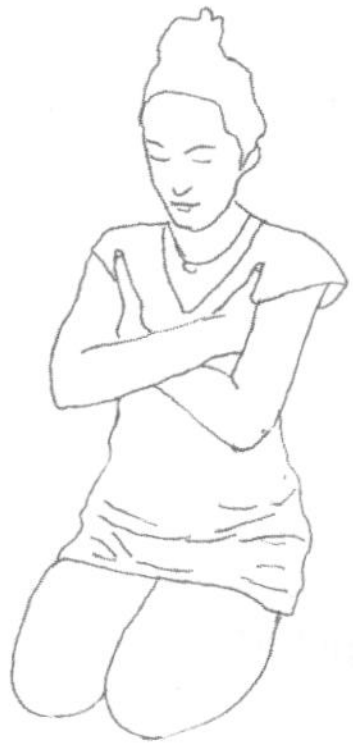

2
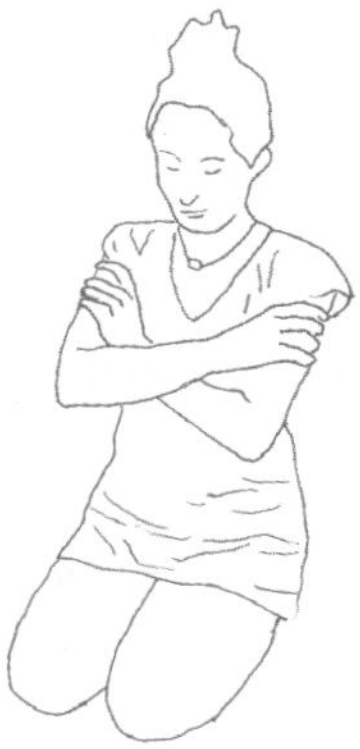

It is the mental focus upon the balancing of the breath that makes this practice most effective. If your arms get tired, just release the hands down by the sides. You can also balance the breath lying down. Bear in mind that if you lie on the right side, the breath will tend to flow on the left nostril, and if you lie on the left side, the breath will tend to flow in the right nostril.

You can also do this practice in a chair. It can be very inconspicuous, so you can experience the calming benefits when travelling. Even a couple of minutes can create a calm and attentive frame of mind.

Sonic massage (*bīja mantra* massage)

In yoga, every place in the body has a *bīja mantra*, a seed sound that contains and expresses the energy at its location. The humming resonance of these sounds energises and soothes, bringing the attention within to the energy centres in the body and naturally extending the exhalation. These short *mantras* have no literal meaning, but their sound is associated with the elements earth, water, fire, air and ether, or space. In the tradition of yoga *tantra* from which this practice is derived, these elements are located in the energy body at specific centres known as *cakras*, or spiralling wheels of energy. Each *cakra* has its own element and its own Sanskrit name, which is given after the English translation in the instructions below. For a good introductory discussion of *cakras*, see 'Psychic Physiology of Yoga' in Swami Satyananda's *Asana, Pranayama, Mudra, Bandha*, pp.513–24.

If you find it helpful to locate the energy centres with a physical trigger, then follow the extra instructions [in brackets] at the start of each section below.

For each energy centre:

1 Sit or lie comfortably, with eyes closed.

2 Establish full yogic breath (pp.131–2) or *ujjāyī* (pp.134–5).

3 Exhaling, bring mental focus to the level of each *cakra* described below.

4 Follow directions for *bīja mantra* at each *cakra*, sounding three repetitions, and resonating the 'mmm' part of the *mantra*.

5 Return to three rounds of your chosen quiet breath between each energy centre.

Earth centre (*mulādhāra cakra*)

Bring mental focus down to the base of the spine. [Gentle *mūla bandha* (p.474) gives a useful connection to this area]. Hold mental awareness here, repeating *mantra* '*Laṁ*'.

Water centre (*svādhiṣṭhāna cakra*)

Move awareness higher up, resting attention in the centre of the body at the level of the pubic bone. [Drawing *mūla bandha* higher towards the cervix can be an effective way to bring the focus of mental attention into the pelvis]. Hold awareness here and move attention in towards the womb, repeating *mantra* '*Vaṁ*'.

Fire centre (*maṇipūra cakra*)

Move awareness higher up, resting attention in the centre of the body at navel level. [Gentle abdominal breath and/or resting thumbs at navel with fingers pointing down can be a vivid focus to connect to this area]. Hold awareness here, breathing into the belly, then move attention back to the spine at this level, repeating *mantra* '*Raṁ*'.

Air centre (*anāhata cakra*)

Move awareness higher up, resting attention in the centre of body at the level of the shoulder blades. [A big expansion to open chest sideways on inhale, lifting sternum, provides helpful focus for this area.] Hold awareness here repeating *mantra* '*Yaṁ*'.

Ether/space centre (*viśuddha cakra*)

Move awareness higher up, resting attention in the centre of the neck at the level of the base of the throat. [Drawing *ujjāyī* breath right up to collarbones and feeling movement at the base of the throat – or even touching fingertips there – can be a clear connection with this area.] Hold awareness here, repeating *mantra* '*Haṁ*'.

Beyond elements (*ajña cakra*)

Move awareness higher up, resting attention in the centre of the head at eyebrow level. [It can be easier to connect with this centre if you lick your thumb and touch the point between the two eyebrows, feeling the cool damp spot at the 'third eye' centre.] Hold awareness here, repeating *mantra* '*Aum*'.

Universal connection (*sahasrāra cakra*)

1 Move awareness higher up, resting attention at the crown of the head.

2 Hold awareness here, repeating *mantra* '*aum*'.

3 At the end of last '*Aum*', exhale, breathing awareness back down to base of spine.

4 With slow *ujjāyī*, for the next seven breath cycles let the focus of attention flow down the spine with each exhalation, from crown of head to tailbone. Let inhalations take care of themselves, and focus all attention on the downward movement of energy and awareness, beginning each exhalation at the top of the head and letting awareness move down to reach the base of the spine at the end of every exhalation.

5 Complete with seven full yogic breaths and no specific focus of awareness, just resting with the easy rhythm of breath.

Focus on the 'mmm' part of the *mantra*s. The resonance of the sound in your body is more important than a loud, outwardly directed voice. Each person finds awareness of these energy centres in their own way, and the locations described above may not precisely match your own experience. With practice, and sensitive awareness you can learn to refine your perception of the precise points of resonance

You can repeat the *bīja mantras* out loud, or hear them silently. If you are voicing sound, then you can do it slowly, with one sound lasting the length of the exhalation, or more rapidly, with repetitions for the length of the exhale. You can also alternate long and short repetitions. A shift in the pitch of the humming sounds can enhance embodied understanding of the energy centres. Settle on a note at the bottom of your voice range for the first centres, and progress upwards, raising the pitch a tone at a time. If you have time, at the end of the last '*Aum*', reverse the process, and chant back down to the base of the spine. These are powerful sounds. If you experience strong physical or emotional responses to any or all of them, it can be reassuring to speak about your experiences with a yoga teacher who has an understanding of the effects of these *mantras*.

It is very delightful to practise this Sonic massage with babies, placing the lips directly on their bodies at the energy centre points to create a warm buzzy massage. This creates a pleasing continuity because the babies recall hearing the sounds of their mother's voice during their time in the womb. Even babies who only hear these sounds for the first time outside the womb find this sonic vibratory massage very soothing.

Humming bee breaths (*bhrāmarī prāṇāyama*)

Bhrāmarī lowers blood pressure, and the feelings of tranquillity that it promotes make it an ideal *prāṇāyama* to do before any relaxation practice. Classic yoga texts claim the most noticeable effect of this breath is to induce a feeling of happiness. It certainly makes most people smile as they do it. Because of its tendency to promote feelings of contentment and well-being, *bhrāmarī* is a useful tool during times when your emotions feel volatile or unsettled.

1 Sit comfortably, eyes closed, and establish a complete yogic breath.

2 Inhaling, raise arms, drawing elbows out wide at shoulder height.

3 Block ears (with heels of hand, index fingers or thumbs, whichever you prefer).

4 Exhaling, resonate a humming sound. It is felt more than heard, so don't strain to make it loud.

5 Focus awareness of sound vibrations in centre of chest.

6 Allow for sound to fade at end of exhalation, then start again.

7 Either keep hands in position throughout however many rounds you choose to do (seven or eleven is good to start), or raise and lower hands as necessary: for example, after every third cycle, or after every cycle if arms feel tired.

Tibetan *bhrāmarī*

This is a beautiful variation of traditional *bhrāmarī* breath.

1 The hands start palms together in front of the chest. As the exhaling hum begins, move the palms of the hands upwards, resting the fingertips initially on the chin,

and then separate the hands and slide the palms of the hands up across the face, up into the forehead.

2 As the hands move across the face, feel that you are washing your face in the sound.

3 Continuing the exhalation, slide the hands up over the top of the head.

4 At the end of the hum block the ears with heels of hands and take the focus within.

5 Allow for the sound to fade at end of exhalation.

6 Then lower the hands back down and bring the palms of the hands back together in front of the chest and inhale.

7 Do as many rounds as feels comfortable (eleven makes a good number to start with). Focus on the sensations of the sound, for yourself and inside the belly where the baby experiences the vibrations as a sonic massage.

With both these forms of *bhrāmarī*, never compromise the easy rhythm of your breath. If you feel the need, simply pause in the practice to take a few rounds of full yogic breath.

Cooling breaths (*śītalī* and *sitkarī*)

These practices require two types of tongue rolling. If you are able to roll your tongue lengthwise by bringing the long sides into the middle to make a tube, than you can practise the first breath (*sītalī*). If your tongue doesn't roll this way, then practise the second breath instead (*sitkarī*), that is done by tucking the tip of the tongue under the back of the front teeth and rolling it backwards and widthways, so that the ends of the tube are on the right and left side instead of at the tip of the tongue.

Cooling breath *(sītalī)*

1 Sit comfortably, and establish an easy rhythm of breath. Close the eyes and watch the rhythm of the breath.

2 Stick out your tongue and roll it lengthwise.

3 On the next inhale, draw the breath slowly in through the end of the 'straw' of the tongue.

4 At the end of the inhale, relax the tongue, bring it inside the mouth and close the lips.

5 Exhale through the nose.

Hissing breath *(sitkarī)*

1. Sit comfortably, and establish an easy rhythm of breath. Close the eyes and watch the breath.
2. Roll back the tip of your tongue and tuck it under the back of the top teeth. If it's comfortable, you can work the tip of the tongue further back into the roof of the mouth.
3. Pull the corners of the mouth back slightly so that air can get in through both ends of the tongue roll.
4. On the next inhale, draw the breath slowly in through both open ends of the 'straw' of the tongue, making a hissing noise
5. At the end of the inhale, bring the tongue inside the mouth and close the lips.
6. Exhale through the nose.

For these practices, it is best to repeat for only three to five cycles of breath before taking a pause and returning to an ordinary breath. Keeping the tongue rolled for any longer than this can make it cramp or ache, especially if the action is unfamiliar. With practice this rolling can become more comfortable, but even so, if you require the sustained benefits of the cooling breaths it is advisable to alternate five cycles of a cooling breath with seven cycles of any breath in which the tongue rests. This way the cooling effects of the breath can be experienced over a longer period without straining the tongue.

Healing breath

For details of this breath, please see page 482.

CHAPTER TWENTY

energy locks and seals (*bandhas* and *mudrās*)

AWAKENING THE FEET AND HANDS (*PĀDA BANDHA, HASTA BANDHA*)

These practices awaken the awareness of the feet and hands as '*prāṇa* nets' to catch energy. Essentially, broadening and lengthening the feet and the hands in any practice will maximise your capacity to energise yourself.

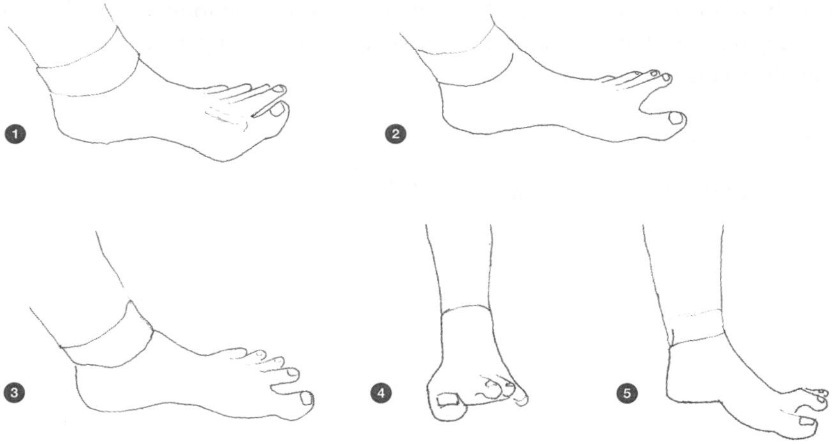

Awakening the feet (standing)

As you inhale, work actively with the muscles of your legs and feet to press the balls of the feet into the floor and spread your toes, lifting them up and out (1).

Be aware how pressure through the balls of the feet with big toes lifted strengthens and lifts the inner arches of the feet. As you lower the big toes to the ground, maintain and deepen the lift of the arches above the inner ankle bones by also pressing down into the backs of the heels and the outer edges (little toe sides) of the feet (2).

Keep spreading out the toes as they all come down to the floor (3). Feel the little toes pressing down into the floor. With each exhalation, press strongly down with active legs and toes, keeping the inner arches of the feet lifted.

Create as much distance as possible between the little toes and the big toes, encouraging the three middle toes to lift (4). Be aware of the spaces between the toes. Be very attentive to pressing down the balls of the feet and the backs of the heels (5).

Energetically, as the arch of the foot lifts, and the feet and legs become active (*pāda bandha*), a supportive and uplifting flow of *prāṇa* comes up into the pelvic muscles. This may naturally result in the experience of a vaginal lift and squeeze as the exhale leaves the body (*yoginī mūla bandha*, see p.474), or it may be that nothing much happens in the pelvic muscles, and that you can consciously encourage the lifting and squeezing as you exhale. Explore what feels supportive for you and your pelvic organs.

Awakening the hands

If your hands are on the floor (e.g. in Cat pose), work actively with the muscles of your arms and hands to press the pads of the index fingers into the floor and spread your fingers up and out.

Be aware how the pressure through the pads of the index fingers with the fingers and thumb lifted strengthens and spreads the hand. As you lower the fingers to the ground, maintain and deepen the lifting of the dome of the palm of the hand by also pressing down into the thumb and the little finger. Keep spreading out the fingers and thumbs as they all come down to the floor. The wider apart the fingers spread, the less stress there is in the wrist. Create as much distance as possible between the little finger and the thumb. Be aware of the spaces between the fingers. Feel the webbing heat up.

If the hands are not on the ground, all of the previous awakenings are helpful. Additionally, sense that the skin on the palms and the backs of the hands is equally spread, so that the hands are evenly spread, front and back, in whatever practice you are doing. Feel how the open and awakened hands expand the capacity to breathe fully.

A NOTE ON TERMINOLOGY: PELVIC MUSCLES AND THE MYTH OF THE "PELVIC FLOOR"

The practices described below work directly to increase, liberate and redistribute energy from the pelvis to the rest of the body. In the instructions that relate to the pelvic sphincters, I do not use the term pelvic floor because in my experience, the idea of there being a muscular floor to the bottom of the pelvis perpetuates an unhelpful misconception about the anatomy of the pelvic muscles in relation to the angle at which the pelvis is held. In fact, when the pelvis is tilted at the optimal angle for female pelvic organ support, then the pubic bones are positioned beneath the body, and it is these bones that provide the most secure support for the pelvic organs.

This means that the pelvic muscles are in fact more accurately described as 'back pelvic walls' rather than pelvic floor. The pelvic muscles closest to the sacrum in the back of the pelvis create a more vertical 'wall' than those muscles closest to the pubic bones. From the point of view of optimising support for the female pelvic organs, the sling of muscle that runs between these two points is really more helpfully considered as a pelvic 'back' than a pelvic floor. It is in this sling of muscles that the sphincters described below are positioned. For more detailed explanations of the importance of pelvic tilt to the support of female pelvic organs, see chapter twenty-one.

VAGINAL ROOT LOCK FOR USE WITH EMPTY WOMB (*YOGINĪ MŪLA BANDHA*)

NB Not suitable during menstruation, and only suitable for occasional therapeutic use during pregnancy, for example to provide a sense of support in cases of pelvic organ prolapse.

Mūla bandha, or the 'root lock' is a standard component in many approaches to *haṭha* yoga. For women to be able to practise accurately, it is important to understand that our 'root' is not the anus, but the vagina. Contraction of the vaginal walls is the *yoginī's mūla bandha*. Appropriate practice of *mūla bandha* for women also takes into consideration the stage of the menstrual cycle, and whether or not a woman is pregnant. This version is suitable for all women except those who are pregnant and menstruating. For a practice appropriate to these times, see below.

Practice of the root lock is synchronised with breath and whole body awareness. It is not the same as a 'Kegel' exercise, which does not include breath awareness. Done with yogic awareness, the *yoginī*'s *mūla bandha* provides gentle but energising, toning and release for the muscles of the pelvic walls, abdomen and the lower back too. Whilst the practice is useful in most poses and movement sequences, to begin with it is most effectively practised from Child's pose, kneeling, with the head and torso resting forward. Some women find lifting the buttocks in the air helpful as a way to connect with this practice in the beginning stages.

1. Establish a comfortable full yogic breath.
2. Exhaling, sense the natural drawing inwards and upwards of the vaginal walls towards the cervix (*mūla bandha*). A movement in the vulva is also usually noticeable. If this movement does not happen spontaneously, then actively draw the vaginal walls inwards and upwards as you exhale.
3. Feel first outer and then deep layers of muscles moving in and up: so there is more of a lift than a squeeze at the end of the inhale.

4 Follow the exhaling breath to lift up as high as feels comfortable.

5 Release this lift as you inhale.

The intention of the root lock is to use the upward movement on the exhalation to *reverse* the flow of downward-moving energy (*apāna*). This means it is a helpful practice to lift a 'dragging' feeling in the uterus and vagina, and can be especially powerful as a means to support positive posture and vitality. It also means that there are good reasons to avoid *mūla bandha*s during menstruation and usually also during pregnancy (except for occasional practice of this technique to support pelvic organ prolapse during pregnancy).

MENSTRUAL AND PREGNANCY ROOT LOCK FOR USE WITH FULL WOMB (*GARBHA MŪLA BANDHA*)

When the womb is fuller than usual, for example during pregnancy or at menstruation, then it is more helpful to connect with downward-flowing energy (*apāna*), than it is to seek to reverse this flow. So at these special times, the upward lift on exhale that defines classic *mūla bandha* is not helpful. Instead, the following practice still works to keep tone in the pelvic muscles, whilst using the breath to encourage a natural and easy flow of *apāna* downwards.

1 Exhaling, bring mental awareness down to the base of the spine and move it forwards until it comes to rest midway between the pubic bones and the tip of the tail bone.

2 Focus attention in the walls of the vagina.

3 Inhaling with awareness here, draw the walls of the vagina in and up.

4 Feel first outer and then deep layers of muscles moving in and up: so there is more of a lift than a squeeze at the end of the inhale.

5 Follow breath to lift up as high as feels comfortable, and then, exhaling, release lift, and let go, down into the support of whatever you are sitting on.

6 Following the easy rhythm of natural breath, let this lifting and lowering movement continue: breathing in, moving up, and breathing out, lowering down.

7 Continue for a few more cycles of rhythmic breath, keeping awareness at the very centre of the pelvic outlet and squeezing and lifting the muscles on inhale, and releasing them on exhale.

UPLIFTING LOCK WITH ROOT LOCK (*UḌḌĪYĀNA BANDHA* WITH *MŪLA BANDHA*)

NB Not suitable during menstruation; only suitable during pregnancy for occasional use to support pelvic organ prolapse (generally better to use the pregnancy lock, p.475). Use only with caution if you have an IUCD in place, and/or if you are seeking to conceive but experiencing difficulty.

This combines the benefits of the root lock with the additional uplift of *uḍḍīyāna bandha*. It is best practised in a soft squat, resting slightly forwards with the heels of the hands on the thighs and the feet and hands fully awakened (pp.472–3).

1 Establish a comfortable full yogic breath (pp.131–2). As breath rhythm settles, notice the soft hollowing of the belly at the end of exhalation. Feel also (or create) a gathering inwards and upwards of the vaginal walls.

2 With the next exhale, more actively draw the abdominal wall diagonally up and back towards the spine and upwards at the same time as the muscles in the vaginal walls move upwards and inwards.

3 As the exhalation completes, allow all these inward and upward movements to result in a sense of uplift that remains whilst the breath stays out. If the bandha is completed, there will be a sense of uplift also in the throat.

4 As you inhale, release the hold on the abdominal and vaginal wall muscles, and return to two or three rhythmic breath cycles.

To begin with, just practise two or three repetitions. With practice increase to seven.

RECLINING UPLIFTING LOCK (*SUPTA UḌḌĪYĀNA BANDHA*)

NB Not suitable during menstruation; only suitable during pregnancy for very occasional use to support pelvic organ prolapse (generally better to use the pregnancy lock, p.475). Use only with caution if you have an IUCD in place, and/or if you are seeking to conceive but experiencing difficulty.

For instructions for this practice see the pelvic support practice section (chapter twenty-one).

HORSE GESTURE (ANAL SQUEEZE) (*ASHVINI MUDRĀ*)

This practice brings the focus of squeeze and release around the anus. The same base positions as for the vaginal lock (p.474) can be used to explore this practice, but once you are familiar with it you can use it in most poses.

1 Exhaling, bring awareness down to the base of the spine, let it rest there, close to the tailbone and around the anus. (If you are sitting upright with support beneath you, or on a ball, then tilt or roll slightly backwards until you can feel some pressure as you sit back towards your tail).

2 Inhaling, squeeze tight the muscles around the anus as if you wanted to hold in a tiny fart.

3 Once you can feel this ring of muscle closing, exhale and release as if you could let go of the imaginary fart.

4 Continue for a few more rounds of rhythmic breath, keeping awareness at the anus, squeezing muscles there on inhale, and releasing on exhale.

PSYCHIC GESTURE (URETHRAL SQUEEZE) (*SAHAJOLĪ MUDRĀ*)

This practice brings the focus of squeeze and release around the urethral opening or pee hole. The same base positions as for the Vaginal lock (p.474) can be used to explore this practice, but once you are familiar with it you can use it in most poses.

1 Exhaling, let mental attention move forward to the pubic bone, right at the very front close to the clitoris. (If you are sitting upright with support beneath you, tilt slightly forwards until you can feel some pressure coming towards the pubic bones).

2 Inhaling with awareness here, squeeze those muscles that would stop an imaginary flow of urine. Imagine that by squeezing tight these muscles you have completely stopped this imaginary flow.

3 Exhaling, release these muscles. Sense how this release would allow the imaginary flow of urine to resume its flow.

4 Continue for a few more rounds of easy rhythmic breath, keeping awareness around the urethral opening and squeezing the muscles there on inhale, and releasing them on exhale. As you squeeze and release these muscles, you may feel a ticklish sensation as the hood of the clitoris is moved by the referred action of the squeeze on the urethra.

URINE DRINKING (*AMAROLĪ*)

NB Not recommended during pregnancy.

Amarolī is included in this "locks and seals" section because it retains and redistributes energy in essentially the same way as the pelvic locks and seals or the hand gestures. It also can bring a profound shift in attitudes and patterns of behaviours towards care of the physical body, particularly in relation to food and drink. Even to consider the concept is to recognise the possibility of a fully conscious relationship with the physical body, a relationship based on an authentic awareness of the truth that everything we ingest becomes a part of who we are. Practising *amarolī* acknowledges this very directly. If you are even thinking about drinking your own pee you become naturally averse to consuming anything that makes it smell or taste bad, for example alcohol, meat or caffeine. You clean up your act, because you are literally planning to swallow the consequences.

1. To start with be sure you are well hydrated and your diet is entirely sattvic: wholesome, fresh and free from meat, alcohol and caffeine.
2. Collect only the mid-stream flow of the first urine you pass in the morning after you wake up. Don't collect the beginning and end of the flow.
3. Only take a sip or two the first time you do *amarolī* and monitor how you respond and its effects.

A major part of the value of *amarolī* is the process of preparation and the shifting attitudes to your body and its fluids that the practice promotes. It is not about drinking a lot of pee, it is about reconnecting to the natural functioning of the body and realising the value of clarity and simplicity and radical recycling. Monitor your own responses and see for yourself what changes in terms of vitality, immunity and attitudes to self-care. For further information and testimonials read Coen van der Kroon's *The Golden Fountain* (Gateway, 2001).

FIVE ELEMENTAL HAND GESTURES (*HASTA MUDRĀS*)

These are utilised in the sequences honouring the elements in chapter seven, but may be included wherever feels natural, or whenever a connection and rebalancing of the relevant element is required, during *asāna*, *prāṇāyama* or meditation.

Earth gesture / *pṛthivī mudrā*

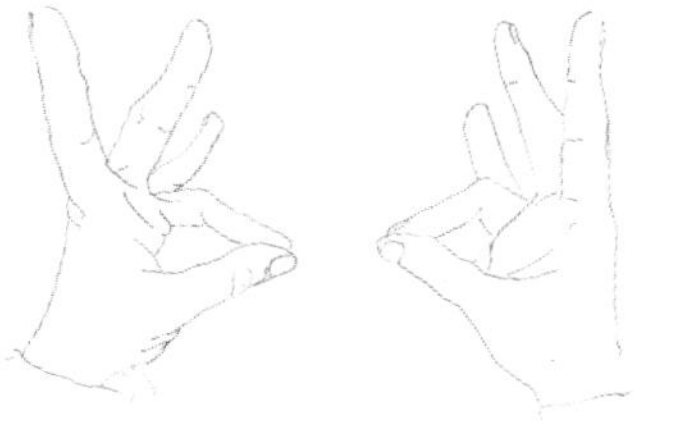

Thumb tip touches tip of ring finger.

Water gesture / *āpas mudrā*

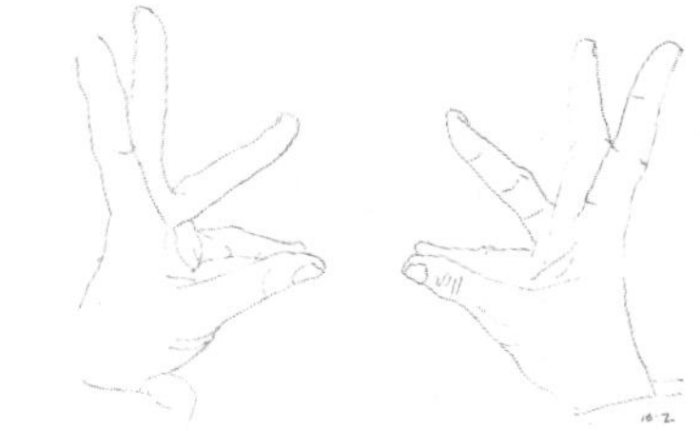

Thumb tip touches tip of little finger.

Fire gesture / *agni mudrā*

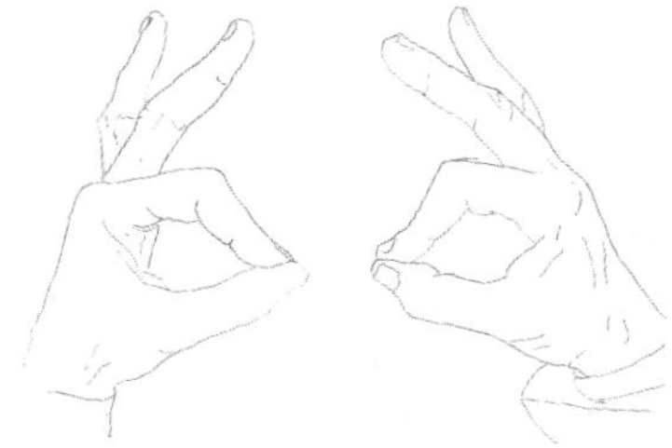

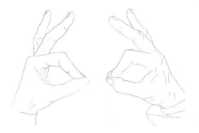

Thumb tip touches index finger

Space gesture / *ākāśa mudrā*

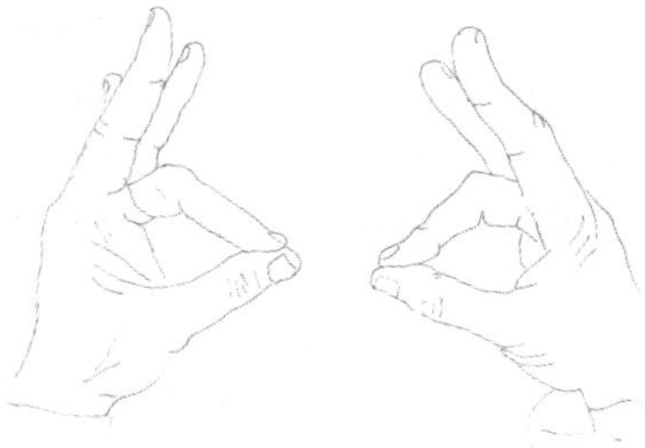

Thumb tip touches tip of middle finger

Heart space gesture (relating to element of air) / *hṛdaya mudrā*

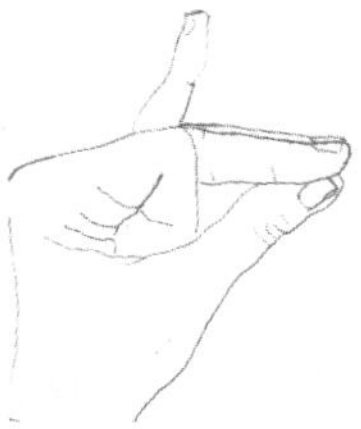

Index finger is tucked into root of thumb. Thumb tip touches the tips of the middle and ring finger together. Little finger is free.

FURTHER READING AND RESEARCH

For further information about *amarolī*, and testimonials, read **Coen van der Kroon**'s *The Golden Fountain* (Gateway, 2001), or visit:
www.universal-tao.com/article/urine_therapy.html
www.yogamag.net/archives/1981/ajan81/amar.shtml
www.aypsite.org/amaroli.html
www.heartlandhealing.com/pages/archive/urine_therapy/index.html

CHAPTER TWENTY-ONE

support and nurture: security and uplift for the pelvic organs

NB Please note that none of these explorations are very comfortable or advisable during menstruation. They are not a great idea in pregnancy either, unless you have the guidance of an experienced yoga teacher to ensure that you practise safely and appropriately, for example to use the techniques to help support pelvic organ prolapse during pregnancy (see guidelines below). If you are experiencing pelvic organ shift it is best to wait until after you have finished bleeding to experiment with these practices.

Women of all ages can experience pelvic organ shift but it is especially prevalent postnatally, during perimenopause and in the years after menopause, which is why you will find the extended discussion of the effects of pelvic organ prolapse in the perimenopause section in chapter fifteen.

The practices described below can assist us to explore and encounter the effects of holistic breath and movement in relation to our pelvis and the organs within. This process can really clarify exactly what we can be doing to help ourselves manage the sensations of pelvic organ shift in daily life. These practices develop an awareness of a positive pelvic angle to support the organs within. They also encourage an active use of the Healing breath (p.482) and can also be helpfully combined with that technique.

APPLICATIONS

The levels of awareness promoted by these practices are vital to promoting postnatal recovery and well-being. They are also the vital foundation of a positive response to the experience of pelvic organ shift at any time in our lives. When we know what's where in our own pelvis, and we start to direct the energy of breath and focus around it to create the optimum pelvic tilt to provide maximum organ support, decompress the organs and relieve pressure on the perineum, anus and vagina, then we can begin to gain a full understanding of the state of our pelvic health. This kind of understanding gives us confidence to know clearly when something isn't right – and to seek help to fix it. It also gives us confidence to build strength and increase vitality.

The work of Christine Kent (2006, and see bibliography) has done much to raise consciousness of the crucial importance of the angle of pelvic tilt as a means of providing life-long support for female pelvic organs. Positive posture is the foundation of good pelvic health. The 'Whole Woman' posture developed by Kent, like a number of other approaches to natural movement that seek to minimise lower back pain (e.g. the Gokhale method), is intended to provide optimal conditions of support to female pelvic organs by developing a naturally comfortable but supported lumbar (lower back) curve that tilts the pelvis forward and lets the pelvic organs rest above the pubic bones. As explained in the previous chapter on locks and seals (pp.473–4), experiencing this posture reveals the idea of the pelvic *floor* to be a myth: for when we stand in such a way as to maximise support for our pelvic organs by settling the pubic bones beneath them, then the pelvic floor is in fact more like a back pelvic wall. It is this basic premise that underpins all of the following yogic practices for pelvic organ support. I am grateful to Lindy Roy, yoga teacher and Whole Woman instructor, for clarifying my understanding of the importance of this posture to women's pelvic health.

INTEGRATION OF PELVIC ORGAN SUPPORT AND POSITIVE POSTURE INTO DAILY LIFE

Take time to experience these practices, and to clarify your embodied knowledge of your body today. Feel what it is you know about how best to position your pelvis in order to experience maximum support for the pelvic organs. Use everything at your disposal to optimise the support you need: the angle of the pelvis, the living vitality and connection of the feet to the earth, the undulating movements of your spine and hips, the lift of your arms and expansion of the rib cage, the effects of your breath and the movements of the abdominal and pelvic muscles. When you feel secure in your understanding of this knowledge, begin to utilise the strength and support that it brings to daily activities. As with the Healing breath using *mūla bandha*, the sense of lift and support through pelvic 'decompression' can be very helpful to relieve any sense of downward pressure on the pelvic walls, such as that which comes when rising to a standing position whilst lifting a heavy weight (like a baby or a bag of shopping), or while driving or working at a computer.

We are all different, and the state of our pelvic health tells our own unique story. Some support practices work better for some of us than others. The only way to discover what works best for you today is to explore how you respond to the exercises, and then to integrate what works for you into your daily awareness.

The exercises on the following pages will help you explore the effects of pelvic angle on pelvic organ support, enabling you to enlist optimal support for the pelvic organs. As you move through the explorations, gradually adding new elements, sense how the arches of the feet, and the angle of the pelvis in relation to the lower back, as well as the contraction and lifting of the pelvic muscles, are all working together to create an optimal, full mobilisation of every type of conscious muscular, breath and energetic support available to the pelvic organs.

HEALING BREATH: LIFTING UP TO HEAL AND ENERGISE

NB Avoid during menstruation and pregnancy.

This is the most helpful breath to use during all of the following practices. It was originally devised to support postnatal recovery but has proved very helpful in the management of the sensations of pelvic organ prolapse. Initially it is easiest to practise from a semi-supine position with a gentle arch in the lower back.

1. Establish a comfortable full yogic breath (pp.131–2).
2. Inhaling, let awareness flow up body from base of spine to crown of head.
3. Exhaling, let awareness flow down body from crown of head to base of spine.
4. As breath rhythm settles, notice soft hollowing of belly at end of exhalation, and how lower back eases down towards floor as belly 'sucks down'.
5. Let rhythmic cycle of breath draw awareness more towards exhalation, feeling that this hollowing of belly and lowering of lumbar spine to floor is building a connection to movement of pelvic muscles. Inhale softly.
6. With next exhale, sense the drawing inward and upward of vagina towards cervix (*mūla bandha*). If this movement does not happen spontaneously, then actively draw muscles in vaginal walls upwards and inwards as you exhale.
7. Keep a gentle grip on this squeeze as you inhale.
8. As you next exhale, lift higher and squeeze tighter, feeling the action of these muscles quite high up inside.
9. Repeat this cycle once more.
10. On next inhalation, release hold on muscles, and return to two or three rhythmic breath cycles.

Work with awareness of pelvic muscles and breath together, so that comfortable, rhythmic lengthening of breath increases muscle strength. To start, tilt pelvis with breath, keeping buttocks on floor, lifting tailbone on exhale and arching lumbar spine a little away from floor on inhale. Connect with the hollowing of the belly (especially low down, close to pubic bone) and the lifting of pelvic muscles.

Once you are familiar with these feelings, then keep breath moving, but stop pelvic tilting, and develop awareness of internal movements. The instructions above take you through one full round of healing breath (i.e. two exhales and two inhales). Once you are comfortable with this, gradually increase the number of exhales which you make while the pelvic muscles are lifted. When you are settled with a comfortable number of exhales per lift, stay with this, and alternate rounds of healing breathing with a rhythmic cycle of full yogic breath. The two key sensations to observe when doing the healing breath are the feeling of the pelvic muscles lifting up as the belly moves in. These two sensations work together simultaneously as you exhale to promote the strength and tone that is healing and revitalising.

SEMI-SUPINE PRACTICES

NB These two explorations are not advisable if you are currently experiencing pelvic organ prolapse. Move straight to Explorations in Decompression (pp.484–8).

The practice which opens this journey of self-discovery offers a yogic perspective on an exploration that was initially devised by Christine Kent, whose life's work on the effects of postural change on pelvic organ prolapse offers invaluable resources and support for women.

Explorations with a flat lower back (counter-nutated pelvis)

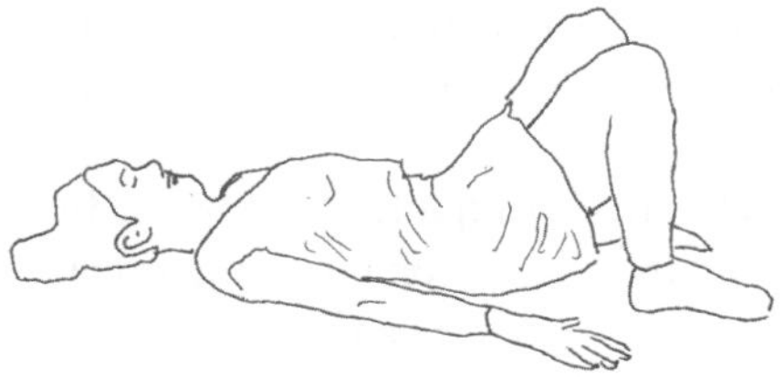

1. Lie down, bend the knees and put the soles of the feet on the floor.
2. Inhale. Begin to exhale and contract the walls of the vagina, and the muscle that runs from your tailbone to your pubis (pubo-coccygeal muscles), feeling how by this action the tailbone draws closer to pubic bone. Contract rectus abdominus and push the back of your waist flat against the floor, flattening out the lumbar curve.
3. Now maintain this position as you continue to exhale and bear down as if you are pushing your pelvic organs to the vaginal opening. Feel how in this flat back (tailbone tucked) position, the pubo-coccygeal muscle offers no resistance (a moderate prolapse will come easily down).

Explorations with an arched back (nutated pelvis)

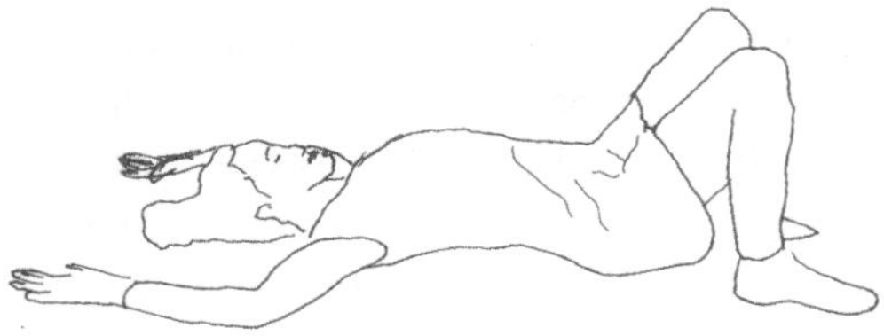

1. Now arch the small of your back. Inhale and lift arms overhead, resting elbows on the floor. Feel your pelvic diaphragm tighten across the middle as it lengthens from pubic bone to tailbone and tightens. During the inhale, allow the belly to lift up and out and over pubic bone. This stretches rectus abdominus (the top layer of abdominal muscles). At the same time, feel the contraction of the transverse abdominus, the deep muscles across the lower belly.

2 Now maintain this position as you begin to exhale and bear down, as if you are pushing your organs to the vaginal opening. Feel how with the pelvis in this position, the organs are being held at the front of the body (above the pubic bone) and can have the boney structure beneath them to help resist the downward forces of intra-abdominal pressure.

It can sometimes be very helpful in these exercises to feel the workings of the inner thighs as an additional source of support. To do this, place a yoga block or a folded blanket pad about (about ten centimetres thick and thirty centimetres long) in between the thighs and squeeze the inner thigh muscles gently in order to hold the prop in place. If this feels as if it helpfully engages supportive muscles through into the lower back and the pelvic walls then it can be a good idea to practise at least some of the time with this prop in place, at least for this exploration, but also possibly for the standing work too.

It can sometimes be a lot easier and more effective to explore this practice by pushing the soles of the feet together and letting the knees drop out to the side in Butterfly pose. If the heels are very firmly pressed together it can be easier to feel the shift in the lumbar curve, and also to lift the inner arches of the feet.

Christine Kent observes that the feeling we get when we arch the pelvis and sense the support of the pubic bone beneath the pelvic organs is a clear encounter with what she describes as '...the dynamics of pelvic organ support created and sustained by natural female standing posture'. 'Natural female standing posture' that best supports the contents of the female pelvis is a posture that supports the natural curve of the lower back, not the tail tucked under. We'll come back to that later on. For the moment, simply note that there is not a great benefit in practising so called Kegels (pelvic muscle exercises) when the lumbar curve is flattened because in this position the contractions do not lift the muscles up, they only move them slightly forward: 'The key to maximising the benefit of pelvic outlet contractions is to do so while keeping the lumbar curve in place. Try it both ways, pelvic tilted forward and pelvis tilted back, and you will see for yourself that ...the (pelvic muscle exercise) is a lot less effective in the backward tilt... (Kent 2006: 153).

Explorations in decompression of pelvic organs

I find the previous exercises work well in combination with the 'Decompression of the pelvic organs' as set out in *Mother's Breath* and based on the experiential physiology of Calais-Germain's *The Female Pelvis* (pp.135-8). Calais-Germain recommends the practice of decompressing the pelvic organs as an antidote to the adverse effects of standing upright most of the time. She observes that the support and suspension systems that hold the pelvic organs in place, as well as the perineum on which all the organs rest, can all become damaged by the effects of compression, and that this can cause pain and discomfort.

Postnatally, or perimenopausally, when the perineum and the support and suspension systems for the pelvic organs may all be in a vulnerable state, the practice of decompression may aid healing and certainly assists in encouraging the pelvic organs to return to the places from which they were shifted during pregnancy or birth, or over years of postural challenges. Allied with yoga breath and awareness, as they are presented here and in the Healing breath (p.482) these decompressing practices bring powerful benefit postnatally and during experiences of pelvic organ shift later in life.

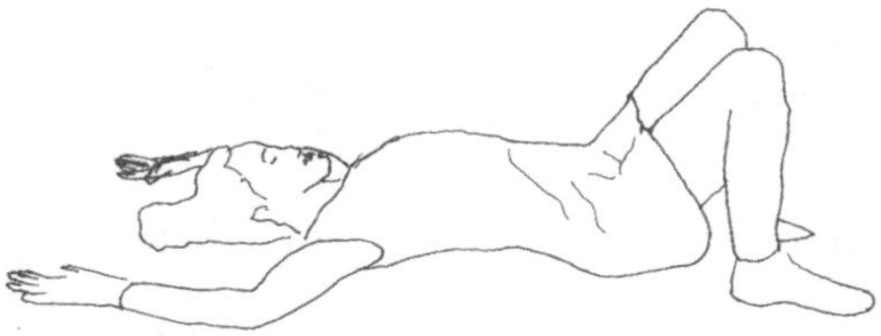

Chest breath decompression

1 Position yourself as for the previous exercises, with the feet flat on the floor and the knees bent, but this time spread your arms out to the sides, your elbows at shoulder height. Have the arms bent if that feels more comfortable. Drop the chin gently to the chest and establish a comfortable rhythm of easy full yogic breath.

2 On your next inhalation feel as if the breath fills the middle part of the chest, opening up space between each rib and its neighbour. Sense the ribs moving out sideways. Also feel the expansion from front to back.

3 As you exhale, feel the ribs moving back to their starting position. Let the rhythmic cycle of the full yogic breath carry you through a few further cycles until you are familiar with the feeling of ribcage expansion on the inhale and contraction on the exhale.

Tip: *The spontaneous settling of the ribs back into the starting position at the end of the exhale is caused by the lungs retracting as they empty. The practice enables you to focus on the strength of the elastic recoil of the lungs, which pulls the ribs back on the exhale.*

Abdominal decompression (*supta uḍḍīyāna bandha*)

This practice employs the basic techniques of the previous practices to focus on the abdomen. If time permits, it works well to do the practices in sequence, letting this one follow on from the previous two.

1 Ensure that you have a full understanding of the chest breath practice above.

2 Drop the chin gently to the chest and establish a comfortable and easy rhythm of full yogic breath.

3 On your next inhalation feel as if the breath fills the middle part of the chest, opening up space between each rib and her neighbour. Sense the ribs moving out sideways. Also feel the expansion from front to back.

4 As you exhale this time, try to maintain the ribs in this fully expanded position, by pushing the elbows down into the ground. This will probably feel very

strange, because it alters the natural response of the ribcage to the elastic recoil of the lungs. Keep the ribs as open as you can by securing the elbows on the ground until the end of the exhalation.

5 On the next inhalation, encourage the full expansion of the ribcage again. This time, as you exhale, not only try to maintain the ribs in the expanded position, but endeavour to push them further apart. Keep opening the space of the chest as you exhale.

6 Repeat the practice a couple of times, and then return to the full yogic breath.

Tip: *This practice uses the maintenance of the open ribcage during exhalation to create an abdominal vacuum: because the ribs are prevented from moving back down in response to the elastic recoil of the lungs, the abdominal mass is drawn upwards instead. This hollowing of the belly is an effect of the elastic recoil of the lungs. The vacuum this creates 'sucks' the pelvic organs up away from the pelvic walls, decompressing them. It also leads to a natural engagement of* mūla bandha *as the anterior pelvic muscles lift. It's a gentle, but immensely restorative, energising practice for postnatal recovery and can help to create sensations of uplift at any time when the pelvic organs feel dropped and draggy.*

If you are familiar with the yoga practice of *uḍḍīyāna bandha* (p.476), you will recognise the sensations that this practice creates. In yoga terms, the abdominal decompression is in fact *supta* (lying down) *uḍḍīyāna bandha*. Whilst these practices are first learnt lying down, their most useful application in daily life requires a shift into the vertical plane. The action of *mūla bandha* twinned with a well-angled pelvis and practised simultaneously with a drawing in and up of the abdominal muscles works to support the pelvic organs and the lower back. This is especially important when lifting and carrying babies or other heavy things. The most effective way to harness this practice in daily life is to use the exhalation as a cue to draw the pelvic muscles up and the abdominal muscles in prior to and during any lifting action. The cue from the exhalation works best if it comes together with a pressure from the heels and the balls of the feet down into the floor: as the feet press down on the exhalation, the pelvic muscles lift up. This cue can be learnt whilst practising in the lying down position described above, and then can be more easily applied when standing upright (see further practices below). As well as providing support and toning for the pelvic muscles, the practice of bringing *mūla bandha* into play at the end of the exhalation can be very energising.

'Aiming the Zone of Decompression'

This is the helpful name that Blandine Calais-Germain gives to a practice that directs the toning and decompressing effects of the previous practices into different layers of the abdomen.

1 Use the same base position instructions as for the abdominal decompression described above.

2 Then imagine that the abdomen is divided horizontally into three layers:
- Upper layer, above the navel,
- Middle layer, below the navel,
- Lower layer, right down to the groin.

3 With the next incoming breath, expand the ribs fully and exhale to create abdominal decompression (*uḍḍīyāna bandha*). Direct the zone of decompression into the upper level of the belly (the most difficult place to activate).

4 Inhale and pause, exhale.

5 On the next inhale, expand the ribs fully and then exhale to create abdominal decompression (*uḍḍīyāna bandha*). See if you can direct the zone of decompression into the middle level of the belly.

6 Repeat, and access the contents of the lower pelvis, decompressing the organs. Gently does it.

7 Return to full yogic breath, and then repeat the practices when you feel ready.

Once you are happy with this aspect of decompression, then you can work to decompress one organ at a time. For this practice, you need a clear image of exactly which organs are where. It is helpful to consult good diagrams that show you visually where everything is (e.g. Blandine Calais-Germain's *The Female Pelvis*, or Pauline Chiarelli's *Womens' Waterworks*), but an embodied understanding is even better. And if you have practised yogic pelvic muscle practices (chapter twenty), then you will already have a pretty clear sense of the positioning of the organs, situated as they are, above the site of the different yoga *mudrā* and *bandha* with which you are already familiar. As a reminder, the bladder and urethra are the organs you connect with when you practise *sahajolī mudrā* (the Clitoral tickle); *mūla bandha* (the Root lock) lifts your awareness up into the uterus and vagina; and *ashvini mudrā* (the Horse gesture) has awareness in the rectum and anus. Following the instructions for the previous practice, you can now begin to direct the zone of compression so that on the next exhalation you can close and lift up one of the following openings:

- The bladder and the urethra (without contracting the abdominal muscles)
- The uterus and the vagina (take care to relax the muscle which lifts the anus)
- The rectum and the anus (keep the buttocks relaxed).

Tips: *Since much of the healing effect of these practices depends upon the vacuum that 'sucks up' the pelvic organs in order to decompress them and relieve pressure on the pelvic muscles, it is important to ensure that other muscles aren't getting in on the act. Calais-Germain issues some clear guidance on the issue of suppressing neighbouring effects (synkinesis): 'You've probably noticed that other muscles come into play to pull up the pelvic organs. These are the abdominal muscles, the levator ani muscle (that lifts the anus), and the gluteal muscles (buttocks). Try to locate and relax them whenever you can in order to concentrate on the traction of the pelvic organs by the lungs alone' (Calais-Germain: 137).*

Not everyone is entirely convinced by Calais-Germain's contention that the drop in intra-abdominal pressure is responsible for any sense of decompression that may be experienced in the pelvic organs located low down in the pelvis. There is a sense of lifting of the intestines as a result of the 'vacuum' caused by the decrease in intra-abdominal pressure created by these practices. It could be that any effects on pelvic organs are in fact due to the contraction and lifting of the pelvic muscles rather than the drop in intra-abdominal pressure. But the combined effect certainly creates a welcome sense of relief, lightness and re-energising of the contents of the pelvis that can be a very welcome element of postnatal healing and support for pelvic organ shift later in life.

Combined explorations with decompression and arched back

Once you have some familiarity with the effects of the decompression exercises described above, then it can be very helpful to utilise the expansion of the rib cage (with elbows wide and pressed into the ground) in combination with different angles of the pelvis to find out what feels most secure and supportive for your pelvic organs. Follow the breathing instructions above to combine these explorations with differently angled lumbar curves.

Explorations in foot arch support (*pāda bandha*) for vaginal lift (*yoginī mūla bandha*), pelvic lift and pelvic organ support

These explorations follow helpfully from the previous explorations and can be done in two positions. It is easiest to start lying on your back on the floor, with your knees bent and feet flat on the floor about hip-width apart, with your ankles directly beneath your knees. Find a comfortable angle in your pelvis by alternately arching and flattening your back, until you rest in a way that feels like it best supports your pelvic organs.

As you breathe in and out, feel that you really have a deep connection with the Womb breath (p.153) and that there is movement in the belly with each breath. Connect this with the movement of the feet into the 'Foot lock' (p.472–3) to maximise uplift from the ground up. Lift the toes.

Feel how all this activity in the legs and feet, pressing down into the earth, encourages a feeling of lifting in the pelvis. Do nothing active to lift the pelvis, simply explore how conscious exhalation and active strength down through the feet and legs to push against the earth will work to lift the pelvis and the pelvic muscles.

INVERTED PRACTICES

NB Avoid during menstruation and only use occasionally during pregnancy (ideally with the support of an experienced yoga teacher) for the support of pelvic organ prolapse.

The value of these inversions is that they give immediate relief from the sensations of descent in the pelvic organs, and also create opportunities to experience ways to maintain a sense of supported lift through the breath, pelvic angle and feet and leg activity, all of which are easy to mobilise in an inversion. If you enjoyed the sensation of working with a block between the thighs in the semi-supine poses then make use of that in these explorations too. Everyone is different, so see what works for you.

Pelvic tilts with feet against wall

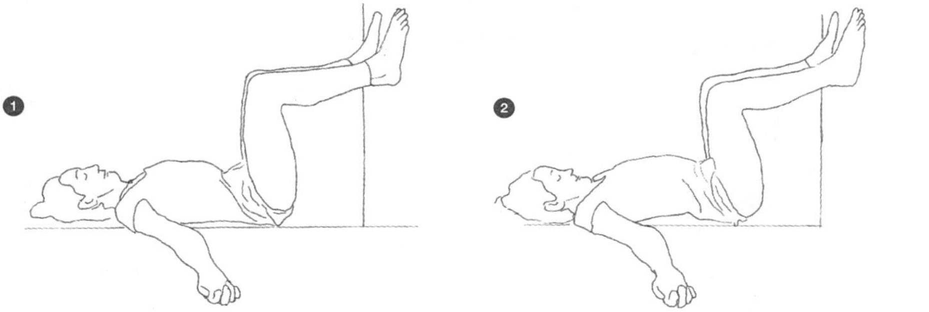

1 Place your mat perpendicular to the wall and lie down with your head away from the wall, your bum about fifty centimetres from the wall, and your knees bent. Place the soles of both feet onto the wall, about hip-width apart, with the toes pointing up to the ceiling. Ideally if you have the distances right, then the shins will be parallel to the floor and at a ninety-degree angle to the thighs. Move further up or down your mat until you can rest comfortably with your feet on the wall. Your hands can rest in *yoni mudrā* over your womb or be by your sides, with the elbows out wide as for the pelvic decompression exercises, whichever feels best for you. It may also be comfortable to clasp the hands behind the head.

2 As you exhale, activate your legs and push the heels and the balls of your feet into the wall, lifting and spreading out the toes. Keeping your lower back on the floor, let the tailbone lift a little as you explore what happens when you tilt the pelvis back, encouraging the lumbar curve to flatten against the mat (2). Then reverse the tilt as you inhale, so that you are arching the back (1). Feel all the while that these movements of the pelvis are in fact originating in the feet as they push against the wall on your exhale.

3 Repeat several times, keeping the bum on the floor, and then experiment with what degree of tilting and arching you can experience if you lift your bum just a little way up off the floor. Feel which of these positions seems to provide the most effective support for your pelvic organs.

Rolling pelvic lift with feet against wall

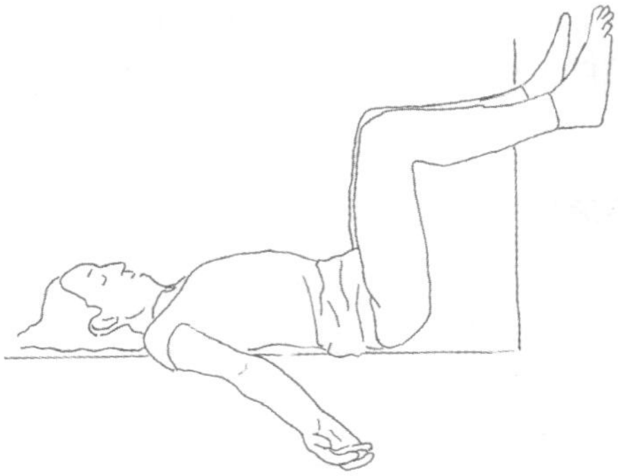

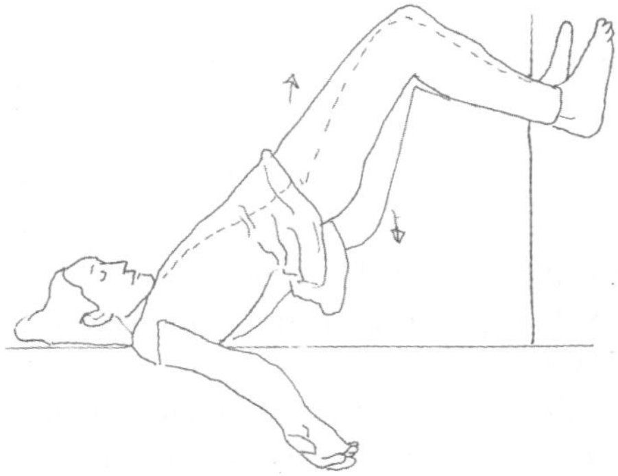

This is a real treat for pelvic organs that feel draggy and low. It proceeds further from the previous practice and uses the same basic position. It is usually easiest with this variation to bring the arms out to the sides and use the downward pressure of the elbows to help with the lift, or even to clasp the hands behind the head, but it can be more comfortable to have the arms down by the sides. See what works for you.

1 Use an exhalation and push the feet into the wall so strongly that the action of the feet and the legs lifts the pelvis and then the whole spine up away from the floor.

2 Inhale in this position and then use an exhalation combined with a healing breath as you lower the spine to the floor. It can be helpful to press the arms, wrists and hands into the floor to assist on the lift.

3 Repeat in this rhythmic way several times: exhaling as the pelvis and spine lift up, and inhaling in the inverted position. Exhale on the descent. When you find an angle of inversion that feels comfortable to you, remain there, breathing freely for as long as you can and maintain sufficient activity in the feet and legs to support the inversion. You may find that to stay comfortable in a longer hold you need to move your feet further up the wall.

Supported restorative pelvic lift with feet against wall and in Butterfly pose

This option provides support to maintain the previous posture in a restorative manner that requires no effort. The basic position is the same, but once you lift your bum up off the floor, put a bolster underneath the lower back to support the sacrum so that you can rest in the inversion as long as you like without effort. Sometimes it feels good to raise the height of support so that there is more of a sense of inverting the pelvic organs. If you make the pelvic support higher you may feel the need for an additional prop like a rolled blanket to support the lower back. Experiment with what works for you. Once you have a comfortable height you can remain for as long as you like, using all the breathing and decompression exercises described previously. It can also be helpful to shift the leg position by dropping the knees out to the sides and pressing the balls of the feet together as you exhale.

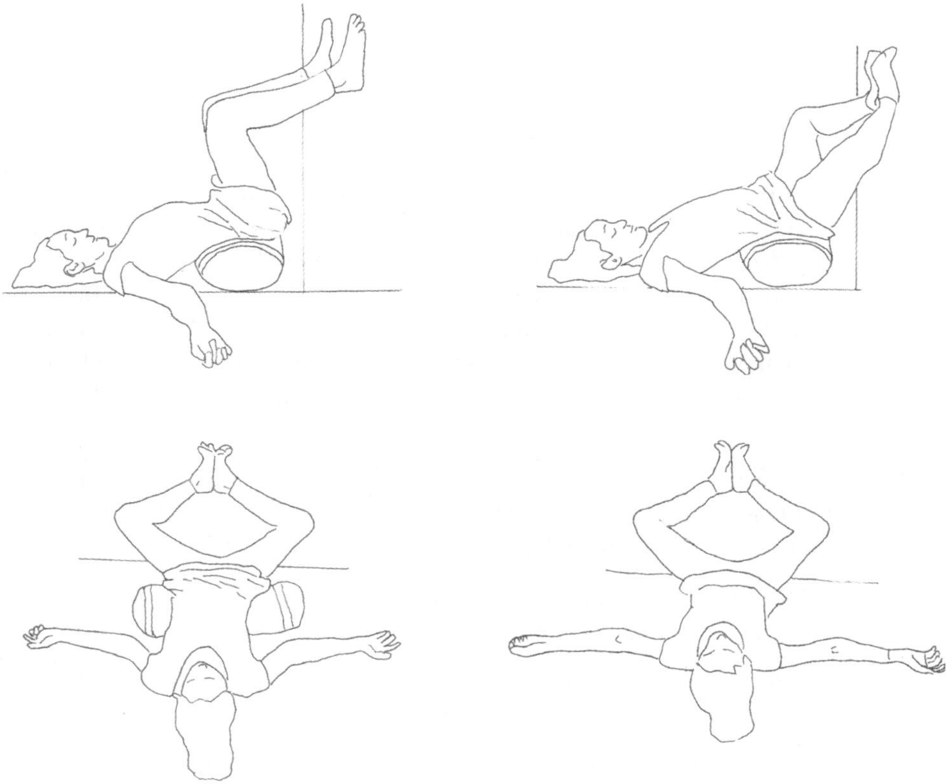

STANDING PRACTICES

Standing cat with *agnisāra kriyā*

NB Unsuitable during menstruation, pregnancy and the immediate postnatal period.

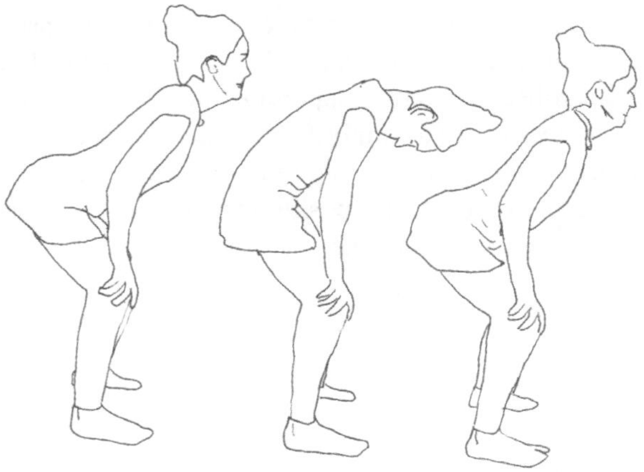

This practice combines powerful breath work with a rhythmic arching of the lower back. It is based on a practice originally devised by Christine Kent with the intention of maximising the beneficial anti-gravitational forces of inter-abdominal pressure created in the essence of fire purification practice (*agnisara kriyā*). Kent calls this 'Whole Woman Fire Breathing' and it integrates the pelvic tilt of the Cat pose with an uplifting exhaling lock that is known in yoga as *uḍḍīyāna bandha*. It is helpful to support her original practice with conscious use of the legs and the arches of the feet to direct supportive energy up into the pelvis.

1. Stand with your feet over hip-width apart and your knees bent. Lean very slightly forward and press the palms of the hands, and also the bases of the index fingers, onto the tops of the thighs, with the fingers pointing out to the sides.
2. As you inhale, lift your heart forward and arch your back, lifting your tailbone and allowing the abdominal muscles to move forward and down.
3. As you exhale, use your hands to create a very rounded back, and allow for the pelvic muscles and the pelvic organs to move upwards and inwards.
4. Start slowly with three repetitions and build up over a period of three weeks to a maximum of twenty breaths.

Pelvic tilts exploration and rolling pelvic lift with back against wall

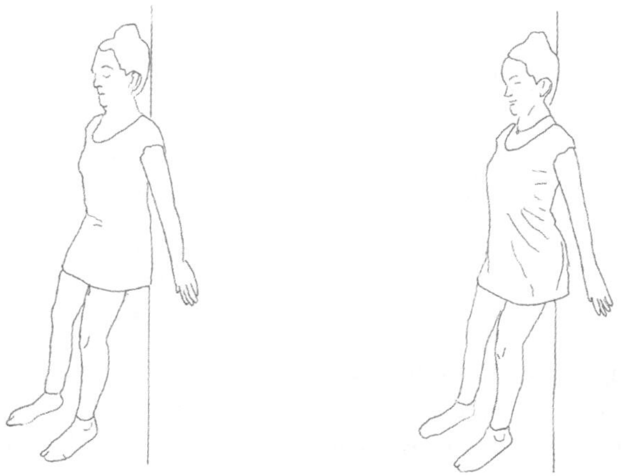

The basic position for both these practices is to stand with your back against the wall, feet hip-width apart and about fifty centimetres away from the wall, and knees bent to a level that activates the feet and legs without tiring them (usually a greater than ninety-degree angle is most sustainable). Have the back of the head and shoulders and the buttocks resting directly on the wall. Whatever natural lumbar curve is there, let that be present. It can be a helpful addition to place a yoga block (or a folded blanket pad about ten centimetres thick and thirty centimetres long) in between the thighs and to squeeze the inner thigh muscles gently in order to hold the prop in place. If this feels as if it helpfully engages supportive muscles through into the lower back and the pelvic muscles then it can be a good idea to practise at least some of the time with this prop in place, at least for this exploration, but also possibly for the semi-supine work too.

1 Circle the back of the sacrum around a few times to find a comfortable relation with the wall. Activate the toes and the arches of the feet by bringing the consciousness and energy into the feet. As the big toe, little toe and heels push into the floor on the exhalation, allow for the arches of the feet to lift and carry energy up into the pelvis. On the next exhale, push down into the heels and toes, and strengthen the legs in the bent position. Let the movement of the pelvis come directly from the feet.

2 For the pelvic tilts, allow for the exhalation to bring the natural lumber curve closer to the wall, and the inhalation to allow the back to arch a little more deeply. Play with the relationship between the curves and the tilts, using the exhalation to initiate the movement which brings the spine closer to the wall and the inhalation to arch the back, with the same quality of feeling as was present in the supine version of this exercise. The point of the exploration is to discover what feels like the most comfortable spinal curve for you and how best that can be supported by the action of the legs and the breath.

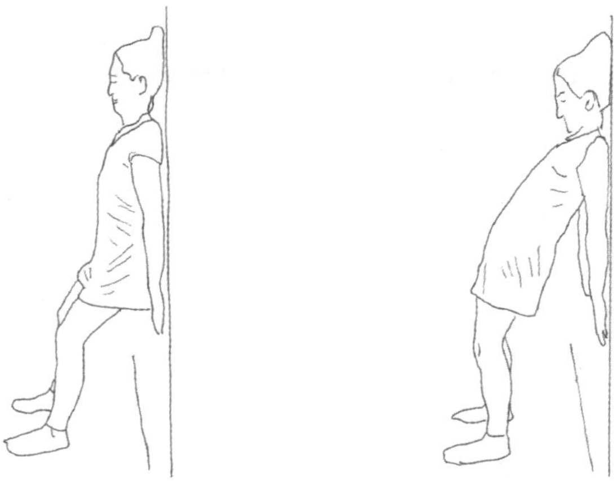

3 After the tilting explorations, for the rolling pelvic lift use the same combination of actions from the feet and the legs and the exhaling breath now to lift the pelvis up away from the wall and forward and up as far as is comfortable. Let the chin descend as this happens and keep the heels firmly pressed into the ground. When you have lifted the spine and pelvis as far away from the wall as feels comfortable for you, take a pause and, keeping the legs strong, breathe in. Use the exhaling breath to let the spine lengthen away from the back of the neck and return to contact with the wall, noticing any changes that may have occurred to the sensations in the pelvic organs on the way down. Repeat as often as feels comfortable for you, noticing what you learn about which angles of the pelvis and which level of lift feel more or less supportive for your pelvic organs.

Dynamic *taḍāsana* (Mountain pose) for pelvic organ support

For this practice, come away from the wall so you have space in front and behind you. Start by awakening the feet (pp.472–3): if our feet are alive and vital and breathing then so is the womb and her two sisters, the bladder and rectum. Living, breathing feet nourish and support the pelvic organs.

1 So, have the knees soft and the feet apart, at whatever width feels most comfortable for the pelvis. Tune into the rhythm of the breath. On the exhale, drop the weight into the backs of the heels. Especially be aware of dropping weight into the outer back curves of the heels and the little toe sides of the feet. Inhale and lift up all the toes, spreading them wide but keeping the ball of the big toe firmly grounded. Exhale, spread out all the toes and put them back on the ground, one at a time if possible.

Let your feet breathe in this way for a few rounds of breath, with the knees soft, until you get a clear sense of the outer boundaries of the feet: the back portions of the heels and the little toe side edges of the feet and the pads of all the toes. Imagine the footprint that your feet would leave if you were walking along the wet sand at the very edge of the ocean: a very clear, deep print from the heel, and a deep imprint also from the ball of the foot and the pad of the big toe. Feel how this footprint would leave a trace of the little toe edges of the feet and that the pad of each toe would be clearly marked in the wet sand, but there would be no print along the inner arches of the feet because they are so beautifully lifted, so from the deep print of the ball of the foot to the clear imprint of the heel would be an open space. Breathe into the arch of the foot and feel the inner ankle lifting and energy travelling up the inside of the legs into the pelvis. As the rest of the foot, the ball and the toe pads and the heel, all press firmly into the ground, the arch rises up, strong and powerful. Perhaps even have the big toes slightly turned inwards, and the heels a little wider, if this feels to you to help the vitalising function of the feet.

2 As you push down into the outer back heels of the feet, begin to notice what happens to the shins and the knees. If they roll in very slightly, notice this, and notice the action moving up into the thighs, so that there is a subtle slight inward rotation of the thigh bones that moves right into the pelvis. Track how this comes up into the back of the pelvis. Let the movement of this effect start from the feet, travel through the knees and then, as the thighs begin to roll slightly inwards, notice what happens to the joints on either side of the sacrum. Do they move outwards, to create a feeling of breadth across the sacrum? And what happens to the tailbone as this happens?

3 Track a train of movement, a river of connection between the activities in the feet, and the inward rotation of the shins, knees and thighs right up into the sacro-iliac joints. Notice what all this does to your tailbone. Does it move out a little? What happens to this tiny little remnant of your tail? Imagine, were you to have a great plume of a fluffy tail like a delighted young collie dog, how it would be lengthening and lifting out proud and free behind you. Can you feel how this creates freedom across the lower part of the belly, giving space for the womb and the other pelvic organs as the tail moves out behind, shifting the angle in the pelvis? Recall the experiences at the start of the semi-supine explorations when you felt the security that comes to the pelvic organs if the feet and legs are really actively engaged in transmitting energy and strength up into the pelvis, and carrying the weight of the pelvis at precisely the most comfortable angle to give optimal support to the organs within.

4 With the knees slightly bent, but the legs feeling strong and the feet fully alive, allow now for the lengthened tail to drop and spaciousness to open out between the sacrum and the last lumbar vertebrae – letting the space in the deepest curve of the back be open and fluid. And then allow the spine above to extend towards the heavens, even as the heels and the balls of the feet connect well with the earth. Be aware of a dynamic relation between the earthing of the feet and the upward lift of the skull. With this awareness allow the pelvis to move freely into its optimal angles, perhaps not even settling completely into stillness.

This basic exploration of pelvic angle in standing position forms the foundation for standing womb salutes, for example Snake circles the womb (pp.168–9) and Standing womb pilgrimages (pp.170–2) in chapter six.

CHAPTER TWENTY-TWO

nurturing and freeing energy

BREAST CARE AND ENERGY NURTURE PRACTICE (DEER EXERCISE)

NB Not recommended during menstruation or pregnancy.

This Taoist practice provides a practical and effective self-help remedy for pre-menstrual stresses, period pain, troubling hormonal fluctuations at perimenopause, and infertility. It is described in detail by Lisa Bodley in her book, *Recreating Menstruation*, and also appears in Pope and Bennett's *The Pill* (see further reading and resources at the end of this chapter).

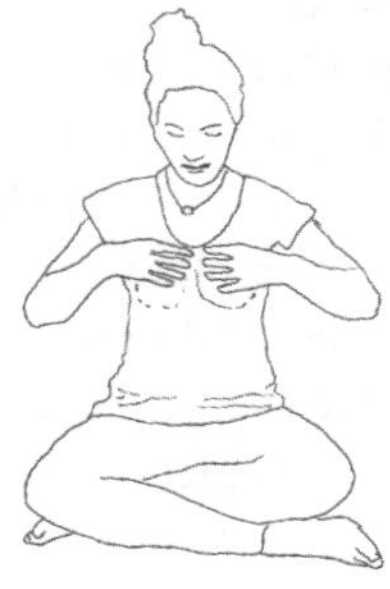

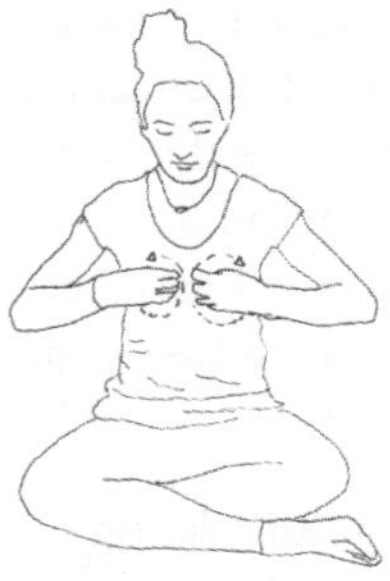

1 Sit with the heel of one foot tucked into the vulva, or kneel on a bolster so as to bring slight pressure into the vaginal opening.

2 Warm your hands by rubbing them vigorously together. Place them over the breasts. Pause to feel warmth coming into the breasts. Bring mental focus inside the breasts. Send awareness out through the breasts to meet the warmth coming in. Repeat up to three times until consciousness is fully in breasts and the breasts feel warm.

3 Lightly rub fingertips in upward and outward circles, in time with the breath, around the breasts, avoiding the nipples. The hands travel together up the inside of the breasts toward the face, then outwards, downwards, inwards, and upwards again. Opinions vary about the best numbers, but Pope and Bennett (following Lisa Bodley) suggest minimum 36 and maximum 360 circles of the breasts. Start with the minimum number to gauge the effects of practice on you at this time. Ultimately, it is more enjoyable not

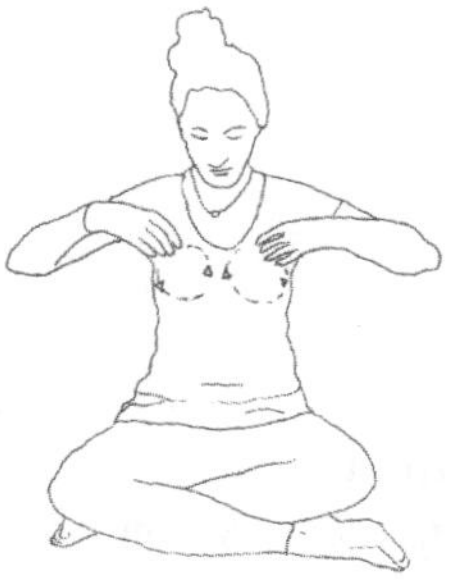

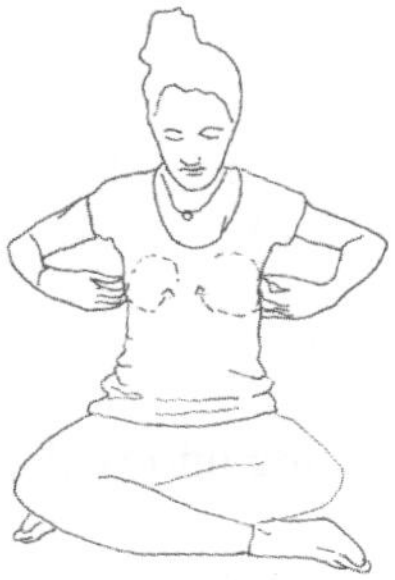

to bother counting, but to set a timer or to listen (or sing) to a piece of music that lasts the right amount of time for your chosen number of rounds.

4 After completing the desired number of breast circles, rest your hands in your lap. Make two fists by encircling thumbs in the other fingers. Exhale, practise Vaginal root lock (*mūla bandha*, p.474) and bring the focus of mental attention up to the third eye (between the eyebrows). During the contraction, try to keep the anal sphincter and stomach muscles relaxed while squeezing and lifting only the vaginal muscles. At end of exhale, relax the root lock and breathe easily.

5 Return to step one and repeat whole practice once more. It can be done twice a day.

COMPLETE LIBERATION OF ENERGY SERIES (*PŪRṆA PAVANAMUKTĀSANA* OR PPMA)

This remarkable sequence combines three approaches to PPMA: its basis is the series first taught by Paramahamsa Satyananda, founder of the Bihar School of Yoga and it includes refinements and improvements developed by Mukunda Stiles, originator of Structural Yoga Therapy. It also includes several additional therapeutic practices developed by an inspirational and very humble yoga teacher who wishes to remain anonymous, and a couple of versions derived from the Shadow yoga warm-ups. What follows synthesises the best of all these approaches.

The sequence is best experienced as a whole, working through each movement in turn to energise the entire body. It is possible also to focus on a specific area. For example, if your neck and shoulders are stiff, work with the practices for that part of the body (pp.506–7). At a physical level, these practices can be used as effective remedies for localised aches and pains.

Each practice usually involves a pair of movements synchronised with breath. The actions bring every joint of the body through its full range of motion, while the breath synchronisation focuses the mind and releases blocked energy. The breath synchronisation and mental focus are just as important as the movements, so before beginning each practice, establish an easy rhythm of full breath. *Ujjāyī* breath (pp.134–5) is the ideal accompaniment for PPMA. Repeat each pair of movements up to seven times in time with your breath.

The movements are grouped around a recommended base position, but if an alternative pose feels more comfortable (for example if you prefer to work from a chair), then do what suits you best.

A: From stick pose

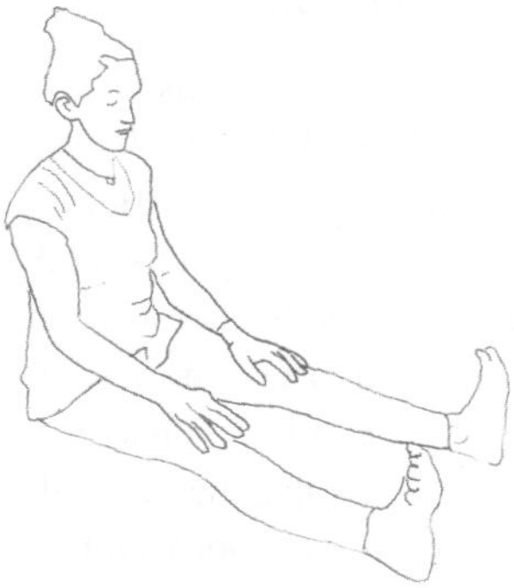

Sit with your legs straight out in front of you, feet relaxed, hands resting on your knees. Sit on a bolster or block if needed for correct alignment of the lower back.

Toe stretching / curling

INHALE, spread toes as wide apart from each other as possible, pushing into heels.

EXHALE, curl toes under and squeeze.

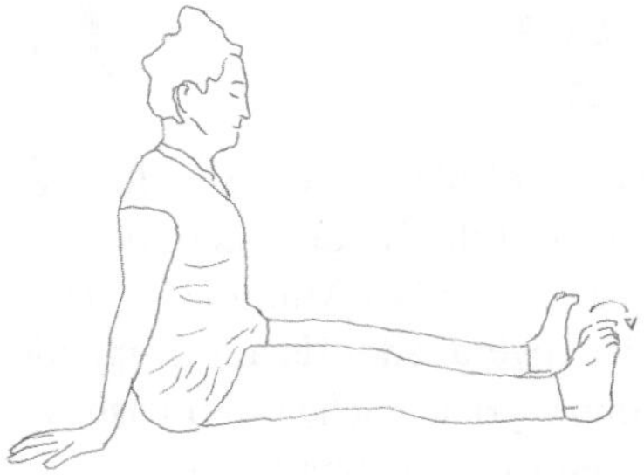

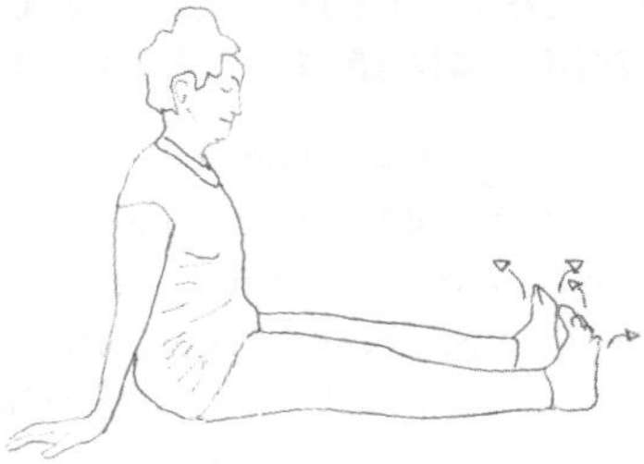

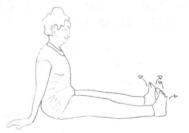

Ankle stretching / bending

INHALE, push into heels and draw fronts of feet back towards head.
Toes are relaxed.

EXHALE, draw heels towards back towards pelvis and stretch fronts of feet.
Toes are relaxed.

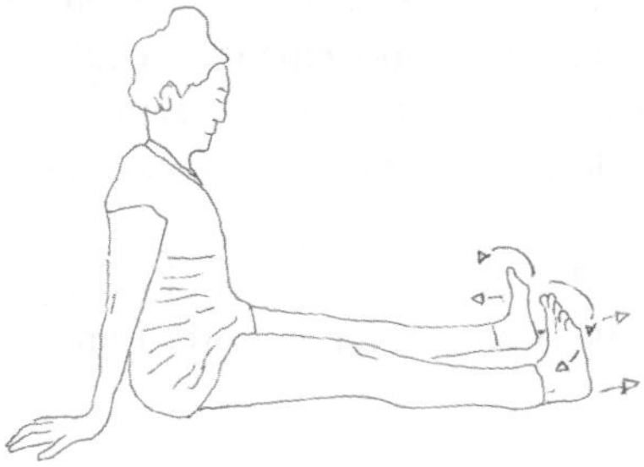

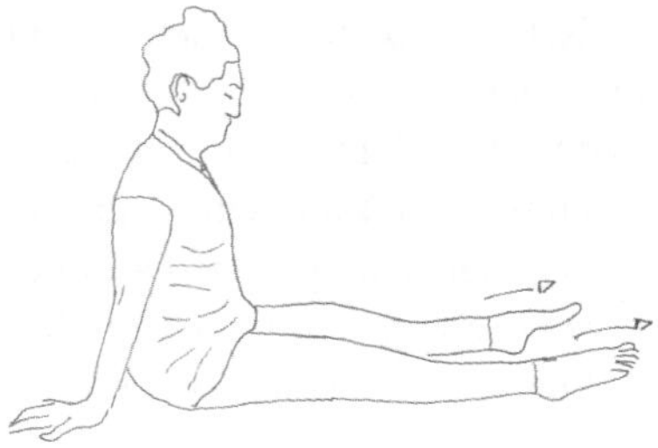

Ankle eversion / inversion

Keep heels pushed away and feet upright.

INHALE, draw outsides of feet towards each other, bring inner arches closer together and stretch outsides of ankles, keeping big toes vertical.

EXHALE, push inner arches of feet away and draw outsides of feet back towards head, feel strength along outsides of legs, keeping big toes vertical.

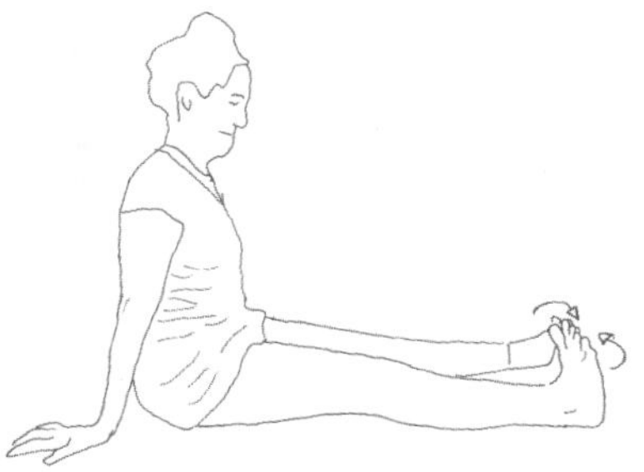

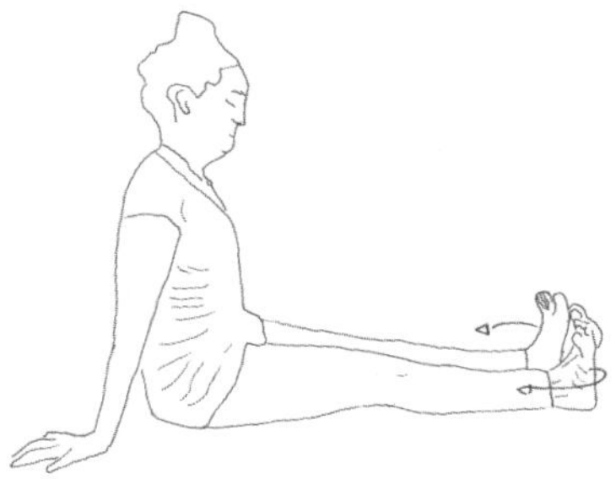

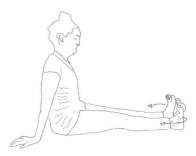

Ankle rotation

One round of breath (inhale and exhale) completes one complete circle.

INHALE, draw semi-circle with toes, both feet moving clockwise towards head, heels pushing away.

EXHALE, draw semi-circle with both feet moving clockwise away from head, toes pointing down.

After seven rounds, repeat in opposite direction.

If time permits, this can also be repeated with the feet moving in opposite directions (as if one of the clocks was going forwards and one was going backwards)

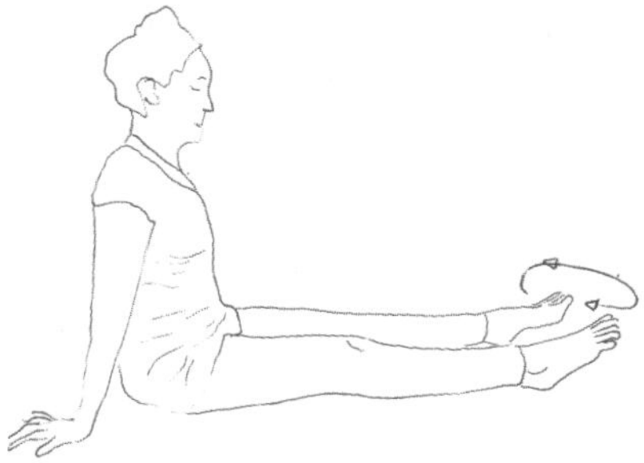

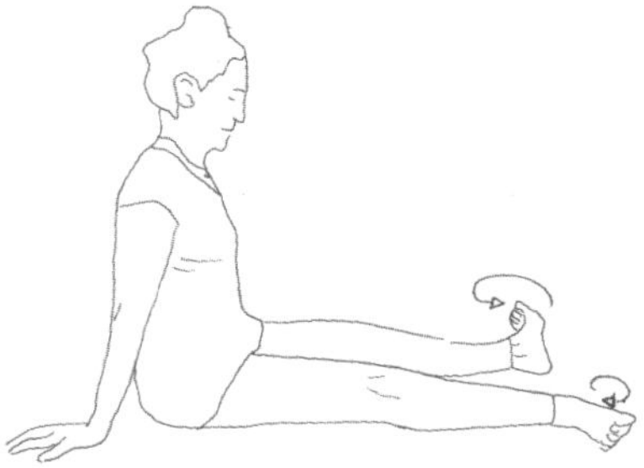

Knee flexion / extension

EXHALE, bend knee, hold thigh close to knee with both hands from beneath and draw heel towards buttock, moving thigh towards outer side of belly.

INHALE, continue to hold leg as knee straightens and push into heel.

After seven rounds swap sides.

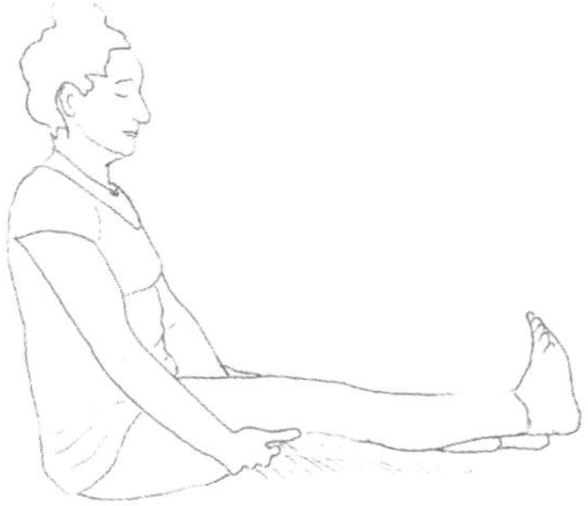

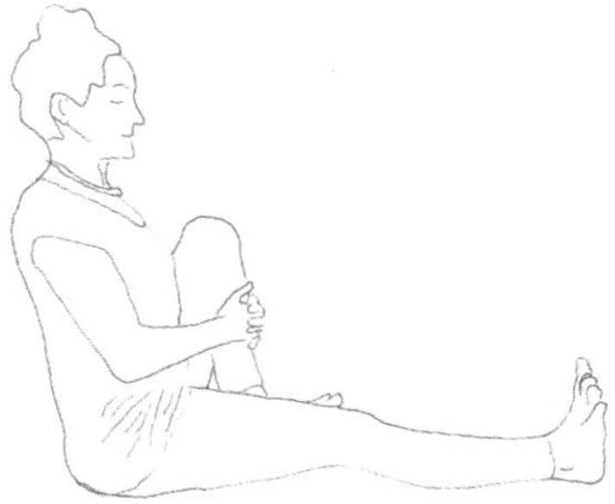

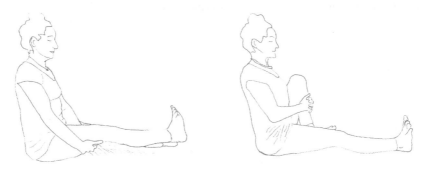

Hip external / internal rotation

Bring hands to floor behind you to provide support and lean back.

Externally rotate left leg so outside edge of foot moves towards floor.

INHALE, slide leg outward, keeping foot flexed, with outer edge close to floor and knee straight.

Internally rotate left leg so inside edge of foot moves towards floor and left buttock lifts from floor.

EXHALE, slide leg inwards, back to the start position, keeping foot flexed, with inner edge close to floor and knee straight.

Repeat up to seven rounds on left and then swap sides.

If strength permits, practise with the leg held a little above the floor throughout. To build strength and stability in this range of movement, fully engage buttock muscles.

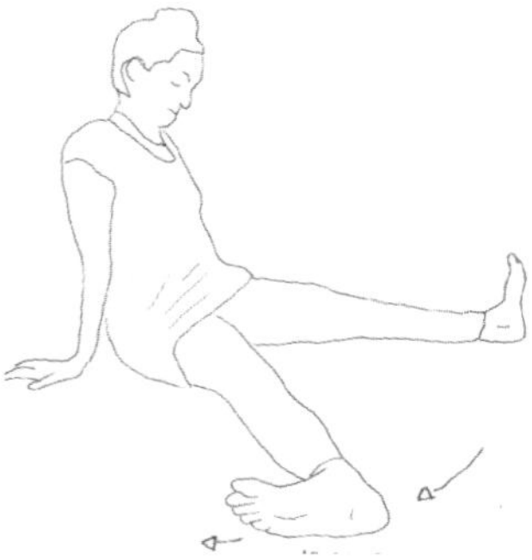

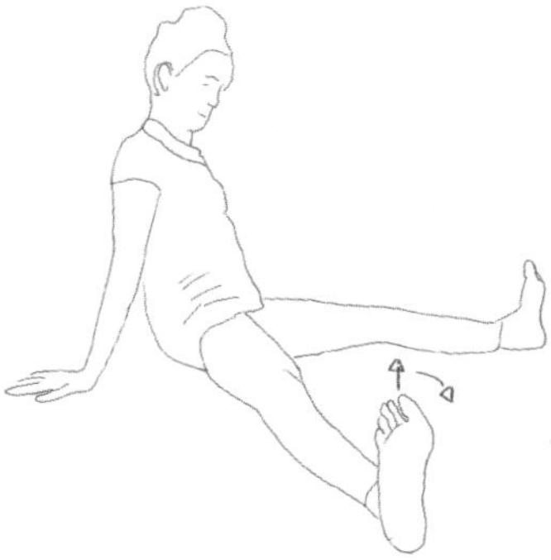

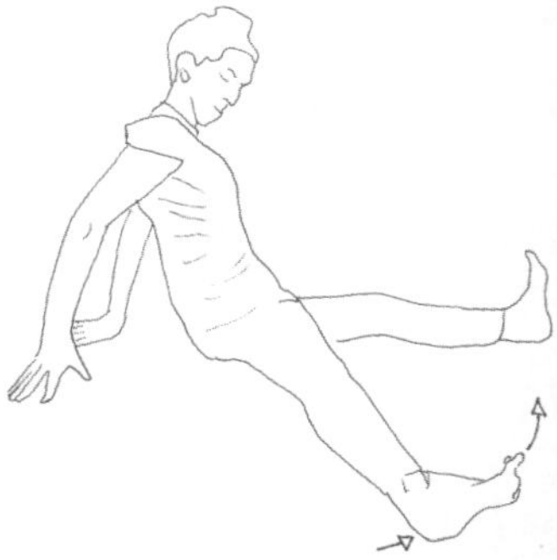

Rocking boat

Bring legs and feet close together and sit tall with knees straight and feet flexed. Squeeze inner thighs together.

INHALE, rock weight into left sitting bone and lift right side of pelvis by contracting waist on right side. Exhale, release and lower pelvis to floor.

INHALE, rock weight into right sitting bone and lift left side of pelvis by contracting waist on left side. Exhale, release and lower pelvis to floor.

Repeat seven times.

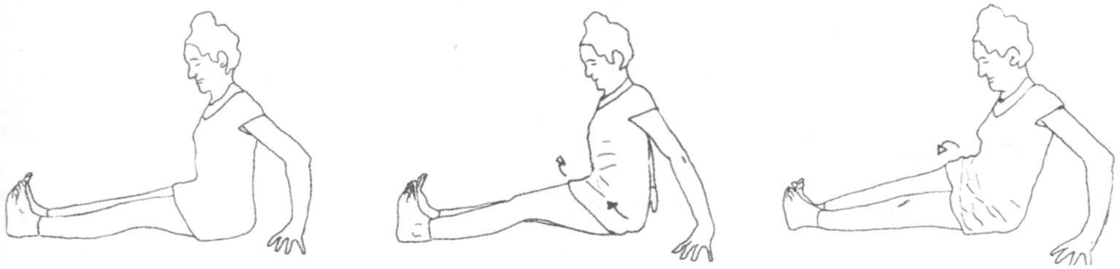

B: From Butterfly pose

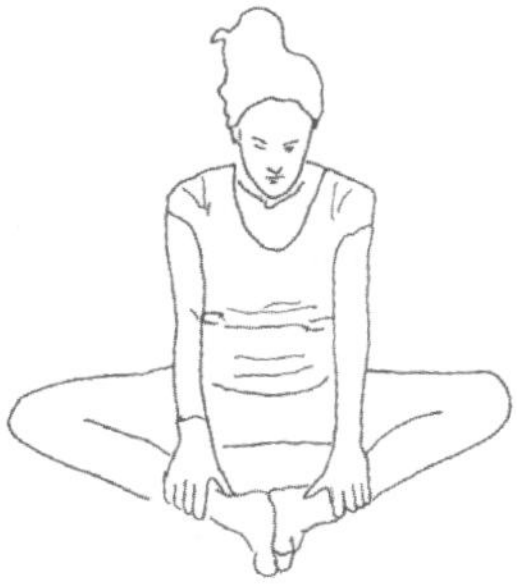

Bring soles of feet together at whatever distance from vulva is comfortable. Hands rest on feet or hips.

Butterfly circles

Add in the full Butterfly womb pilgrimage (p.167) at this point. Combine feet breathing (pp.166–7) with hip circling on a second round of repetitions if time permits.

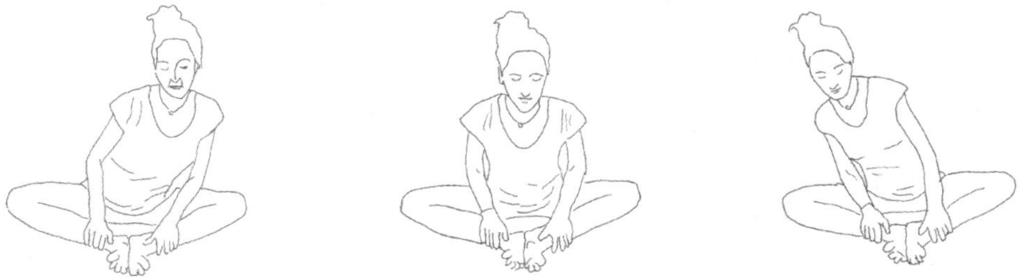

Rocking baby

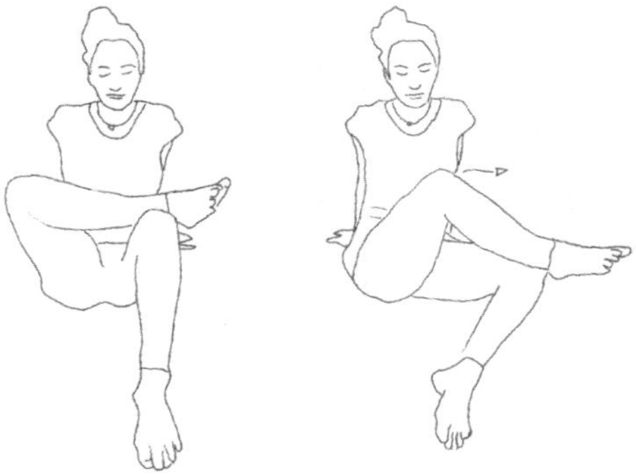

Bend right knee, place sole of right foot on the floor. Lean back and support weight on hands on floor behind buttocks.

Bend left knee and rest outside of left ankle on right thigh, or knee.

Keep spine straight.

INHALE, rock right leg over to right side.

EXHALE, rock right leg over to left side.

Repeat seven times then repeat on other side.

C: From Cat pose

Spinal flexion and extension on all fours

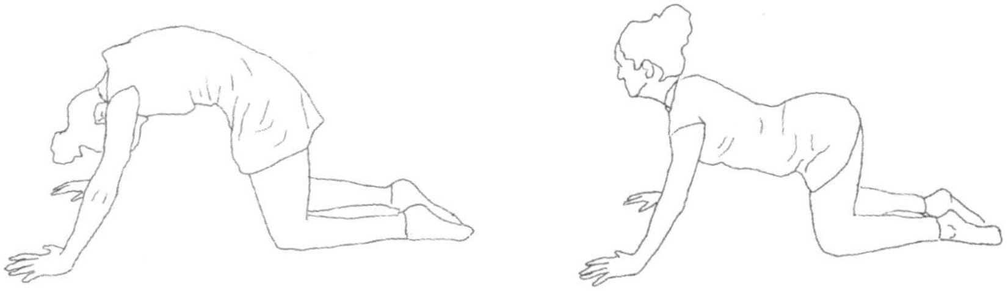

Have the hands slightly ahead and wider than shoulders. Elbows slightly bent. Knees are hip-width apart. Fingers are spread wide.

EXHALE, round back, lengthen spine and tuck in chin.

INHALE, lift heart, lengthen and arch spine and roll tops of shoulders back and down.

Hip and knee flexion and extension

Use the same base position as for flexion and extension above.

EXHALE, round back, tuck in chin, bend knee and tuck it in towards belly.

INHALE, straighten leg out behind you level with the pelvis, keeping foot flexed.

Repeat on the other side.

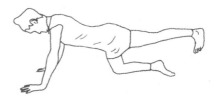

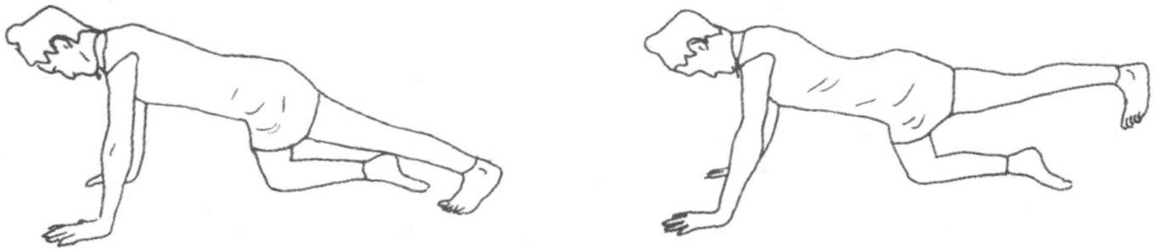

Hip adduction / abduction

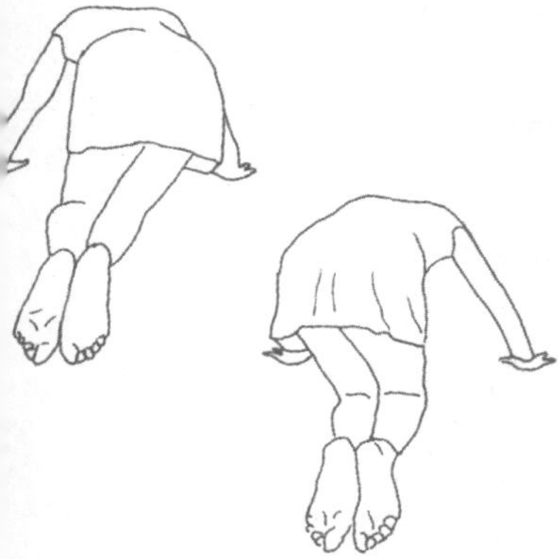

Use the same base position, but squeeze knees and thighs together throughout this practice.

INHALE, lower hips to right side, keeping buttocks in line with knees.

EXHALE, raise hips back to start position.

Repeat on left side.

Alternate between left and right sides for seven rounds.

D: From kneeling

Kneel back on your heels or on a bolster, with your knees together.

Hand stretches / clenches

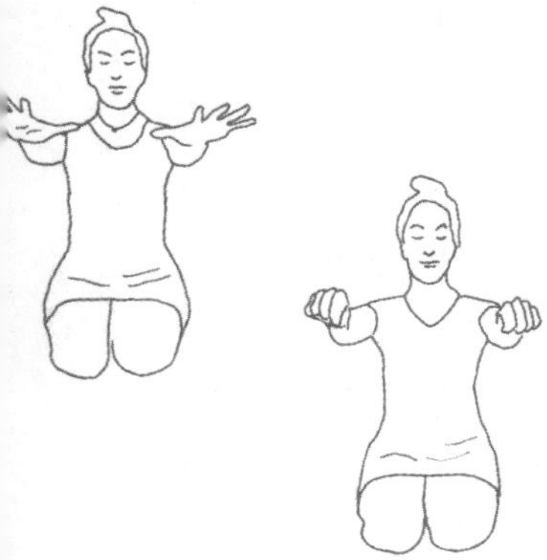

Maintain arms as close to shoulder height and width as is comfortable for you throughout.

INHALE, spread fingers and thumbs as wide apart as possible.

EXHALE, tuck thumb in and clench fingers around it, squeezing tight. Hold for one round of breath (inhale and exhale), then release.

Wrist bends

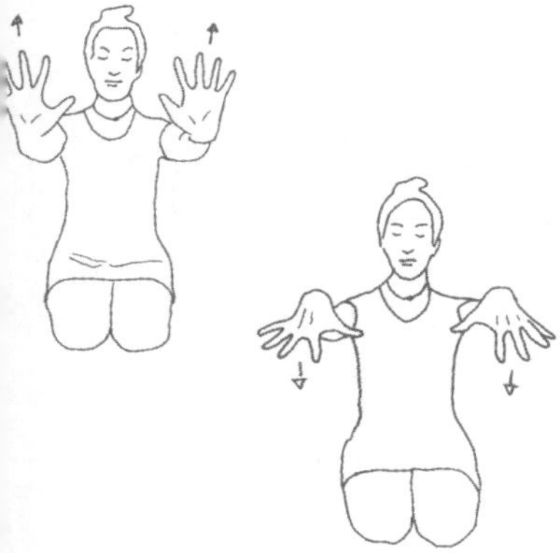

Maintain arms as close to shoulder height and width as is comfortable for you throughout.

INHALE, push into heel of hands and point fingers and thumbs upwards.

EXHALE, point fingers and thumbs downwards.

Repeat up to seven rounds.

Wrist side bends

Maintain arms as close to shoulder height and width as is comfortable for you throughout, palms facing down, fingers straight.

INHALE, draw outer edges of hands (little finger sides) towards outer edges of forearms.

EXHALE, draw inner edges of hands (thumb sides) towards inner edges of forearms.

Repeat seven rounds.

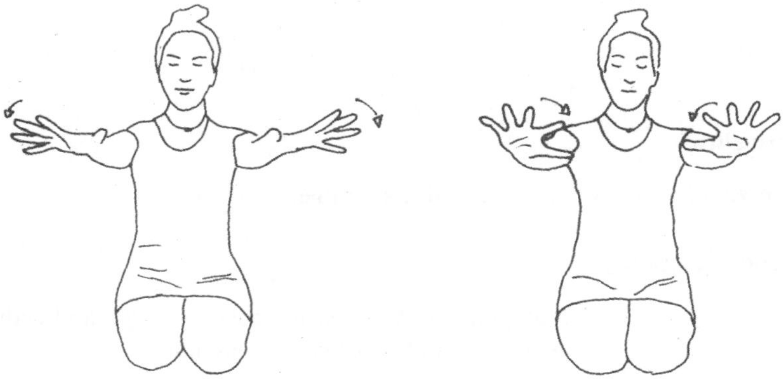

Wrist rotations

Maintain arms as close to shoulder height and width as is comfortable for you throughout, thumbs tucked in and fingers curled around thumbs.

One round of breath (inhale and exhale) completes one complete circle.

INHALE, move fists in semi-circle downwards and outwards.

EXHALE, move fists in semi-circle upwards and inwards.

After seven rounds, repeat in opposite direction.

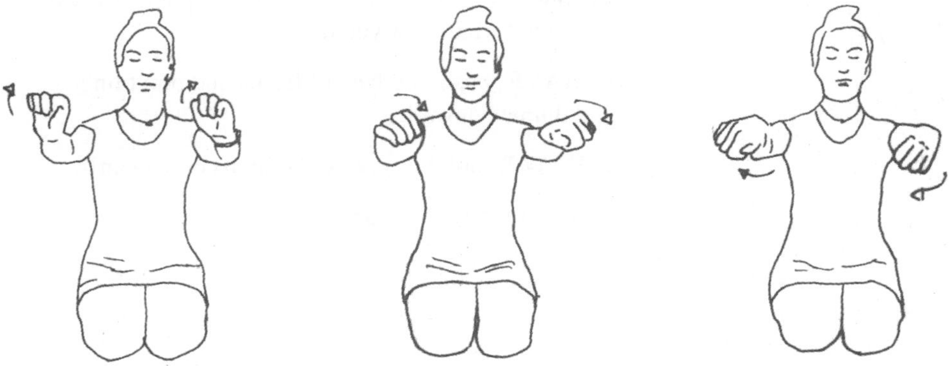

Intense wrist bends with shoulder circles

Hold both arms out straight. Make two fists with thumbs inside.

EXHALE, bend the wrists in towards each other.

INHALE, keeping wrists bent at ninety degrees, inhale and open arms out wide, bring arms behind back at shoulder height.

EXHALE, inwardly rotate shoulder and bend elbows, still keeping wrists at ninety degrees. Draw fists forward under armpits to return to start position.

Repeat seven rounds, keeping wrists bent throughout.

Elbow bends

Maintain elbows as close to shoulder height and width as is comfortable for you throughout.

INHALE, straighten elbows to bring hands to shoulder height, palms up.

EXHALE, bend elbows to bring fingertips to shoulder tops.

After four repetitions, include an additional exhale and soft release as the elbow, come into the straight position. Repeat three further rounds.

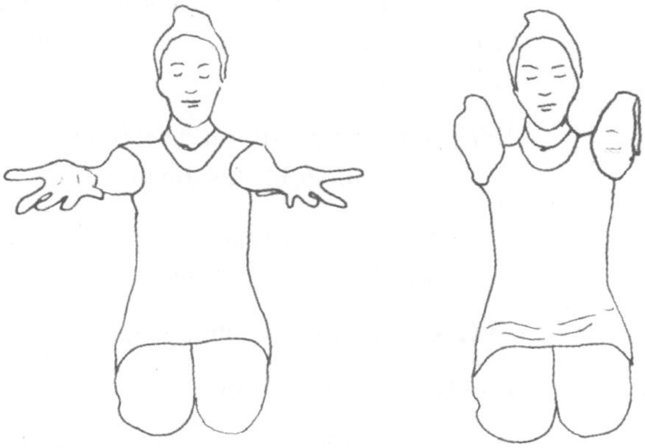

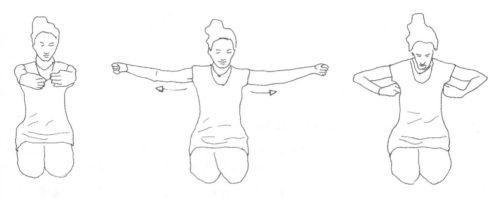

Shoulder circling

Maintain elbows bent with fingertips lightly resting on edges of shoulder tops throughout. One round of breath (inhale and exhale) completes one complete circle.

INHALE, bring elbows together in front of chest and lift as high as possible. Exhale, as elbows lower bring them wide out to sides and then as close together behind back as possible.

After seven rounds, repeat in opposite direction.

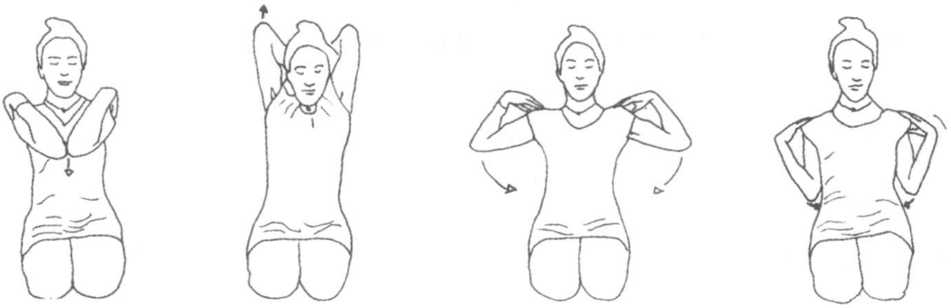

Shoulder external / internal rotation

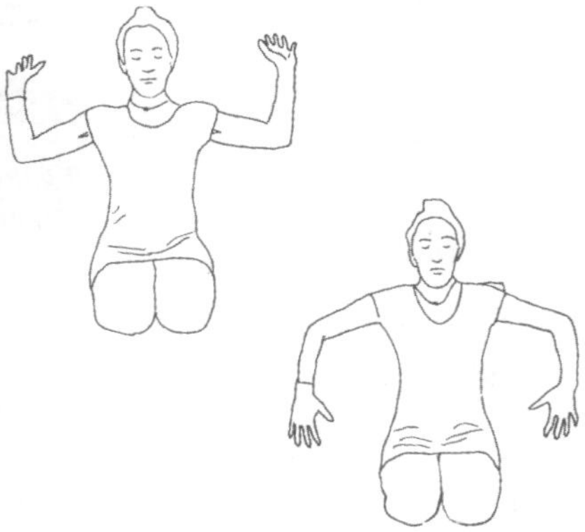

Maintain elbows wide out to sides as close to shoulder height as is comfortable for you throughout.

INHALE and bring forearms vertical with hands (palms facing forward) above elbows, at right angles to upper arms.

EXHALE, lower hands, keeping forearms vertical at right angles to upper arms.

Repeat seven rounds.

Shoulder extension / flexion

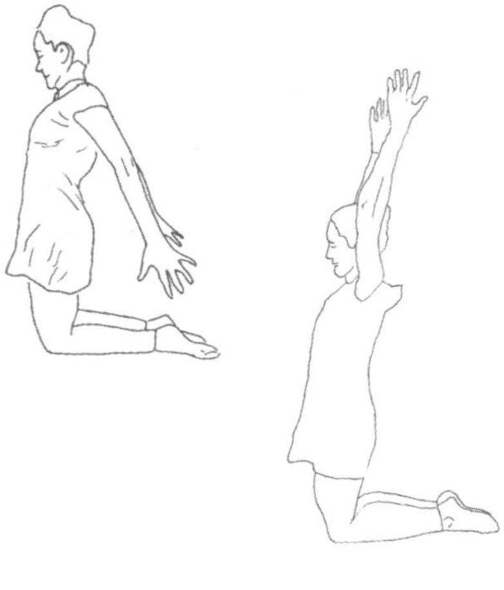

Rise up on knees to give clearance for hands. Keep arms straight at shoulder width throughout. Palms face each other.

INHALE, lower arms and bring them behind back, drawing shoulder blades together.

EXHALE, move arms in a forward arc, reaching arms above head, aiming to bring them in line or behind ears.

INHALE as arms reach highest point.

EXHALE to lower arms.

Repeat the whole exercise three times.

Shoulder-opening arcs

INHALE, squeeze shoulder blades together and down the back. Reach into fingertips with palms facing forwards, and extend arms out to the sides and above head, keeping arms back behind ears and shoulder blades squeezed together throughout.

EXHALE, lower arms down to side, keeping arms back behind ears and shoulder blades squeezed together throughout.

Repeat three rounds.

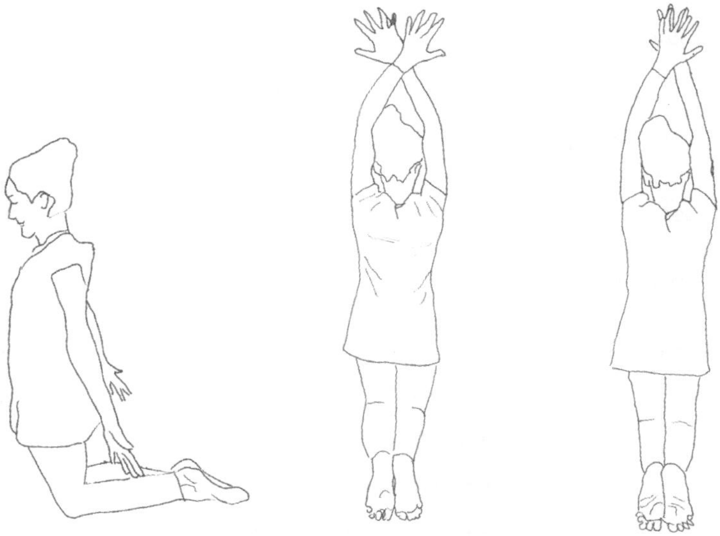

Shoulder releases with sound

INHALE, squeeze tops of shoulders right up to ears. Hold tight.

EXHALE, release shoulders down with a loud HA!

Repeat three times.

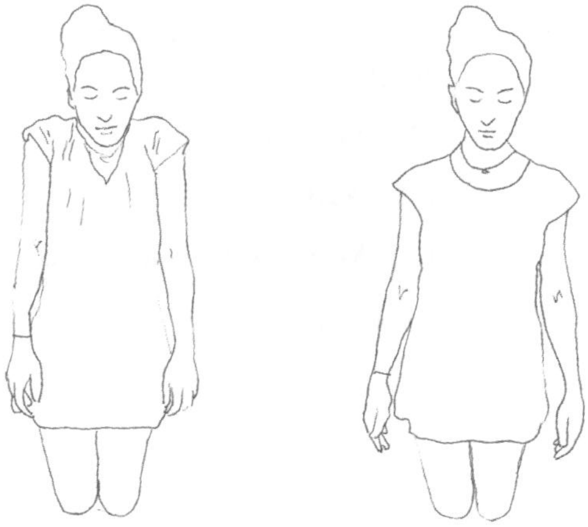

E: From easy cross-legged pose

Cross legs so that leg corresponding to currently dominant nostril breath is in front.

Spinal flexion / extension

Rest hands on knees.

EXHALE, tuck in chin and tailbone, round spine.

INHALE, lifting breastbone and head, move spine forward.

Repeat seven rounds.

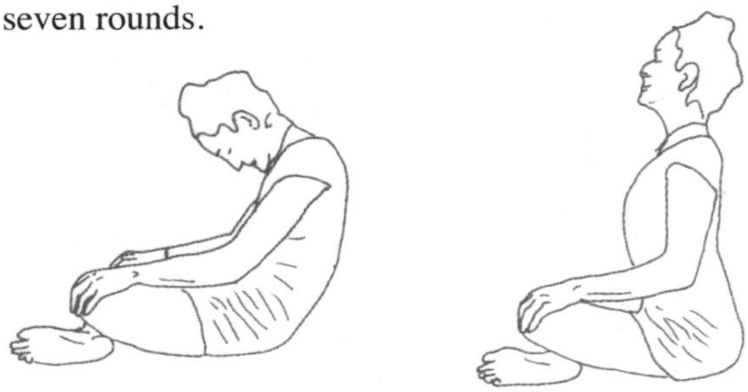

Spinal side bends

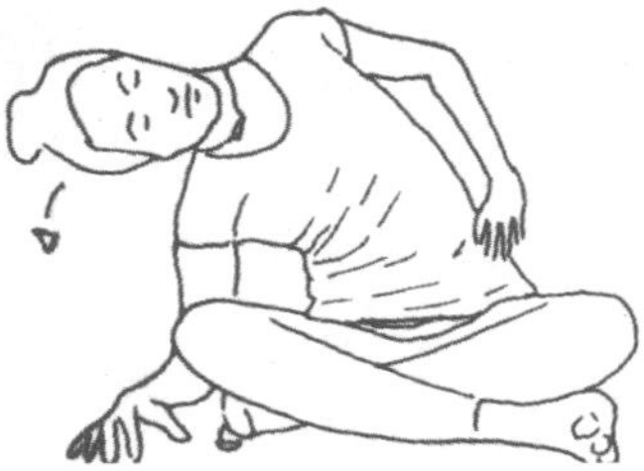

Place right hand on right hip and left hand on floor at left side.

INHALE, sit tall.

EXHALE, bend to right side, keeping chest open and right hand on the floor.

Swap hands and repeat on left side.

Alternate between sides to repeat seven rounds.

Spinal rotation

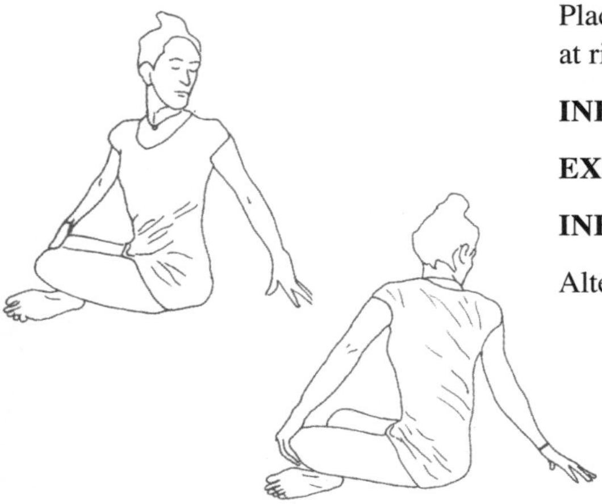

Place left hand on left knee and right hand on floor at right side.

INHALE, sit tall.

EXHALE, twist to right side, keeping chest open.

INHALE, return to start position.

Alternate between sides to repeat seven rounds.

NB at this point, it is wise to swap the cross of the legs.

Neck flexion / extension

INHALE, sit tall, lift chin and lengthen neck.

EXHALE, drop chin to chest.

Repeat seven rounds.

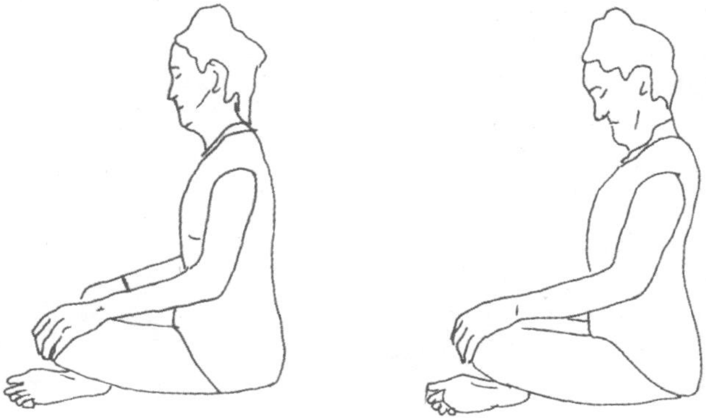

Neck side bends left and right

INHALE, sit tall, lengthen neck.

EXHALE, bend neck, lowering right ear towards right shoulder while keeping face forwards. Inhale return to central position.

Alternate on each side to repeat seven rounds.

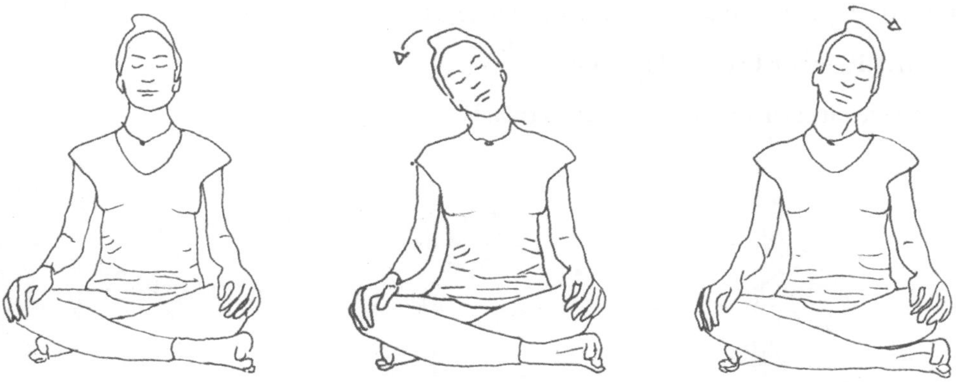

Arm-assisted neck side-bends

INHALE, sit tall, lengthen neck and extend arm corresponding to dominant nostril breath high above head. Exhale, bend elbow, cradling crown of head in crook of arm. Hook middle finger into ear hole,

EXHALE, bend neck slightly forwards very slowly indeed, allowing weight of arm to arc downwards and across body towards opposite side. Wait at lowest comfortable point of arc. Breathe up to five rounds of breath. Inhale, very slowly return to central position.

Repeat on other side.

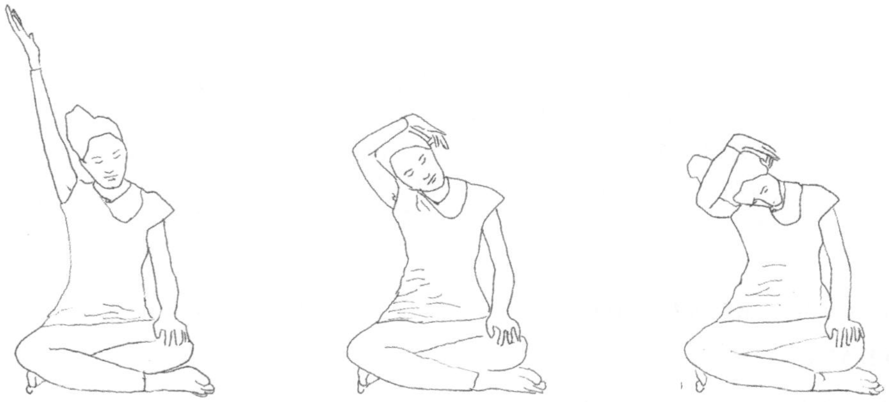

Neck rotation

INHALE, sit tall, lengthen neck.

EXHALE, turn head to right, keeping chin level.

INHALE, return to central position.

Alternate on each side to repeat seven rounds.

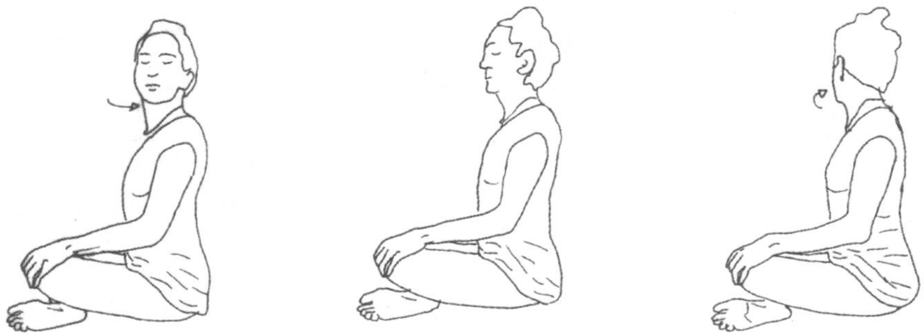

POSES TO UNBLOCK THE LIFE FORCE ENERGY (*ŚAKTI BANDHAS*)

These rhythmic movements free stagnant energy from the core of the body, build strength and promote mobility and vitality. Use *ujjāyī* breath (pp.134–5) with the practices and repeat up to seven times or more if the mood takes you.

Womb pilgrimage (*cakki calanāsana*)

This first and most effective energy block release practice is described on p.164.

Pulling the rope

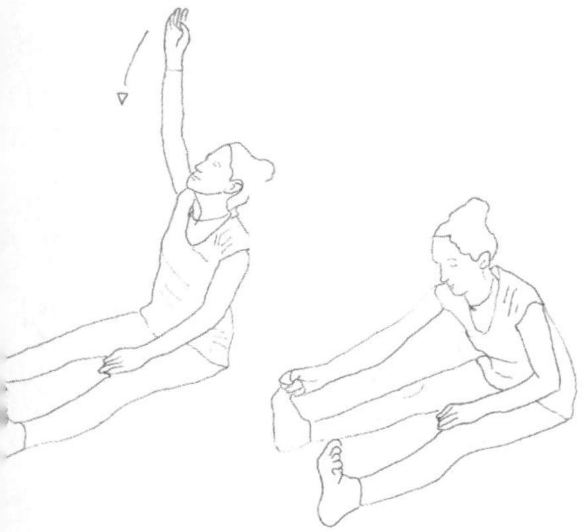

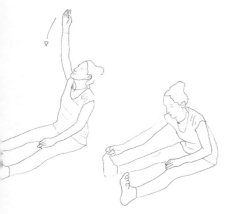

Sit with legs out straight and feet flexed. Keep arms straight throughout.

INHALE, reach right arm forward and straight up, clenching fist as if grabbing a rope.

EXHALE, draw right arm down strongly.

Alternate on both sides to repeat seven rounds.

Dynamic spinal twist

Sit with legs out straight and feet flexed, or if lower back is not comfortable, bend the knees. Keep arms straight throughout.

INHALE, sit tall.

EXHALE, reach right arm across the body towards left foot.

INHALE, come back to centre and sit tall.

EXHALE, reach left arm across the body towards right foot.

INHALE, come back to centre and sit tall.

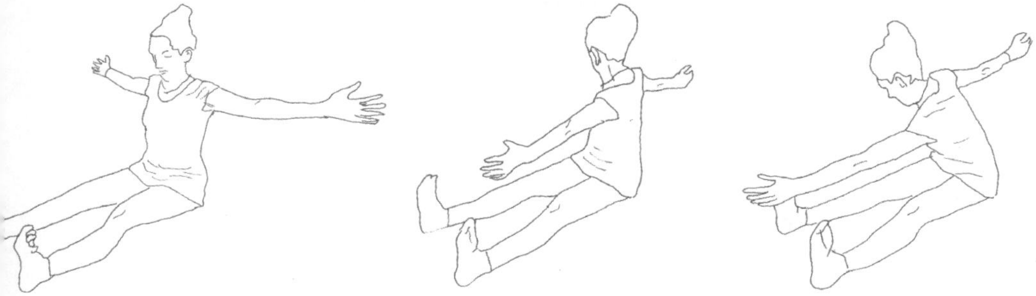

Rowing the boat

Sit with legs out straight and feet flexed, or if lower back is not comfortable, bend the knees.

Bend elbows and clasp hands as if holding oars.

INHALE, sit tall.

EXHALE, reach both hands forward until arms straighten.

INHALE, come back to centre and sit tall.

Repeat with a rowing action, seven times.

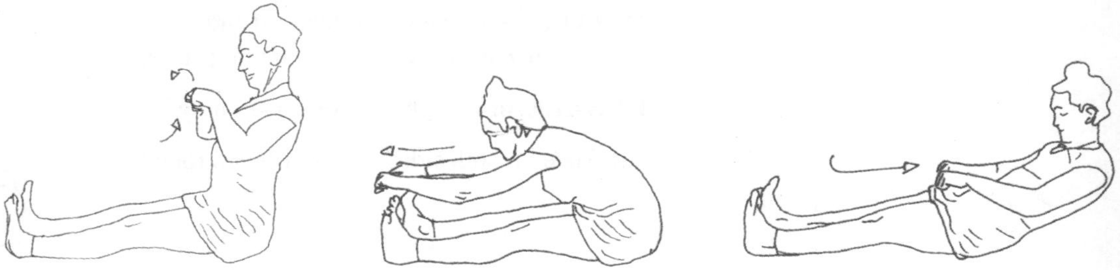

Pumping water (easy version)

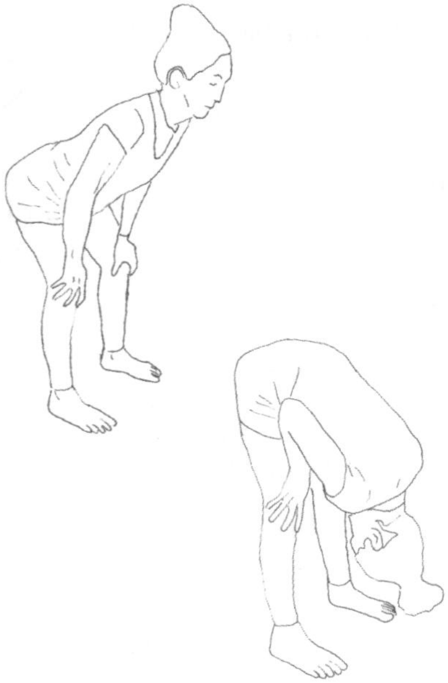

Stand with feet hip-width apart or wider, parallel or very slightly turned out (as if at 'five to one' on the clock).

EXHALE, bend knees and lower into a comfortable squat with hands on knees, elbows bent.

INHALE, lower bum, lift head and chest, lengthen spine, look up, straighten elbows. Knees stay bent.

EXHALE, lower head and chest, bend elbows, look down. Knees stay bent.

Repeat up to seven times or more.

Pumping water (deeper version)

Stand with feet hip-width apart or wider, parallel or very slightly turned out (as if at 'five to one' on the clock).

EXHALE, bend knees and lower into a deep squat with hands holding insides of feet, fingers tucked under arches, elbows bent.

INHALE, lower bum, lift head and chest, lengthen spine, look up. Heels and outsides of feet stay in contact with floor.

EXHALE, raise bum, lower head and chest, straighten elbows, look down. Knees stay bent. Heels and outsides of feet stay in contact with floor.

Repeat up to seven times or more.

Greeting squats

Stand with feet hip-width apart or wider, parallel or very slightly turned out (as if at 'five to one' on the clock)

EXHALE, bend knees and lower into as deep a squat as allows the heels and the outside edges of the feet to remain on floor.

INHALE, bring palms together at chest in *namaste*. Lift head and chest, lengthen spine, look up, lower bum. Heels and outsides of feet stay in contact with floor.

EXHALE, reach arms out straight in front of head, arms either side of ears. Lift bum and lengthen spine. Knees stay bent. Heels and outsides of feet stay in contact with floor. Inhale.

EXHALE, raise bum, lower head and chest, straighten elbows, look down. Heels and outsides of feet stay in contact with floor.

Repeat up to seven times or more.

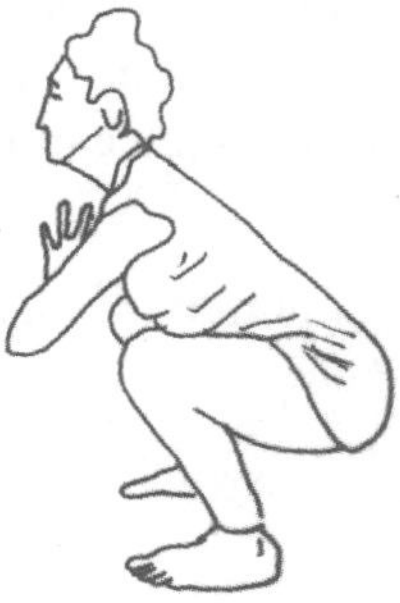

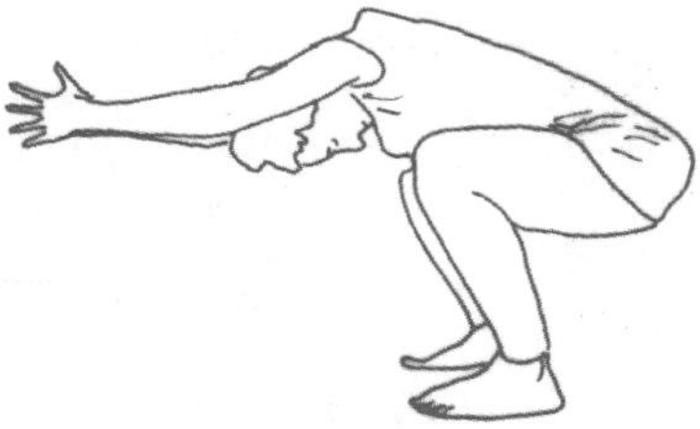

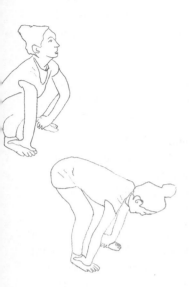

Rocking and twisting mermaid (sacro-iliac joint-stabilising practice)

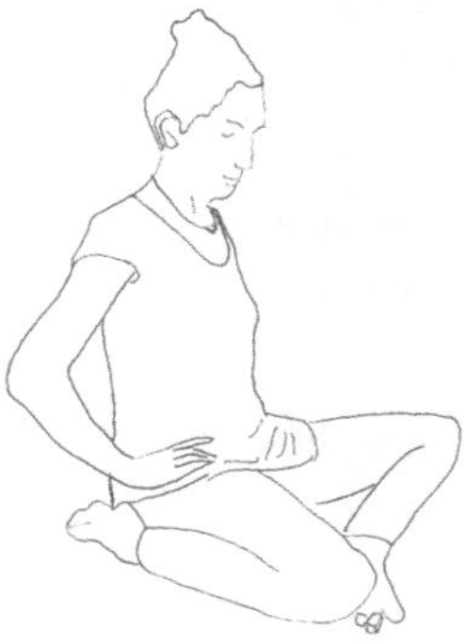

This rhythmic sequence was devised by yoga therapist Mukunda Stiles to manage lower back pain. To be most effective, it needs to be done in the order set out below.

Sit on floor with legs in front.

Bend right knee and draw toes in to touch inside of left knee, externally rotating right hip to allow right knee to drop out sideways.

Bend left knee up and take left foot to outer side of left buttock, so that front of left foot and ankle rest on floor, and toes of left foot point straight back behind, tucked in towards side of left buttock. This is an uneven sitting base so weight will feel as if it is mostly on right sitting bone. To settle, circle pelvis gently.

If you do not feel stable on the floor, or if the pose causes discomfort in your ankles, knees or lower back, then sit on a fairly high support (a block or folded blanket under both sitting bones) and gradually reduce height as your back and hips gain strength and mobility.

Part one: rocking mermaid

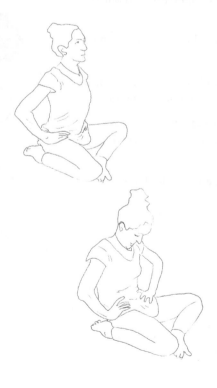

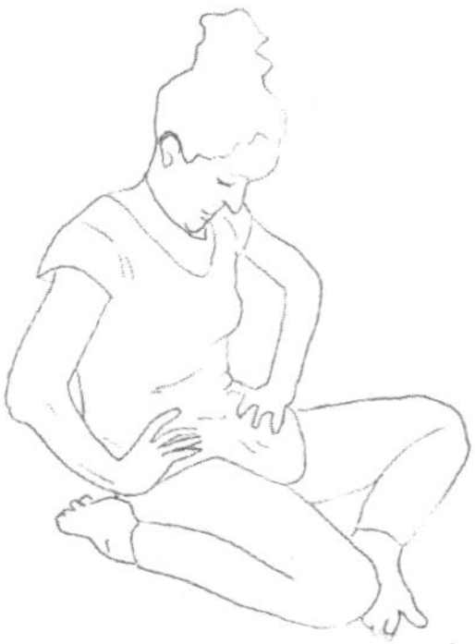

Be in mermaid seat as described above, with right foot in front and left foot tucked back behind, using whatever props are necessary for comfort.

Place hands on hips, with fingers to front and thumbs pointing back in towards spine.

EXHALING, contract transverse abdominal muscles and tuck tailbone under, rounding spine backwards, as if fingertips were pressing back to tilt top of pelvis.

INHALING, reverse movement, contracting lower back muscles, lifting ribcage high and bringing curve of lower back forwards, as if thumbs were pressing pelvis forward and up.

Alternate between these two movements, exhaling to round spine and inhaling as front of body lifts forward and up. Feel that the source of movement is the pelvis.

Repeat fourteen times, or until movement feels smooth and easy, whichever takes longer.

Move on to part two before switching leg position.

Part two: twisting mermaid

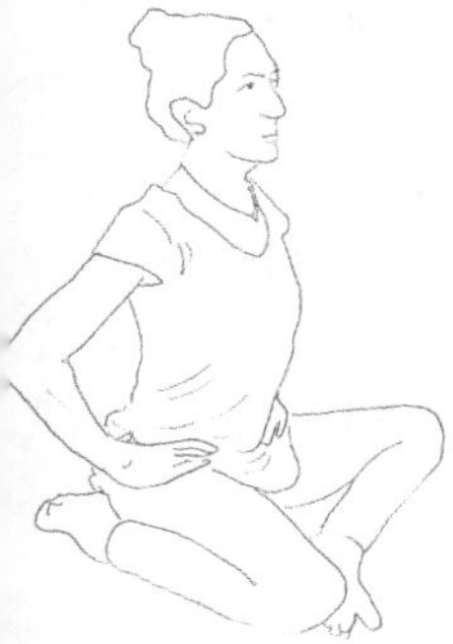

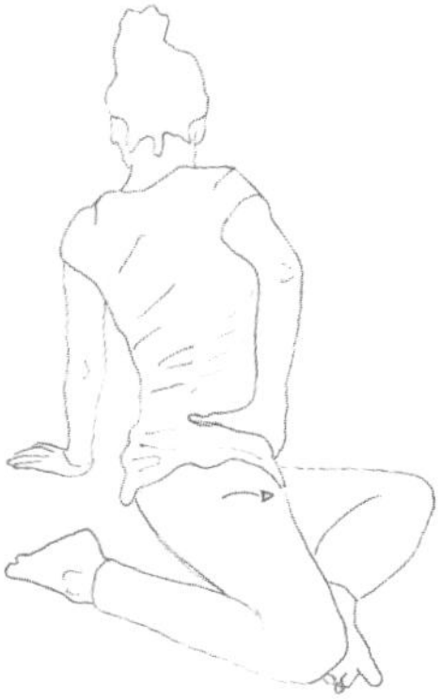

Be in mermaid seat with right foot in front.

Rest left hand on left hip.

EXHALING, contract left buttock.

Continue to contract left buttock until left thigh inwardly rotates and lifts left buttock from floor. As this happens, bring right hand to floor behind you and twist gently, powered by the contraction of the buttock. Opening chest, roll left thigh inwards, and turn to look over right shoulder.

INHALING, release twist and return to start position.

Alternate between these two movements, exhaling as you twist and inhaling as you return.

Feel that the source of movement is the contraction of the left buttock that inwardly turns left thigh, to turn pelvis.

Repeat fourteen times, or until movement feels smooth and easy, whichever takes longer.

Switch leg positions and return to repeat part one before repeating twists on other side.

CLEANSING PRACTICES (*KRIYĀ*)

Like the *śakti bandhas* above, these techniques use rhythmic breath and movement to free the body and mind from feelings of being 'stuck'. Additionally they bring a tangible experience of clarity and luminosity.

Essence of fire cleansing (*Agnisāra kriyā*)

NB Avoid during menstruation or pregnancy or if you are seeking to conceive. Practise with extreme caution if you have an IUCD in place.

Stand with your feet over hip-width apart and your knees bent.

Lean very slightly forward and press the palms of the hands, and also the bases of the index fingers, onto the tops of the thighs, with the fingers pointing out to the sides.

INHALE, lengthen spine.

EXHALE, allow for the abdomen and pelvic muscles to move swiftly upwards and inwards. Keep the breath out and 'flap' the abdominal wall in and out, feeling that the movement works upwards from the pelvic muscles and the base of the abdomen around the pubic bones.

Start slowly with three repetitions of the 'flapping' to get a sense of how this pumping or bellows action builds heat and uplift in the body. Build up over a period of three weeks to a maximum of twenty breaths.

Close the practice with *uḍḍīyāna bandha* (p.476) and *mūla bandha* for as long as the out-breath can be comfortably held.

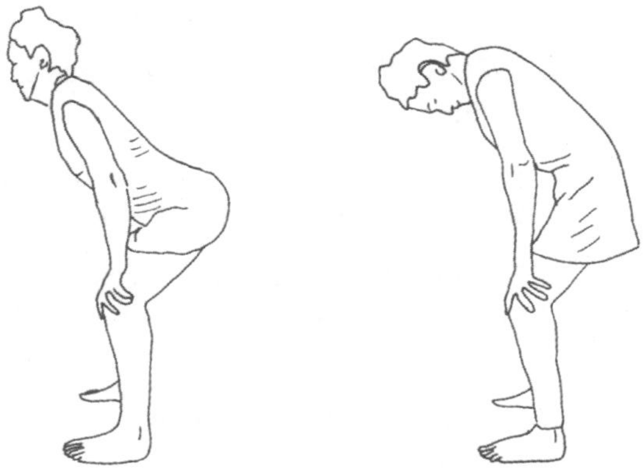

Shining skull breath (*kapālabhāti*)

NB Avoid during menstruation or pregnancy. Practise with extreme caution if you have a IUCD in place or are seeking to conceive.

Sit in a comfortable and stable meditative posture for example kneeling or cross-legged. Inhale, lengthen spine.

EXHALE, allow for the abdomen and pelvic muscles to move swiftly upwards and inwards. Release the belly forward on a passive inhale: simply allow for the breath to come in as the belly releases outwards. There is no need to make efforts to breathe in, the breath will enter without you doing anything.

Start slowly with three repetitions to get a sense of how this pumping action builds heat and uplift in the body. Add additional pumps a couple at a time to build up steadily to a maximum of fifty breaths per round. Exhale steadily and rhythmically at a pace that is sustainable to you. It does not have to be super fast to get effects.

Close the practice with *uḍḍīyāna bandha* (p.476) and *mūla bandha* for as long as the out-breath can be comfortably held. Then breathe normally.

BEING IN THE CYCLES / THE DANCE OF LIFE

This beautiful and accessible movement sequence promotes a powerful connection between the heart and the earth. It is an adaptation of a native American ritual dance ceremony known as the Cherokee dance of life and it has similarities in effect to some of the yoga sun and moon salutations (in chapter twenty-three). It is identified as a *kriyā* or cleansing practice because, in this version, the focus is upon cleansing and releasing from whatever weighs you down and holds you back. The practice also powerfully reconnects to the experience of being part of the cycles of life. It fosters our own capacity to keep energy moving healthily through us, to build a conscious link with all of life. It is best practised outside, barefoot on the earth, offering the movements in turn to each of the four directions, but it is also effective when done inside, for example in a circle of other *yoginīs* in a studio.

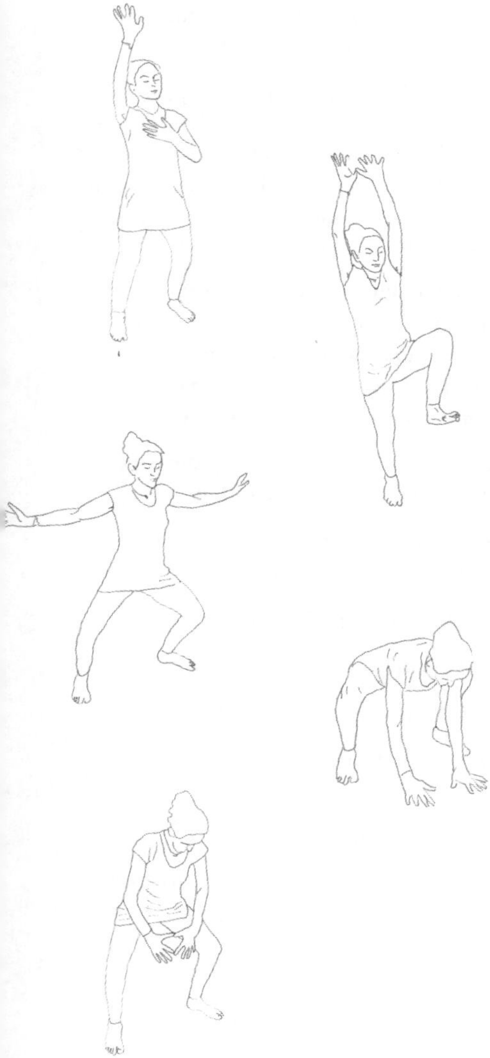

Stand facing east, feet over hip-width apart. Place left hand on heart, right palm stretched up to the light.

Take weight on right foot, bend and lift left knee and step out to left, externally rotating left hip, opening to the feminine side.

Reach arms above, out to the sides and down as you step the left foot down.

Bend knees into a squat and circle palms over the earth.

Bring the thumb and index fingertips together into *yoni mudrā*, and draw the *mudrā* up the centre line of the body.

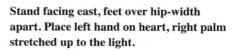

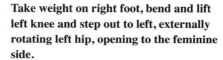

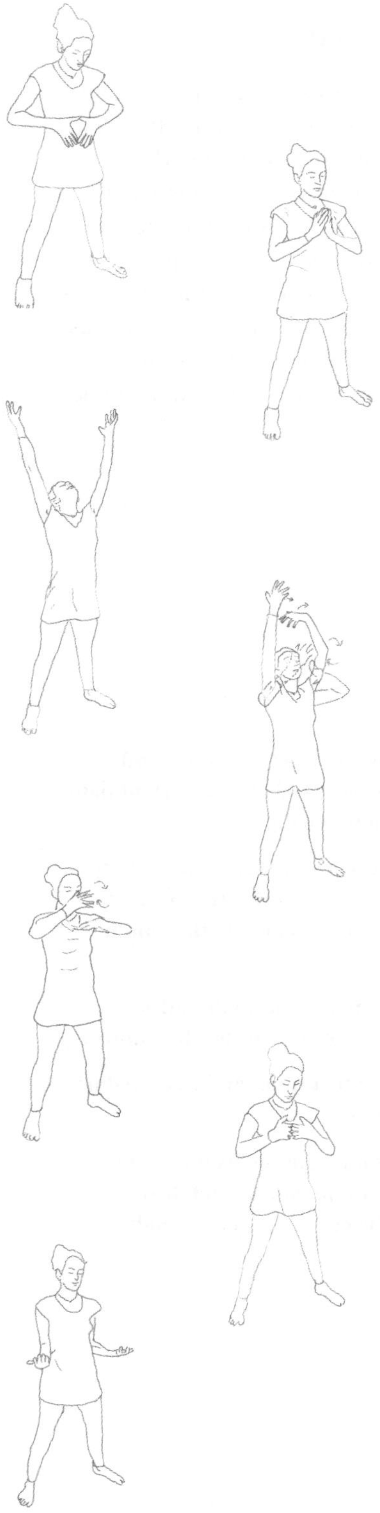

Draw *yoni mudrā* **up the body, and pause with hands in** *namaste* **at the heart.**

Then stretch arms up to greet the heavens.

Circle the hands one over the other moving down towards the heart, keeping the wrists fluid. Integrate energy in the heart.

Stand with hands to the side, palms up, at womb level, ready and willing.

Now repeat the actions from the previous page on the other side: take weight on left foot, raise up right knee and step out to right, externally rotating right hip, opening to the masculine side. Reach arms above, out to the sides and down as you step right foot down.

Bend knees into a squat and circle palms over the earth. Bring your hands into *yoni mudrā* **at the belly, then** *namaste* **at the heart, then up to greet the heavens, and then to integrate in the heart.**

Stand with hands to the side, palms up, at womb level, ready and willing.

The song that accompanies this first part of the movements is:

Amatikewa-ah **(left side out)**

Nyohey **(squat to salute the earth)**

Oh Shona **(raise hands to salute sky)**

Hi-i no, Hi-i no **(circling down hands into heart)**

Hey-i yaah **(hands open)**

Repeat the song and sequence twice – first to the left, then to the right.

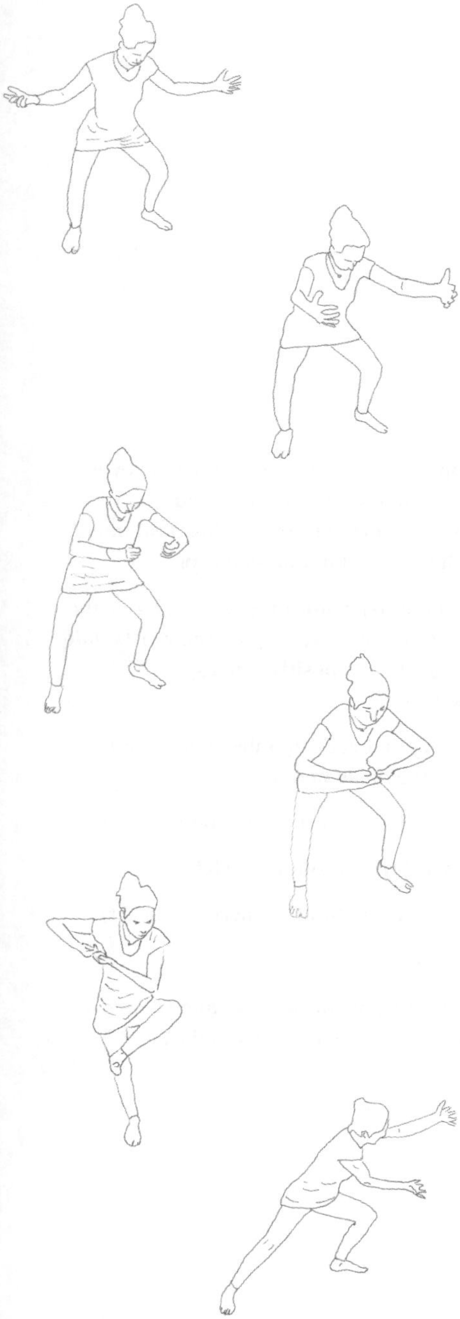

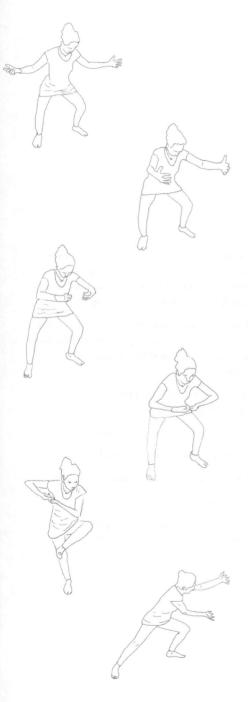

Stretch out your arms to the sides, palms open.

Gather from in front of you and out to the sides, everything you wish to be free from: energies, qualities, anything you can think of, bring all this negativity in.

In a flowing movement, raise up onto the ball of the right foot, keeping toes well spread, swinging the gathered negative energy up to the right with elbows lifted. Then reach out to the left, throwing out everything you have gathered that you wish to be released from. To counter-balance this movement, bend your left knee and extend your right leg.

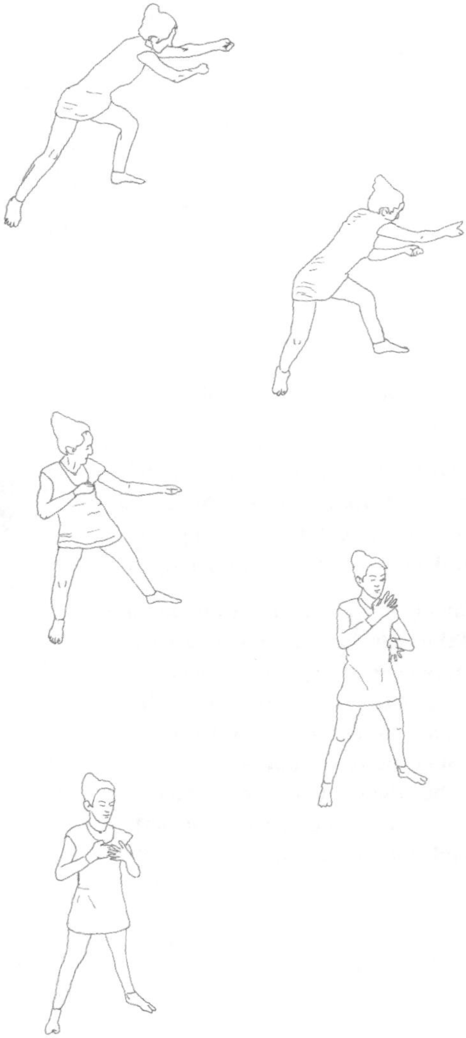

Keeping your right leg extended, draw in from the left all the energies and qualities you wish to bring into your life. Pull hand over hand as if hauling in a rope.

Returning to a wide, even stance, circle the hands towards you, keeping the wrists fluid, to integrate this positive energy in the heart.

The song that accompanies this second part of the movement is:

***Hey-ey, Hi-i no* (gather unwanted energy)**

***HEYAH!!* (throw out to the left)**

***Hi-i no, Hi-i no* (pull in energy to heart)**

***Hey-i yaah* (hands open)**

Repeat this part of the song and sequence twice, first to the left, then to the right.

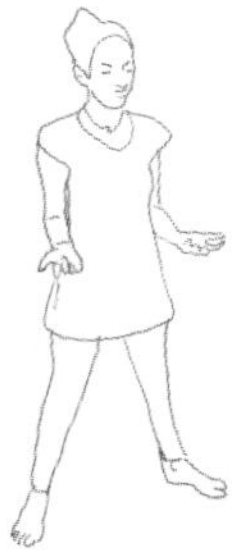

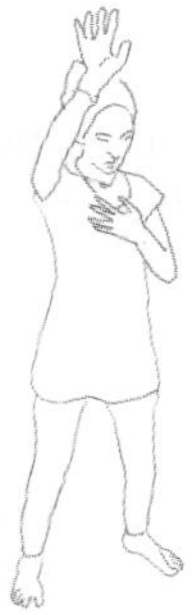

Stand ready and willing, palms open and facing upward.

Complete the full sequence by placing your left hand on your heart and stretching your right palm to the sky.

Turn ninety degrees right to face south and repeat the whole sequence in each direction with the song.

Repeat the entire sequence a third and final time, once to the left and once to the right. but this time in silence.

FURTHER READING AND RESEARCH

For more information on the Deer exercise, consult **Lisa Bodley**'s *Recreating Menstruation* (Gnana Yoga Foundation, 1995).
There are many inspiring testimonials to its efficacy here:
www.shemiranibrahim.com/eliminate-pms-deer-exercise/
The Deer exercise is also described in **Alexandra Pope** and **Jane Bennett**'s book *The Pill* and on a number of Taoist websites including **www.umaatantra.com/female_deer_exercise.html**

To hear the song that accompanies the Dance of Life, visit **www.wombyoga.org/resources**
To watch a video of a version of the Dance of Life sequence, visit **www.yonishakti.co**

CHAPTER TWENTY-THREE

integrations

SEQUENCED POSES WITH GESTURES (*ĀSANA-MUDRĀ-MANTRA-VINYĀSA*)

These sequences bring together flowing postures with hand gestures to create engaging and accessible sequences that resonate with different aspects of lunar and feminine energy.

Full moon salute (*pūrṇa candra namaskāra*)

This adapts a classic yoga sun salutation (*sūrya namaskār*) to provide more space for expanded movement and energy awareness. Use *ujjāyī* breath (pp.134–5) throughout if comfortable.

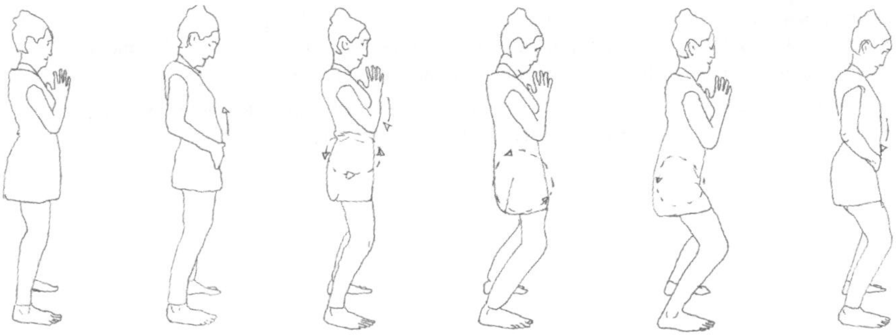

Stand in Mountain pose with hands in prayer position and do three Snake circles the womb (pp.168–9) with Standing heart-womb river greetings (pp.172–6).

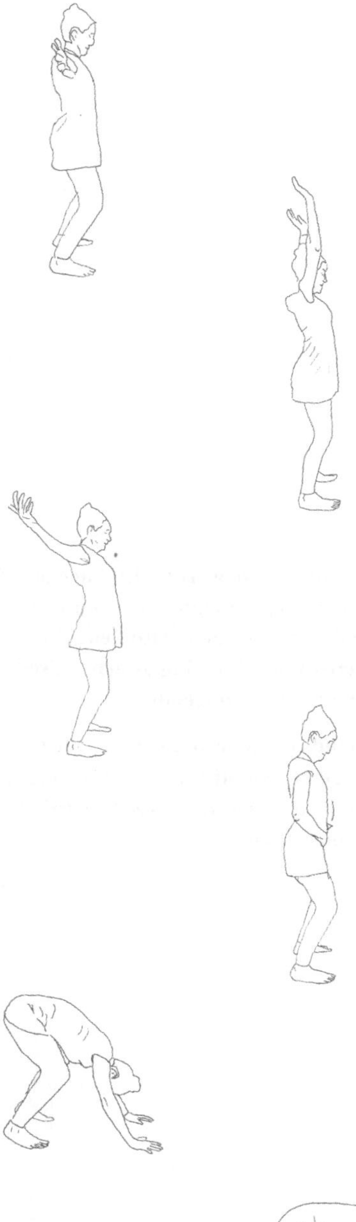

Inhale and lift the arms, circling them out wide to come to rest back at *yoni mudrā* (p.150). Repeat three times.

Bend the knees, then fold at the waist and come down to all fours. Inhale and exhale in Cat pose, three repetitions (p. 502).

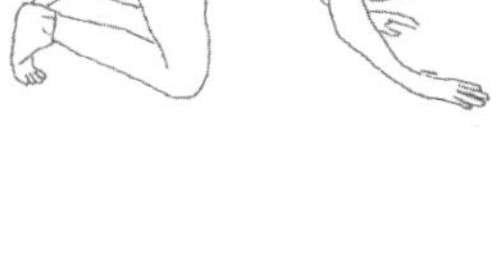

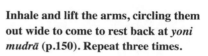

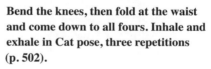

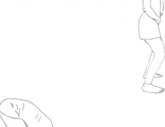

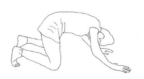

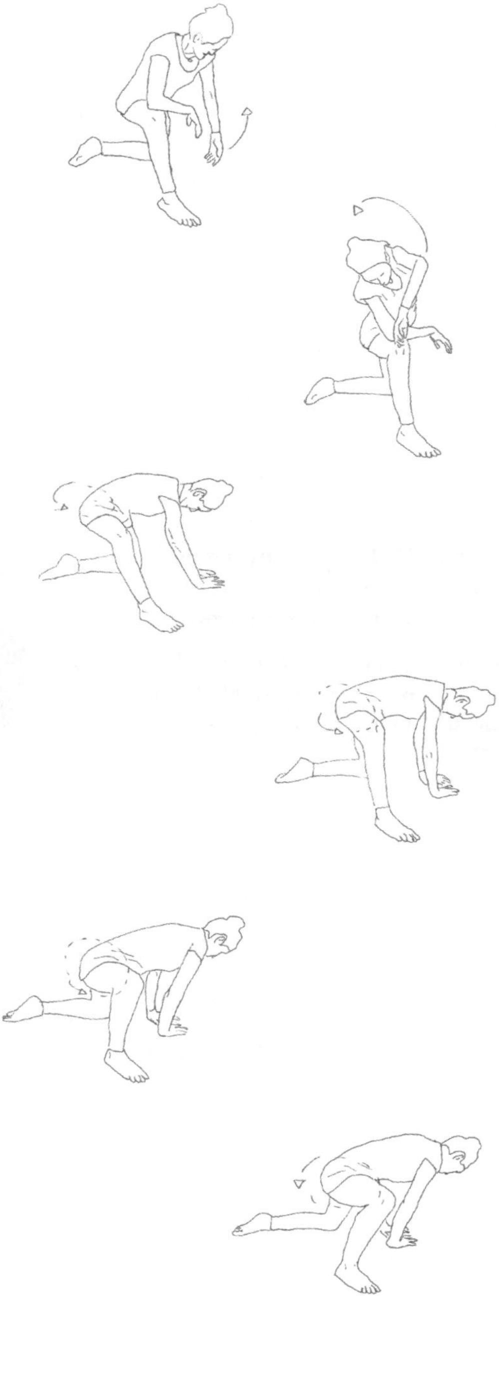

Bring right foot forwards with knee at ninety degrees, rest right elbow on right knee and circle left arm with bent elbow, three repetitions, inhaling as arm raises and exhaling as it descends.

Place hands on floor and bend left leg, placing right foot off the side of the mat to make half squat circles, three repetitions in both directions.

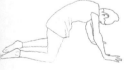

Then do half-moon variation with right leg straight (p.540) and left knee on the ground, with three rounds of breath.

Then return to all fours and practise three repetitions of Cat pose.

Do Hare pose, and rest as long as necessary (p.553)

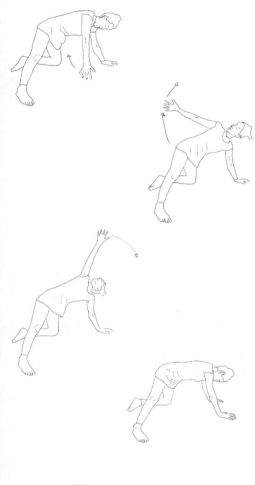

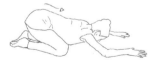

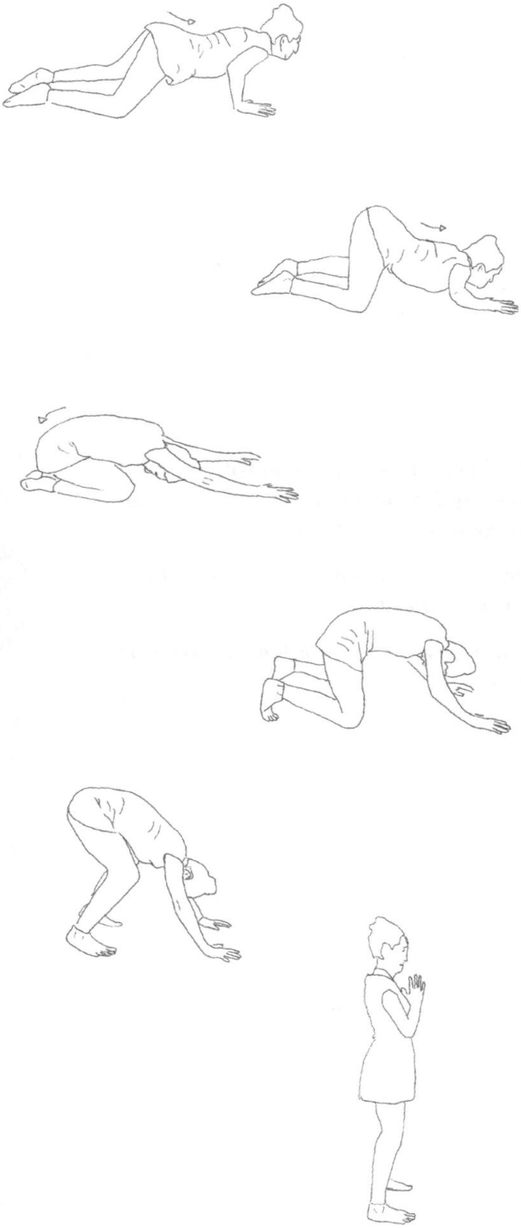

Rising snake sequence: inhale forward and exhale back, three repetitions (p.543).

Transition from all fours to standing in Mountain pose. Then practise three repetitions of Snake circles the womb (pp.168–9) and Womb greetings (pp.143–6) (not illustrated).

Pause, then repeat entire sequence again with left foot forward.

Moon phase salute (*candra namaskāra*)

This lunar flow sequence encourages fluidity of movement and sustained self-awareness. It re-energises and releases the pelvic area and it is best done with conscious awareness of the present position and cycle of the moon. All the movements are done on the exhalation. It is a good idea to have a folded blanket or cushion under the knees throughout this practice.

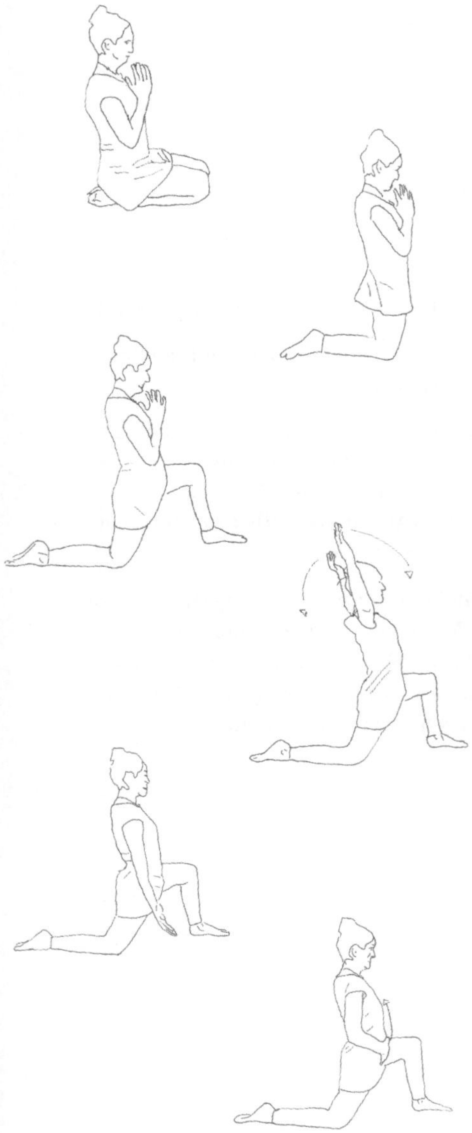

Start from kneeling. Bring hands into prayer position. Press heels of hands together. Exhale.

Inhale, contract buttocks to raise up on your knees. Position the knees about hip-width apart.

Exhale, step left foot forward. Allow the knee to bend at a ninety-degree angle so that left knee is directly over the left ankle. Inhale.

Inhale, reach arms up from prayer position and exhale out and down either side to trace the form of a complete circle, ending with *yoni mudrā* below the navel. Repeat three times.

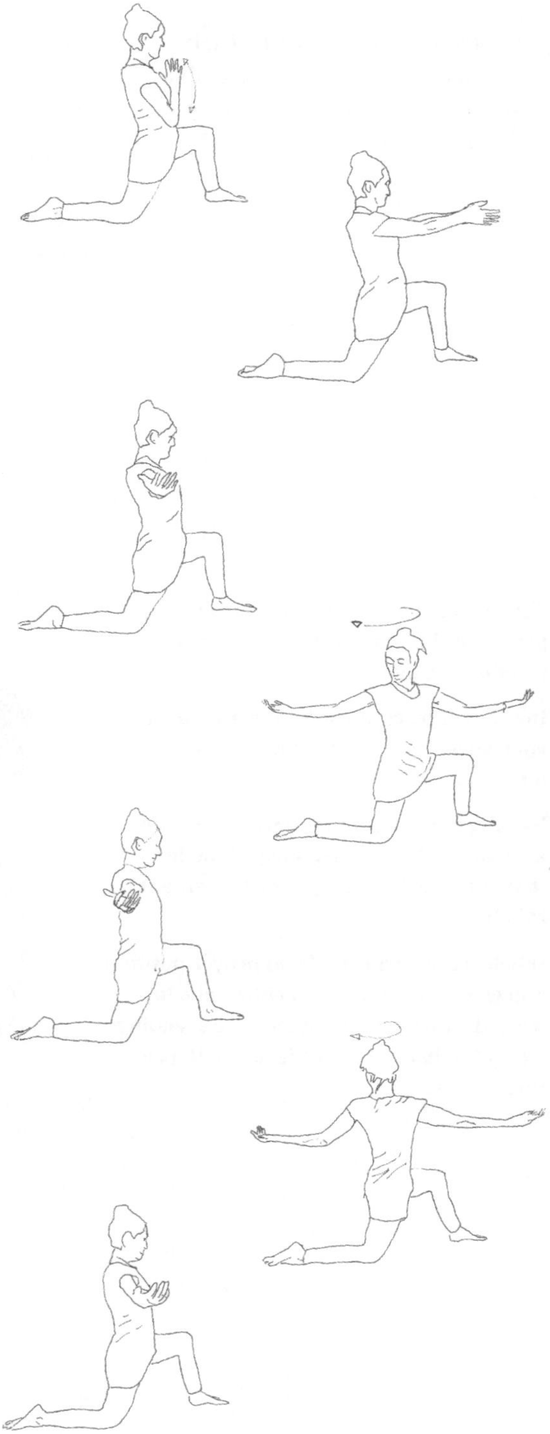

Exhale to return hands to prayer position.

Inhale and bring the arms out in front of you, palms together.

Then exhale and twist to bring the right arm back behind. Look along length of right arm. Keep both arms out at shoulder height with elbows softly bent. Inhale as you return to front.

Exhale as you twist to bring the left arm back behind you. Look along length of left arm. Keep both arms out at shoulder height with elbows softly bent. Inhale as you return to front. Exhale.

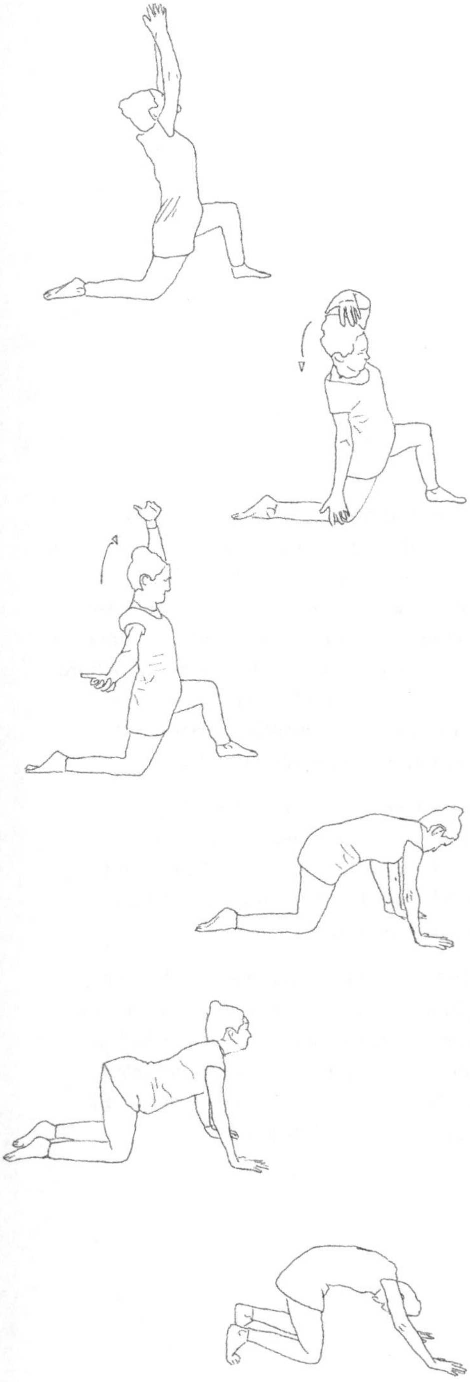

Inhale, reach up, palms together. Exhale, bend sideways at waist to lower the right arm, reaching fingertips down towards the floor (there is no need to touch the floor, just reach towards it). Bend left arm, stretch elbow up, keeping a long line from right elbow to left fingertips.

Inhale, return to centre, arms wide.

Exhale to repeat on the other side.

Bring the hands to the floor and come down onto all fours for the Cat pose. Have palms flat on the floor, ahead of shoulders with fingers well spread and pointing forwards. Inhale fully as you look forwards and slightly up, lengthening through whole spine as it arches slightly. On an exhalation, tuck chin down right into chest, round the lower back and suck belly up to spine. The back should be rounded right over. Press heels of hands down into floor and open up a space between shoulder blades. Inhale and look forwards again, arching back slightly

(NB during pregnancy do not arch the back in this pose).

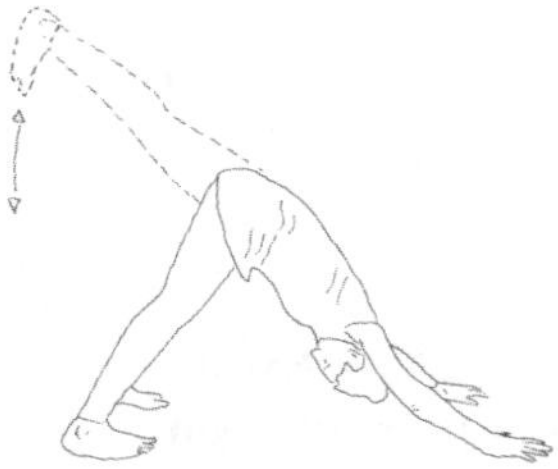

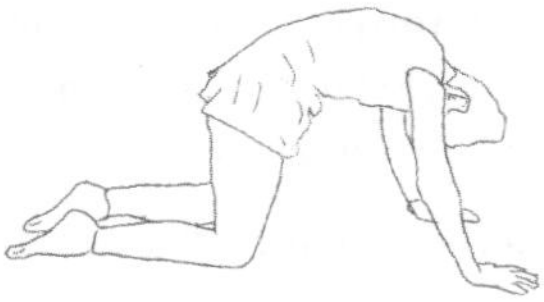

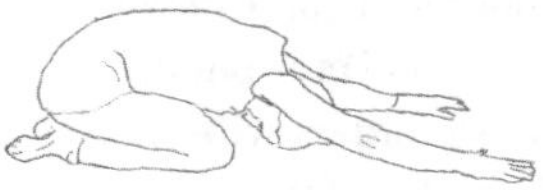

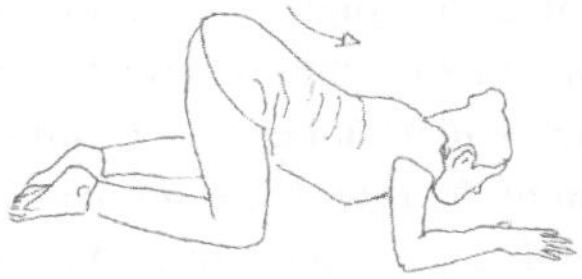

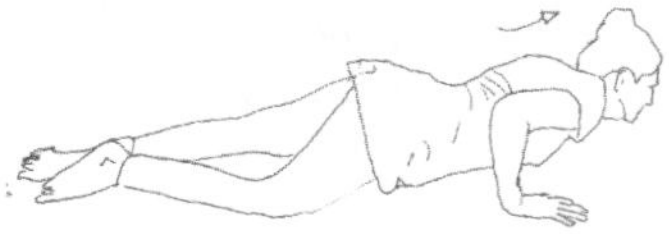

Dog pose and variations (these are best avoided during menstruation or pregnancy). Exhale, tuck toes under and swing your tailbone up into the Dog pose. Inhale, raise right leg up behind. Exhale, place it back on the floor. Inhale, raise the left leg up behind. Exhale, place it back on the floor. Inhale. If you enjoy incorporating circles and snakes in this pose, then go ahead.

Exhale bend knees and lower down to floor into Hare pose. Lower head to the floor and extend arms out in front at shoulder-width. Move the knees wider to make this easier.

Rising snake pose variation (p.543). Keep the hands and knees firmly rooted into the ground as you creep chest forwards, low along the ground, slowly bringing front of body into contact with the ground, and lifting chest into Cobra pose.

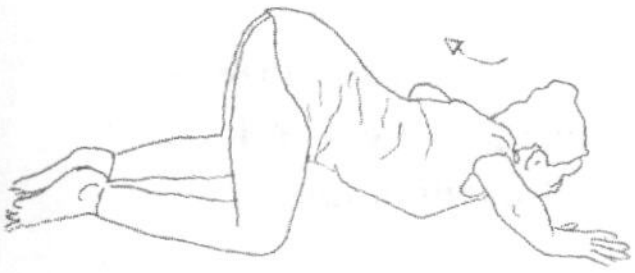

Return the same way you came, pushing backwards a little way up from the floor to return to the Hare pose.

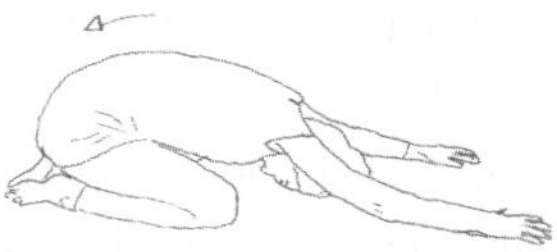

Return to the start: inhale and roll up through spine, raising arms and upper body back to vertical, keeping ears between arms, so that there is a continuous line from tailbone to fingertips.

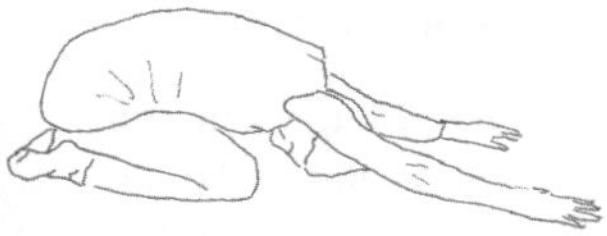

Keep sitting back on heels, exhale, move hands back into prayer position, pressing heels of hands together.

Then repeat the sequence with the right foot forwards, starting each pair of movements with the right arm moving instead of the left arm. Start and finish kneeling with hands in prayer position.

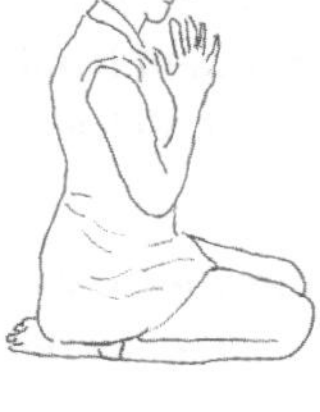

Swaying palm tree with Womb greeting sequence (*taḍāsana vinyāsa* with *yoni mudrā*)

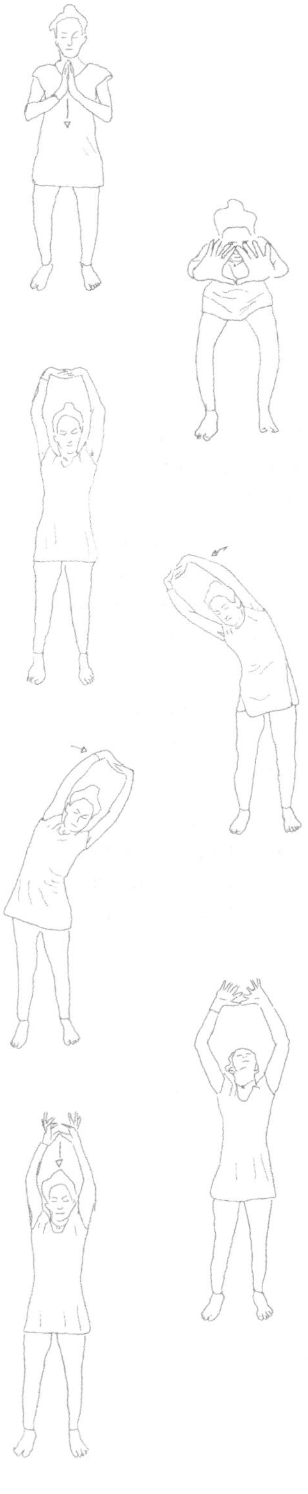

Stand with feet about hip-width apart, with soft knees and hands in *namaste*. Do three pelvic circles in each direction (Snake circles the womb pp.168–9) with three Heart-womb river greetings (lotus-ocean form pp.145–6).

Interlock hands so that dominant nostril (see p.462) hand fingers are on top, push palms out. Inhale and raise them up above head. Do one pelvic circle in each direction (Snake circles the womb) with one Heart-womb river greeting (lotus-ocean form).

Release arms down to return to *yoni mudrā*, change cross of hands and repeat previous step with the opposite interlock of hands. Release arms down to return to *yoni mudrā*.

Interlock hands so that dominant nostril hand fingers are on top, push palms out, and up above head. Inhale and rise up on balls of feet end exhaling, do one pelvic circle in each direction (Snake circles the womb). Inhale, extend palms to sky and exhale, drop heels back to earth.

Release arms down to return to *yoni mudrā*, change cross of hands, and repeat previous step with the opposite interlock of hands. Release arms down to return to *yoni mudrā*.

One pelvic circle in each direction (Snake circles the womb) with one Heart-womb river greeting (lotus-ocean form).

Interlock hands so that dominant nostril hand fingers are on top, push palms out, and inhale them up above head. Exhale and side-bend to dominant side. Inhale back up and exhale over to the other side. Return to centre, do one pelvic circle in each direction (Snake circles the womb).

Release arms down in front, change cross of hands. Inhale, push palms out, and up above head, and repeat previous step with the opposite interlock of hands, moving to non-dominant nostril side first. Release arms down to return to *yoni mudrā*

One pelvic circle in each direction (Snake circles the womb) with one Heart-womb river greeting (lotus-ocean form).

Complete the sequence with Full hands womb energy pilgrimage (pp.176–8) and Eternal fountain of energy invocation (pp.178–9). Return to stand with feet about hip-width apart, with soft knees and hands in namaste. Do three pelvic circles in each direction (Snake circles the womb) with three Heart-womb river greetings (lotus-ocean form).

Postnatal sun salute

This modifies a basic *haṭha* yoga sun salutation to provide more support for the lower back and more opportunity sto trengthen the upper back and promote good posture.

NB Only suitable for women for whom a lifted mūla bandha *feels secure and comfortable, i.e. minimum four to six months after birth.*

NB Use the healing breath (p.482) throughout this sequence.

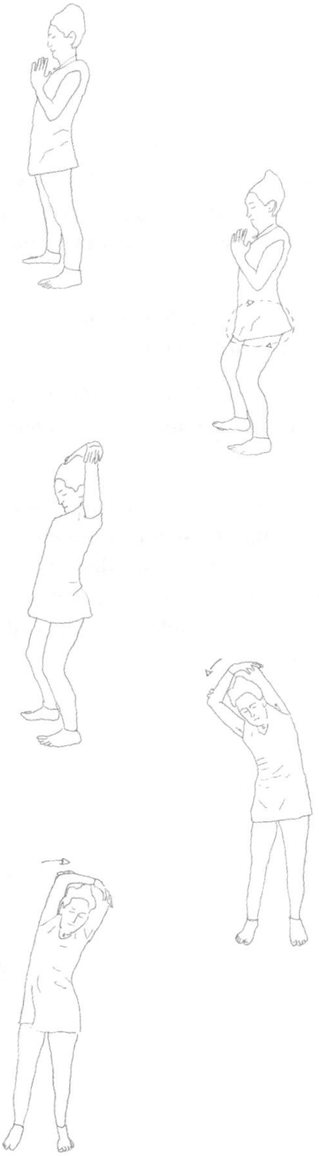

Stand in Mountain pose with knees bent. Do three Snake circles the womb in each direction (pp.168–9). Inhale, reach up overhead with hands and hold elbows with opposite hands to keep chest open. Draw shoulder blades together and down.

Inhale, push elbows up into hands. Exhale, bend sideways to the right.

Inhale, return to centre and push elbows up into hands. Exhale, bend sideways to the left.

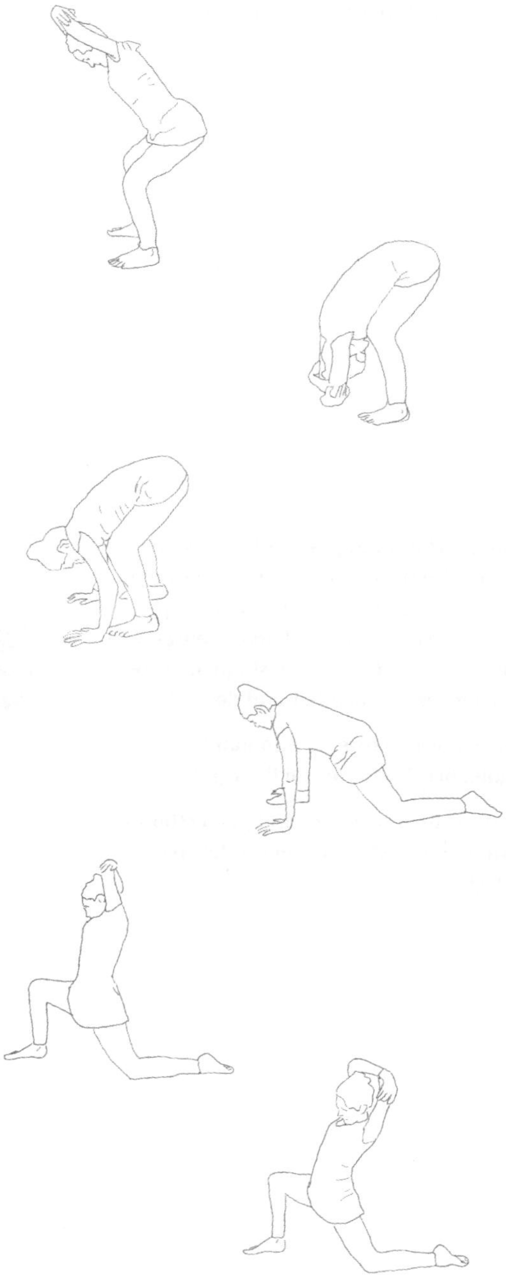

Inhale, return to centre and push elbows up into hands. Exhale, bend forwards and down with knees bent on descent to protect lower back.

Three rounds of breath in standing forward bend with bent knees.

Inhale, place palms of hands on floor, step back with left foot and maintain a ninety-degree angle at the right knee.

Inhale, bring torso to vertical and grasp elbows in the opposite hands. Push elbows up into hands. Exhale, bend sideways to right. Inhale, return to centre and push elbows up into hands. Exhale, bend sideways to left.

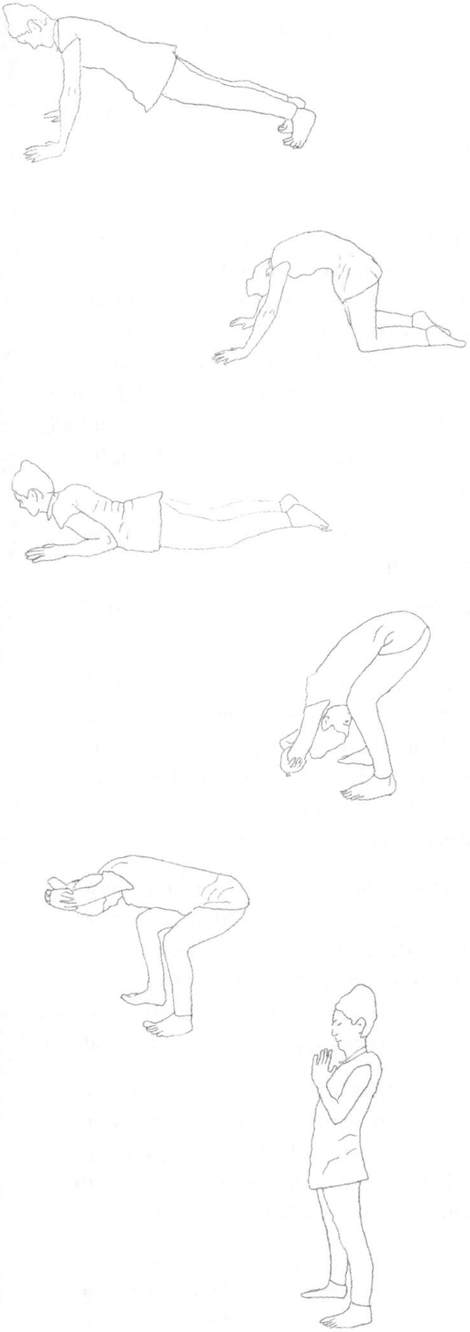

Inhale, bring hands to floor and step back into plank, with hips, spine and legs aligned. Be sure to hold plank steady with the back and backs of legs in a straight line.

Exhale into Cat pose (all fours). Take three rounds of breath with the spine moving in Cat pose (p.502).

Inhale into Sphinx, with elbows and fore-arms on the floor, legs straight out behind and chest lifted.

Exhale, push back into Cat pose (not illus-trated) and then walk hands back towards feet to return to standing forward bend with bent knees.

Inhale, hold elbows with opposite hands and push elbows forwards and up to return to standing.

Repeat whole sequence again with right foot moving forward and back.

Feminine strength: spiritual warrior dance

This sequence takes the usually fixed warrior poses and frees them up to allow a fluid flow of movement and energy in the pelvis. In contrast to the classic wide-legged warrior stance, this modification uses a shorter stride, giving the option to shift from bent knee to straight as you need.

The sequence works very well in a pair if you face your partner and place the palms of the hands together as you move the upper body.

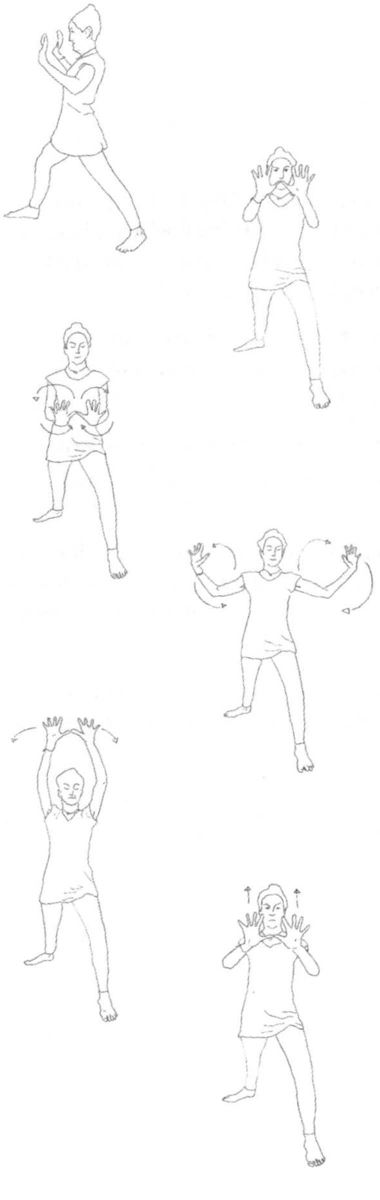

Stand at front of mat, legs about hip-width apart and feet parallel. Bend knees, let shoulders and heels drop. Inhale, bring palms together at chest. Exhale, step left foot backwards, maintaining hip-width between legs and only taking a short stride. Have right knee slightly bent, and left leg straight. Pivot on ball of left foot to angle toes out slightly to right, keeping arches lifted.

Inhale, lengthen back of body from left heel through to top of head.

Exhale, feel weight descending through both heels.

This is the base position. From here, experiment with pelvic circles and movements, e.g. Snake circles the womb (pp.168–9), and the same pelvic circles as can be done from all fours (p.541). Combine these movements with arm lifts and circles as follows:

Inhale and reach arms up above you, elbows bent. Exhale, turn to right and open arms out straight at shoulder height. Inhale, return to arms reaching up, and exhale around to the other side, arms out straight at shoulder height. (NB this part of the sequence is not illustrated.)

Now trace circles around you in time with the breath. Moving hands in opposite directions, take four circles in each direction, gradually increasing the size of the circles. Inhale as the hands arc up and exhale as they move down.

If you are working with a partner, his/her stance should mirror yours. Press your right palm to his/her left and your left palm to his/her right, and make the circles together.

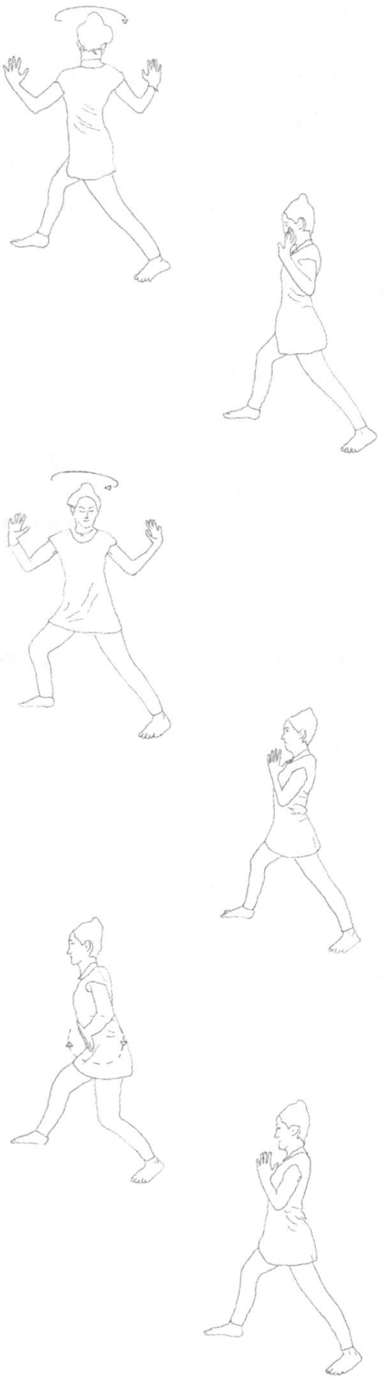

Then move into twists. pushing one hand straight forward and drawing the other arm back behind you, elbow bent.

If you are working with a partner, then press palms together so that one partner has right hand forward, one has left hand forward. Synchronise the movement with the breath, exhaling into the twist and inhaling to move out of it.

Complete the practice with three rounds of Snake circles the womb (pp.168–9).

Release arms to side, swap legs around and repeat again with the left foot forward.

If you are in a pair to do this practice, then complete the sequence as follows:

Stand in Mountain pose, about arm's length away from your partner.

Take your legs slightly wider than hips (about yoga mat width is a good guide), bend knees very slightly and have feet either parallel or slightly turned out.

Each partner takes a firm grasp of the other's forearms and straightens the arms.

Step back if necessary, so that straightening the arms causes the upper back to round. The upper back should feel open and stretched so each partner can lean their weight back, trusting the hold of their partner.

INHALE as you alternately pull forward and back on each arm, dropping shoulders and bringing a soft rhythmic twist into upper back.

EXHALE, push into heels and move buttocks out behind, and round out lower back curve. The whole spine should feel in a comfortable curve.

EXHALE, bend knees deeper, keeping the lower back rounded and a strong sense of support in the upper back as you lean back against your partner's weight. Descend on exhale only so far as you can comfortably go with heels remaining in firm contact with the floor.

INHALE and straighten knees to ascend.

Repeat up to five times, exhaling down and inhaling up. Take pauses between rounds if that feels more comfortable.

Greet each other with hands in prayer position to complete the practice.

BALANCING POSES

Fierce goddess and Lord of the dance *vinyāsa* (*śiva/śakti: devījai utkaṭāsana-naṭarājāsana vinyāsa*)

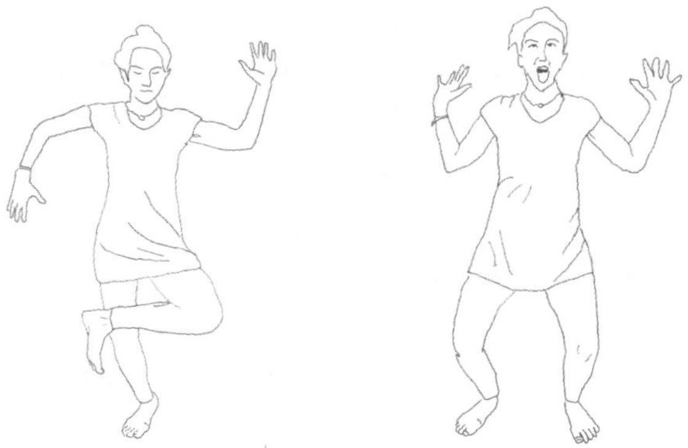

This pair of poses is an energising expression of the creative force of feminine energy, alternated with the still consciousness of masculine energy. Moving between them makes a pleasing contrast between the earthy descent of Fierce goddess and the spacious airy poise of Lord of the dance. The combination works best if the Fierce goddess pose comes between left and right side balances of Lord of the dance.

Lord of the dance

Stand in Mountain pose, feet at a comfortable width for squatting.

INHALE taking elbows wide to side at shoulder height.

EXHALE and drop deeper into squat, taking weight into right foot.

INHALE and raise left leg, taking left knee to side and lifting left foot to bring shin towards horizontal at knee height. Keep breath even as you balance with elbows wide, raising left hand to push palm forwards, fingers pointing up.

Let right wrist bend, and fingers of right hand point down towards earth.

EXHALING, release hand positions, keeping elbows out to side and bringing left foot back to ground, returning to squat, and then move into

Fierce goddess

INHALE, straighten legs, raising arms up straight up above head, wider than the shoulders, with fingers spread wide.

EXHALE loudly through mouth, bend knees and elbows to drop straight down towards earth. The louder the exhale, the more energising the pose. On descent, stick out tongue as far as it will go and roll eyes up and back.

At end of exhale, return to start position and do the other side of **Lord of the dance**:

INHALE taking elbows wide to side at shoulder height.

EXHALE and drop deeper into squat, taking weight into left foot.

INHALE and raise right leg, taking right knee to side and lifting right foot to bring shin towards horizontal at knee height. Keep breath even as you balance with elbows wide, raising right hand to push palm forwards, fingers pointing up.

Let right wrist bend, and fingers of left hand point down towards earth.

EXHALING, release hand positions, keeping elbows out to side and bringing left foot back to ground, returning to squat.

Repeat up to seven times, alternating between left and right sides with the **Fierce goddess** in between the two sides. At the end, return to Mountain pose for a few rounds of breath.

Tips: *If you get confused about coordination, remember that the lifted hand corresponds to the lifted leg. Keep transitions between one side and the other smooth and even. The experience of balance and poise is more secure if you keep your eyes focused on a still point ahead of you. Being mindful of the meaning of the gestures deepens your experience of the pose: the raised hand with palm forward signifies 'fear not', while the fingers pointing to the earth draw attention to the ground of our being and the need for a down-to-earth connection even as we dance in the air.*

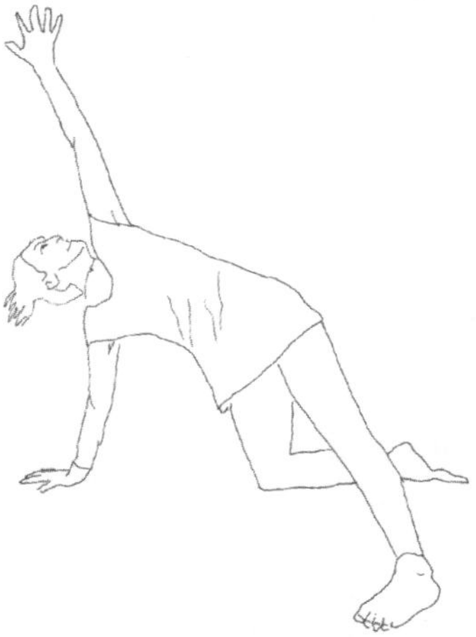

Half moon pose: easy version

From Cat pose, step left foot off to side of your mat, and straighten left knee so the side of the foot is resting on the floor.

INHALE, reach left hand forward and straight up above into the air, turning head and chest to look up at the hand.

EXHALE and reach the arm forward and down, stretching forward with the arm forward along left ear before putting hand back on the floor.

Return to Cat pose (p.502) for three rounds of breath and then repeat this pose on the other side.

FURTHER READING AND RESOURCES

To watch a video of the Swaying palm tree with Womb greeting sequence (*taḍāsana vinyāsa* with *yoni mudrā*), visit **www.yonishakti.co**.

CHAPTER TWENTY-FOUR

spirals and snakes

SEQUENCES FROM CAT POSE AND KNEELING

Circles and spirals

These rhythmic movements optimise mobility, relieve stiffness and have a calming, hypnotic effect.

Breathe fully in all-fours position, with padding under knees as needed. Imagine the central point of a circle between the knees, and slowly circle hips clockwise around this point, letting the size of the circle increase or decrease as feels comfortable.

After about ten rounds, change direction and repeat.

Pause, shift movement up body so that the imaginary central point of the circle is now between the hands. Circle shoulders and upper body clockwise, and then anticlockwise, moving freely and easily.

Connect shoulder circles with hip circles, as if drawing a figure of eight by moving hips in one direction and shoulders in the other. Feel central crossover point in figure of eight, and savour moments when lower circles cross into upper and vice versa.

When you have moved enough in one direction, change direction and repeat.

At end of the sequence do one round of Cat (p.502) and rest in Hare pose, supported as needed (p.553).

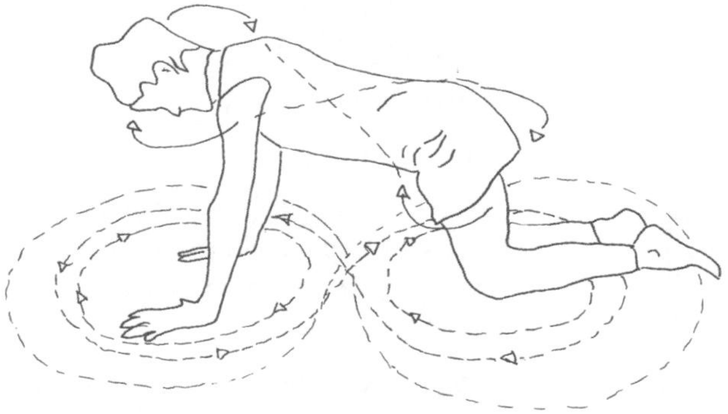

Kneeling salutations (*vajrāsana namaskāra*)

These simple spinal movements are energising and revitalising, and are especially valuable in the postnatal period when babies can be laid in front of mothers and still be close enough to see them whilst they move. Be sure to put padding under the knees. If you are practising with a baby present, you can click your fingers and clap your hands in order to entertain the baby for long enough to complete the sequence (see *Mother Nurture* DVD for a demonstration of how this technique works).

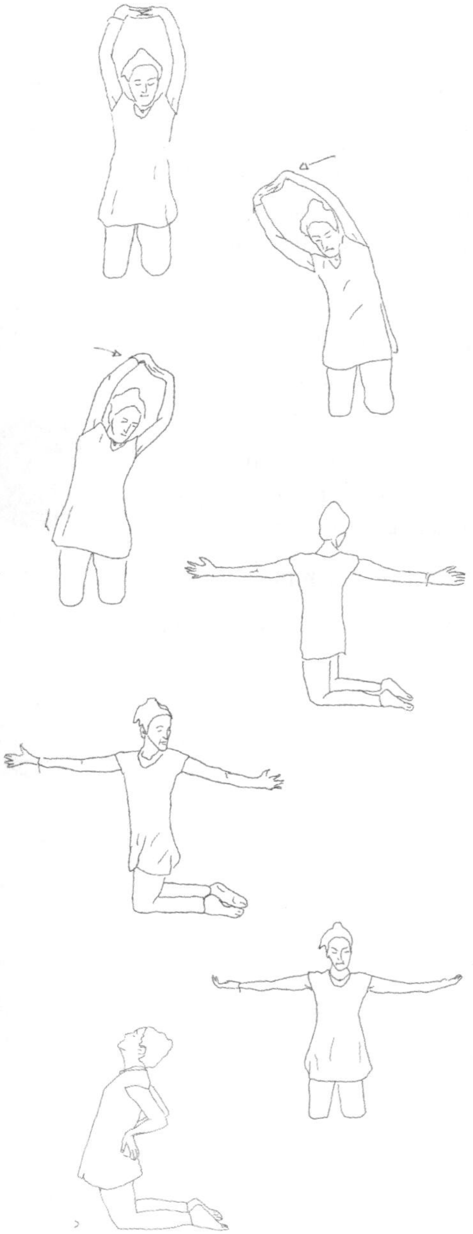

Start from kneeling. Use a bolster under the buttocks if you cannot easily rest buttocks on heels.

EXHALE, contract buttocks and rise up, with hips and torso above knees. Thighs are vertical and knees hip-width apart. Have your toes tucked forwards and the balls of the feet on the floor.

INHALE, lengthen the spine and reach arms above head. Interlock hands. Exhale, side bend to one side, and inhale back to centre. Repeat on the other side.

INHALE, return to centre and reach arms up above head and out to the side at shoulder height.

EXHALE, keep arms out-stretched and twist to left, inhale to centre and exhale twist to right.

Camel pose modification

INHALE, come to centre, place your palms on your buttocks, fingers pointing down. Breathe into the abdomen and chest. Keep your spine extended and slowly move the hands down as far as is comfortable for you. Only go as far down as you can whilst maintaining the thighs vertical. Encourage the front of the chest forwards with a big inhalation, and keep your shoulders down away from your ears.

EXHALE, release hands from your back and return to vertical.

INHALE and lengthen spine. Let arms hang loose and swing shoulders from side to side, with arms wrapping softly around yourself as in Standing twist (p.544).

EXHALE, fold forwards into the Hare pose and lengthen the spine. Breathe into the belly and feel it moving against the thighs.

Rising snake series (*kuṇḍalini vinyāsa, śaśāṅkabhujaṅgāsana*)

This is a flowing rhythmic alternation between Hare pose and Cobra pose, running them together into one smooth movement in time with the breath.

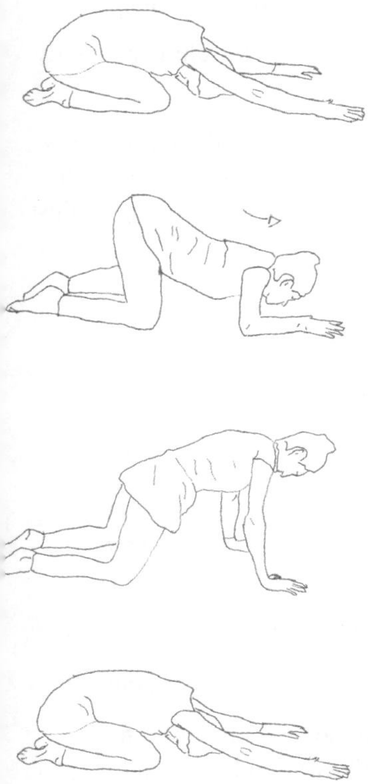

Begin in all fours. Move knees a little wider apart, with enough space to take your belly forward between them easily. If it feels more comfortable, let toes move closer as knees move wider. Breathe fully. Let rhythm of breath determine pace of movements.

EXHALE, round back. Keeping spine rounded, maintain firm connection between hands and mat, continue to exhale and lower buttocks towards heels. At end of exhale, sense you have moved as far back towards heels as is comfortable (Hare pose).

INHALE, bend elbows and move forwards, keeping as low to mat as you can. When you reach thumbs, straighten elbows, lifting body back into flat-back position.

EXHALE, round spine and drop back towards buttocks.

Continue for a couple of rounds, exhaling with rounded spine as you move back to heels, and inhaling with a flat back as you move forward to hands.

After three repetitions, pause, evaluate your response and either rest, or repeat up to ten rounds.

Rest in Hare pose, supported as needed (p.553).

Tips: *As elbows bend to support forward motion of body, there are two directions in which they can move. Letting elbows stick out sideways gives more freedom of movement but less strength; tucking elbows into sides of body challenges range of movement but builds strength. Choose whichever option seems most appropriate, or alternate between the two. If dropping buttocks back to heels feels awkward, and you do not get very far, it can be more comfortable to have a support to sit on as for Hare pose, so place a stack of blocks (two or three) or cushions between feet.*

Snake pose variation

If you experience painful menstrual cramps, you may find that this version of the Cobra pose provides relief.

Lie flat on your front with your forehead on the floor and your arms by your sides. Have your legs straight, your heels together. Bring your arms behind your back, moving your elbows as close together as you can. Place the palms together and interlock the fingers.

Roll your shoulders down and back away from your ears, squeezing your shoulder blades together. **EXHALE.**

INHALE, lift your head and raise the front of your chest up away from the floor.

EXHALE, slowly lower the arms back down onto the back, tuck in the chin and gently rest the forehead on the floor.

Move freely with the breath, up on the inhale and down on the exhale. If the pose suits you at this time, remain in the chest-lifted position for up to seven breaths. Keep your neck long and your ears well away from your shoulders. Feel your belly moving against the floor as you breathe fully.

TWISTS

Extended heart space twist

See part one, p.159 for illustration and instructions.

Standing twist (*katicakrāsana*)

This is a beautiful completion for any standing pose sequence. Let the breath flow however feels natural and let the arms be very soft.

Stand with feet hip-width apart, knees soft and arms hanging loose.

Gently swing shoulders from side to side, with arms wrapping softly around yourself.

Start with the hands at hip level and then swing the arms higher and higher each time until they are higher than the shoulders and then the elbows can bend to allow you to pat yourself on the upper back, with hands reaching over the top of the shoulders and down to the shoulder blades.

Continue swinging but let the hands come lower and lower to return to the starting level.

Slowly come back to stillness.

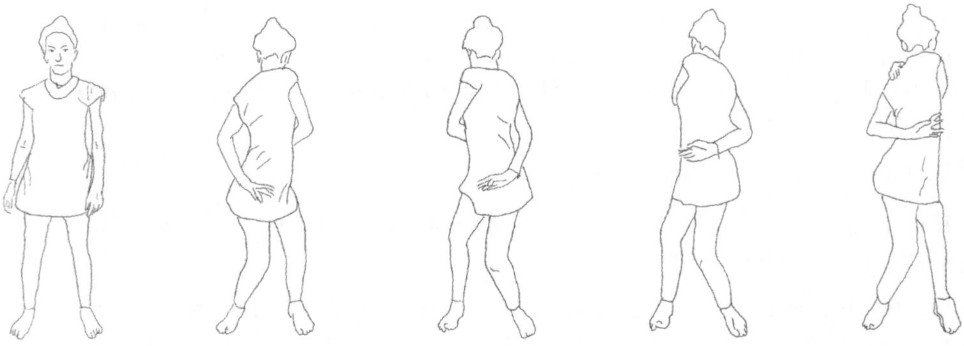

CHAPTER TWENTY-FIVE

nourishment

INVERSIONS

Legs up wall with support and knees bent, supported pelvic lift

See pelvic organ support section, pp.489–91 for instructions.

Half shoulderstand flow (*viparīta karaṇī mudrā*)

NB Avoid during pregnancy and menstruation

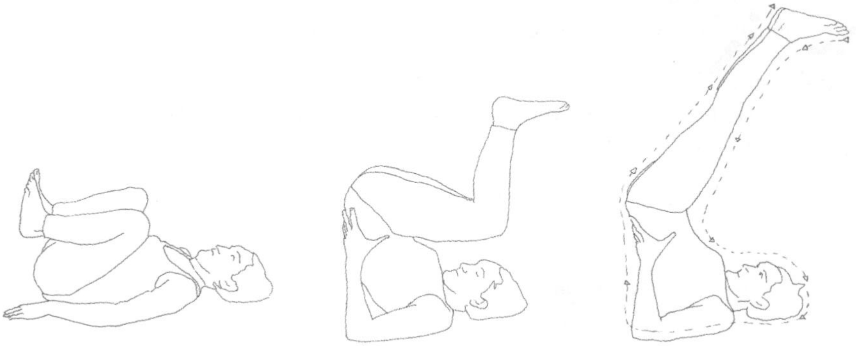

Place a folded blanket under your spine. Lie on back, tucking your knees into belly.

Use hands to support the hips, with thumbs at the sides and fingers pointing up the lower back.

Let the weight of the legs and buttocks transfer down through the elbows into the floor. As you feel comfortable, lift your knees up away from your belly and let the legs straighten so they are held upwards at an angle of about forty-five degrees over your head.

Breathe fully in the pose. To come down, bend the knees into the belly and roll back to the floor.

Once you are familiar with the feeling of the posture, then focus to allow the flow of breath to trace an energising circuit: inhale and breathe awareness down from top of toes, along front of body to top of head, exhale and breathe awareness along back of body, from top of head, up the back of the legs to the heels.

SUPPORTED POSES AND RESTORATIVES PART 1

Wall as teacher sequence

Working against the wall gives a unique combination of resting and strengthening options to improve posture and build strength in supported poses. This group of poses works well as a coherent series, but each pose can also be done alone.

Ladder against wall

This upright resting option uses the wall for support, comfort and privacy. It is an upright version of *praṇāmāsana* (p.555) which is more comfortable for pregnant and breastfeeding mothers, or those women who get pain from fibroids when lying on their bellies.

Stand in Mountain pose, about 50cm away from wall, with feet hip-width apart and parallel.

INHALE and reach arms up above head, palms facing the wall.

EXHALE, shift weight into balls of feet, tilting body forwards until hands and arms come into contact with wall. Connect your fingertips in *yoni mudrā*.

Breathe fully, sweeping mental awareness from heels to head on inhale, and from head to heels on exhale. Settling into pose, creep elbows higher up wall to bring length and space into sides of body.

Rest here as long as you need, and then follow with next pose.

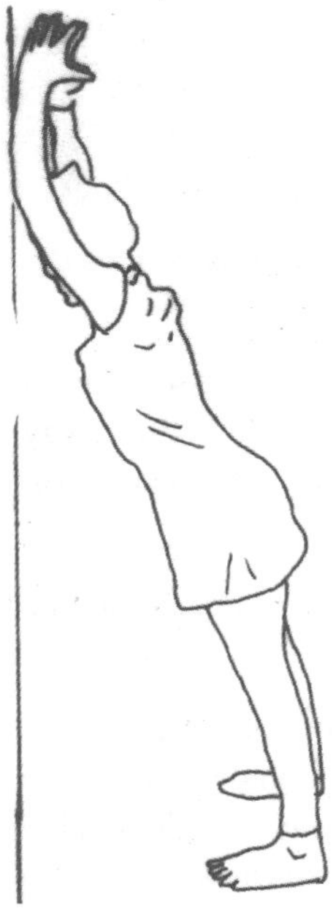

Chair against wall

This is a useful pose to relieve lower backache, counteract stooping shoulders and strengthen lower back, feet and legs.

Stand in Mountain pose, with your back about 50cm away from wall, feet parallel, hip-width apart, arches well lifted.

INHALE, reach back to bring palms of hands flat on wall.

EXHALE, let arms take weight of body as you slowly ease spine to wall. When spine is resting against wall, bring hands onto your belly in *yoni mudrā*.

INHALE and lengthen spine, keeping tailbone, head and shoulder blades in contact with wall.

EXHALE, bend knees slightly, sliding spine a little down wall.

INHALE and arch lower back a little away from wall while maintaining contact between back of head and wall.

EXHALE and lengthen the curve of the lower back, bringing it closer to wall and squeezing the buttocks together.

Keep feet strong, arches lifted, and breath flowing freely as you continue to tilt pelvis in time with breath for up to seven or eight rounds.

To complete, straighten legs, press palms against wall and push back to starting position. Rest in Ladder against wall (see p.532) for a few rounds of breath.

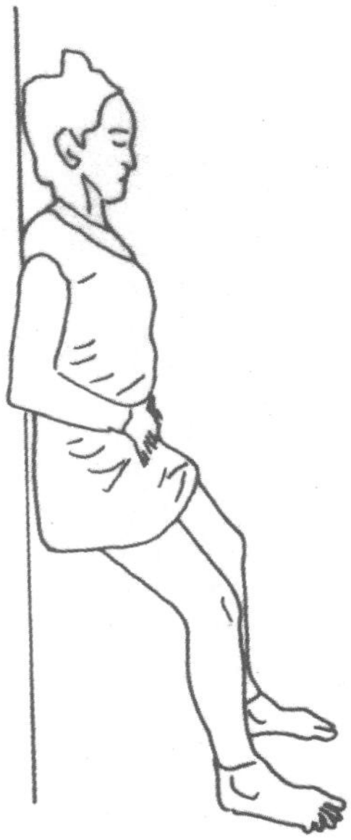

Side stretch at wall

This is the best pose for creating space and openness along the sides of the body.

Stand in Mountain pose, with right side about arm's length from wall, feet parallel, hip-width apart.

INHALE, raise right hand to shoulder height and press palm into wall. If necessary, adjust distance from wall so that right arm can be held straight at shoulder height.

EXHALE and push back of left heel firmly into floor.

INHALE, raise left arm above head, with elbow straight or bent.

EXHALE, push right palm into wall and heel of left foot firmly down into floor, letting head and neck tilt slightly to right and feeling descent of left heel freeing movement through left side of body.

INHALE, breathe fully into open space around left armpit and ribs.

With each inhalation, reach left arm higher up. With each exhalation, press right palm firmly against wall and left heel down into ground. Continue for up to five rounds.

To come out, inhale right arm back up above head, and exhale both arms down to sides.

Pause for a round of breath in Mountain pose before reversing position to repeat on other side.

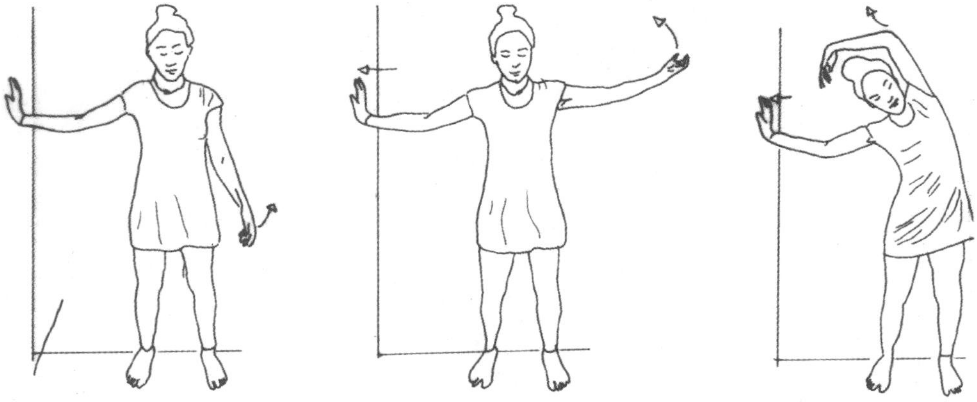

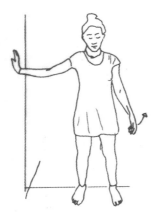

Dog against wall

This works well in sequence with the previous pair of poses. Three rounds of Dog followed by a period of active rest in Chair and recuperation in Ladder is an effective way to realign the spine. This is also a useful option to use during menstruation or pregnancy when the full Downward-facing dog may not feel very comfortable.

Stand in Mountain pose, facing wall at arm's length distance.

INHALE, reach arms above head to place palms on wall, shoulder-width apart.

EXHALE, press weight into heels, keeping arches lifted. Keeping breath even, slowly walk palms of hands down wall, no lower than hip height.

Step feet back away from wall little by little to create length in spine. Keep knees bent and move only as far away as enables you to keep hips straight above ankles, with strong hand contact on wall. Do not step further back than this. Keep feet hip-width apart and parallel, arches lifted and weight pushing down into heels. If your back feels comfortable straighten the legs.

Spread fingers wide and keep strong pressure from heels of hands into wall.

INHALE, lengthen sides of body, pushing heels of hands into wall.

EXHALE, lengthen spine towards tailbone, pushing heels of feet into floor.

Breathe here up to five rounds.

To come out, slowly walk hands up wall and step feet in towards wall. Rest for a few rounds of breath in Ladder against wall (p.546).

If you enjoyed the pose, repeat twice more.

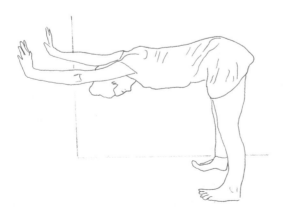

SUPPORTED POSES AND RESTORATIVES PART 2

Simple and super deluxe five-star corpse pose (*savasana*)

The Corpse pose is the classic yoga relaxation pose, in which the physical body lies flat out on the back, dead still. Often it is more comfortable to bend knees to reduce strain in lumbar spine. The most comfortable way to do this is with support under knees. These two options provide different levels of support.

You will need: a pillow or two for your head and either a chair (the seat of a sofa works well), or a beanbag and/or bolster to support lower legs.

Simple version

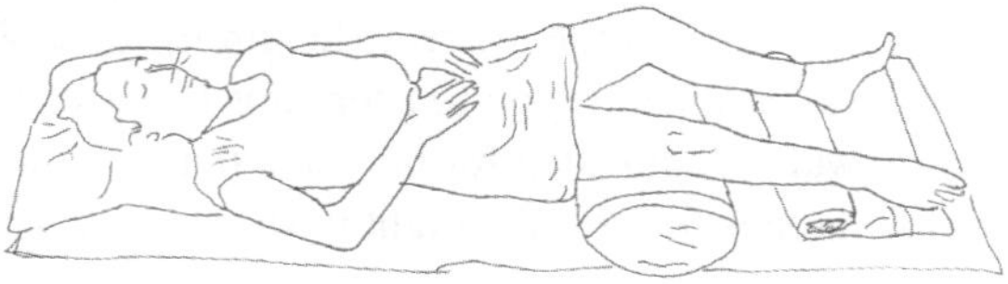

For lower level of support, simply place prop under knees to create a comfortable bend. The height of support directly impacts on lumbar (lower back) curve, so experiment to find what suits.

When bend in knees feels right, place pillow under head.

Super deluxe version (or semi-supine rest with chair)

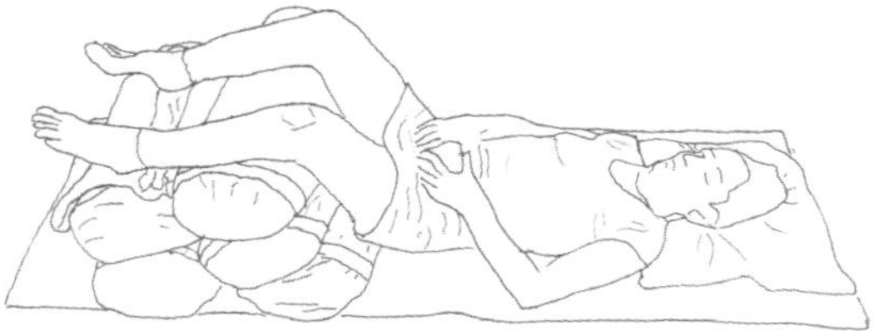

For higher level of support, have a higher prop like a chair (the seat of a sofa works well), so you can bend knees and lift feet and lower legs up higher to rest the whole of the calves on the support. Ensure backs of knees are in contact with front edge of support. Be sure higher prop is at a level that can support back of knees. If it feels too low, raise top edge of prop by adding a rolled blanket under knees.

Either place feet close together and allow knees to drop to either side or keep feet hip-width apart and shins parallel.

For both levels of support, slide tops of shoulders down away from ears and either have hands resting by sides, palms up, a little away from body or bring palms to rest on belly. If your elbows do not touch the ground, then place cushions beneath them. *Yoni mudrā* is often comfortable in this pose.

Supported side-lying

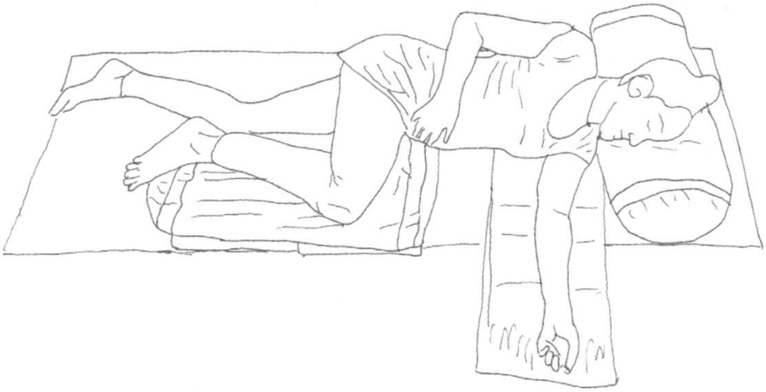

If lying on your back is uncomfortable, then this supported side-lying is an excellent replacement.

You will need: a pillow or two for your head, and either a bolster or stack of yoga blocks (six is optimal) to support top leg. It is a good idea to have an extra blanket so that your hip doesn't stick into the floor. Also, if you are pregnant, you will need an extra pillow to put under your bump.

Ensure leg support is high, firm and long enough to support the entire lower leg (from above knee right down to ankle) at hip height. This means leg support should be at least as high as your hips are wide. Check this by placing a hand on either hip and then comparing distance between your two hands with height of prop.

Lie on your side (whichever you prefer, or in late pregnancy, ideally on your left). Have the underneath leg either straight, or slightly bent. Bend top leg and support it so that whole length of lower leg, from just above knee to foot, is resting on top surface of support.

Once legs are comfortable, if required place pillow under belly to support weight of bump, and adjust arms and head.

Place the underneath arm in whichever of the following four positions feels most comfortable: out in front, resting on floor at shoulder level; out in front, bent and tucked in under the pillows beneath your head; stretched up above head, underneath supporting pillows; or extended slightly behind body, so that there is a slight roll in front of body. If the underneath hand is out in front, or back behind, then position pillows one under shoulder and one between ear and shoulder to support neck.

Slide shoulders down away from ears and gently tuck in chin. Allow body to settle into supports.

Open flower (*supta baddhakoṇāsana*)

Instructions are as for the inhale position in the Seed-flower pose (pp.154–5). Remain in this pose and breathe freely.

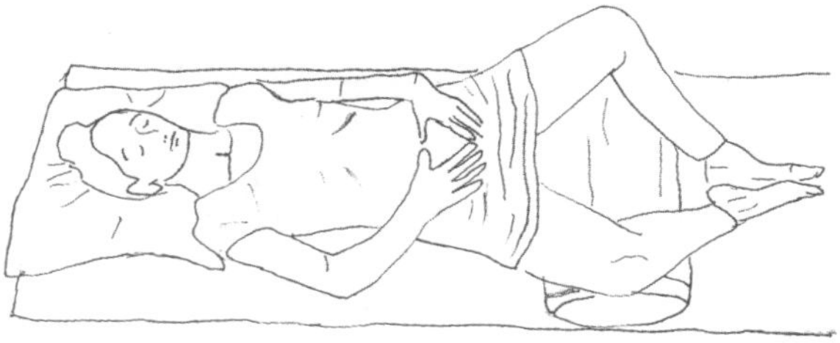

In the golden cosmic womb (Queen's pose) (*hiraṇya garbha* / supported *supta baddhakoṇāsana*)

This is a blissful restorative pose, giving complete support and protection to the back of the body to promote an attitude of receptivity, acceptance and contentment. It offers the essential openness of the Open flower above, without any physical effort. It can take a while to set up and uses lots of props but is well worth the effort because once you are in the pose, you can breathe, rest or do meditative practices in total comfort for up to forty minutes or longer if you are comfortable.

You will need: a mat, cushion or folded blanket to sit on, a belt to support sacrum, a bolster or two plus a wall or bean bag to provide inclined support, and bolsters or cushions for thighs and elbows. Additional cushions for head support can be useful, plus blanket and eyebag.

Set up back support first, putting one end of bolster on cushion and leaning bolster against wall, using blocks, cushions or a bean bag to create a comfortable angle of around thirty degrees. Place bolsters either side of knees so they are easy to reach.

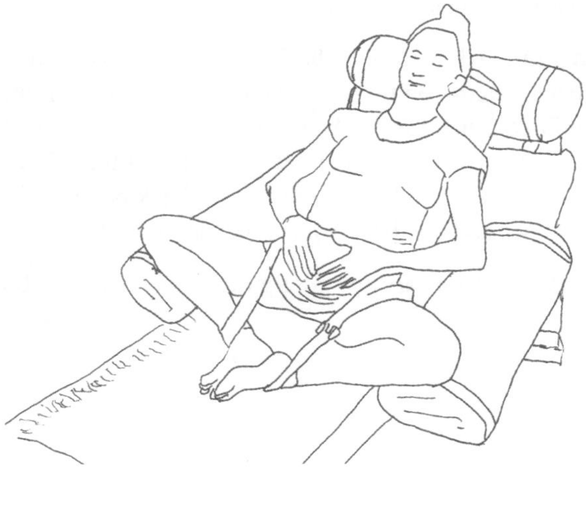

Sit on cushion in front of bolster in full Butterfly (p.167). Place belt around lower back, just across sacro-iliac joints (either side of flat part of lower back), bringing ends around to inside of your legs. Take belt underneath feet so that soles are held together without any effort. Adjust distance between heels and buttocks until it feels easy, and then secure belt to hold feet in this position. Place belt buckle so that it does not stick in your leg.

Now lean back, ensuring whole length of spine is supported by upright bolster.

Move cushions or bolsters in to support thighs and elbows.

Use additional cushions or folded blankets to support head and neck if necessary.

Cover with a blanket if you are planning to be in the pose for more than a few minutes, and cover eyelids with eye bag or scarf.

Rest hands either on supports, or over your belly, whichever you prefer.

When you feel ready to come out, move slowly and gently. First uncover yourself and draw knees inwards, supporting outside of knees with palms of hands.

Hare pose (*śaśāṅkāsana*) with fists and blankets

From Cat pose, move knees a little wider apart, with enough space to take your belly forward and down between knees easily. If it feels more comfortable, let toes move close together as knees move wider apart.

Exhaling, round spine.

Move buttocks back towards heels, keeping hands in place.

Rest buttocks on heels and allow forehead to rest on support.

If comfortable, remain here for up to ten breaths, or as long as feels good. If there is any discomfort, then come out and adjust as described below.

Tips: *Whilst Hare pose is calming and restful for many pregnant women in early pregnancy, many women prefer higher support as the bump grows. A stack of blocks*

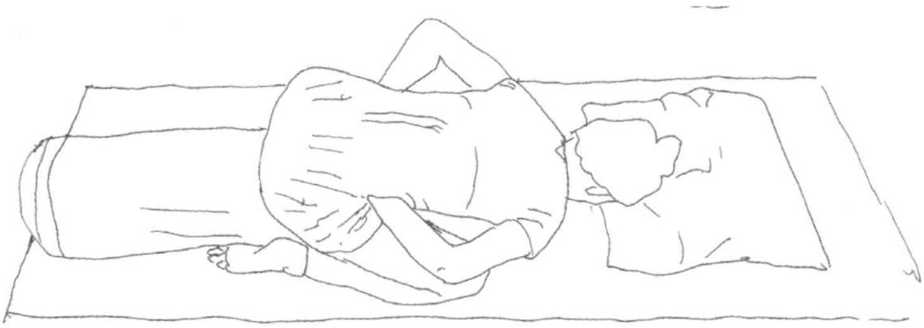

(two or three) or of cushions between the feet provides a higher resting place for buttocks. A cushion, bolster or folded blanket gives a higher resting place for the head. Adjust height until it feels right: instead of being horizontal, the body rests on a slight forward incline, using a chair, bean bag, or even the seat or the back of a sofa. This higher support is very necessary if the standard pose tends to induce nausea, and/or aggravate heartburn or breathlessness. If knees or ankles feel uncomfortable when buttocks drop back, then place cushions or a blanket behind knees before moving buttocks down.

Supported forward bend

Resting with the forehead supported brings a sense of deep tranquillity.

Sit on the edge of a folded blanket or cushion, with your legs out straight as on page 164, and place a chair in front of you between your legs so that you can rest your head forward on the seat of the chair. Put a bolster or cushion on the chair seat to make it the right height (when it is exactly perfect your lower back is completely comfortable). If it is too high, then use a bolster on the floor instead.

If it does not feel comfortable to have your legs straight, then bend the knees and put the feet on the floor. An alternative or additional variation is to have the legs crossed. If using this variation, swap the cross of your legs half way through the practice.

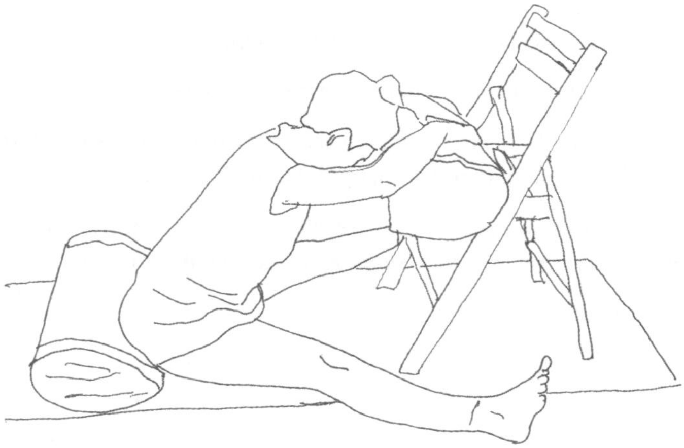

Surrender and worship (*praṇāmāsana*)

NB Avoid during pregnancy, or if you have fibroids in the womb that are painful under pressure. During menstruation this may or may not feel comfortable; explore it gently for yourself.

This is a powerful physical gesture of surrender. It puts the front of the body in direct contact with the earth, and promotes a clear experience of the full yogic breath.

Begin in Hare pose (p.553). Reach out the hands and slide forwards until the front of the chest and belly come into direct contact with the mat / earth.

Stretch out the legs behind and let feet rest with big toes touching. If this is uncomfortable, let the heels be touching instead.

Ideally, bring forehead to the floor, if necessary with a folded blanket underneath. If this is uncomfortable, turn head to side and swap half way through to other side.

Reach arms out along floor in front of head and either bring hands to prayer position, or rest with arms at shoulder width and palms facing up or down

Breathe with *ujjāyī* (pp.134–5) and full yogic breath. Let the weight of the body settle down into the ground on every exhale.

Be here for a couple of minutes as a minimum, up to as long as you feel comfortable. This is the perfect pose in which to contemplate or to hear the story of Sitā (pp.508–9).

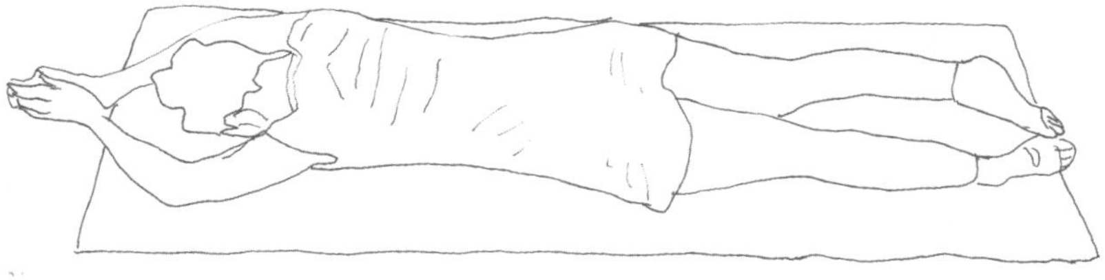

CHAPTER TWENTY-SIX

connection and flow

SUGGESTED SEQUENCING FOR PRACTICE AND CLASSES

For uplifting spirits and energising:

1 greeting the womb with love seated practices (pp.143–147)

2 being in the cycles (pp.517–521)

3 moon phase sequence (pp.527–31)

starry night pure *yoga nidrā* (pp.435–41)

4 five dimensions of being (pp.183–7)

5 extended heart space twist pose figure (p.159)

1

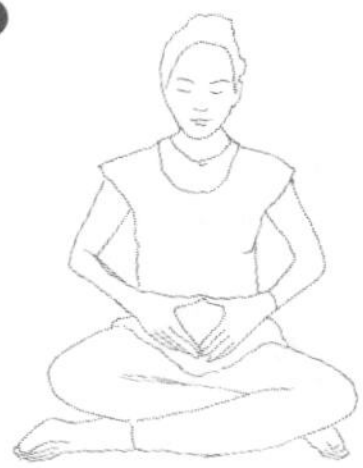

2

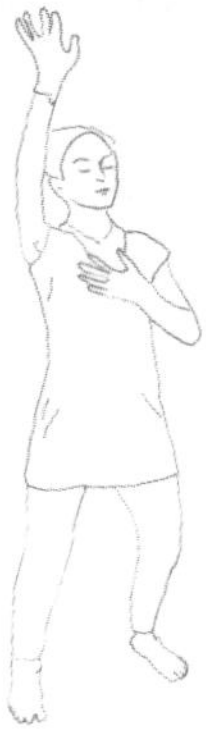

3

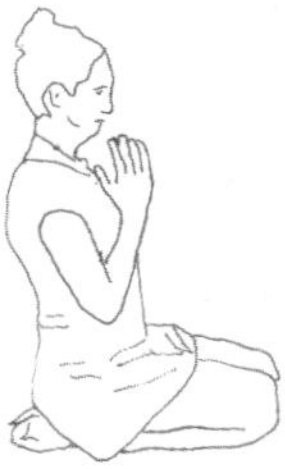

4

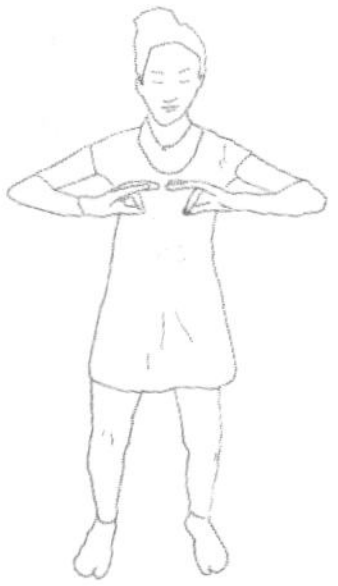

5

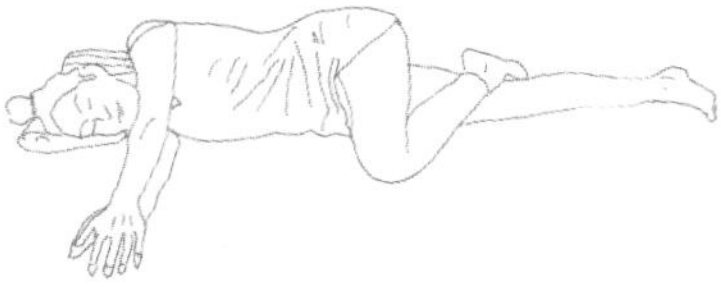

1
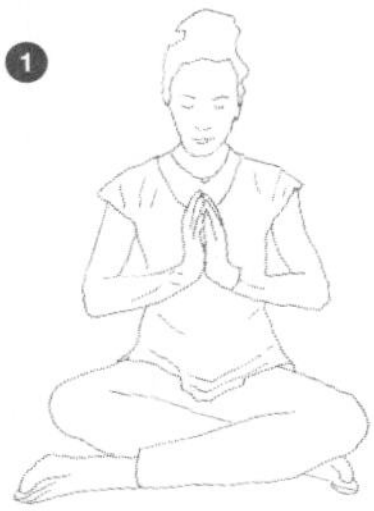
2
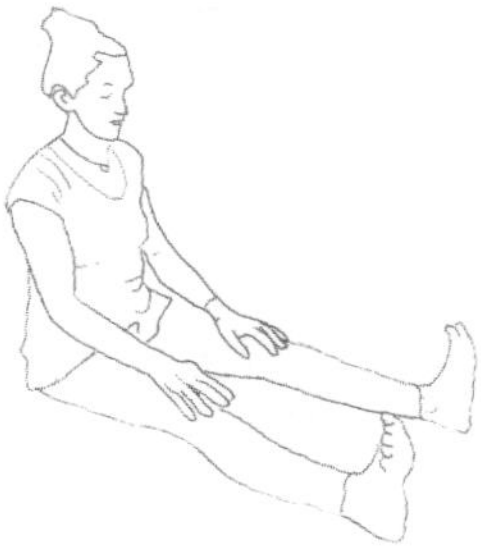
3
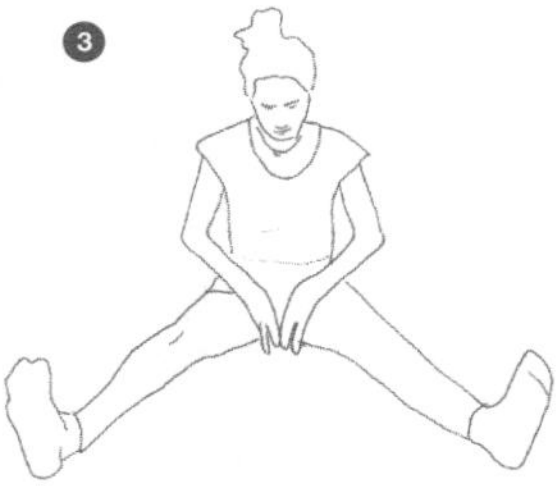

For calming and grounding:

1 greeting the womb with love seated practices (pp.143–147)

2 complete liberation of energy sequence (pp.497–510)

yoga nidrā: an invocation to *yoni śakti* (pp.17–21)

3 honouring the elements with sound and gesture (pp.189–99)

For reconnection and self-acceptance:

1 honouring the elements with sound and gesture (pp.189–99)

2 five dimensions of being (pp.183–7)

3 womb elevation bridge sequence (pp.155–8)

4 greeting the womb with love seated practices (pp.143–147)

1
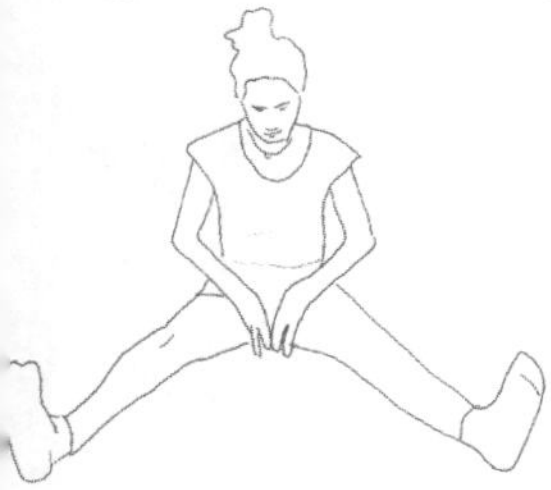
2
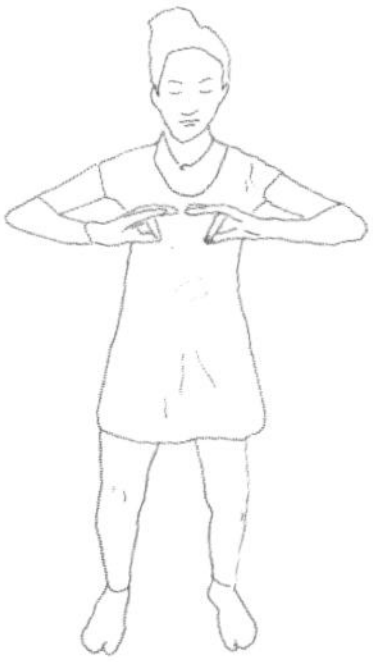
3
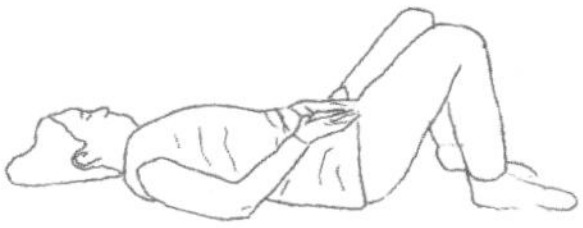
4
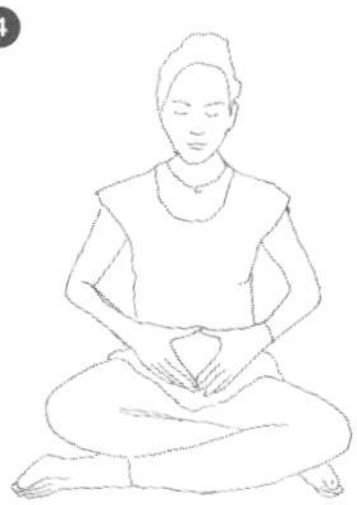

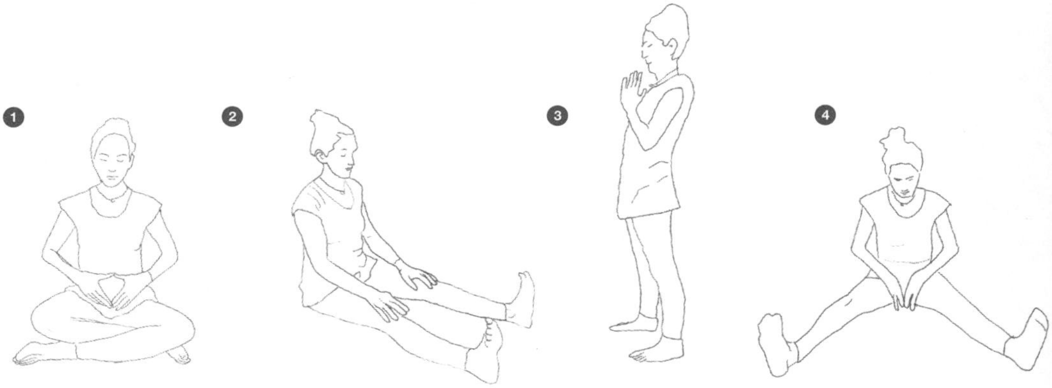

To nourish and strengthen:

1 greeting the womb with love seated practices (pp.143–147)

in the *yoginīs'* temple *yoga nidrā* (pp.454–9)

2 complete liberation of energy sequence (pp.497–510)

3 postnatal sun salutation (pp.533–5)

4 honouring the elements with sound and gesture (pp.189–99)

To get unstuck and move on:

1 *śakti bandhas* (pp.511–5)

2 being in the cycles (pp.517–521)

cyclical wisdom *yoga nidrā* (pp.443–6)

3 greeting the womb with love seated practices (pp.143–147)

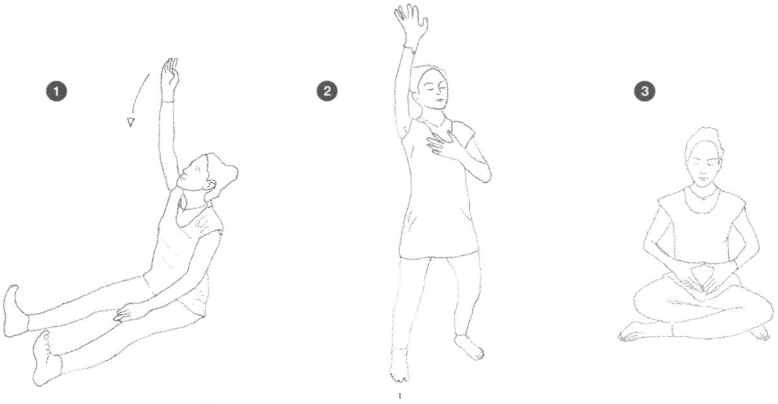

1
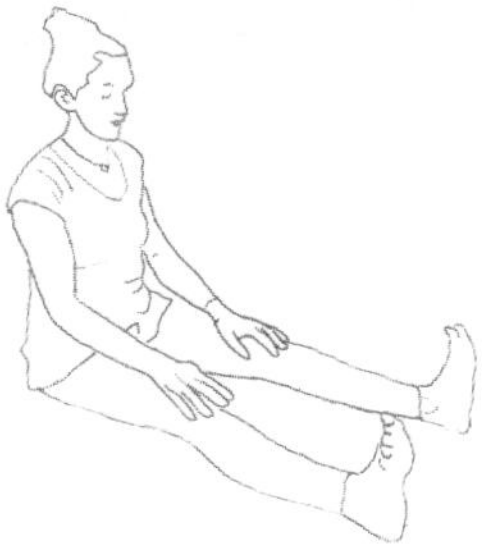
2
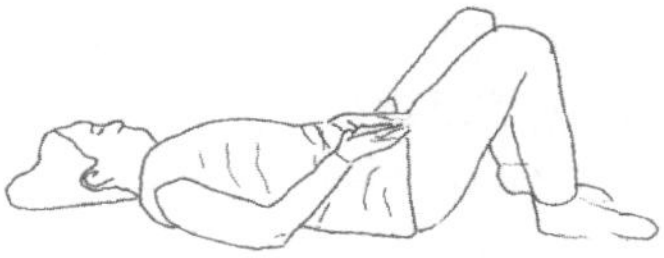
3
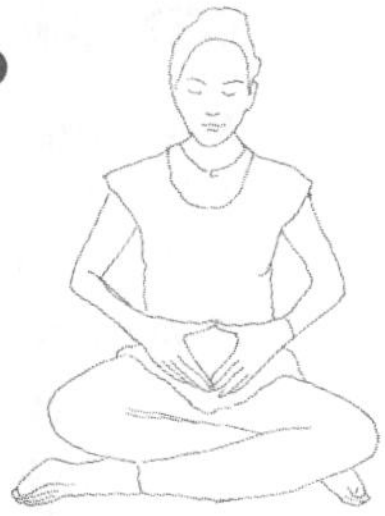

To become cool, collected and quietly energised:

Cooling breaths (pp.470–1)

1 complete liberation of energy sequence (pp.497–510)

2 womb elevation bridge sequence (pp.155–8)

3 greeting the womb with love seated practices (pp.143–147)

in the *yoginīs'* temple *yoga nidrā* (pp.454–9)

To build sexual and creative energies:

1 greeting the womb with love seated practices (pp.143–147)

2 *śakti bandhas* (pp.511–5)

3 swaying palm tree with womb greeting (p.532)

4 womb elevation bridge sequence (pp.155–8)

in the wild garden, joyous freedom to flow *yoga nidrā* (pp.445–6);

5 extended heart space twist pose (p.159)

1
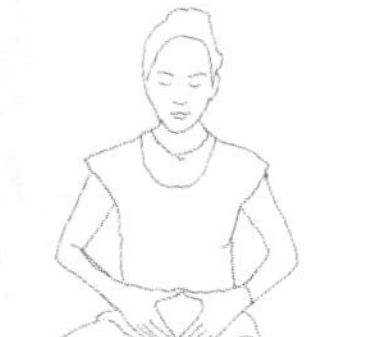
2
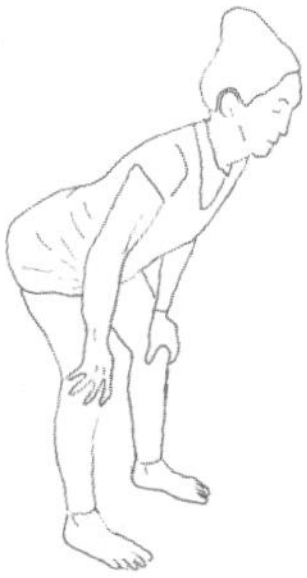
3
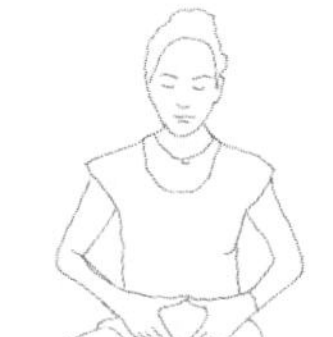
4
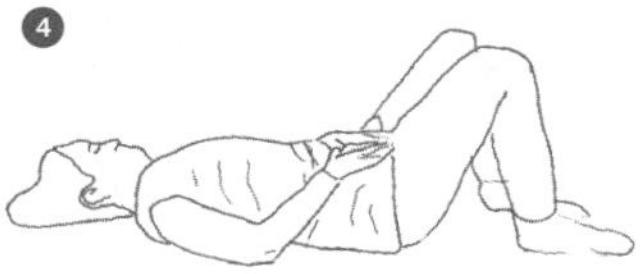
5
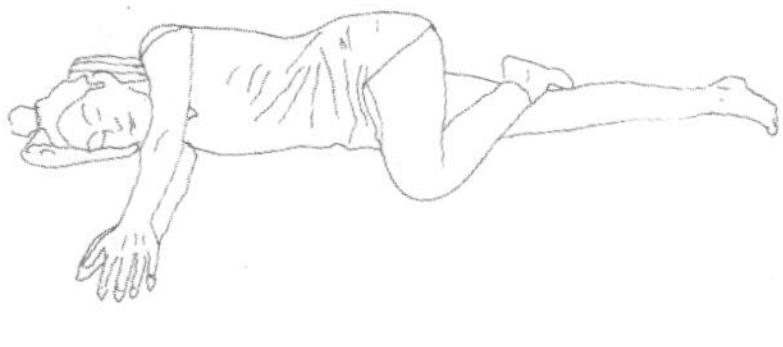

MENSTRUAL AND FERTILITY *MĀLĀ*: CIRCLE OF PRACTICES TO PROMOTE A HEALTHY MENSTRUAL CYCLE AND TO SUPPORT FERTILITY

Nine core practices:

1 Full yogic breath in super deluxe savasana *(p.550)*
2 Open flower (p.552)
3 Śakti bandhas *(pp.511–15)*
4 Moon phase salute (pp.527–31)
5 Supported forward bend (p.554)
6 Extended heart space twist (p.159);
7 In the golden cosmic womb (Queen's pose) (p.552)
8 Yoga nidrā *(pp.443–4 or pp.446–8, as appropriate to where you are in your cycle, see below) (not illustrated)*
9 Greeting the womb with love seated practices (pp.143–7)

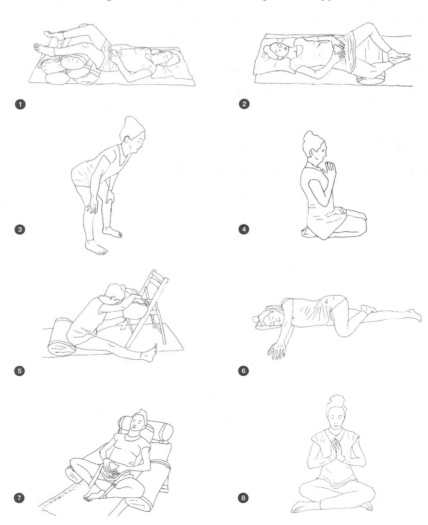

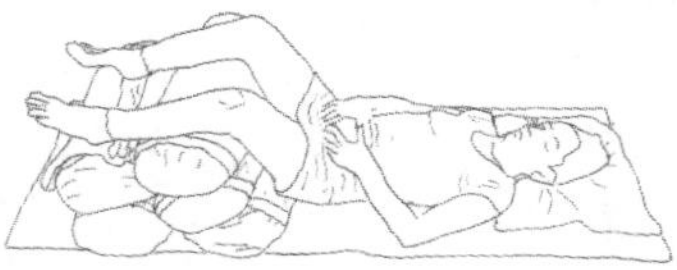
1

2

3

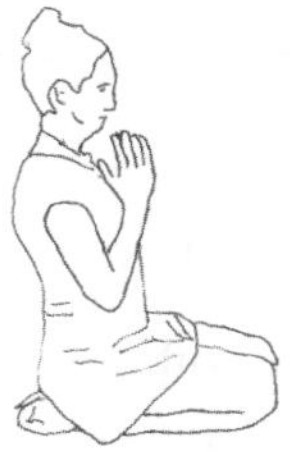
4

5

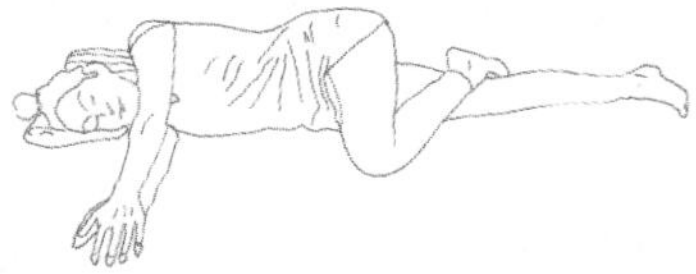
6

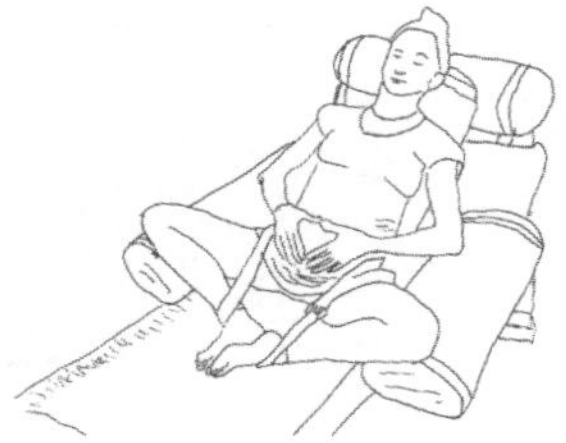
7

8

A *mālā* is a circular string of beads used for meditation: each time a bead is passed through the fingers, another *mantra* or prayer is recited (audibly or mentally). It is similar in function to a rosary: the beads serve to count the number of repetitions and to keep the mind focused on the practice. The *mālā* beads can be used with lightness and ease, passing rapidly around the circle, flicking swiftly from one bead to the next to provide an almost subliminal source of familiar comfort; or the beads can be used with great intensity, holding tight to each one as the *mantra* or invocation is repeated, to provide strength and support in a time of challenge. Because the beads are strung in a circle, the practice is always cyclical, bringing the practitioner back to a fresh start at the end of each cycle, just like our menstrual cycle. With each repetition of the cycle we grow in understanding and awareness.

This circle of yoga practices can function like a *mālā*: as a circular string of relaxed practice to create balance and ease on the journey through the cycle's monthly rhythm. The individual yoga practices can also be used in a more focused manner, to assist with the difficult physical or emotional passage at a particular point, perhaps a place that causes struggle or pain, during which time it is helpful to focus more on certain practices that provides relief. So you can keep the circle of practices ticking over throughout your cycle or you can focus on practices to bring relief at certain points, or (most likely) you can do a mixture of both.

Whether you are using the practices for the creation of a general balance in your cycle, or to relieve difficulties associated with certain parts of that cycle, the circle of yoga practices brings benefits by focusing your mind on the practices suited to each part of your cycle, and by deepening your awareness of the cyclical nature of menstruation. There is nothing linear about it. The arc of the circling cycles holds us within its rhythm, and this yoga practice gives us the opportunity to deepen our connection with the rhythm of life itself. As deeper understanding grows through the practice of yoga we learn that certain experiences during our cycle simply need conscious management and support: for example deeper rest, finer awareness through meditation, or more profound release through breath and movement.

And so at the centre of the circle is a set of core practices to provide balanced support for menstrual health throughout the cycle. The central programme is a month-long commitment, in that it is suited to most days. They include a range of active and passive practices to create balance throughout the cycle, building a harmonious relationship between times when we are more able to give out (energy, emotions, focus, activity) and times when we need to focus more within, to be protective of our quiet space and inner life.

But there is no sense of rigidity: no need to do all of it every day. Be aware of the circular nature of the cycle and recognise that there will be days when you feel like doing less, but other days when you feel engaged with the more active practices. The deep aim of this circle of women's yoga practices is to enable you to accept and honour the rhythms of your monthly cycle.

The maximum amount of time you might want to spend on this whole programme would be 110 minutes for a full leisurely practice. An abbreviated version could take fifteen minutes, or a short complete version would be about half an hour. There are suggestions for modifications and adaptations to suit your cycle below.

Tailoring the core practice programme to your changing needs

The nine key practices on page 560 form the heart of a feminine practice of yoga that is safe and supportive through your whole cycle. The sequence promotes fertility and also is safe whilst pregnant, even if you are in the very early stages of pregnancy. However, it is likely that at certain points in the cycle you will wish to modify this basic sequence. You can modify the basic practice in two ways:

If you need to make changes because of pressure of time, then it is best to follow this guidance: practices 1, 7, 8 and 9 are always worth making time for, but they can be shortened to take less time. Instead of spending five minutes with practice 1, do two minutes. Practices 7 and 8 work best in combination, and are effective even if you spend only ten minutes.

If you need to make changes because of how you are feeling in response to your cycle, then you can adapt the basic sequence to meet your needs. You can do this either by making use of the restorative variations (for example if you feel less inclined to be active, use the supported version of the forward bend, p.554, and the still versions of the lying twist, p.159), or by removing or adapting practices 2, 3 and 4 and replacing them, or by expanding your focus within the practices according to the cycle-specific recommendations described below.

Choose your *yoga nidrā* practice appropriate to your needs, too. If the intention is to support healthy menstruation, use the Cyclical wisdom practice on pp.443–4. If the intention is to support fertility and promote conception, then use the Nourishing growth practice on pp.446–8.

The key to gaining positive benefit from your practice of yoga is to focus your attention within: practice 1 is always the place to start. Gauge your own needs and respond to the cyclical changes by honouring the place you are in.

Yoga during pre-ovulatory phase

The focus for yoga practice here is to nourish and grow. Give full attention to your full yogic breath and allow *yoni mudrā* to help you connect with your ovaries, nestling just beneath your palms. This can be the time to focus your attention on a sense of growth and expansion: pay attention to the receptive feeling of the Open flower position, and extend into your fingertips as you practice *candra namaskāra* (Moon salute, pp.522–6).

This can be a good time in the cycle to experiment with strengthening and opening practices such as the Half moon pose (p.540). Add three or more repetitions of this pose during the Moon salute. It is also a good time to work with the Rising snake series (p.543). The Camel pose (p.542) can also feel good at this time of the cycle, and fits well in the Moon sequence, just before the final forward bend.

This stage can also be a helpful time to use a therapeutic inversion: Half shoulderstand (*viparīta karaṇī*) (p.545).

Yoga during ovulation

The focus for yoga practice at this time can helpfully be to nourish and release potential. During this part of the cycle, the Half shoulderstand (p.545) can be enjoyable, and some of the more opening, liberating movements of the Dog pose and its variations (p.530) are appropriate. Alternating the Cobra (p.530) with Dog can also be very strengthening and vitalising at this time, and if you enjoy the Camel pose (p.542), then include that in your programme too.

For meditation practice, let the seated womb greetings (pp.143–7) guide your awareness within. If you experience pain on ovulation, then *praṇāmāsana* (p.555) and adaptations of the Hare pose (p.553) may afford relief.

Yoga during the pre-menstruum

Let the focus of your yoga practice during this part of the cycle be to nourish and grow. Gentle but rhythmic repetition of the *śakti bandhas* (pp.511–15) can help to dissipate any physical congestion. Be sure to allow sufficient rest periods, and if you are feeling edgy, then use the Golden thread breath (p.462) to release physical and mental tension. In addition, Balancing breath (p.466) and Triangle breathing (pp.464–5) can help to cope with the demands of mood swings or turbulent emotions. Use them at the end of your yoga programme, just before meditation.

Yoga during menstruation

Let the focus for your yoga practice at this time be to nurture, release and cleanse. Avoid all inversions. Be prepared to be still. But if movement feels right, use soft rhythmic repetitions. Use the *śakti bandhas* (pp.511–5) softer and more rhythmically, and only do those elements of the Moon sequence (pp.522–6) that feel right to you. Often the Hare pose (p.553) feels comforting, and if you experience pain during this time, then these Hare pose variations can be helpful: make two fists with your hands and settle them into the groin area before you fold forwards, to bring warmth and pressure into the ovaries; and/or place a blanket over your lower back and have a friend hold the ends of blanket firmly down either side of your hips, bringing even pressure and warmth into the lower back. If you are practising alone, then using the weight of a sand bag on the lower back can have similar benefits. If you don't have a sand bag then use a large bag of pulses or beans, or a warm hot water bottle.

Also, it can be comforting to rest on the back and hug the knees into the chest, drawing the thighs in close to the belly on the exhalation [*apanasana*]. Supported forward bends (p.554) can also provide comfort and relief. For some women, painful menstrual cramps are better relieved by backward bending than forward bending. It is best to experiment for yourself to find what works for you. The Camel pose (p.542) and Rising snake (p.543) are both backward bends that may be helpful in the relief of pain during your bleeding time, as can *praṇāmāsana* (p.555), but it is also likely that regular practice of these poses throughout the rest of the cycle may help to prevent or lessen future suffering of this kind. So if you regularly experience pain during menstruation, endeavour to practise these poses as part of the core programme. They fit well within the Moon salutation sequence, just at the end before the final forward bend. If you feel in need of balance and comfort during your bleeding time, you may find the Triangle breaths (pp.464–5) and Balancing breath (pp.466–7) helpful.

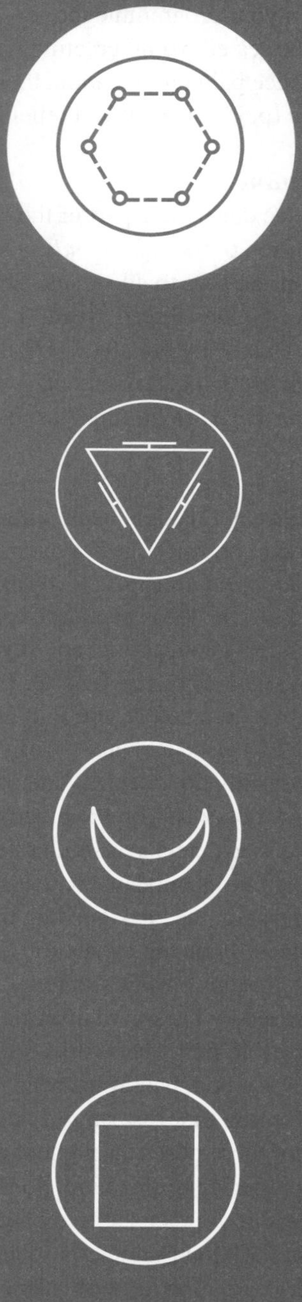

PART FOUR
EXPANSIONS

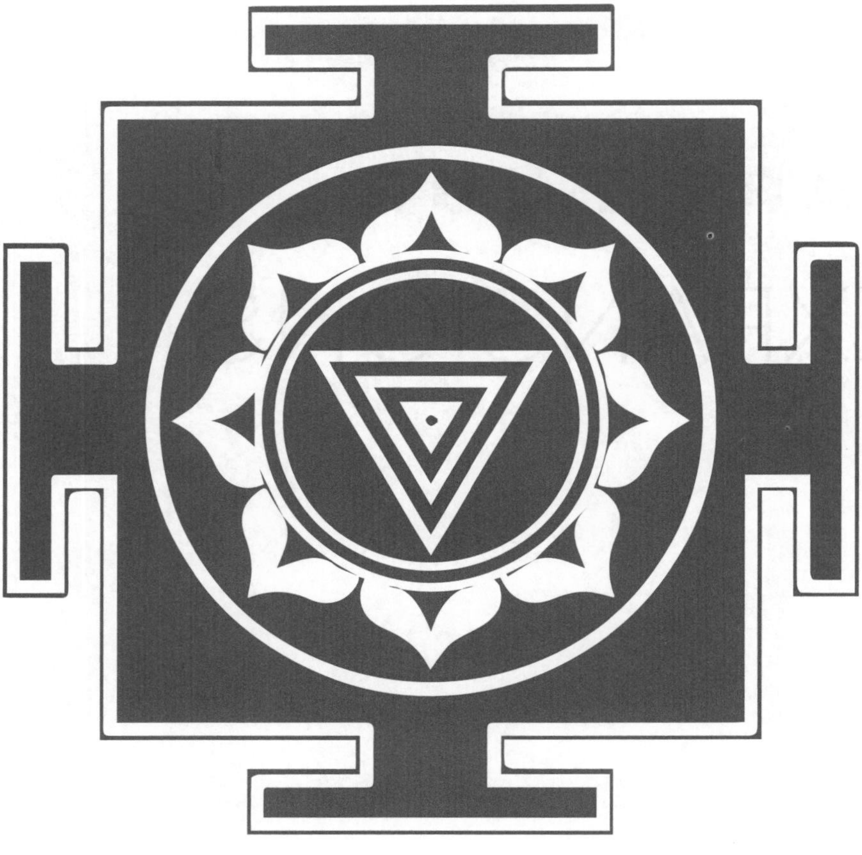

CHAPTER TWENTY-SEVEN

world as womb: womb ecology, eco-feminism and yoga activism: a powerful force for change

What if ... our negation of the feminine principle were responsible for climate change? ... The shock [of disconnection from the earth] needs to melt so that the locked up energy is made available to the creation of the world we actually want. If we don't feel it, if it doesn't become personal, then nothing will change. This vital, ancient and very present grief is the lubricant of behaviour change. Feel it, and you will no longer be able to collude with it. (Clare Dakin, Founder of Tree Sisters)

To take back control of our health and stop these egregious [environmental] crimes, we have got to reclaim the primordial feminine force ... we must take appropriate steps to honour and preserve the maternal energy known as Mother Consciousness. This energy is being fractured every moment. This hurt reflects deep into the womb of every female of every species. Mother's womb of life exists far beyond the uterus of her female species; it is stretched to the forest, ocean, skies and into the core of the earth itself. (Mother Maya Tiwari 2011: 15)

Be in the world as a womb,
Know the womb as world.
Both are places of nurture and creativity,
Spaces for nourishment and growth.
The wombs in the world are worlds within.
(Uma Dinsmore-Tuli 2012, Womb Yoga training manual)

Links between women and the earth as mother have deep mythic origins across many cultures. The perception of our womb as a microcosmic world within us has a truly powerful contemporary resonance in relation to the present ecological crisis. The practice of yoga that honours the cycles of womb life has a special place in raising awareness of the urgent need to honour the earth as mother, our world-womb. In this chapter I set out the old tales, and explore the current wave of eco-feminist awareness and yoga activism that grows from women's personal responses to global climate change and natural disasters.

Rooted in the ancient traditions of India (in the *Mahābhārata*, the *Taittirīya Saṁhitā*, the *Purāṇas*, and in other places too) are tales that tell how the earth's seasonal changes are evidence of her menstrual cycles. The story goes that Indra, the king of the Gods, murdered a Brahmin called Vṛta. To murder a Brahmin was a heinous sin. But because Indra was the top god, he avoided the dire punishment for his great crime by dividing the 'stain' into three parts and passing it on. One third of the punishment was transferred to human women, one third to the trees of the forest and one third to the mother earth herself (White 2003: 68 and Samuel 2008: 91). All three of the recipients of Indra's punishment are seen to contain fissures (women have vulvas, trees have clefts in their bark, whilst the earth herself has caves, and cracks in her body of rock and mountain), and all three of the recipients are connected through their experiences of cyclical change (women menstruate, trees lose their leaves, and rivers ebb and flow through fissures and channels). So the earth's seasonal changes are seen to be her menstrual cycle. All these cycles are also seen to be a punishment. The ill-effects of such a negative valuation of menstruation were explored in chapters nine and ten, so we won't go over all that again here.

This myth clearly links women's experience of menstruation directly to the seasons of the earth. But this link has resonances which go beyond the mythical. At a practical level of menstrual awareness, the seasonal understanding of our cycles has been helpfully reclaimed and positively utilised by a number of contemporary menstrual awareness writers and activists (see Pope 2001 and Gray 2009). At the level of global ecological awareness, the connection between women and the earth is profound. The increase in women's health problems is matched today by a global environmental crisis. There is a powerful link between women's health and the health of our planet. The growth in women's involvement in yoga has been paralleled by an increasing awareness of green issues. Yogic awareness of the spiritual interconnection of all life is a form of environmental consciousness. Since so many of the people on this planet who practise yoga are women, the growth of eco-feminist projects around the world is being well nourished by a spiritual perspective on ecology that is a natural outgrowth of the practice of yoga. The deep ecology movement, and the global activism around what many call 'the great turning', is founded on recognising that a shift in consciousness, combined with practical efforts to repair ecological damage to the earth, are both key to global change and healing. Before turning to celebrate the intentions and achievements of projects that bring together yoga, women and ecology, it is helpful to see how the framework of yogic understandings can provide a sound foundation and inspiration for practical eco-activism at the level of personal and global change.

The roots of the *tāntrik* reverence for *śakti*, the feminine energy of the life force, are rooted in the language of those Indian philosophies that also form the framework of the yogic project. The very words that are used to describe women's bodies in these traditions signify power, spiritual dignity and cosmic connections. The word *yoni*, which carries the meaning womb, vulva, and vagina, as well as the sense of a 'place of rest, or homecoming', is understood to be the cosmic gateway through which the power of *śakti* enters the world—both in terms of giving birth, and in terms of the creative powers of manifestation, of the *prāṇa śakti* working her way into our world through women. In the *Ṛg Veda*, the oldest of the Indian sacred texts, the goddess Aditi squats down to give birth to all the gods through her *yoni*, and this cosmic gateway to immense creative power is embodied in every woman. The *jagad yoni*, the universal *yoni*, or great cosmic vulva of space and time, is embodied in every woman's womb. A reverence for the womb as a creative power is present also in the Sanskrit term *garbha gṛha*, which literally means the 'womb house,' and refers to the innermost space of any temple, the holy of holies, the inner sanctum. The same word *garbha* is also present in the concept of the *hiraṇya garbha* or the golden cosmic womb of consciousness, the universal mind in which the whole of creation is held. In the philosophical bedrock of yoga and *tantra* is a reverent respect of the balance of life, the cosmic eco-system of which our womb consciousness is a part. The energy of *yoni śakti* is the energy of the whole creation.

In human terms, this means that the well-being of women is foundational to the health and happiness of the whole family, of the whole community, of the whole planet. If we see each womb as a 'world' then we can see that the environment of the womb is the creative space for future life, and for the powerful, healing, creative projects of women around the world. When we see the whole planet as mother, we see that we live in her womb. If we see the world herself as the womb in which we live, then we can understand how important an ecologically responsible attitude is to the creation of positive health in women. In terms of the health of our planet, our 'womb', we are at a turning point now. Shame, guilt and disgust at the natural healthy functioning of women's menstrual cycles has already created an ecological disaster because of the 'discreet' disposal into our rivers and oceans of toxic, non-biodegradable products from the sanitary protection industry. In the UK, the use of tampons, pads and applicators generates more than 200,000 tonnes of waste per year, most of which ends up out at sea. The average UK woman throws away 124–150kg of pads and tampons during her lifetime. According to a 2010 BeachWatch survey, for every kilometre of beach, over thirty items of discarded sanitary protection were found: twenty-two sanitary towels/panty liners or backing strips, and nine tampon applicators (Women's Environmental Network [WEN] sources).

Sanitary protection is a profitable industry, with combined annual sales of nearly £350 billion. This industry has caused an expensive and unnecessary ecological mess. The products are often toxic, both in their production and to their users. (For re-usable non-toxic alternatives that don't pollute, see the resources at the end of this chapter). In addition to environmental pollution caused by the disposal of sanitary products, synthetic hormones from hundreds of millions of contraceptive pill users worldwide have already polluted our drinking waters and created intersex fish. Even as western ideas about what is necessary to live as a woman (i.e ready supplies of the contraceptive pill and disposable sanitary protection) pollute the environment, everywhere on the planet women are exploited, abused and underpaid. It is time to awaken to the connection between our wombs and our world: to see that the way we care for our planet mirrors the way we treat our women and girls. The mirror works two ways: the rape and destruction of the natural resources of our planet are expressions of the disrespect in which women and our bodies have been held.

The practice of yoga now helps us to understand that women's bodies, minds, hearts and souls are living reflections of the painful experiences of the mother earth herself. Viewing our current circumstances with a yogic consciousness gives us the clarity of awareness to see how the global crisis in women's health is an expression of our global ecological crisis. Our planet's natural rhythms and patterns have become disrupted and her beauty and spaciousness have become damaged by the crowded over-development and stripping of natural resources that have accompanied the relentless pursuit of economic growth. As the usual rhythms and functions of the earth's unfolding seasons and temperatures have begun to be disrupted, so too do we observe globally striking increases in the difficulties that our women's bodies have in functioning as they have evolved to do, as creative and fertile echoes of the seasons of the earth, as rhythmic teachers for the depths of cyclical wisdom.

Many women now experience menstruation as a painful trial, or at best an annoying inconvenience that can be controlled by synthetic hormones, so that a large proportion of women are not really experiencing ovulation or a full cycle of menstrual rhythms at all. The long-term serious damage that menstrual suppression does to woman's bodies is only now becoming evident (Rako 2003). Doses of synthetic hormones suppress the natural seasonal shifts of our endocrine systems not only during our menstruating years, but also at menopause. Many of us are struggling to conceive, and if we do conceive naturally or with assistance, then we can be so overwhelmed by the power of birthing energy that we require a phenomenal array of medical interventions and supports in order to give birth. The global numbers of caesarean births are soaring as fast as the breastfeeding figures are plummeting. There is a very direct and alarming resonance between the disrespectful and distrustful attitudes to women's bodies that are at the heart of medicalised western birthing culture, and the industrialised farming practices of agribusiness, as Michel Odent identified in his visionary work, *The Farmer and the Obstetrician* (2002).

But it is not just in our experiences of birth that we can feel such resonances. We have an epidemic of menstrual problems, prolapse and hysterectomies. All aspects of women's health worldwide are in deep crisis. There are many complex reasons for this. Many circumstances and histories have brought us to this place. In the previous chapters, which addressed the cultural restrictions and disempowerments encountered at every stage of a women's life, I have considered how this may have come about. In summary, the current crisis in women's health is all about disconnection, and this same experience of disconnection is at the root of our environmental crisis. As Clare Dakin, founder of the women's environmental project Tree Sisters writes,

When you devalue the Mother and curse her womb as dirty and sinful you break the strongest link there is to who we are and where we come from both in terms of our human and planetary Mothers... The wound of this desecration in both men and women is so shocking and alien, that we slip into a survival state of disconnection to cope with the lostness and grief incurred by dislocation from our Mother root. The disconnection ensures that we can collude with the system that rapes our Mother, the earth and barely feel the consequences. We are dominated, and become unconscious dominators unable to meet the gaze of the Mother who still provides for us even as we destroy her ....

It is because we have become so disconnected from our *yoni śakti* that yoga offers us such a powerful tool for healing. The very root of the meaning of the words *yoni* and yoga is *yuj* – the yoking, or connection that brings us to the experience of union or oneness. To practise yoga is to re-connect. In a supremely practical, physical, emotional and spiritual way, yoga connects us with the experience of unity.

This route to unity is vital at this time of crisis in the health of women and the health of the world. So many of us have become so dissociated from our muddy roots as creatures of the earth that we no longer have our true bearings. Yoga offers a sure way to reconnect with our real nature. Initially, that reconnection needs to be at a personal level, with our own elemental make up, and the recognition of ourselves as microcosms, composed of the same elements that make up the cosmos: the elements of earth and water, fire and air, all held in space. Yoga practice can give us the tools to understand and respect those aspects of our own being which connect us with the qualities of stability and nurture which we experience as earth; with the qualities of fluidity and creativity which we experience as water; of brightness and heat which we experience as fire; and of movement and spaciousness which we experience as air and space. This elemental awareness can empower us to realise that an holistic, elementally connected practice of appropriate yoga is a healing force for the support of women's health. Yoga supports the unfolding of cyclical wisdom. Seeing the whole cycles unfolding in a woman's life can move us naturally to an understanding that places this whole picture in the broader context of a planetary life cycle. As our world moves towards a healing crisis, and as human consciousness changes as part of this planetary evolution, a revaluation of feminine consciousness and power is crucial.

The yogic reverence for *śakti*, the power of the life force, is rooted in an embodied understanding of the elemental connection between everything that lives on, in and around our planet. Everything that is alive is made of the same elements. The experience of connection, of embodying the power of these elements, is available to men as well as to women, but it is especially and readily accessible to women through our experience of the female *siddhis* as described in chapter three. Conscious awareness of the female *siddhis* can invite a naturally occurring encounter with timelessness, and with the experience of the power of the elements at play within the physical form of a human female body. For example, women who have had normal physiological labours and births, or who are aware of altered states of consciousness at times of menstruation or orgasm, often report vivid encounters with undifferentiated time, as the intensity of these *siddhis* demands full attention. What we can encounter at these moments is the power of connection to the source: *yoni śakti*. These experiences of *yoni śakti* can show women how the very flow of our blood, and the open awareness of our bodies hold within them the wisdom to connect consciously to the cosmos and our place within it.

All the other female *siddhis* provide similar opportunities at different points in the life cycle, offering an unfolding range of insights and awareness to deepen spiritual wisdom as a woman ages. The first bleed opens the gates to this wealth of wisdom, and moments like birth, female orgasm and breastfeeding provide us with opportunities to experience at a visceral, physical and emotional level the abundance of the universe flowing through our bodies in the form of blood, vaginal juices, milk and babies. As a woman's body ages and her wisdom deepens, this personal encounter with the raw play of elements within her – for example the raging fires of hot flushes, the drenching night sweats, or the unfolding spaciousness of the relaxed and accommodating wisdom of the postmenopausal woman secure in her knowledge and experience – all navigate a woman's consciousness towards the lived experience of yoga.

These experiences of elemental connection are, of course, open to men, and there are many technologies and programmes of spiritual discipline to bring male consciousness to these same encounters via different routes. The point is not that men are excluded from these experiences, for they are the birthright of all conscious humans; the point is that the nature and rhythms and capacities of female bodies offer women direct access to heightened awareness and sensitivity that can lead straight from the experience of being female to an experience of unity consciousness. For the essence of what the female *siddhis* have to offer is the seed of this unified experience of connection: the rhythmic patterns of a woman's hormonal shifts connect her to her sisters' cycles, to her baby's experience of hunger, to her children's need for comfort, and to the lunar rhythms which create tidal flows in oceans and wombs. To inhabit a body whose intelligence is shaped by cyclical flows naturally empowers us to embody a higher wisdom guided by cosmic rhythms and elemental patterns.

Alexandra Pope, in her inspirational work on the spirituality of the menstrual cycle, describes how the capacity for spiritual insight and wisdom is literally encoded in the cyclical rhythms of women's bodies. But if this wisdom is encoded in our bodies, why do we need books to explain how to connect to this understanding? And what does all this have to do with eco-feminism? These questions bring us back to the problem of disconnection. The womb yoga practices in *Yoni Śakti* offer a means to re-connect. I observe and experience that many women, although our bodies may be offering the clues to elemental connection and wisdom, do not experience these cues as signals to spiritual insight and awareness. The womb yogas in *Yoni Śakti* are practical exercises in re-tuning our consciousness to pick up these cues, which we may be missing because of many multiple layers of powerfully obscuring, encultured attitudes of fear, shame and disgust. Our presently patriarchal culture oppresses and exploits women and the natural world. It has established certain attitudes towards the use we make of the earth's resources, and it has structured our expectations and understandings of what it is to be a woman, so that it is very hard for us to read the cues which point us to our inner wisdom, or to feel our living connection to the earth herself. Shame, embarrassment, disgust, and the wholesale medical control of nearly every aspect of women's hormonal rhythmic cycles and capacities for insight have stolen from women our birthright.

My understanding of what has happened to women's embodied knowledge and spiritual wisdom is this: in the beginning, women naturally had the insight that connected them to their power, and it was acknowledged (Knight 2006), worshipped and honoured in societal structures rooted in reverence for the mother earth, and reverence for the cycles of the women's bodies whose rhythms manifested the cosmic ordering of the elements. Men who honoured mother earth treated the human women who embodied her power with great respect. For many complex and contradictory reasons, this respect was transposed into fear and resentment, and the honouring of women's power, and the desire to protect and nourish the vulnerability and sensitivity that was part of her power, was replaced by a desire to possess and control that power. At the heart of patriarchy was a fearful inadequacy: violence reflected impotence, and the systematic disempowerment of women expressed inadequacy and profound fear of disconnection, which of course has became a self-fulfilling prophecy. The frameworks of thought that support eco-feminist understandings of the whole unsustainable structure of capitalist economics, and exploitation of the earth's resources, including women and children, all reveal that the patriarchal project has largely succeeded in convincing most people on the planet that material success is the only thing worth having.This patriarchal project has been long in the making, and will not disappear overnight. Any amount of fighting and complaining about it will not restore this birthright of conscious elemental connection with the planet on which we live. The only way to reclaim this experience is to take the long route around the back, to delve into the depths of consciousness and each woman's personal experience of her menstrual cycle, and to reclaim our understanding by stealth. By reconnecting with our own cycles we reconnect to the mother earth.

This is the time for reconnection. It is inspiring that there are so many ecologically aware projects working towards planetary healing from a feminine perspective. There are also projects that bring this global consciousness together with yogic practice to make the link between personal transformation and planetary change. The green initiatives of the "Embracing the World" project are a positive example of how a *bhakti yoginī* of global standing can create change at a grassroots level. The South Indian spiritual leader Amritanandamayi Devi, most widely known as Ammaji, the 'hugging saint', has poured the immense resources donated by her devotees into many traditional charitable projects such as orphanages, hospitals and disaster relief work. Her international collective of charitable foundations have also made women's empowerment and green initiatives a top priority. Vocational training and start-up capital for women's employment co-operatives have enabled thousands of Indian women to generate income to support their families though small businesses and co-operative farming. These projects are part of a wide range of incentives that include a global grassroots environmental movement called Green Friends, that has organised the planting of more than one million trees worldwide since 2001, including thirty thousand saplings along the Keralan shoreline hit by the 2004 tsunami.

Ammaji uses her high international profile and spiritual authority to prioritise the concerns of women and the environment as a major focus of global reconnection. Her spiritual practice of *bhakti* yoga, and her environmental message are the same: 'Embrace the World'. With an international travel schedule that brings her on the road for many months every year, Ammaji is literally embodying her message. Mother Maya (previously known as Maya Tiwari and Srī Swami Mayatitananda), the founder of the Wise Earth School of Ayurveda and the Mother Om Mission, has also committed her own energies to demanding international tours in recent years. Mother Maya has devoted the past twenty years to developing materials and trainings for an earth-reverent, women-centred approach to *āyurveda*, and since 2001 her focus has been to connect this practice of environmentally respectful health care with a message that seeks to foster the inner harmony from which deep global healing will flow. 'Living *Ahimsa*' offers ritual and practice to empower individuals to develop inner harmony. Her intention is that taking a vow of *ahimsa* teaches us to '...transform violence, disease and despair into harmony, wellness and joy. 'Living *Ahimsa*' embodies and shares the deepest value of peace and harmony in every person who strives to do the inner work to cultivate personal awareness.' The 'Living *Ahimsa*' project is all about re-connection: to each other, to our inner world, and to the earth herself.

Other well-known women in the international yoga world have used their fame to put across a similar message of re-connection as a path to personal and global healing. For example, Los Angeles-based celebrity yoga teacher Seane Corne founded 'Off the Mat (OTM) and Into the World' to link yoga practitioners with projects for social and environmental change worldwide. OTM's intention is to 'use the power of yoga to inspire conscious, sustainable activism and to ignite grass roots social change'. Corne offers US-wide leadership trainings entitled 'Yoga, purpose and action' to empower American yoga practitioners (mostly women) to 'discover the connections between the yogic path and the way of divine service or Seva'. The shifts in consciousness that such trainings facilitate lead directly to practical activism. Yoga teachers and practitioners working with OTM have used grass roots outreach and local community building activities in the US to raise hundreds of thousands of dollars through annual 'Global Seva Challenges' to initiate and sustain projects around the world. These include building a birth centre for HIV-positive women in Uganda, funding refuges and support for survivors of sex-trafficking in India, and replanting trees, removing rubble and rebuilding communities in Haiti.

OTM uses social networking and community outreach work to build a global *sangha* of yoga practitioners who are committed to extending their own experience of transformation out into the world to make changes for the better at social and environmental levels: 'Why stretch when you can reach?' is their motto. Many of the connections which are being made between individual yoga practitioners to effect global change are through internet sites, webinars, and synchronised meditative events all over the world. These are the tools that are being used by California-based international yoga teacher Shiva Rea, whose Global Mala Project links eight hundred separate events across fifty different countries to synchronise awareness of the rhythms of the earth's cycles, for example by sharing meditation at equinoxes and solstices. Rea's Yoga Energy Activism (YEA!) projects have also raised funds to plant over 350,000 saplings in partnership with Trees for the Future reforestation projects. The global community of yoga practitioners who are involved with the YEA! projects participate in 'energy regeneration days' by reducing their own use of electricity, 're-energising' through the practice of yoga, and 'clearing up' through fasting (from food / technology) and producing zero waste.

The projects initiated by globe-trotting saints such as Ammaji and Mother Maya, and the work of high-profile international yoga teachers such as Shiva Rea and Seane Corne are the most visible, large-scale and popular aspects of a global spread of yoga-inspired efforts for planetary healing. The on-going reflections and resources shared through organisations such as the Green Yoga Association also serve to support a growing global community of eco-conscious yoga practitioners, the vast majority of whom are women. Increasing numbers of yoga studios and retreat centres embrace practical ecological responsibility through action and education. Grass roots, small-scale initiatives are sprouting every day. A selection of recent local events and projects in the southwest of England that link an eco-feminist environmental consciousness with yogic awareness include: the womb yoga International Women's Day celebration in Bristol that combined a seasonally-attuned *śakti*-blessing practice of womb yoga with a screening of *Yoga Woman*, and a set of full-moon womb-yoga-with-womb-blessing workshops in Glastonbury, Welshpool and Bristol. In the Forest of Dean, sacred sexuality facilitator, yoga practitioner and women's *tantra* activist Jewels Wingfield has established the Earth Heart Centre to bring her work with women's spirituality into a living relationship with the principles of deep ecology; and in the countryside near the city of Bath, Carla Esteves, a somatic movement therapist, doula, shaman and *yoginī*, has created Somaterra, a profound healing modality that integrates her support for women's health and well-being with an eco-somatic approach to movement and the feminine as a gateway to the natural world. All these many individual initiatives that are seeded from an awareness of (yogic) connection create a network of positive support that builds, little by little, into global change for women's lives. For example, the props used in the womb yoga sessions and trainings are sourced from Yoga United, a small UK business run by a husband and wife team that imports yoga props and bags and runs yoga holidays and retreats in South India. Everything Yoga United sells is fair traded through personal connection with Yoga Malai, a network of women working in Tamil Nadu whose livelihoods are supported by the Yoga United imports. At the level of fairtrade, the Somerset womb-*yoginīs* are actively supporting the right livelihood and low-impact business of their sisters in Tamil Nadu.

Whilst the combination of yoga, eco-feminism and environmental activism is a relatively recent but growing phenomenon, there are numbers of eco-feminist environmental projects that have been bringing about planetary change in the fields of women's health and environmental awareness for many years. The following selection of women-led projects gives an inspiring flavour of what a few of these initiatives are achieving. Although they are not specifically connected to yoga practice, many of these achievements have been motivated by personal shifts of consciousness that lead to an awareness of the need for global change. Contact details for all of these projects are provided at the end of the chapter.

For the past twenty years, the Women's Environmental Network (WEN) has been working for environmental justice through feminist principles. Past successes of WEN include highlighting the presence of risky chemicals in cosmetics, the Real Nappy Campaign, and an effective raising of global consciousness about what WEN describes as the Sanitary Protection Scandal. The WEN website continues to provide an overview of environmental issues from a woman's perspective, together with many valuable resources for further reading and links.

Tree Sisters is a project that mobilises women's networking skills and capacity for nurture to accelerate global reforestation and the shift to sustainable living. The aim of founder Clare Dakin is to create a network of women to reforest the tropics within ten years, and the organisation has grown from her own work with reforestation projects in India. At the heart of the project is a spiritual, ethical and emotional framework that resonates with yogic ethics and philosophy. Clare explains it in these terms:

> *Tree Sisters is based around a framework of five choices, that sit like the head, arms and legs of a woman around the womb at the centre (in effect, a five-pointed star). The choices of consideration, encouragement, intimacy, responsibility and courage represent the human capacities to live in humility, unity, love, gratitude and generosity. They sit around the womb, because the womb represents our capacity to create, nurture, respect and protect life, both in terms of our own relationship to the life that lives us (self-knowledge), and the planetary mother who sustains us. If we lived consciously with all our capacities and orientations stemming from connection to our source, then we would be incapable of harming her. As it is, money currently sits at the centre of our human map, and acquisition of this temporary form of wealth is driving the destruction of our ecology. The point of Tree Sisters is to explore how women can help reinstate the value of the feminine back into human awareness. How can we help bring the planet, the womb of all life, back to the centre of our human map so that all our activities seek to serve rather than dominate life?*

The support of women's empowerment and global sustainability that motivates the Tree Sisters is also at the heart of the global changes being created by the training projects of the Barefoot College based in Rajasthan, which reach 125,000 people worldwide. Their projects include training illiterate village women from eighteen different countries including India as Barefoot Solar engineers, hand-pump mechanics and recycling professionals to bring power, safe drinking water and sustainability to their villages.

Also based in India, the MATRIKA project (Motherhood and Traditional Resources, Information, Knowledge and Action) has been working with traditional birth attendants (*dai*) since 2002 to document and promote indigenous birth knowledge as a cultural resource. Although MATRIKA may not seem to be an eco-feminist project, if we broaden our understanding of 'environment' to include the cultural environment of indigenous knowledge and women's blood wisdom, then the efforts to share and promote such knowledge comes from the very same intentions as the reforestation projects of Tree Sisters, for example. MATRIKA grew out of Janet Chawla's work with antenatal preparation amongst middle-class women in Delhi. She saw how the mothers' experiences of birth were compromised by a medicalisation of women's bodies that was disconnected from indigenous, traditional approaches rooted in the cultural environment of respect and honour for *yoni śakti*. This inspired her to bring together grass roots reclamation projects to value and promote traditional midwifery practices that support safe birth. An eco-feminist perspective values both cultural and biological diversity.

The protection of biodiversity, indigenous seeds and organic farming is at the heart of *Navdanya* ('nine crops'), a woman-centred movement for the conservation of biological and cultural diversity in India. Its co-founder, Vandana Shiva, is perhaps the most well known, globally active eco-feminist. Her calls for earth democracy, sustainable agriculture and food rights have always been linked to her recognition of the central role of women in farming in India. Her work takes the consciousness of women's direct experience of inequality and exploitation as a starting point for the desire to support and conserve biodiversity and to protect the environments in which it can flourish.

The deep ecology projects of eco-feminist activists like Vandana Shiva, Joanna Macy and Clare Dakin inspire many women to work together for the health of our planet. Small grassroots projects make a big difference: the inspiration of eco-feminist activism is that it works from the microcosm to the macrocosm. When we acknowledge our own relationship as part of the web of living beings that includes mother earth herself, then we are inspired to take action to protect her rights. Polly Higgins' proposal to the United Nations in 2008 for a Universal Declaration of Planetary Rights utilised our existing legal framework to create a new paradigm of environmental protection founded on principles of deep ecology. When viewed from the perspectives of yogic ethics and philosophy, deep ecology is the logical outcome of a personal experience of connection. In *Yoga for a World out of Balance*, Michael Stone convincingly presents yogic teachings on ethics and social action as an urgent moral imperative for all those practising yoga to take personal responsibility to 'follow through' on environmental issues. He rightly encourages *yogis* and *yoginīs* to move forward from the development of a meditative, yogic awareness of the need for personal change, into an engagement with personal, grass roots, community action for global change.

The experience of reconnection that we gain from our own yoga practice resonates with the deep ecology that teaches us that care of the earth and care of ourselves are one and the same. We see that our personal choices help global changes happen. Switching to a re-usable menstrual cup or washable pads, for example, immediately reduces the amount of sanitary protection waste we create in our lifetime. As well as making us feel good about ourselves as eco-activists, menstrual cups and washable pads also save money, and can create a much more positive relationship with menstruation, and with our own menstrual blood flow. It's an eco-feminist choice with multiple benefits every month of our menstruating lives. And womb yoga can work in the same way; it is also an eco-feminist project for planetary healing. To practise womb-friendly yoga fosters positive womb ecology. Creating balance in the inner ecology of our womb life is a personal key to global change. The evolution of feminine spirituality through yoga is one sure (and very pleasing) way to promote a sustainable green consciousness worldwide. The place to start is with our own well-being, and the foundation of a woman's well-being is most often her womb energies. These energies are not necessarily focused solely in the organ of the womb, but in the energies of nurture and creativity she represents.

This chapter began with those ancient Indian stories that spoke of a deep resonance between the earth's seasons and the cyclical rhythms of women's blood wisdom. The *śākta tāntrik* reverence for the *yoni* as cosmic life-source grew along with these stories, and both now serve to nurture contemporary yoga practice that is womb-friendly. From this practice, and nourished by these roots, it feels natural to honour the womb as a literal embodiment of the mother earth's capacity to create and nurture, so that the womb energy of each woman is seen as a microcosm, a whole world within. One key to healing our planet is to attend to the world we carry within us, and to respect the rhythms of the womb as a reflection of cosmic patterns. If we can positively embrace the rhythms of our own cycles, then womb life can be honoured as a source of intuitive wisdom, a valuable resource for personal and world healing.

There is an enormous turning of the tides right now: millions of yoga-practising women are awakening to a higher consciousness of the importance of their own health, self-esteem and spiritual wellbeing as a positive step towards planetary change. Things are truly shifting. And women's immense involvement and passion for yoga is a truly vital part of this change. We can encourage, support and assist women as they practise yoga by sharing those practices that best nurture and nourish the power of the life force in women. We can practise and teach yoga with respect and honour for women's cycles. And as we cultivate conscious awareness and respect for our own life cycles, then we naturally desire to honour the cycles of the natural world and bring profound healing to our planet. We are healing the world, one womb at a time. We are assisting at the birth of a new consciousness that respects and honours the cycles of the life force, in women and all beings. Yoga is a revolutionary force for spiritual and practical change, and promoting women's health and freedom is the key to a future of peace and co-operation, respect and honour. We start one womb at a time, one woman at a time. And then we need to get together. Together, in circles of power and love, we are helping each other to support positive change. What happens when women bring their experiences together to share is explored in chapter twenty-nine: *Śakti* Circles.

RESOURCES FOR YOGA AND ECO-FEMINIST ACTIVISM

Barefoot College: **www.barefootcollege.org**

Deep ecology and the work that re-connects: **www.joannamacy.net**

Earth democracy and planetary rights: **www.pollyhiggins.com**

Earth Heart Centre / Living Love: **www.jewelswingfield.com/ecology-environment.php**

Embracing the World, Amritanandamayima's green initiatives:

www.embracingtheworld.org/environment

Flow (portal for resources on water issues worldwide): **www.flowthefilm.com/takeaction**

Green Yoga Association: **www.greenyoga.org**

MATRIKA (Motherhood and Traditional Resources, Information, Knowledge and Action): **www.matrika-india.org**

Living *Ahimsa* (Mother Maya's peace vow): **www.mypeacevow.org**

Menstrual cups (re-usable alternatives to tampons and sanitary pads): **www.mooncup.co.uk** and also **www.divacup.com**

Mother Om Mission: **www.motherom.org/home.html**

Off the Mat and Into the World: **www.offthematintotheworld.org**

Tree Sisters: **www.treesisters.org**

Wise Earth School of Ayurveda: **www.wisearth.com**

White Ribbon Alliance for Safe Motherhood: **www.whiteribbonalliance.org**

Women's Environmental Network: **www.wen.org.uk** See the resources section for downloads on sanitary Protection and the environment.

Shiva Rea's Sacred Activism: **www.shivarea.com/sacred-activism**

FURTHER READING AND RESEARCH

The Women's Environmental Network publication, *Sanitary Protection Scandal* (1989), by **Alison Costello, Bernadette Vallely** and **Josa Young** is a complete and shocking exploration of the environmental disaster that has been caused by disposable sanitary products worldwide. **Elizabeth Arveda Kissling** has done a remarkable job of exposing the financial exploitation of women's menstrual cycles in *Capitalizing on the Curse: the Business of Menstruation* (2006). The polluting effects of contraceptive pills are described in **Pope** and **Bennet** (2008) and also discussed here: **www.huffingtonpost.com/susan-kim/birth-control-water-and-w_b_385532.html**, **www.nationalreview.com/articles/224265/pill-pollutant/iain-murray** and **www.mnn.com/local-reports/south-carolina/local-blog/birth-control-pill-endangers-fish-populations**

For a full exploration of the Indian menstruation myths in relation to seasonal cycles, see **Julia Leslie**'s chapter, 'Menstruation Myths' in her book *Myth and Mythmaking* (1996: 87–105).

Michael Stone offers a helpful exploration of the practice of yoga as a means to awaken environmental responsibility in *Yoga for a World out of Balance*.

For a full exploration of the subtle and powerful eco-feminist analysis of precisely how and why patriarchy is doomed to failure I warmly recommend the work of **Vandana Shiva**. Her book *Earth Democracy* communicates the author's powerful vindication of the rights of the earth.

The ecological consequences of meat consumption are lucidly set out in the European Vegetarian Union pamphlet of the same name (2009).

Bunker Roy's TED talk offers his passionate advocacy of the transformative power of a grass roots global grandmother network through the Barefoot College. **www.ted.com/talks/bunker_roy.html**

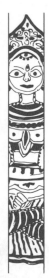

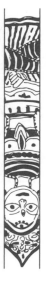

RUNNING TO GROUND, GOING HOME TO THE EARTH: THE STORY OF THE BIRTH AND DEATH OF SITĀ

This story is derived from tales of Sitā in the great Indian epic poem *The Ramāyana*. My intention in re-telling it here is to share a deep sense of our belonging to the earth: she is our mother and we are her daughters.

In the visionary work of Alexandra Pope, the experience of menstruation is understood to comprise four chambers: the chamber of Separation (from everyday consciousness), the chamber of Surrender (to the process of the bleed itself), the chamber of Renewal (as we come to the end of the bleed and sense the beginning of a new cycle), and the chamber of Clarity and Direction (whereby the spiritual experience of menstruation offers guidance and insight).

In Womb Wisdom retreats, I share this story as part of a menstrual yoga sequence; it forms an important part of the process of becoming conscious of menstruation as a holy time of reconnection to the earth. I settle the women into the *pranamāsana* posture, resting on their bellies (p.555) and tell the story whilst they breathe into the earth. To experience the tales of Sitā's earthing in this way, listen to the download on **www.yonishakti.co** whilst you rest on the earth. Enjoy!

Imagine now, as you lie face down on the earth, that the front of your body is resting on the bare earth, in a deep furrow in a newly ploughed field. Feel how you are lying in this groove, like a seed planted in the earth, with the sides of the furrow nestling either side of you.

It was in just such a furrow that the much loved goddess-queen Sitā was born. The name Sitā literally means furrow, and she was born when the two sides of a furrow in the earth parted like an open cunt, giving birth to a baby girl. The earth gave her as a gift in response to the prayers of her parents, who had long been desirous of a child. King Janaka, was out walking his lands one early morning when he saw the infant in the furrow as the answer to his prayers.

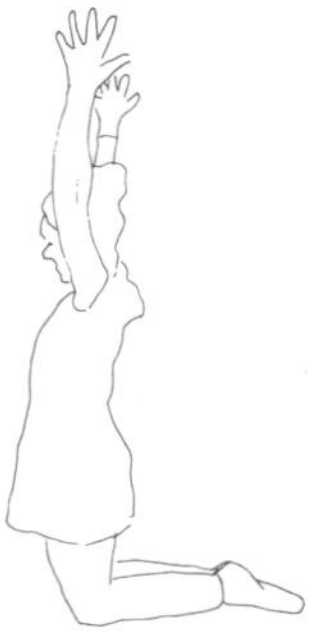

And so Sitā began
her life in the world as a tiny
infant lying in the arms of her mother
the earth, the sides of the furrow keeping
her safe. And King Janaka, he knelt down in the
furrow, scooped up the muddy little baby girl and
brought her home to the royal palace, where she grew into
a beloved and beautiful young princess.

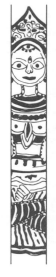

Sitā's troubles began after she met and married her soul-mate, the god-king Rāma. Through a twist in fate, Rāma was deposed and the newly-weds were were banished to the jungle, from where Sitā was abducted by a ten-headed demon and flown through the air on his aerial chariot all the way down to Sri Lanka.

There she was kept his prisoner until the monkey god Hanumān and Rāma's mighty army came to rescue her. Her sexual integrity questioned, she underwent trial by fire. Although she passed the trial, Rāma's subjects continued to doubt her, and she was banished again to the jungle. Alone and far from home, Sitā gave birth to twins, with no one to help her but hermits and ascetics.

At the end of her life Sitā was faced with a final deep challenge to her integrity and her honour. There was nothing she could do: neither to defend herself, nor to contest the unfairness of the accusations levelled at her. Pushed to her limit, she had no choice but to surrender. There was nothing to be done. Beyond all hope, Sitā fixed her gaze on the earth beneath her feet. She gave up her struggle. 'Mother', she called, and for Sitā, to call for her mother was to call out to the very earth herself. 'Mother!' she called, 'Mother, if I am blameless, take me home.' And beneath her feet a great furrow opened up, just as it had when Sitā had been given to the world as a baby girl. The furrow in the earth widened out and out like a birthing cunt. The sides of the furrow rose up around Sitā and enveloped her completely. And the sides of the furrow were the loving arms of a mother embracing her child. And the arms of the mother earth drew her daughter back down into the heart of the world. Sitā disappeared. She went home to the earth.

And as you breathe and rest in the arms of the earth, you too can
give up the struggle. Nothing to do, nowhere to go, no-one
to be. There is nothing to be done. Surrender the body
to the earth. Come home to yourself. And in that
homecoming, realise your very body is the
earth herself.

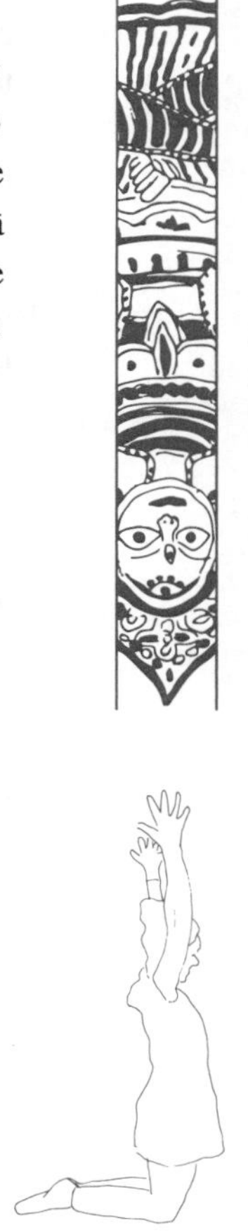

CHAPTER TWENTY-EIGHT

a womb-friendly yoga manifesto

Foundation

Above and beyond all else, to practise womb-friendly yoga is to support and encourage women in their experience of appropriate yoga practice. To that end, it is crucial not to support financially, or in any other manner, any organisation or individual known to exploit or manipulate women under the guise of teaching yoga.

PART 1
THE NEED FOR WOMB-FRIENDLINESS IN THE YOGA WORLD

Most of the people on this planet who practise and teach yoga are women. Most of these women have wombs. And many of these women have little clear understanding of the effects of yoga practice upon their wombs. This is because yoga was originally developed by men for men's bodies, and has been, until recently, transmitted through exclusively male lineages. Traditional forms of teaching yoga are thus likely to have zero womb awareness, so there is much ignorance and confusion in the yoga world about what happens to our wombs when we practise yoga.

The aim of the womb-friendly yoga manifesto is to ensure that every woman who practises and teaches yoga is fully informed about the key techniques to avoid at certain times, so that she may fully respect and honour the health of her womb throughout her life. When a woman has correct and complete information then she has the power to make appropriate yoga choices for herself. The information provided overleaf sets out the aims and effects of certain yoga techniques and outlines the effects of these practices on the womb.

Why bother?

The healthful energies of a woman's womb are key to her life-long well-being and vitality. In the yogic anatomy of the energy body, the womb is the seat of creativity, fertility and capacity to nurture and grow new life, new ideas – to manifest. It is literally the cosmic gateway for *śakti* (power) within. Yoga is all about refining awareness, of body, mind, breath, emotions and energies: it is about 'union' or re-connection with the source of all life. To pay no attention to the changing needs of womb cycles is to neglect the very place within that is the source of vitality and well being. Respect for womb cycles is the foundation of a refined and sensitive yoga practice for women. I encourage you to make the inner harmony and health of your womb your first priority. I encourage you to practise womb-friendly yoga!

PART 2
THE INFORMATION

'Caution please—wombs present'

The following practices need to be handled with caution for female yoga practitioners at many times in their lives.

Inversions

One of the key purposes of inversions in *haṭha* yoga is to reverse the flow of *apāna*. Reversed *apāna* does not effectively release menstrual flow, so practising inversions during menstruation can increase the length of time that you bleed. Practising inversions during pregnancy has an unquantifiable effect on the blood flow to the womb. Since rectus abdominal muscles in pregnancy are necessarily stretched, they are unable to contract sufficiently to provide the usual source of lower back support during inversions. Postnatal women rarely have the necessary abdominal strength to provide adequate lower back support for accurate practice of inversions.

Bandhas

The purpose of *bandhas* (locks) in yoga is to alter and contain the flow of energy (*prāṇa*) in the body. *Mūla bandha* (root lock) when practised in the classical fashion with a lift on exhalation, is intended to reverse *apāna*, and this is the energy responsible for the release of menstrual blood flow and also the flow of blood during healing after birth. (There are alternative breath patterns which can be used to support this flow). Practising a strong or continuous *mūla bandha* during pregnancy can create a thickening of the pelvic muscles that may obstruct the passage of the baby in second stage labour.

Uḍḍīyāna bandha (abdominal lift) brings a powerful physical uplift to all the abdominal and pelvic organs, with the intention of reversing the flow of *apāna* and with the same effects on the release of blood from the womb as described above. This bandha, like *jālandhara bandha* (chin lock) works synergistically with the pelvic muscles so that when *uḍḍīyāna* and *jālandhara* are practised correctly they tend to involve a simultaneous *mūla bandha*, which will lift the vulva and vagina and reverse the flow of *apāna* within.

Mahā mūdra is a combination of all three previous locks practised at once or in close connection to each other. The effects of all three locks when practised together are more intense then when they are practised singly.

Pumping breaths (*Kapālabhāti*, *Bhastrika*, 'Breath of fire')

All these breaths use rhythmic abdominal and pelvic muscle contractions to facilitate forced exhalations (*kapālabhāti)* or forced inhalations and exhalations (*bhastrika*). They often activate rhythmic lifting and lowering of the pelvic muscles and are frequently followed in yoga practice by application of the *bandhas* described above to maintain a longer pause after exhalation (*bahir kumbhaka*). The accurate practice of these breaths both builds upon and requires abdominal strength, and so it can be impossible to practise them correctly during pregnancy. The action of these breaths directly and rhythmically compresses, lifts and releases the womb. This has an unquantifiable effect on the baby inside the womb, and upon the oxygen and carbon dioxide levels in the blood circulated to the placenta and the baby. It also has the effect of reversing *apāna*, so the same comments about menstrual flow made in relation to the *bandhas* apply to these breaths.

Hot and/or fast yoga

The practice of yoga *āsana* sequences which build heat, or which are done in a greatly heated environment, are intended to promote greater flexibility and range of motion in the joints during *āsana* practice. This can be problematic premenstrually, during pregnancy or postnatally, especially when lactating, when hormonal changes promote softness in ligaments. Pregnant women tend to be several degrees hotter than usual anyway, and their resting heart rate is much higher than normal, so speed and heat are not particularly nurturing or comfortable at this time. Some perimenopausal women find hot yoga practice helpful in 'burning off' excessive heat, and others find it profoundly enervating and depleting. For women who are seeking to conceive but experiencing difficulties, then intense heat and speed in *āsana* may have a 'drying effect', depleting their vital energies and compromising fertility. Hot and/or fast yoga during lactation can impact adversely on breast milk production and postnatal recovery.

YOGA AND WOMB LIFE: SPECIAL TIMES

At these special times the practices described above can be especially inappropriate.

When menstruating

During menstruation the womb is under the influence of a special *prāṇa* (or energy flow) called *apāna* that, amongst other things, controls the downward release of menstrual blood. The practice of vigorous pumping breaths and *bandhas* which reverse *apāna* can lengthen the time it takes to release the blood. Menstruation is a time when *prāṇa* naturally gravitates to the uterus to effect the shedding and renewal of the womb lining, so often before and during menstruation there is simply less available *prāṇa* to put into a more externalised yoga practice such as *āsana*.

When your menstrual cycle is very erratic, or absent, and you are seeking to re-establish a more regular rhythm

At these times it can be wise to avoid fast and hot yoga, and to focus the energies towards nourishing the body. This will encourage the menstrual cycle to return or to become more regular.

When using an IUCD (intra-uterine contraceptive device)

The correct positioning of an intra-uterine contraceptive device is not only essential for its effective functioning, but also for comfort. Pumping breaths and *uḍḍīyāna bandha* can sometimes dislodge IUCDs from their correct position, causing pain and/or bleeding.

When seeking to conceive, or during early pregnancy

A woman who is seeking to conceive requires all of her energies to be available to nourish her womb and maintain her health. Very hot and fast yoga practices can compromise the rhythms of the cycle and deplete the *prāṇas* needed for conception. Strong practice of *uḍḍīyāna bandha* can also be disruptive of these energies.

At the time of conception and during the first three months of pregnancy, all of a woman's *prāṇas* are mobilised in the astonishing job of creating new life. It is a delicate time. Great powers are at work within the womb, and so very little *prāṇa* is available for anything else. Nurturing yoga is needed.

During pregnancy (after 14 weeks)

As the pregnancy becomes securely established, many physiological adaptations are made by the mother's body to accommodate the growing baby. They affect every system of the body, and most significantly in terms of yoga practice, the cardiovascular system and the musculo-skeletal system. This means that specially modified yoga practices are best, either in yoga for pregnancy classes, or with a skilled and experienced teacher who has respect for the massive changes that occur in the mother's body, breath, mind and heart during pregnancy in preparation for birth and motherhood.

During the postnatal period

However her baby/ies arrived, a woman who has just given birth is in a deeply vulnerable state, physically, emotionally and physiologically. Her joints may be unstable, her abdominal and pelvic muscles very weak, her emotional state very sensitive and her vitality low. Sleep deprivation and the displacement and malfunction of pelvic organs are also widespread experiences at this time. Yoga practice during this period can bring many healing benefits, but it needs to be handled very carefully indeed by knowledgeable teachers who are aware that standard approaches to *āsana* and *prāṇāyāma*, including most of the practices on the 'Caution please—wombs present' list, can often do more harm than good. The same sensitive awareness should also be held during periods following miscarriage or stillbirth.

During lactation

In relation to yoga practice, it is important to know that the hormones which control milk production and let-down can make ligaments very lax. Fast and heating practices can adversely affect milk production.

Perimenopause

In this time of uncertainty when menstrual cycles may be very erratic, very heavy, or sometimes continuous, yoga practice needs to be responsive to changing, sometimes rapidly changing, needs. Although some of the practices on the 'Caution please—wombs present' list, for example inversions and some pumping breaths, can certainly be beneficial outside of bleeding times, it is important to understand that responses to menopause are highly individualised. For example, fast and heating practices may be superbly helpful for some women but deeply depleting for others.

Postmenopause

Yoga *āsana* (done slowly and steadily) is of proven benefit in the prevention and management of osteoporosis, and many of the pumping breaths and *bandhas* are of value in optimising vitality. Practice of inversions and fast or hot yoga needs to be cautiously evaluated according to the capacity of the student and her previous experience and encounters with the preceding 'special times' (in particular her experiences with pregnancy/ies, the quality of her postnatal recovery/ies and the nature of her menopause) which all influence the choice of appropriate yoga after menopause.

At-a-glance table for womb-friendly yoga practice

Times of a woman's life / times in the menstrual cycle	Types of Yoga: *Pumping breaths*	*Mūla bandha*	*Uḍḍīyāna bandha*	*Jālandhara bandha*	*Inversions*	*Hot or fast āsana*
During menstruation	☹	☹	☹	☹	☹	☹
When menstrual cycle erratic / absent and you are seeking to restore balance	☹	☺	(!!)	(!!)	(!)	☹
When you are seeking to conceive (including during IVF)	☹	(!)	☹	(!)	☹	☹
During first trimester of pregnancy	☹	(!)	☹	(!)	☹	☹
During second trimester of pregnancy	☹	(!)	☹	(!)	(!!)	☹
During third trimester of pregnancy	☹	(!)	☹	☹	☹	☹
During immediate postnatal recovery period (first twelve weeks)	☹	(!!)	☹	☹	☹	☹

Key: ☺ = ok; ☹ = avoid; (!) = with care; (!!) with extreme caution

At-a-glance table for womb-friendly yoga practice

(Continued)

Types of Yoga

Times of a woman's life / times in the menstrual cycle	Pumping breaths	Mūla bandha	Uḍḍīyāna bandha	Jālandhara bandha	Inversions	Hot or fast āsana
During extended postnatal recovery period (up to two years)	!	!	!	!	!	!!
During lactation	!	!	!!	!	!	!!
With an IUCD in place	☹	!	☹	!	!	!
Following miscarriage	☹	!	☹	!	☹	☹
With prolapsed pelvic organs	!!	!	!	!	☺	!
During perimenopause	!	!	!	!	!	!!
Postmenopause (age, desire and agility permitting)	☺	☺	☺	☺	☺	☺

Key: ☺ = ok; ☹ = avoid; ! = with care; !! with extreme caution

A VOICE FROM THE WOMB

Hiya! It's your womb talking. Glad of your attention. Now, I won't be long. I'm absolutely delighted you're practising yoga, for certain it's the wise and healthy choice. I just wanted you to know though, that some of that stuff you're doing can make me and the old ovaries feel pretty weird at certain times of the month. I get on with things the best I can, but to be honest ... some of those things aren't so great for me.

So, here we go: You know that thing you do, uḍḍīyāna bandha, *when you breathe out and suck your belly right in and up? And then your bumhole and vagina come right along with it? Well, when I'm trying to empty stuff out, that feels pretty, well, really strange – like I'm trying to clear the old lining through the cervix, and you're busy counteracting the forces of gravity, and everything gets sucked back in and up again. Can you leave that one out? At least on the heavy days when I'm a bit bogged down here in the flow – it's just going take me longer to clear the old lining out, love, and it's a long enough job as it is.*

And the upside-down things? Same story. I just find I can't get on with the job of the flow. I'm doing my best here, but it really holds me up, if you know what I mean. I love the whole upside-down thing the rest of the month, though – makes me feel ten years younger!

And the leaping around really fast? I can tell you really love it, and most of the time, so do I. But I could do with some of that energy in here on the big days, you know. I've got a monthly clear-out to sort. Just take the day off. I can sort things out better with a bit of peace.

And there's a sort of pumping thing you do with the belly moving in and out super-quick. Sometimes that feels fabulous, but it kind of lifts me up at the end when you hold your breath out – and if it's a big red day, then I struggle. Give it a rest on my big red days, can't you?

And if you want that IUCD to stay put, girl, then I think you need to tone it down a bit with those uḍḍīyāna bandhas. *Heard about one the other day that got lodged way up high and was a devil of a job to get it out again. Don't fancy the sound of that myself.*

That's about it. Except to say, if you're ever thinking of inviting guests, maybe a baby or two, then I'd really be glad if you could just give me some time to get settled down here. I'll need a lot of energy to prepare before they arrive. You don't want me all worn out and the place in a mess before they get here now do you? And while they're here I'd be glad if you could leave off the pumping and sucking malarkey for a bit – it's not going to help me keep everyone happy here. You can always go back to it later, once they're safely out.

Other than that, you're doing a fine job. Keep up the good work!

SHARING THIS INFORMATION

– Do you go to yoga classes?
– Are you a yoga teacher?
– Do you run a yoga studio/s?
– Do you employ yoga teachers in your gym or health club?
– Do you train yoga teachers?
– Do you recommend yoga classes to your female clients or patients?

If the answer to any of these questions is yes (or even 'sometimes'), then you owe it to yourself and/or the women in the yoga classes you teach, provide or recommend, to be sufficiently informed about the effects of some yogic techniques upon the womb in order to respect the need for caution at certain times in a woman's life.

If you are a yoga teacher trainer, then you have a special responsibility to ensure that your trainings make space to share this information with the teachers you are turning out; the health, well-being and self-respect of thousands of women can be supported, compromised or seriously undermined by their choice of yoga practices, and their capacity to choose wisely depends upon their access to good information, which they may depend upon their yoga teachers to provide.

Simply ensure that all the women in your classes / yoga studio are provided with the previous information when they come to class, for example by including it as part of any registration document or health questionnaire they may complete prior to taking the class. If possible make the information available on your website (or by linking to **www.wombyoga.org**) so that women can engage with it before they arrive, and ideally have hard copies to distribute at the reception desk before women go into class.

There are many ways to share this information: for example, the points as set out on the previous pages, a summary table, or the 'voice from the womb' story on p.589. You know the women who come to your classes, and what they're likely to respond to the best, so choose which version is most appropriate for your students / clients.

REVEALING THE COSMIC GATEWAY

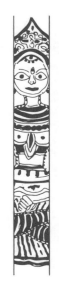

Once upon a time there was a city with nine gates. The people who lived in the city were thoughtful and dedicated spiritual practitioners: they were *yogis*. In their experience of the state of 'union' or oneness that is yoga, they understood that their city was a metaphor for their own physical bodies, and they saw that the gateways to the city were like the orifices of the human body: the eyes, ears, nostrils, mouth, anus and urethral openings.

The *yogis* who lived in this city were men, and it was the men of this city who created the texts and practices of *haṭha* yoga. In these texts there were many references to the nine gates of the yogic city, and many ways were taught to contain the power of conscious awareness within the walls of the city of the human body for the purposes of enlightenment. So the male *yogis* passed the precious practices and texts down, from teacher to student, in an unbroken lineage or *paramparā*, enabling millions of *yogis* over thousands of years to benefit from the wisdom and learning that had been created and tested in the nine-gated city.

The city was a beautiful place, full of light and wisdom, and most of the people within it were illumined souls. They meditated singly, and sometimes gathered together in a gracious light-filled temple in the centre of their city. Such was the aura of contentment that exuded from the city, that many people were drawn to come and practise what the *yogis* were doing.

One day, a woman came to the city and asked to be given access to these practices. It was an unusual request, since the city had been built for the men and there had never been, so far as anyone in that city could remember, a woman within it. Some of the ancient inhabitants recalled that in fact women had originally been prohibited from entering the city. But by this time the *yogis* were so far advanced in their knowledge and wisdom that they could recognise this seeker as a genuine soul in search of guidance and light, so they let her in and taught her and she proved herself to be a very adept and worthy *yoginī*.

More women came and studied in the city, and they became accomplished *yoginīs*. They loved yoga and they were keen to spread the word. Women can be very good networkers. So their sisters came, and their daughters and cousins and nieces and aunties and friends, and in a very short time, the nine-gated city of *yogis* got so full of women that there

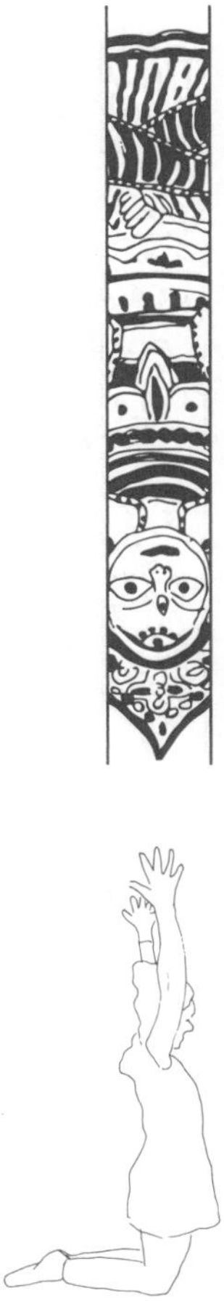

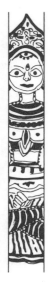

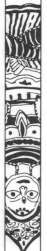

simply wasn't enough room for everyone inside the walls. It got a bit cramped.

What to do? Since it was the very walls of the city itself which had given rise to the central metaphor holding the whole yogic tradition together, it didn't seem quite right to knock down those walls. So little encampments of *yoginīs* grew up around the nine gates outside the city. And meanwhile more people were coming.

From the top of the walls of the city, one of the *yogis* noticed a huge cloud of dust in the distance. It was moving towards the city. A young woman with very sharp eyes squinted into the cloud and saw that it was raised by the feet of hundreds of thousands of women all running towards the city of *yogis*. Lots of them looked as if they were pregnant, she said, and she figured some of them could even be in labour, but they seemed to be running to the city of yoga anyway and she reckoned they'd be arriving pretty soon. The accommodation problem was about to become very urgent. It wouldn't be right to have the pregnant ones camping outside the gates.

And so the *yoginīs* decided to build another new city just outside the gates of the first one. Possessed now of magical powers as a result of long yogic practice, the women in the nine-gated city created with great rapidity a beautiful city for the new arrivals. It was a short walk to the first city, but it was a separate place of its own.

And in that new city remarkable things began to happen. The pregnant ones grew larger and began to go into labour. And some were doing yoga practices when they gave birth. And then the women with the babies were practising yoga with their infants, whilst they fed and played with them. And the women who'd been living in the old city were intrigued and inspired, and began to notice some interesting things happening to human bodies that no one in the old city had ever really pointed out before. Blood was flowing down and milk was flowing out.

'We need more than nine gates' said the women in the new city. 'We have extra gates'. So they created a garden around their new city, and the garden had twelve gates. It was a beautiful and abundant place.

Some of the women in the old city said all this was nonsense. They viewed the extra gates as mere distractions, and took no notice of the voices in the new city. But some of the old *yoginīs* came out of the old city and helped the new arrivals with their garden. Before long, the garden grew so huge that it surrounded not only the new city, but also the old,

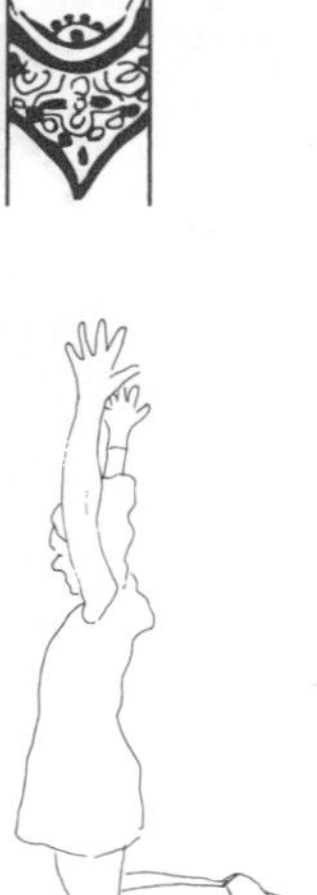

and all the encampments around it. Parts of the garden were wild and free, and others were formal and tidy. It was fruitful, abundant and richly fragrant. And in and out of its twelve gates all day long flowed hundreds and thousands of women. As the garden expanded and spread and grew, there were women in it who never even knew about the ancient city of the nine gates around which the garden had grown.

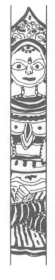

And then one day, one of the older *yoginīs* who had lived in the nine-gated city and was now happily residing in one of the wilder corners of the garden, noticed a strong energetic field emanating from an interesting hole at the base of a tree. It was as if the earth was singing to her through that hole. She had an especial affinity with this particular hole because it was the place where she used to pour her menstrual blood into the earth, in a ritual offering to feed the tree and the earth in which it was rooted. Over the years, the tree had begun to thrive and grow abundantly, and the *yoginī* had begun to revere and honour her bloodroots to the earth.

This particular morning, she felt inside the hole and noticed ridges and whorls as if they had been carved in the stones in the earth. She called her sisters and they began to explore, feeling with their bare hands, and clearing away stones and earth. Slowly at first, but then more rapidly, they began to uncover an astonishing cavern. The cavern led down into the heart of the earth and expanded underneath the garden, deep and low and warm and slightly damp. Its walls were carved with swirls and whorls and curvilinear mandalas of great beauty.

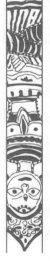

As more *yoginīs* assisted in the excavation, a magical under-garden emerged, vast and gorgeous. The women flooded into it, admiring the astonishing scale and stupendous beauty of the structure that felt as if it had grown rather than been made.

And then the realisation dawned.

Right in the centre of the huge under-garden cavern was a vast hall. Shaped like a *yoni*, the cosmic gateway through which the blood and babies were arriving in the garden above, this enormous hall was clearly the energetic focus of the entire cavernous under-garden. The floor of the hall was a deep red, stained with the menstrual flow of the ancient *yoginīs* whose ritual practices and observances of the lunar rhythms of the womb had been conducted in this very space.

Built right above this hall, towering and tall, was the old city of nine gates. And the foundations of the old city were now

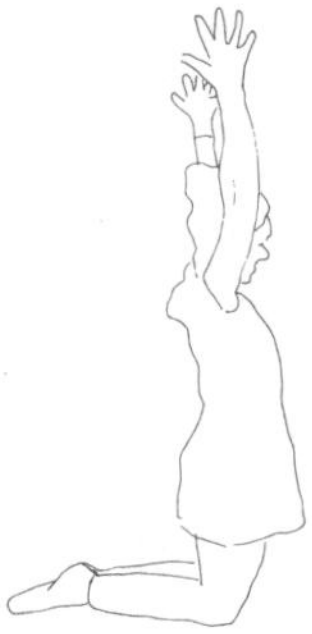

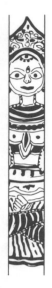

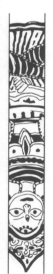

clearly visible; they were the caverns of the women's under-garden: the earth herself. The nine-gated city was built above the cosmic gateway of the women's under-garden. The ground on which was once revered the naturally arising union states of the women's bodily rhythms and flows, this was at the very roots of the yogic edifice. The nine-gated city of *yogis* was built on this foundation. The roots of the city were in the women's under garden, and everything practised within it was intended to promote the states of being which naturally arose in the bodies of the women who had for so long been absent from the nine-gated city.

And so it became clear to the women that the *yogis* in the nine-gated city had spent thousands of years developing conscious practices of control and restraint to access those very same powers of ecstatic trance and higher consciousness which had been worshipped as rhythmic cycles naturally occurring in the bodies of the women who had created this astonishing earthen cavern.

Now this is a fairy story, and so it has a happy ending. For, once the *yoginīs* in the women's garden that had grown to surround the nine-gated city realised the power of the ritual space in the great under-garden, they ran to tell the *yogis* and *yoginīs* inside the nine-gated city. It was still a beautiful space, that old city, and the residence of many illumined souls, who were intrigued and excited to hear about the discoveries in the garden. Everyone in the nine-gated city flocked to the central temple space in the middle of the city and began to dig. And everyone in the ritual earth space beneath the temple looked up and started to clear a circular space in the central dome of the ceiling.

And so it was that by the time the moon rose full in the sky that night, her light was able to shine down on the nine-gated city, and pour through the gracious temple of the old *yogis* to create a lake of moonlight on the floor of the newly uncovered ritual space in the women's under-garden.

This was cause for great rejoicing in the new and old cities and in the garden surrounding them both. Men and women danced together in the moonlight, and the powerful rhythms of the earth cycles that had been honoured in the cosmic gateway of the cavernous under-garden raised up with effortless grace the consciousness of all the *yogis* and *yoginīs*. By the time the sun began to rise, all the spirits of the men and women were in celestial ascent, singing together in a joyous throng, like larks high in the dawn sky.

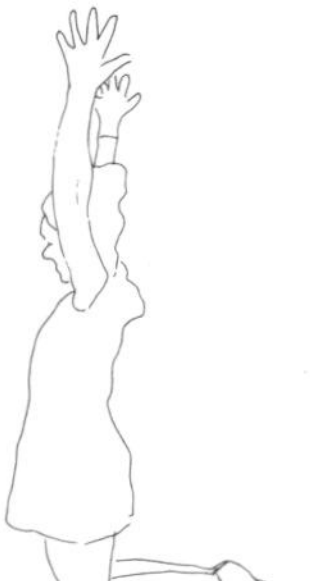

CHAPTER TWENTY-NINE

conclusion and beginnings: *śakti* circles

Patriarchy sustains itself by keeping us apart. (Lee Flinders 1998: 322)

... the most deeply damaging aspect of patriarchy has been how it has locked women out of themselves. (Alexandra Pope, Womb Wisdom Retreat, Hawkwood College, UK. February 2012)

Many women have discovered in themselves the capacity to devise beautiful, satisfying ceremonies for personal or group use, which please them more than the traditional posturing of self-styled spiritual fathers. This form of creativity now pours forth with immense vitality from those women who have rediscovered its inner wellsprings, who have found courage to reject patriarchal habits in favor of their own emotional and aesthetic instincts. (Barbara G Walker 1990: 17)

This chapter on '*śakti* circles' comes at the end of *Yoni Śakti*. But in fact it is a whole lot of beginnings. The book starts and finishes at the same place, but with a changed consciousness of the nature of that place. It's a place of synthesis: a place that honours the great healing power of gathering, of bringing together, of women's circles. In the introduction I complained that the only reason I needed to write this book in the first place was because all the useful information and experiences I had found to support our understandings of *yoni śakti* were hidden away in such very separate places that there was no communication between them. Nobody had the big picture because all the pieces were so far distant from each other. My research for *Yoni Śakti* has been a great ocean voyage, bringing home many disparate sources and stories, and circling them together in the interests of women's spiritual empowerment. Writing the book was a process of rounding up all the relevant material, regardless of its provenance, into a great circle of reference and support for the spiritual journeys of women now. *Yoni Śakti* has brought together yoga practices and scholarly histories, fairy stories and feminist commentaries, testimonies and spiritual autobiographies, all within the great circle of their relevance to the possibility of women's freedom now. The intention of this powerful gathering is to create the possibility for healing that leads to women's lives lived in genuine freedom.

A circle of women of all ages and backgrounds can create healing by sharing. Such sharing increases each woman's power. So too, the gathering together in *Yoni Śakti* of all these different voices within one circle has created a resource for transformation that is more powerful than any single stream of information. A circle of sources that includes practice and poetry, personal testimony and scholarly resource, ritual and reference is a powerful force. Above all, the combination of perspectives and practices that circle around the subject of women's experiences in *Yoni Śakti* is a testimony to the power of acknowledging cyclical wisdom as it plays out in the cycles of women's lives. This cyclical wisdom is a feminine way of knowing, a way of understanding that often requires us to revisit and return, to circle back on ourselves to gain a clear perspective, to circle around in a wider arc to encompass other perspectives and sources before coming home to ourselves, and sometimes to circle in on ourselves and to wait in a state of uncertainty as we feel for the next great cycle of experience to reveal another circle of connection. Such cyclical wisdom is never about following doggedly a single line of progress, advancement or improvement: it is always about spiralling around and back and into experiences that frequently surround us. We don't drive straight through menopause or motherhood or menstruation: these experiences are states of being that encircle us, and whose power lies in teaching us that sometimes you just have to watch things circle back home, and surrender to the cycle that is unfolding, before you understand anything about what you were meant to learn from it. These are the patterns of women's lives: month by month, pregnancy by pregnancy, from one uncertain perimenopausal insight or outburst to another, the circles of power intersect and overlap. There are no straight lines.

The circular patterns of the cycles in women's lives are reflected in the shape of this book. Its circular structure echoes the interconnected circles of cyclical wisdom that it has sought to honour and support through yogic means. This arc of return to the starting point of the circle demonstrates that when we open to an understanding of the true nature of cyclical wisdom then we may notice something very important: even though we seem to come back to the same point, our consciousness of its significance changes, because the journey of the cycle has changed us and how we see things.

But a circle is not simply a structural device. It is a tool for transformation. This book began with a story about how a circle of *yoginīs* gathered in meditation was able to change the construction of their reality. When the Islington *yoginīs* responded to being called 'CUNTS' by punching the air and affirming 'YESSS!' they changed expectations, both of the lads who had thought they were insulting them, and the women who had previously been distressed by receiving similar insults in the past. The collective power of the *yoginīs*' focused energy and conscious awareness as they sat together in a circle had the force to make change happen.

This means to focus the spiritual power of an encircled collective of women is ancient. Miranda Shaw observes that the earliest *tāntrik* texts '... trace the origins of this movement to circles of women practising together in the countryside... These intrepid women assembled in non-hierarchical circles, feasted together, and shared their spiritual insights with one another... they empowered one another as women and as spiritual seekers' (Shaw 1996: 3). But the power of a circle of women is also alive in contemporary practices of spiritual, political and ecological consciousness-raising and activism. I have described some of the many contemporary women's circles of transformative power in this book. The ecological activism of Tree Sisters, the global projects for improvements in women's health and well-being such as Women's Quest, the White Ribbon network, and Seane Corne's 'Off the Mat and Into the World' projects, as well as many real and virtual networks for the spiritual growth and support of women and girls worldwide, such Alexandra Pope's Women's Leadership Apprenticeship Trainings and Miranda Gray's World Womb Blessings, and the Red Tent movement worldwide are all grounded in circles of women's sharing. These circles are powerful forces for growth and change. Their power is rooted in the experience of reconnection. When women sit together in *satsaṅg* [a yogic 'congregation'], practise cycles of healing yoga together, sing together in the practice of *bhakti* yoga, or simply listen to the experiences of other women in the circle, then things change: consciousness alters, energy is shifted, burdens are lifted. Women feel better about themselves because they feel part of a community of shared interests and understandings. This is truly a yoga that reconnects us to the deepest power that is our true wealth: our shared experiences of cyclical wisdom.

This is power and wealth that increases by sharing. It is very different to the model that patriarchy has given us, which teaches us to build power and wealth by keeping as much of it as possible to ourselves. Within the history of yoga lineages, secrecy and exclusivity were often emphasised as a means to maintain the hard-won powers of the yogic *siddhis*. The spiritual wealth attained by concerted efforts and disciplined practice was considered so precious that the means by which it had been achieved was kept a closely guarded secret. The idea was that once you knew how to attain such power you did not pass it on to anyone, except a very few suitable initiated adepts. The secretive and power-protective hierarchies that have grown up around yoga trainings and schools reflect this basic belief.

But the female *siddhis* function in the opposite way: secrecy depletes and disavows the power of the female *siddhis*. The initiatory experiences that open the possibility for the discovery of women's spiritual power are naturally arising. The powers that can be realised by bringing these experiences into the light of conscious awareness are freely given. And sharing these experiences is part of the process of bringing them to conscious awareness. Generosity and openness, not secrecy, is the means to protect and expand the spiritual power of the female *siddhis*. Sharing our encounters of the female *siddhis* enables women to affirm and understand that our experiences are initiations to access sources of power. So long as there are circles of other women with whom to share and affirm the great powers of the female *siddhis*, then the consciousness of these physical experiences can be raised to perceive them as spiritual gateways for transformation and wisdom. When women support each other in respecting and honouring our experiences, then this respect and honour makes it possible to understand these encounters as *siddhis*, to see them as part of an unfolding of the cyclical wisdom of the deep feminine.

The great triumph of patriarchy has been to establish men's definitions of femininity as the basis of women's understanding of our own experiences, and thus to define women's experiences only in relation to men. This has the effect of separating women from each other so that we are unable to share our experiences. Thus we encounter the physical challenges of these *siddhis* as suffering, without ever becoming conscious of the true nature of their power. Because our culture has removed opportunities for meaningful spiritual connection with other women, it is hard to see our experiences from the broader perspective of the cyclical wisdom that communion with other women helps us to recognise. When we are separate from each other we are locked out of ourselves. From a feminist perspective, the most potent revolutionary act is to establish a heartfelt communion of women and girls: '... Everything we know about the history of patriarchy suggests that ... [it] sustains itself by keeping us apart' (Lee Flinders 1998: 322).

When we are locked out of ourselves in this way then we become so desperate to return home that we buy into the hierarchies of secrecy and separateness that further cut us off from each other. This is why acknowledgement of the spiritual power of the female *siddhis* has gone underground: they have been denigrated and overlooked and made the object of distaste and revulsion, the focus of medical control, and some have been almost eradicated. For without the circles of women's sharings and support these *siddhis* have no lifeblood. Women listening to each other—this is the lifeblood which feeds the consciousness of the female *siddhis*. When they are not shared, the consciousness of their power fades, and they are no longer understood to be *siddhis*. When they are shared, then the consciousness is raised to re-connect with the understanding that they are *siddhis*. What has kept women apart is what has all but destroyed our awareness of the female *siddhis*. But what brings us back together has the capacity to retrieve the consciousness of the power of these female *siddhis*. I say retrieve, but it is in fact the case that they have never really been lost, they have just been hidden from the light of our consciousness. The gift of yoga now for women is that it has the capacity to illuminate that aspect of our consciousness, and this illumination is a direct result of us coming together to share in circles.

In the *yoginī* feasts of Hindu and Buddhist *tantra*, *yoginīs* were treated with respect and awe as powerful entities in and of themselves. But it was when they circled together that their spiritual power was amplified. The same magnification of power continues to be experienced by contemporary women who gather for womb-friendly yoga practice, or indeed any activity that connects women together with the conscious intention of linking to the guidance of our higher selves for the benefit of ourselves, our communities, or the healing of our planet. A circle of women has a collective force and potential that no individual carries alone. It is a *śakti* circle: a circle of power. To be part of such a circle imbues the individual women with the power of the whole circle. Circles of women are powerful healing forces because they create opportunities for women to share. Opportunities for women to share are crucial to our well-being because they help to affirm our understanding of the female *siddhis* as gateways to great spiritual power. Without other women with whom to share, we can feel isolated, misunderstood and confused. This isolation and confusion is disempowering. But within the circle, a clarity and genuine empowerment can be accessed, through supportive connection with other women.

I have been privileged to witness innumerable occurrences of the healing power of women connected in a circle to practise the yoga of *satsaṅg*. I have seen the relief in the faces of young women who arrived at a 'Creating Menstrual Health' circle almost unable to move because of crippling menstrual cramps, but who discovered the intense sensations lifting as the other women around them honoured and acknowledged the reality of their deep suffering: 'My pain is gone' they announce part-way through the day. The circle moves it on. I have heard great sobs of sadness lifting from women as they shared their dawning recognition of resentments and anger they had been carrying for decades as a result of the suppression of their menstrual cycles: 'For fifteen years, I have been cut off from my own cycles,' they say, and then a light comes into their eyes as they connect with a deepening sense of their inner wisdom and power. 'I didn't know the harm I was doing to myself. Now I know I can reconnect with my inner life.' The sharing within the circle links them into this reconnection. I have felt the great warmth which thaws forty years of frozen fear and shame as grandmothers have shared the humiliating or disrespectful experiences they encountered when birthing their children: 'I never spoke of this to anyone before now. I am glad it doesn't have to be this way for you'. The warm welcome of the circle supports their healing, and it seeds learning for future mothers. I have seen the grief pass from the bodies of women who have held their experiences of multiple miscarriage or stillbirth hidden in their hearts and wombs for years as they reach out to support some other woman in the circle with a simple affirmation: 'I know how painful that can be'. The circle creates the sharing, and the sharing heals. And I have watched in awe the lightness and freedom that flows through women of all ages, from all over the world, as they acknowledge in the circle each other's beauty and power and strength to survive the suffering of what it is to be a woman in a culture that has locked us out of ourselves, and kept us separate from each other. Coming together in a circle we set this right. We reconnect to each other, and the *śakti* rises and moves. Transformation happens.

As *Yoni Śakti* closes, I return to the circles of women, and to an understanding of how these circles of women support the cycles of our life experiences, and honour these encounters as female *siddhis*. When we create supportive circles of women around us then change is possible. We can change fierce rage and grief into acceptance and resolve. We can access creativity and power. We can honour once more what has been dishonoured and reviled. We can change how we feel about ourselves and the world, and we can change how we respond to the cycles and circles of our lives by seeing them in the light of conscious awareness. In this way menstruating women can return to our moon-time each month with a different perspective, an opportunity to evaluate and consider the lessons learned through the previous month, and the chance to start afresh. In this way, menopausal women can return to the wounds and hurts of the girls they once were, and see how these experiences can be integrated within the circle of understanding that heals and transforms. In this way, mothers can watch our little daughters discovering themselves and the world, and choose to give them different answers, different words, and different perspectives from those our mothers were able to give us, because we can feel how these circles of women reconnect us to our conscious awareness. We can know that our conscious awareness, our practice of yoga, helps us understand that as we return to those points in a cycle that we recognise, then we are empowered to make choices to live in freedom, and to help others to be free also.

When *śakti* circles form, then women heal. We heal ourselves and we heal each other and we heal the planet by honouring the blood wisdom that is deeply coded within our physicality. When we create *śakti* circles, we honour the fact that this deep knowing, this cyclical wisdom, these female *siddhis*, have never really been taken away: all that has been denied is access to the consciousness of the true wealth that this wisdom brings, not just for women but for the whole planet. *Śakti* circles bring us back together with other women so that we may honour each other. When we create connection and sharing through honouring our sisters in *śakti* circles then we rediscover the key to our own inner life: our cyclical wisdom. In *śakti* circles we realise that sharing with other women in this way opens the doors to our own self-understanding. It is this self-understanding and acceptance that is the deepest inner teacher. It is this inner wisdom that holds the greatest power. Creating *śakti* circles invites deep power and great freedom into women's lives. Women with power can choose to live in freedom and to practise the yoga that supports that freedom.

CLOSING RITUAL: GREETING WOMEN'S POWER IN A ŚAKTI CIRCLE

'*NAMASTE* TO YOU, SISTER: AND *NAMASTE* TO YOUR ŚAKTI!'

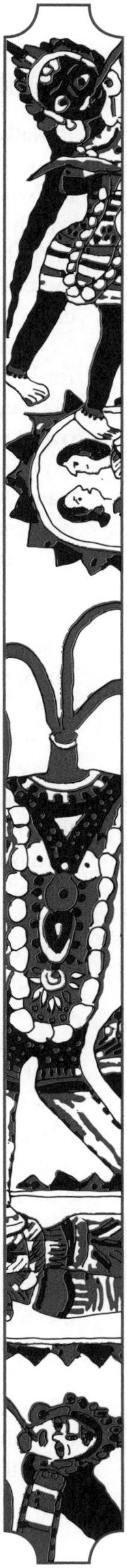

I often open and close classes, retreats, workshops and trainings with this ritual greeting. It honours the power (*śakti*) present in every woman. The ritual has a profound healing power. It extends welcome and support to each woman, and acknowledges the inner power that has brought her to this gathering. To be part of a circle which makes this greeting to all the women within it is to become part of a powerful force for change.

The ritual can be done with any number of women. If there is only you here right now, you can do this ritual facing a mirror and greet your global sisterhood in the form of your self. If you are with other women, then sit in a circle. Look around the circle and catch the eye of each woman in it. Every woman brings her palms together on her breastbone in the prayerful greeting called *namaste*. Settle your hands there as you inhale, sending your attention to your heart to evoke a feeling of warm welcome there. On an exhale, use the river-lotus form of the Heart-womb greeting (pp.144–5) to slide the hands down the central line of the body, down the heart-womb river, bringing them to rest over the womb in *yoni mudrā*.

On an inhale bring the hands back up to *namaste*. Then turn to the first woman in the circle, and working widdershins (anti-clockwise), greet each woman in turn by asking her to say her name out loud. Then, with hands in *namaste* the whole circle responds: '*Namaste* sister [name]', and then, as the hands slide down to cover the womb, '*Namaste* sister [name's] *śakti*!' Then everyone calls a warm and smiling 'Welcome!' to the sister and her *śakti*. At the end of the session / retreat / meeting, repeat the process in the opposite direction, returning to the first woman after having said 'Thank you' to each of the women and each of their *śakti*s. If any women in the group are pregnant, then it is nice to greet the baby/ies in the womb as well, '*Namaste* sister [name], *namaste* sister [name's] *śakti*! and *Namaste* to sister [name's] baby!'

We spread freedom to our sisters when we greet their power.

Hari Om Tat Sat.

A NOTE TO MALE READERS

Initially I conceived this book as being especially for women. My experience as a yoga teacher, trainer and therapist has been almost exclusively with women, and my work as a writer and communicator has always been focused on experiences which are entirely and exclusively feminine, for example, menstruation, pregnancy, birth, lactation and menopause. Because this is the nature of my experience, I do not pretend to understand men and their experiences in the same way that I know that I can understand women and their experiences.

This is not to say that the techniques presented in this book are not suited to men, for indeed they are of great benefit in terms of developing a connection with feminine energy, and of encouraging a lived experience and understanding of a man's own feminine side. I have received very positive feedback about just this kind of experience from the few remarkable men who have attended classes, workshops and trainings with me. Sometimes they came in pairs because it was a bit scary to be the only man in a circle of thirty *yoginīs*: 'Can I bring my friend?' they asked, and we welcomed them both, and welcomed their appreciation at the end of the class: 'We loved that. We think other men would love it too.'

But at this time I can offer no informed guidance as to how appropriate each practice may be to particular male life experiences. I invite those *yogis* who have an interest in these practices, and who seek to foster the evolution of their own feminine side, to experiment with the practices I describe and discover for themselves their application to men's experience.

I would be interested to develop a future form of yoga practice for men and women to enjoy together in celebration of *yoni śakti*. But for the time being I sense that it is important to give women the space and respect to encounter this yoga as a means to explore their own femininity, on women's terms, with women's values, and (usually) amongst other women only. When we have a fully mature respect and connection with the power of our own femininity, then will be the time for the *yoginīs* to return to the men to share our findings. At that point, it would be nice to discover that the *yogis* have been conducting their own experiments and developments, and then we can move forward together.

In the meantime, I feel that much of the discussion and observations presented in this book will be of great interest to men who live with women. As Geeta Iyengar observed in her 'Lecture on Yoga for Women' given in Poland in 2002: 'Although this talk is related to women, it is necessary for men to know it too. Why? Because it is a matter of fact that each man has himself come into existence through the existence of a woman, that is his mother, who menstruated. If men understand their mothers, they will understand their wives also … Men have a great role to play in order to maintain the health of women. As a father a man has to see that his daughter maintains a good health for her womanhood. As a husband he has to learn to respect the health of his wife. Often men do not think deeply about the physical strength, physiological capacity and emotional health of a woman. Often misunderstanding comes… If a man understands… he may be able to help her in a better way. Then life will be adjustable and amicable. Therefore, I welcome the men who are attending this lecture'.

In the same spirit, I warmly welcome male readers to *Yoni Śakti*.

A NOTE ON YOGA LINEAGES AND TRADITIONS

You are probably reading this section because you have an interest in knowing the traditional roots or lineage of the approach to yoga described in *Yoni Śakti*. There is an unhappy relationship between the traditionally patriarchal structures of most yoga lineages and the women inside them. Many traditional yoga schools and lineages headed by male *gurus* have been bedevilled by scandalous tales of sexual exploitation and other abuses of women. This is not to say that all *gurus* and their followers are bad, and that every yoga institution is a thoroughly unsafe environment for our daughters. Certainly there is much for which to thank these lineages. They have certainly preserved and promoted yoga worldwide very well, and have largely supported women's access to yoga practice. I explore the place of women in these traditions in chapters one and two, which deal respectively with the modern and ancient histories of women in yoga.

But it is very important to recognise that if the intention of our yoga practice is to rediscover our own spiritual wisdom and power as women, then a traditional, male-dominated framework of teaching is unlikely to be the best place to look. The intention of womb yoga is to provide women with experiences that lead each of us back home to our inner teacher, our heart's wisdom. There is a direct and intimate link between the heart and the womb at a pranic level (and this book includes many techniques to enable you to experience this for yourself). My experience and belief is that within every woman lies a deep wisdom, a profound understanding that resides in the very blood of the menses, the walls of the womb and the rhythms of a woman's life, and which is, in itself and of itself, a completely clear and true source of guidance and teaching for that woman. The intention of the womb yoga shared in this book is to enable you to encounter practices that provide you with your own experience of being in communion with this inner wisdom and energy, this *yoni śakti*, in order that you may live your life in freedom.

Womb yoga offers ways to allow a profound sense of deeply rooted blood wisdom to fill your heart and live life fully and free. When this living connection with blood wisdom is accessed, then there is a sense of rightness, and a trust in the clarity and understanding that flows through the heart. From this experience comes a quiet but truly secure confidence, a total trust that the heart's wisdom is founded on the deep inner knowing of blood wisdom, evident in the rhythms of the woman's body through her life. The rhythms of the body and the blood wisdom are one and the same: they are in union. In this state of yoga or union, no mediator is needed – no lineage, no tradition, and no outer teacher can come close to the deep sense of wisdom and understanding that flows through a woman who is absolutely and profoundly connected with her own intuitive understanding of what is best for her.

Womb yoga is not about following the teachings of a particular tradition, text or lineage. It is about accessing the route back to the original intuitive wisdom that resides within the womb energies and is experienced within the heart as the 'inner teacher' who guides us to live in freedom.

AFTERWORD

genesis, gestation and birth of *Yoni Śakti*: learning to be fearless

> *Do you want to accept the world as it is? Do you want to accept it and join it and become like that? Do you want to be that? Do you want to conform? Do you know what it means not to conform with something? That means going against the whole structure of society, against the morality, business, religion, the whole culture, which means you have to stand alone…*
>
> *Don't just say, 'I am frightened'. The culture in which we are born makes us conform. Conformity brings fear… If you are frightened, then you are caught forever. But if you say, 'I am not going to be frightened', let's examine it, then let's find out how to live in this world without being frightened, without conforming… If you know how to live that way you will never be frightened.*
>
> *Krishnamurti in dialogue with students at Brockwood Park School 1971 (Krishnamurti 2011: 13)*

Yoni Śakti is the book that I wanted to read when I began menstruating nearly thirty years ago. The feminine and feminist approach to women's practice of yoga set out in the previous pages is what I wish I had known about when I first began attending yoga classes and teaching yoga classes to women. What I have shared in *Yoni Śakti* is slow-grown. The practices within this book are the spiritual baby of over forty years' gestation of yoga practice. The sequences and insights have been nurtured through nearly twenty years of teaching and facilitating groups of women of all ages in urban and rural locations from the west coast of Ireland to the heart of Moscow. In yoga teacher and yoga therapist training courses, on Śakti Rising and Womb Wisdom retreats, in yoga classes and at yoga camps, I have been privileged to serve many accomplished and beginning *yoginīs*, as students and clients, supporting them to use a full range of therapeutic yoga practices to enhance their experience of the female *siddhis* of menstruation, fertility, motherhood and menopause. *Yoni Śakti* has presented these explorations of womb yoga as accessible practices that are intended to inspire you to reveal, through your own encounter with yoga, a means of being in union that best speaks the present truth of your blood wisdom. It is my hope that those who engage with these yoga practices will be encouraged to take a brave and fearless step closer to following the guidance of their own inner teacher.

It took much longer than I expected to write this book because the process of holding, developing and articulating all these powerful ideas was very slow. This slowness was good, because many of the topics presented in *Yoni Śakti* are not neutral: they awaken intense feelings and reactions, and it has been a necessary process to let all the often disturbing and frightening emotions around these topics come to the surface, be examined in detail, and then to set aside some of the troublesome confusions in the interests of clarifying what is most relevant to share. I have taken time to sift through the very angry and fearful reactions and opinions (my own and those of the women whom I serve) that first came to light when I began this journey. What remains, I hope, is a compendium of useful practices and inspiring philosophical reflections that will be of practical benefit to those who encounter them.

In the final stages of gestation, as I was up to my ears in reworking some of the historical arguments and editorial refinements suggested by Mark Singleton, a number of shocking revelations rocked the yoga world. All of these stories related to abuses of power and the sexual exploitation of women by teachers, trainers and other leaders in the wider fields of yoga, including yoga teacher training, yoga therapy and *bhakti* yoga (the increasingly popular yoga of devotional music and song). Whilst I was fiddling with commas and footnotes, attending to the minutiae, the bigger picture of many women's unhappy experiences in the world of yoga came more clearly into focus around me. It was very ugly.

Whilst I was endeavouring to bring harmony and precision into a book celebrating women's empowerment through yoga, all around me disharmony and confusion were revealing just how profoundly disempowered many women had been by the very structures and institutions that purport to promote yoga practice and teaching. I was trying very hard to keep my eyes down and focused on the small picky stuff so I endeavoured not to look too closely at what was being revealed. My priority was to get the book finished. But every day for two weeks I heard yet another sorry tale from a different teller:

Did I know that female volunteers in the service of an international chain of yoga retreats were being sexually abused by renunciates and senior staff? asked a trusted colleague shortly after she returned from a visit to one such retreat.

Had I not heard that devoted young *bhakti yoginīs* had been, just like rock and roll groupies, serving the sexual 'needs' of popular devotional singers touring European yoga centres? asked a concerned musician who had worked on the tour.

I tried not to be distracted by these stories, and I attended to my commas. But then I began to receive emails from disillusioned ex-staff of a globally admired yoga therapy institution, describing how trainee yoga therapists and long-term yoga teachers had been manipulated and controlled by the senior male teacher who had been appointed as their spiritual guide and professional advisor.

The stories kept coming.

I became aware that, despite the resignations of experienced staff and teachers in protest at high-level misconduct, the senior international women tutors of one yoga training organisation had failed to support the claims of sexual abuse raised by young women against their key male mentor. Five years later the stories had come to light again, along with other, more serious accusations that are were being investigated by Interpol.

Dismayed sister *yoginīs* shared with me how trainee teachers and women staff in one yoga *aṣram* were too scared to even enter the rooms of certain swamis because they feared that they would be molested, just as many other younger *yoginīs* had been previously.

One colleague pointed out that even though ten years earlier a *guru* at a huge yoga training and retreat centre had been unceremoniously ousted from his position of power following numerous reports of sexual misconduct with students and staff, this same charismatic yoga pioneer was now back on the workshop circuit, gaining praise and popularity.

Hadn't I heard? enquired a further colleague, that yet another famed yoga *guru* had effectively 'reinvented' himself and had returned to teaching only seven months after some scandalous financial and sexual improprieties had come to light.

Was I not aware? asked my yoga sisters in the subcontinent, of the fact that, even whilst he was under investigation for multiple cases of mental, emotional and sexual abuses, another esteemed yoga tutor was continuing to teach sessions in India.

At first, the more stories I heard, the more I didn't want to listen. I sent out auto-reply emails. I got back to the minutiae of writing. I told people to piss off and leave me alone. I was finishing *Yoni Śakti*. I was working on a celebration of yoga to heal and empower women, I was looking to the future, when women everywhere would be able to find their own power and health through yoga, and it would support them to live in freedom and grace. My mission was to be super positive about yoga as a way for women to connect with their own *yoni śakti*, with their deep source power, with the well-spring of their intuitive knowledge and wisdom.

So just at the point when *Yoni Śakti* was reaching completion, when this huge compendium of positive yogic support for the empowerment of women was almost ready to see the light of day, when after its inordinately long gestation, it was finally ready to be birthed, I was faced with an important choice: whether to include any coverage of these scandals or not.

It simply did not feel right to send *Yoni Śakti* out into the world without any acknowledgment of these stories of the exploitation and abuse of women in the yoga world. But neither did it feel right to re-write the entire book, shifting the focus and tone to a more negative but perhaps more realistic appraisal of the place of many women in yoga now. It was hard to know quite what to do; it was like being about to go into labour and hearing some massive civil disturbance going on outside in the street, so loud and so disturbing that it stalls the process of labour. How to respond?

Initially I simply wrote a new preface on sexual exploitation on planet yoga, expressing my deep disgust at the misogynist abuses that had been revealed to be so widespread. I stuck the preface up front, and hoped that would fix the balance. But even that was not the right strategy. Whilst it was important to acknowledge those very bad stories, it was not a good way to start a book whose purpose was to celebrate women's power in yoga. So in the end, I ditched the outraged author's preface and chose to open with the celebratory invocation to *yoni śakti* that appears on pp.17–21.

So what then is to be done with all those shocking stories? What becomes of all the tales of exploitation and sexual abuse? I have chosen to gather them here at the end, where they put a salutary sting in the tail of an entity that is largely positive and encouraging. For, in the context of a whole book of celebration, it is clear, that on balance, yoga can be very good for women, even if many of the organisations which purport to promote it are rooted in hierarchical and commercial power structures that can foster exploitation and abuse. And we have the capacity to change the power balance here. For at a very practical level, it is a simple matter to make a decision never to support any yoga institution or organisation that condones, accepts or ignores the abuse of the women within it.

In the final edit, I inserted an invitation to this commitment as the first statement of the womb yoga manifesto. Practising what I was preaching, I withdrew my participation as a student from the organisation that had recently been forced to reveal the immorality of its leading male tutor. I simply chose not to pay the next invoice because I sensed that to feed money into any of these organisations is to perpetuate abuses of power and the mistreatment of women in yoga. It is my hope that if other women yoga students and teachers recognise the role that *yoginīs* have to play as agents of social justice, that they too may choose to redirect their money towards individuals and training outfits that do not harbour old fears and new scandals. Without the continued financial support of women, these organisations will not last very long, and then maybe those who exploit and abuse will have have nowhere left to hide.

To attend in detail to the significance of all these stories would take a whole new book of its own. But even just to hear the stories of the women who have encountered abuse in yoga organisations is an important part of healing the hurt caused by those abuses. As I began to lecture and talk about *yoni śakti*, at yoga festivals and gatherings, I was privileged to hear testimonies from many women of their truly shocking experiences at the hands of so-called yoga *gurus* and senior teachers (both male and female) in almost every yoga school of which I have ever heard. But even in the face of abuses and exploitations, these courageous *yoginīs* were empowered by the tangible benefits of their own practice of yoga. They have continued to practise yoga, and it has continued to nourish and support them. What these brave *yoginīs* have done is to encounter fear and to overcome it with the love and positive energy that their yoga practice brings them. It is good that yoga practice builds our courage, because courage is what is needed now.

Courage is needed, because deep in the heart of many of the world's yoga organisations, and in all of the organisations and institutions that are home to these stories of exploitation, the organising principle is basically fear. It is fear that enables these abuses to occur. People, especially women, and especially vulnerable young women, are frightened that if they follow their own intuitive wisdom it might lead them to a place of exclusion or ridicule: if we resist the unwelcome advances of those in power, it may cause us to be excommunicated or ousted from the apparently supportive structures that can be centred around powerful teachers. Dissenters will not be allowed to continue to 'belong'. We may fear isolation and disapproval. The older women who may be in a position to protect the younger ones fear that if they do not continue to support and condone the misogynist and exploitative misbehaviours of those in power, then they may in turn lose their own power within the organisation. Almost everyone is afraid to criticise, for fear they will be cast out. Beyond the current scandals, this fear is almost omnipresent. It is stronger in some places than others, but there is barely any corner of any traditionally structured yoga school or institution that it doesn't reach in some way. If it does not manifest as outright sexual abuse, it is often clearly detectable in other abuses of power within protectionist hierarchies of yoga teaching, for example the exclusion of practitioners and the expulsion of able teachers in the interests of maintaining the status quo.

During the weeks that I was fielding testimonies from colleagues about the deep fear of explusion that permits the exploitation of women in so many yoga institutions around the world, I recollected the faint echo of an expulsion anxiety that I myself had experienced more than a dozen years previously. I recognised the fear which prevented so many people from speaking out about abuses of power within the yoga hierarchies: it was the same fear that had led my younger self to try desperately to please the power-holders of a yoga tradition so that I could remain safe within it. My struggle to maintain my place on a teacher-training course brought me very close to the suffocating stench of this fear: 'Listen!' hissed the top swami of the establishment as I endeavoured to remonstrate that my expulsion from the course was unfair, and that there should be some procedure for redress, 'Shut up and listen! This is important. When you are a trainer, when you are running your own courses, believe me, you will want to be able to treat your students in the exact same way that we have treated you. You will want to be able to expel students and not to give them any good reason. You will need to be able to do this. This is just how it is: this is how to treat students. This is how we have always trained teachers.' When I suggested perhaps that it was time to consider other ways, the response was emphatic: 'I'm too old to change now – we can't change this. And you can't either.'

I was so stunned that at first I did't even recognise the deep fear which motivated this proclamation. But once I identified it, then all desires to remain part of any organisation that perpetuated that kind of fear and resistance to change totally vanished. My radical feminist, agent of social justice, union-representative fire rose up inside me and I looked that swami straight in the eye. I could smell her fear. I spoke to it: 'So you abuse me, as a way to ensure that I might in turn perpetuate these same kind of abuses of power upon my future students? And you believe there is no way to change any of this? And you want me to behave just like you?' There was of course no answer. 'Well, you're wrong. That's not what I want to do.' I left. Once I felt free of the fear of not belonging, I never felt frightened like that again.

It was in that moment of freedom from fear that I first conceived of the seed that became *Yoni Śakti*. I knew yoga to be a force for change. I know that using yoga institutions to resist change, or to maintain existing power abuses, was just plain wrong. The seed that was planted in my heart at that moment was very tiny but very potent: its essence was the desire to liberate the transformative potential of yoga from any limitation that might dwarf or stunt its potentially world-changing capacity to grow and thrive. It took a very long time for that tiny fragile seed to grow into this book. But the desire to nurture the freedom for every woman to practise the form of yoga that most nourishes and honours her at every stage of her life was a powerful motivation, which sustained the gestation and birth process of *Yoni Śakti*. For I believed then, and I know now, that the ultimate aim of any truly good teacher is to enable her students to be better, and more powerful than her. I believed then, and I know now, that yoga is an optimal means for women to encounter their own power. I fervently and honestly desire for all women to have access to those practices and techniques of yoga that most empower and strengthen their ability to honour their own inner teachers, and thus to live in freedom and love throughout the whole of their lives. That is why I persevered through the protracted gestation, long labour and birth of this book.

As a direct result of my desire to be free from the fear that permeates almost every yoga institution I have ever heard of, I have consciously chosen in my work to remain independent from any alignment or affiliation. Even within the apparently open and kind worlds of pregnancy and postnatal yoga, I have encountered a kind of deeply fearful protectionism that manifests as a resistance to allow students from 'other' traditions and schools to learn from each other. I have steadfastly kept the doors of all my own trainings, classes and those of the students who have trained with me, absolutely wide open to *yoginīs* from all traditions. The doors can be open because we have no fear – there is no power structure or hierarchy to maintain, and so there are no abuses of power or fearful, protectionist agendas at work. This is a profound freedom to breathe the fresh air of confidence and power.

Exploitative hierarchies harbour the fear of what happens when people can hear the clear guidance of their own inner teacher, and need no-one to tell them what to do. When we stand unafraid, outside these limiting, old structures, then we are truly free to embrace our diversity of yogic experience. We can be clear and strong, empowered by our own yoga practice to listen to the voice of our inner teachers, and to follow the deep intuitive wisdom that can immediately detect the slightest whiff of something that is inappropriate or harmful for us.

The revelations that so disturbed the completion of this book show us how fear can limit and control us, and lead us into situations where we may be harmed and abused. Once I had found a way to place these important stories in relation to the celebratory and positive tone of the rest of *Yoni Śakti*, then the labour that had been stalled by fear, started up again and the book could be born. My own fearful response to that massive disturbance out in the wider yoga world was quieted: I knew that the positive tales and helpful techniques shared in *Yoni Śakti* were safe to be born: they didn't need to be hedged about with expressions of disgust and horror. The gestation and birth process of this book, long and demanding as it has been, has taught me that we have no need to be afraid of challenging the yogic status quo. Now is the right time, the needed time, to be sharing positive news of women's power and yoga.

So long in gestation, so delayed in labour, and so difficult to birth, *Yoni Śakti* is out alive, and its birth cry is a cry for freedom: the freedom to honour your own inner teacher, the freedom to encounter your power, and the freedom to enjoy an open-hearted and fearless practice of yoga that has full commitment to the evolution of women's spiritual empowerment.

ACKNOWLEDGEMENTS

My first deep debt of gratitude is to my mother for introducing me to yoga at the age of four, and my second debt of gratitude is to all the hundreds of yoga students and teachers who have come to my classes, trainings, retreats and workshops over the past eighteen years. I am fortunate to have been guided by the generous sharings of many yoga teachers, yoga students, friends and colleagues. In particular, I thank the regular *yoginīs* at my Bristol weekly classes, and all those women who have consulted me as a yoga therapist for trusting that my perspective on the therapeutic practice of yoga was of healing value for them. I am especially thankful to Marinella Benelli, Rachel Fleming, Naomi Francis (Hari Pyari) and Ali Woozley, whose passionate enthusiasm for the practice of womb yoga has inspired me greatly.

I thank Swami Satyasangananda Saraswati and the late Paramahamsa Satyananda Saraswati not only for the presentation of *Tattva Śuddhi* and the inspirational translations of *Saundarya-Laharī* and *Vijñāna Bhairavī Tantra*, through whose deep roots this work has been nourished, but also for the support, hospitality and encouragement they both so generously gifted to me and my family since 1997. I am also thankful to my teachers Gyananjan and Gyanmurti at Shraddha Yoga Centre in Italy, and Mukunda and Chinnamasta Stiles in the US, for profound teachings in yoga, *tantra* and *āyurveda*, and for always answering my difficult questions. I offer sincere appreciation to Elizabeth Stanley and everyone at Yogacampus, especially Berenice Wurz, for providing a securely professional and supportive administrative structure from which I have been able to share these techniques with many teachers and trainee teachers.

I offer deep appreciation and a very special thank you to Angela Farmer for sharing her wonderful story of Parvati's invention of yoga, and for her inspirational teaching and practice of yoga to unfold the deep feminine.

Laura Tonello in Rovereto, Italy, Nicole Forman-Levitas at Yoga Form, Antwerp, Katerina Shlyakhova and Anna Shuklova at Birthlight Moscow, Vivi Letsou at NYSY Studio Athens, Angela Georgeson at Yogamum in West Yorkshire, Susan Hopkinson and Sophie Girard-Sequiera at Inspiration Yoga in Brussels, Therese, Fiona and Mary Tierney at Yogaloft in Cork, Trea and Kevin Heapes at the Santosa yoga gathering at Pure Camping in County Clare, Ireland, and Bodil Stentebjerg Olsen at Yogamudra in Copenhagen have all enabled me to present this work in powerful intensive forms that truly helped to crystallise and clarify my understanding of the effects of these practices. Christopher Gladwell and Sarah Harlow at Yogasara Studio in Bristol provided a city home for the weekly explorations in womb yoga during the gestation of this book. I am also very glad to have had the support and encouragement of Dave Brocklebank at Burren Yoga and Meditation Centre, whose ideal retreat space in the wild west of Ireland has provided a superbly nurturing and enlivening environment for women to dive deep into the healing properties of these practices. For all the opportunities and perfect teaching spaces that I have been offered by these generous *yogis* and *yoginīs*, I am very glad.

Many people helped in the preparation of this book, reading chapters and offering helpful feedback. I thank Graham Stanley and Sophie Leek for giving so generously of their time and giving me the huge benefit of their scholarly and editorial expertise, Penny Fuller for testing out the practice instructions, and Alexandra Pope for contributing the foreword, and providing encouragement and reassurance when I felt the project had got too big for me. Heartfelt thanks also to Colette Nolan, Jo MacDonald, Eunice Laurel and Annie Leonard for timely critiques of crucial chapters, and to Lindy and Ranju Roy whose attentive corrections clarified vital sections on history and anatomy. I give deeply grateful thanks to Lucy Crisfield for sorting out my Sanskrit, and to Sandi Sharkey for patiently reading the entire manuscript with great kindness and attention and for offering insightful comments. Paul Walker at Yogamatters / Yogawords was unfailingly enthusiastic about the project for several years, even when it didn't look as if it would ever see the light of day. Ben Jarlett's timely, skilled and cheerful technological and design support was crucial, especially when I was floundering in a sea of gigantic documents. I am deeply thankful for Mark Singleton's scholarly editorial skills, which fine-tuned the text, and his good-humoured encouragement, which maintained my sanity. Zoë Blanc's very welcome arrival at the eleventh hour, along with the design expertise of Allan Sommerville, ensured the whole project actually got finished. Thank you to all these beings.

Special thanks to my husband, Nirlipta Tuli for the many drawings and paintings that bring womb yoga and the wisdom goddesses to vibrant life on the page.

Grateful acknowledgement is made to the Hosking Houses Trust (**www.hosking-houses.co.uk**) for their residency in 2011, without which this book would not have been completed at all.

My husband and children put up with an awful lot. I thank them for their good humour, patience and persistent enquiries about whether it was ever going to get finished, especially when it felt as if it was going to go on forever. Here it is. For any errors, omissions, confusions or oversights I have no-one to thank but myself.

TRAININGS, RETREATS AND LEARNING RESOURCES

In the first instance, for training courses and retreats directly related to the practices described in *Yoni Śakti*, the sites I have developed specifically to support this work offer helpful further information, including dates for currently available retreats and trainings:

www.yonishakti.co
Images, resources and a range of up-to-date links related to this book.

www.wombyoga.org
A home for information about the practice and teaching of womb yoga, including national and international training courses for womb yoga (well-woman yoga therapy), integrated mother and baby yoga training courses and pregnancy and postnatal yoga teacher trainings. Downloadable resources, training dates, workshops, weekly classes, one-to-ones and national and international retreats. This site also lists teachers trained by the author, worldwide.

www.yoganidranetwork.org
Yoga nidrā in Europe: listings and links of teachers from all traditions with skills and training in the delivery of *yoga nidrā*. Workshops and teacher trainings in *yoga nidrā*. Free downloads, further information, tracks to buy and information about local events.

The following websites give contacts for and share valuable information from organisations offering training courses or retreats relevant to the development and expansion of *yoni śakti*. For additional sites and recent updates please visit **www.yonishakti.co**

www.activebirthcentre.com
Workshops and professional trainings from founder Janet Balaskas and colleagues in active birth, hypnobirthing, pregnancy yoga and postnatal support.

www.aspacetobe.co.uk
Yoga, Thai massage and residential yoga holidays in a quiet corner of Northumberland. Family-friendly yoga classes and workshops.

www.birthlight.com
Educational charity founded by Françoise Freedman, offering trainings in UK and abroad in yoga for pregnancy, birth, babies and women's health. International listing of teachers.

www.brightfamily.ru
Bright Family, a centre in the heart of Moscow, offering yoga and aqua yoga for women, their babies and children and their families. Workshops, weekly classes and teacher trainings.

www.burrenyoga.com
Superb retreat and training centre for yoga and meditation in the west of Ireland, in the heart of the Burren. A place to re-energise and dive deep into transformative practices, including yoga for women and *yoga nidrā*.

www.cherishthecunt.com
Workshops, campaign and educational resources including cuntcraft and cunt-positive events.

www.inspirationyoga.eu
Welcoming yoga centre in Brussels, with a supportive community of women practitioners, weekly classes and workshops from visiting teachers.

www.janebennett.com.au
Highly recommended trainings and seminars on the facilitation of positive celebrations and rituals to mark girls' transition to womenhood through menarche. Jane is based in Australia, but offers online support and makes visits to the UK.

www.jewelswingfield.com
Sacred relationship, deep ecology and tantra workshops, trainings and events including red tent days and a year long women's tantra training.

www.louyoga.com
Dublin-based teacher offering classes and workshops in pregnancy yoga, active birth and womb yoga.

www.mirandagray.co.uk
Worldwide womb blessings and moon mother trainings for holding womb blessings and healings.

www.meztlicihuatl-english.blogspot.co.uk
Belinda Garcia Reyes' blog includes one of the most comprehensive lists of links to inspirational websites and women's circles around the world. Many of the sites Belinda recommends offer training and support around topics related to women's spirituality. Hours of happy browsing start here.

www.naturalmysticbhajans.co.uk
Practices and event listings for chanting, mantra, kirtan, shakti dance and more, in London and around the UK.

www.rikhiapeeth.net and **www.yogavision.net/rp/about.htm**
Sources of information about training courses and events in Rikhia, Jarkhand, northeast India, at the home of the late Paramahamsa Satyananda Saraswati.

www.sadhanamala.com
Recommended teacher training courses and support for further intelligent and sensitive development of yogic practice, including retreats, and art of individual teaching courses.

www.santosayogacamp.co.uk and **www.purecamping.ie**
Both these sites carry details of the Santosa yoga camps, where living yoga in beautiful surroundings includes daily chants, yoga nidrā, womb yoga and other delights.

www.shaktidance.co.uk
Teacher-training courses, retreats, workshops and links for shakti dance teachers all over the UK and Europe.

www.specialyoga.org.uk
London-based yoga centre with an excellent and comprehensive teacher-training programme for teaching yoga and meditation to children with and without special needs.

www.theredboxcompany.com
Really useful resources, trainings, workshops, publications and a lively online community of women with a focus on positive attitudes for menstruation, especially for girls and young women.

www.theyogavillage.co.uk
Family friendly Nottingham yoga centre offering workshops and classes for women during pregnancy, postnatal recovery and beyond.

www.theyogarooms.co.uk
Community co-operative yoga spaces in Chorlton and Manchester. Weekly programme includes yoga for pregnancy and postnatal recovery.

www.womensquest.org
Fabulously useful site for connecting with women all over the world who have an interest in the spirituality of menstrual health and related topics. Highly recommended workshops and training courses (in particular, Alexandra Pope's year-long Women's Leadership Apprenticeship), also events and discussion forum.

www.yogacampus.com
Highly recommended, non-dogmatic yoga teacher-training courses, also offers a yoga therapy diploma, workshops and intensive trainings from a wide range of top national and international teachers.

www.yogajunction.co.uk
A long-established, family-run London yoga studio offering courses and trainings in yoga philosophy and yoga for pregnancy. Weekly programme includes pregnancy and postnatal yoga.

www.yogaloftcork.com
Beautiful yoga space in Cork city. Weekly programme includes womb yoga classes and yoga for pregnancy. Also full moon sessions, Bodytalk sessions, trainings and workshops from visiting teachers.

www.yogamudra.dk
A beautiful and peaceful yoga sanctuary in the heart of Copenhagen, offering weekly classes, yoga teacher trainings and intensives with local and international teachers.

www.yogaplace.co.uk
Gorgeous yoga studio in east London, offering classes, courses and workshops including a full spectrum of yoga for women.

www.yogasara.co.uk
Community yoga studio in Bristol offering highly recommended 'immersion' and 'intensive' yoga teacher trainings; also weekly classes including shakti dance, womb yoga and postnatal and pregnancy yoga.

www.yoniversity.com.au
Highly recommended workshops and sessions for women and for men, presented by Laura Doe Harris, who is based in Australia, but makes regular visits to the UK.

Please note that the organisations and studios listed above are specifically only those that offer workshops, trainings and retreats. General information sites, and those selling products or hosting archives are listed in the appropriate further reading sections of each individual chapter. For listings of teachers offering weekly womb yoga classes, please visit **www.wombyoga.org**.

NOTES ON PRONOUNCING SANSKRIT WORDS

I have limited the use of Sanskrit in *Yoni Śakti* to those terms for which I can find no really satisfactory English translation. In practice this means there is minimal use of a range of a few crucial Sanskrit proper names and terms for yoga techniques and aspects of esoteric anatomy.

There are many more letters and sounds in Sanskrit than we have letters for in the Roman alphabet. Depending upon how you define them, there are at least forty-eight letters in the Sanskrit syllabary, compared to only twenty-six in the English alphabet. So writing Sanskrit words in English is always only an approximation of the pronunciation indicated by the original Devanāgarī script. This is why a special set of marks (dots, lines and slashes known as diacriticals) is used to create extra sounds from Roman letters.

It is very pleasing to learn to pronounce these words as accurately as possible: saying the words right creates a special experience of focus and openness, and allows us to savour the feeling of the words in our mouth. This expands consciousness of the range of sounds we can create, and can be very enjoyable, so here is a brief guide to how to pronounce these specially marked letters:

Sanskrit vowels are pronounced very like the vowels in Italian. Vowels are either long or short, and this is indicated by the presence and absence of horizontal lines:

ā is pronounced aa (two beats) as in 'father', and

a is pronounced a (one beat) as in 'cat';

ū is pronounced like the oo in 'noodles',

and u like the u in 'but'.

However, o is always long, as in 'so'; and e is always long, as in 'great'.

ṛ is also a vowel, pronounced halfway between the ri in 'riddle' and the er in 'mother', with the tongue curled slightly back, like the American 'vocalic r' in words like 'purdy'.

c is always pronounced like ch in 'church'.

j is pronounced as in 'jelly'.

The letter transliterated as ñ is pronounced in two different ways: either like the ñ in the Spanish word mañana, or as'gya' in some Northern Indian pronunciations.

A dot underneath any letter indicates that the tip of the tongue should touch the roof of the mouth as it is pronounced (e.g. ṭa, ḍa, ṇa, ṣa).

ś is pronounced sh (said smilingly).

ṣ is pronounced sh (with the tip of the tongue touching the roof of the mouth).

There are also aspirated ('breathed') consonants in Sanskrit that require special attention, since they need to be pronounced distinctly:

bh is pronounced as the join in 'fab hair',

gh is pronounced as the join in 'dog head',

dh is pronounced as the join in 'mad house',

ph is pronounced as the join in 'top hat', and

th is pronounced as the join in 'coat hook'.

I have pluralised some words like *cakras* and *mudrās* and *Mahāvidyās* simply by adding an "s", which is not acceptable to academic Sanskritists, but makes the meaning clearer.

SANSKRIT GLOSSARY OF TERMS

NB in the interests of legibility, unlike elswhere in Yoni Śakti *the Sanskrit words in this glossary are not italicised.*

Aditi: mother of the gods, the Vedic mother-goddess.
Agastya: Vedic sage.
Agnisāra kriyā: 'essence of fire'. Cleansing practice that utilises an abdominal lift and pumping on the exhalation.
Ahaṁkāra: the 'I-maker', or ego-identified consciousness of self.
Ājñā cakra: 'command/control centre', the sixth cakra, located at the third eye.
Ākāśa; space, the fifth element.
Alpapadma: small lotus, a hand gesture.
Amarolī: use of urine for medicinal and spiritual purposes.
Anāhata: the 'unstruck sound', fourth cakra, located at the heart centre.
Ānandamaya: 'made of bliss', the dimension of being relating to the spirit body and the experience of unending bliss.
Aṇimā: primary siddhi, the capacity to become minuscule.
Anna: food.
Annamaya: 'made of food', the dimension of being related to the physical body.
Antar mouna: inner silence.
Antarkaraṇa: the inner instrument, or state of mind.
Apāna: form of energy that flows downwards from pelvis to earth.
Āpas: water.
Āraṇyaka: forest dweller.
Āsana: literally 'seat', generally understood as posture.
Aśvinī: the 'horse seal', or anal sphincter squeeze.
Aṣṭa siddhi: the eight magical powers.
Aṣtanga Vinyasa Yoga: flowing form of athletic yoga sequences taught by K. Pattabhi Jois.
Atharva: the fourth Veda, dealing with magic and healing rituals. The name derives from Atharvan, an ancient Rishi (sage).

Baddha koṇāsana: the Cobbler's pose, sometimes also called titali (Butterfly) pose).
Bagalāmukhī: the 'paralyser', literally 'the face that has the power to control'.
Bandha: a lock, or binding bond.
Bhairava: a fierce form of Śiva.
Bhairavī: feminine counterpart of the fierce form of Śiva .
Bhakti: heartfelt spiritual devotion.
Bhava: inner vision, feeling or intention.
Bhrāmarī prāṇāyāma: humming bee breath.
Bhuvaneśvarī: she whose body is the world.
Bīja: seed.
Brahmā: the creator, as part of the triad with Viṣṇu and Śiva
Brahmacārin: one who observes restraint, in particular often celibacy.
Brahmacarya: restraint, often celibacy or sexual continence.
Brāhmaṇa: earliest parts of the Vedas.
Buddhi: discriminative intelligence.

Cakki calānāsana: grinding the mill posture.
Cakra: literally wheel, or vortex, metaphorically a spinning energy centre.
Candra: the moon.
Candra namaskāra: moon salutation sequence of postures.
Chinnamastā: she whose head is severed, the self-decapitated goddess.
Cin mudrā: gesture of consciousness.
Citta: psychic content of mind.

Ḍākinī: 'sky dancer', goddess or yoginī.
Darśana: literally a vision or glimpse, but also a term to describe schools (perspectives) of Indian philosophy.
Daśa: ten.
Devī: goddess.
Devijai utkaṭāsana: victory pose of the fierce goddess.
Dhāraṇā: concentration.
Dhūmavatī: the widow goddess, grandmother goddess.
Durgā: fierce form of the goddess who rides on a tiger.

Gandha: sense of smell.
Garbha: egg, embryo or pregnant womb.
Garimā: siddhi that confers capacity to become immensely heavy.
Ghrāṇa: nose.
Guru: literally 'heavy', a teacher.

Haṃ: seed mantra for viśuddha cakra.
Hanumān: monkey god, embodiment of courage, devotion and intelligence.
Hasta mudrā: hand gesture.
Haṭha: literally 'forceful', generally referring to physical yoga practice.
Hiraṇya garbha: golden cosmic womb / egg.
Hṛd / Hṛdaya: (spiritual) heart.
Hṛdaya mudrā: heart gesture.
Hṛdaya-yoni nadī: heart-womb river.
Hṛdayākāśa: space of the spiritual heart.

Īśatvam: siddhi, possessing absolute power.
Jagadambe mātāki jai: victory to the great mother of the world.
Jālandhara bandha: literally the lock that 'holds the web', or chin lock.
Jñānendriya: organs of knowledge (sensory organs).

Kāḷī: the black goddess.
Kamala mudrā: lotus gesture.
Kamalātmikā: the lotus goddess.
Kāmarūpa: centre of sexual desire.
Kapālabhāti: 'shining skull', pumping breath.
Kārikā: a doctrine stated in verses, e.g Saṁkhya Kārikā.
Karmendriya: organs of action.
Kathā: speech, narration.
Kaṭicakrāsana: waist-rotating pose.
Kaula: literally 'family' or clan – specifically groupings of tantric sects.
Kāya mudrā: body gesture (as opposed to a hand gesture).
Khecarī mudrā: tip of tongue rolled back against soft palate and up towards naso-pharynx.
Kośa: 'sheath', layer or covering, referring to different aspects of existence.
Kriyā: 'action or effort', also referring to cleansing practices in haṭha yoga.
Kṛṣṇa: Hindu god, incarnation of Viṣṇu.
Kuṇḍalinī: coiled energy in the first cakra, envisioned as a sleeping snake.

Laghimā: siddhi, the capacity to become weightless.
Laṁ: seed mantra for mūlādhāra cakra.
Layayoga: yoga of dissolution, or absorption of mind and breath into the heart space.

Mahā: great.
Mahā bandha: the great lock (combination of mula-, uḍḍīyāna- and jālandhara bandhas.
Mahā mūlādhāra mudrā: the great sacral gesture.
Mahāvidyā: great wisdom, great wisdom goddess/es.
Mahimā: a siddhi, the capacity to become enormous.
Mālā: garland, or rosary.
Mām or mā aham: me.
Manaḥ : mind.
Maṇipūra: 'City of jewels', the third cakra, located at navel centre.
Manomaya: Full of mind, the dimension of being related to thoughts, feelings and opinions.
Mantra: 'instrument of thought' i.e. sound or words containing the energy of spiritual transformation.
Mataṅgī: the outcaste poet goddess.
Mudrā: gesture.
Mūla bandha: root lock, the vaginal squeeze and lift.
Mūlādhāra: 'root support', the first cakra, located for women in and around vulva and the walls of the vagina.

Nadī: river.
Nāḍī: subtle energetic channel.
Namaskāra: greeting.
Namaste: greeting with palms in prayer position, signifying 'the divine light in me greets the divine light in you'.
Nāṭarājāsana: the dancer's pose.
Nāth: 'lord' or 'protective refuge', the name of yogic sect.
Nidrā: sleep.
Nirvikalpa: 'free from change'. Describes the highest form of samādhi. Also a form of Bhairava q.v.
Nyāsa: 'to place or apply in a special way' e.g in *yoga nidrā*, the placing of conscious awareness at each part of the body.

Pāda: foot.
Pādabandha: foot lock, or conscious broadening and lengthening of the feet to lift the arches and spread the toes.
Padma: lotus.
Pañcatattva: five elements.
Pāṇi: hand.
Paramparā: uninterrupted lineage of teachers and disciples.
Pārvatī: consort of Śiva, the mountain goddess.
Pavanamuktāsana: poses that liberate the principle of energy / movement.
Pāyu: anus.
Pīṭha (cf Pīthadhishvari of Rikhiapīṭh): seat / place.
Prajñā: intuition.
Prakāmya: a siddhi, the capacity to realise whatever one desires.
Prakṛti: nature, the manifestations of śakti.
Prāṇa: life force.
Prāṇa śakti: the power / energy of the life force.
Prāṇa śakti pūjā: worship of the power of the life force.
Prāṇa vāyu: the life force in the form of breath, or 'wind'.
Prāṇam / prāṇamāsana: prayerful gesture of humility, greeting and praise, with palms together, standing or prone.
Prāṇāmaya: full of prāṇa, or life force; that dimension of being that is to do with energy.
Prāṇāyāma: expansion or extension of the life force through the extension and conscious control of the breath.

Prāpti: a siddhi, the capacity to be in all places at once.
Pratipakṣa bhāvana: the inner cultivation of opposite perspectives, i.e the conscious use of mind to create elevated attitudes (Yoga Sūtra 2:33).
Pṛthivī: earth.
Pūjā: ceremonial or ritual worship (simple or complex), done with devotional attention to honour deities or elemental forces.
Purāṇas: early Indian narratives including histories, creation stories and tales of deities and demons.
Pūrṇa: fullness, completeness, perfection (complete chant, 'Pūrṇamada').
Puṣpam: flower.

Rahasya: secret mystery.
Rāja: king.
Raṁ: seed mantra for maṇipūra cakra.
Rasa: taste, flavour or sentiment.
Rūpa: outward form or appearance.

Śabda: sound or word.
Sādhana: literally, to realisation, i.e spiritual practice.
Sahajolī mudrā: powerful gesture (female equivalent of vajrolī).
Sahasrāra: crown cakra, with the form of a thousand petalled lotus.
Śākta: relating to energy or power as a goddess, a worshipper of that goddess or power.
Śakti: energy, power, strength or ability.
Śakti bandha: poses to unfasten or unlock energy.
Śālā: hall or school room.
Sāma: equal or matched, the same.
Samādhi: intense absorption in unified consciousness.
Samāna: a form of prāṇa, with equalising balance between upward- and downward-moving properties. Located in the belly.
Saṁhitā: collection of verses or texts; also the force that holds the universe together.
Saṁkalpa: wish, intention or solemn desire.
Sāṁkhya: discriminative or rational, 'about numbers'; school of Indian philosophy.
Sarvam: relating to all.
Satī: Śiva's first wife (also meaning a virtuous woman).
Śaśaṅkabhūjaṅgāsana: hare-cobra pose.
Śaśaṅkāsana: hare pose (child's pose).
Siddha: person possessed of siddhi/s.
Siddhi/siddhis: attainment, fulfilment or magical power.
Śirṣāsana: head balance pose.
Śītalī / sītkārī: cooling breaths.
Śiva: the 'beneficent' or 'kindly one'; the god of destruction and lord of yoga.
Śmaśāna: burial or cremation ground.
Sparśa: touch.
Ṣoḍasī: the sixteen year-old goddess, aka Tripura Sundari.
Śrotra: ear.
-sthāna: a place or site, eg yonisthāna.
Supta: reclining: 'in bed but not asleep'.
Sūrya namaskāra: sun salutation.
Sūtra: thread, verse.
Svādhiṣṭhāna: 'one's own place or abode'; second cakra, located in the pelvis.
Svāmi: 'boss' or 'lord', honorific for renunciates. Commonly spelled 'Swami'.
Svara: flow of air breathed through the nostrils. Svara also means a musical note or tone.

Tāḍāsana: Mountain pose (Iyengar yoga); Palm tree pose (Satyananda yoga).
Tan: to manifest, or extend towards.
Tanmātra: subtle element.
Tantra: text or doctrine, also with the meaning 'loom, fibre, or weave'.
Tāntrik: to do with tantra.
Tāntrika: practitioner of tantra.
Tapasyā / tapas: disciplined ascetic effort, austerity, heat.
Tārā: 'star (f)', one of the Mahāvidyās, also with the meaning 'crossing over' (m).
Tattva / tattva: element, essence or substance.
Tattva śuddhi: purification of elements or essence.
Tattva yantra: geometric form representing / encasing element or substance.
Tripura sundarī: one of the Mahāvidyās, beauty of the three worlds.

Udāna: a form of prāṇa that spirals upwards.
Uḍḍīyāna bandha: upward-moving lock.
Ujjāyī: victorious breath.
Upaniṣad: literally, 'to sit near', philosophical texts, the last part of the Vedas.
Upasthā: reproductive organs.
Uttarabodhi mudrā: gesture of the highest enlightenment.

Vajrāsana: thunderbolt seat (kneeling).
Vajrolī mudrā: thunderbolt gesture (male version of sahajolī mudrā).
Vāk: speech, personified as a goddess in the Vedas.
Vaṁ: see mantra for svādhiṣṭhāna cakra.
Vaśitva: a siddhi, the capacity to control everything.
Vāyu: air, or form of prāṇa.
Veda: ancient Indian scripture.
Vedānta: the 'end of the vedas', Indian philosophical system.

Vibhūti pāda: the chapter of the Yoga Sūtra dealing with magical powers (vibhūti).
Vijñānam: special knowledge.
Vijñānamaya: full of special knowedge, that dimension of being to do with intuition and special, inner understanding.
Vinyāsa: sequenced flow.
Viparīta karaṇī: inverted practice.
Viṣṇu: god of preservation.
Viśuddha cakra: fifth cakra, purification centre, located in throat.
Viveka: discrimination.
Vyāna: form of prāṇa that circulates throughout the body.

Yajur: one of the four Vedas.
Yaṁ: seed mantra for anāhata cakra.
Yantra: geometric symbol, mystical diagram for meditation; any instrument or apparatus.
Yoga: union.
Yogi: one who practises yoga (male).
Yoginī: one who practises yoga (female).
Yoginī śakti ki jai: victory to the power of the yoginī.
Yoni: source, origin, cunt, vulva, vagina, womb. Also means home, or place of rest.
Yoni śakti pūjā: ritual to honour or worship the power of the yoni.
Yonisthāna: place of the yoni.
Yoni-namaskāram: yoni greeting.
Yoni puṣpam: yoni flower, i.e menstrual blood.

SELECT CHRONOLOGY: 50,000 BCE – 2003 CE

A personal selection of key dates, texts, temples and people in the history of women in yoga.

BCE

c 50,000 Neolithic cultures, creating mother goddess and dancing women images in cave art and sculpture: e.g. cave carvings of *yoni* shapes, La Ferrassie, France.
c 30,000 dancing priestess of Galgenberg.
c 27,000 Venus of Willendorf.
c 24,000 Venus of Lausel.
c 30,000 pastoral nomad societies in India.
c 25,000 urban societies merge along banks of Indus river.
c 6000–2000 megalithic dolmen burial sites in Kerala.
c 2200–2000 Harappa at its height.
c 2000–1500 Indus Valley Civilisation declines.
c 1700–1500 Nomads in the Punjab compose the *Ṛg Veda*.
c 1300–1000 proto-Chinnamastā goddess figure, Maharastra.
c 1200–900 the Vedic people compose *Yajur*, *Sāma* and *Atharva Vedas*.
c 1000 cave painting of childbirth scene, in Bhimbheka caves, Sanchi district, Madhya Pradesh.
c 900 Vedic people move down into the Ganges Valley.
c 950 *Mahabhārata* battle at Kurukshetra (the location for Arjuna's debate in the *Bhagavad Gīta*)
c 800–600 *Brāhmaṇas* composed.
c 700 – 600 Early *Upaniṣads* composed.
c 483/410 death of Siddhartha Gautama the Buddha.
c 400 Mother goddess figures carved on ring stones and stone disks in the Punjab and Bihar, north India.
c 400 – 100CE Later *Upaniṣads* composed.
c 300BCE – 300CE *Mahābharata* composed.
c 200BCE – 200CE *Ramāyana* composed.

CE

c 100–200 Pātañjali codifies practice of yoga in *Yoga Sūtra*.
c 100 *Dharma Śāstra* (Laws of Manu) compiled.
c 200 *Sāṃkhya Kārikā* (one of earliest texts of Sāṃkhyan philosophy) composed.
c 300 Sculpture of Harītī 'the goddess who kidnaps infants', in Patna.
c 350–700 Early *Purāṇas* composed.
c 350 *Guhyasamāja Tantra* [Assembly of Secrets] composed (oldest Buddhist *tantra*).
c 400–800 cult of the *Saptamātrikas* (seven mother goddesses) at its height.

c 500 Karaikkal Ammaiyar, Saivite poetess *yoginī* lived.
c 600 *Saptamātrika* (seven mother goddesses) carved in panels in caves in Ellora.
c 650–800 Other early *tantras* composed, including:
c 700 Sahajayoginicinta's *Vyaktabhavanaugata-tattva-siddhi* ('Realisation of Reality through its Bodily Expressions' Buddhist *tantra*)
c 750 *Devī-māhātmya* (part of the *Markaṇḍeya Purāṇa*) composed.
c 700–800 *Saundarya-laharī* composed (*Śākta tantra*).
c 700–800 Height of popularity for pilgrimage to the *Śakti* pithas all over India (sites where Satī's body fell to earth).
c 800 *Vijñāna Bhairava Tantra* (Kashmir Saivite *tantra*) composed.
c 800 Matsyendranāth composes *Kaulajñānanirṇaya Tantra*.
c 800–900 *Bhāgavata Purāṇa* composed.
c 900–1000 *Kubjikā Tantras* composed.
c 1000 emergence of the Kaula (*tāntrik*) sects.
c 945–1031 Khajuraho temples built, Chhatarpur, Madhya Pradesh.
c 975–1025 Abhinavagupta, Śaiva philosopher and interpreter of *tāntrik* ritual, lives in Kashmir, writes *Tantrāloka*.
c 1000 Circular, roofless sixty-four *yoginī* temples built at Hirapur (Bhuvaneshvar), Madhya Pradesh.
c 1000 Circular roofless sixty-four *yoginī* temple built at Rhanipur-Jharial Orissa.
c 1000 Circular roofless sixty-four *yoginī* temples built at Chhatarpur and Mitawali (Naresar), Madhya Pradesh.
c 1100 Circular roofless sixty-four *yoginī* temple built, Bhedaghat, Jabalpur, Madhya Pradesh. Includes carving of *Yoni pūjā* (veneration of the vulva).
c 1200 *Kūlacūḍāmaṇi Tantra* composed.
c 1300–1400 *Gorakṣa Śataka*, *haṭha* yoga text.
1300–1600 *Bhakti* yoga (yoga of devotion) movement thrives in India.
c 1300 Lalla Ded ('Granny Lalla'), Kashmir Saivite ascetic poet composes *Lallavākyāni* 'sayings of Lalla'.
c 1350 *Yoginī Tantra* composed.
c 1300–1400 Svātmārāma composes *Haṭha Yoga Pradīpikā*.
c 1498–1573 Mirābai, Vaiṣṇavite *bhakti* poet lives.
c 1500 *Śiva Saṁhitā* composed.
c 1600 *Mahānirvāṇa Tantra* composed.
c 1650 *Yoni Tantra* composed.
1757 First wave of the British Raj in India.
c 1800 *Gheraṇḍa Saṁhitā* composed.
1813 Second wave of the British Raj begins.
1849 US Transcendentalist Henry David Thoreau describes himself as a 'yogi'.
1853–1920 Sarada Devī, wife of Ramakrishna, lives.
1855–1936 Sir John Woodroffe (aka Arthur Avalon) lives.
1857 Third wave of the British Raj in India.
1863–1902 Swami Vivekananda lives.

1870 Married Women's Property act in UK grants some limited rights to married women to own property.
1875 Helena Blavatsky, Colonel Henry Steel Olcott, and William Quan Judge found the Theosophical Society.
1888–1989 Tirumalai Krishnamacharya lives.
1887–1963 Swami Sivananda lives.
1888 Pierre Bernard (who would later marry Blanche DeVries, who herself became a celebrated yoga teacher) learns yoga from a visiting *tāntrik* master in Nebraska.
1888 Married Women's Property Act (ii) grants further limited rights for married women in UK to own property.
1890 Queen Victoria studies yoga with Shivapuri Baba on his visits to London.
1893 Swami Vivekananda attends World Parliament of Religions in Chicago.
1895 Margaret Noble (Sister Nivedita) meets Swami Vivekananda in London.
1896–1982 Bengali mystic Anandamayi Ma lives.
1897 Swami Vivekenanda founds Vedānta movement in US.
1898 Sister Nivedita travels to India with Swami Vivekananda.
1899–2002 Indra Devi (Eugenie Labunskaia) lives.
1900 Women's colleges of London University admitted as 'schools' of the university i.e women could be awarded university degrees.
1908–1999 Vanda Scaravelli lives.
1911–1995 Swami Sivananda Radha (Sylvia Demitz) lives.
1912 Mollie Bagot-Stack studies yoga-based *āsanas* in India.
1915–2009 K. Pattabhi Jois lives.
1918–2014 B.K.S Iyengar lives.
1918 UK women over the age of thirty given right to vote in national elections
1920–40 Mollie Bagot-Stack teaches yoga-based 'stretch and swing' in London.
1920 US women given right to vote in national elections
1923–2009 Swami Satyananda Saraswati lives.
1928 UK women given equal voting rights with men.
1930 Indra Devi studies yoga with T. Krishnamacharya.
1938 Blanche DeVries opens yoga studio in New York City.
1938–present T.K.V Desikachar, son of Krishnamachrya, lives.
1944–present Geeta Iyengar lives.
1944 *Haṭha Yoga* by Theos Bernard published.
1945 Italian women given right to vote.
1947 Indian Independence. Partition.
1950–60 Vanda Scaravelli studies with Iyengar and Desikachar.
1950 Indian women given right to vote.
1953–present Swami Satyasangananda Sarswati lives.
1953–present Ammaci (Amritanandamayi Mā) lives.
1953 *Yoga for Americans* by Indra Devi published.
1956 Swami Sivananda initiates Swami Sivananda Radha into *saṃnyāsa*.
1956 Magaña Baptiste (student of Indra Devi) opens yoga centre in San Francisco.

1960 *The Complete Illustrated Book of Yoga* by Swami Vishnudevananda published.
1966 *Light on Yoga* by B.K.S Iyengar published.
1972 –1991 Nischala Joy Devi studies and teaches yoga at Swami Satchidānanda's US ashram.
1974 *Prenatal Yoga and Natural Birth* by Jeanine Parvati Baker published. The first pregnancy yoga book.
1977 *Nawa Yogini Tantra* by Swamis Muktananda and Satyananda Saraswati first published. The first yoga book on women's health.
1978 *Kundalini Yoga for the West* by Swami Sivananda Radha published.
1981 *Wise Earth Ayurveda* founded by Maya Tiwari.
1981 *Active Birth Manifesto* published by Janet Balaskas
1983 *Yoga: a Gem for Women* by Geeta Iyengar published.
1991 *Awakening the Spine* by Vanda Scaravelli published.
1998 Birthlight Trust founded by Françoise Freedman
2000 *Living Your Yoga* by Judith Lasater published.
2003 *Bringing Yoga to Life* by Donna Farhi published.

(A compilation of dates based on Wendy Doniger's Hindus: an Alternative History*, pp.683–4, David White's* Kiss of the Yoginī*; and a variety of sources for other dates).*

BIBLIOGRAPHY

Where relevant, first edition dates are shown in parentheses.

Amazzone, Laura. 2010. *Goddess Durgā and Sacred Female Power*. Hamilton Books, Lanham, Maryland. An astonishing amalgam of feminist scholarship and spiritual autobiography. The form and worship of Durgā and the collective power of the *yoginīs* are presented as a force for personal and planetary transformation.

Angier, Natalie. 2000 (1999). *Woman: An Intimate Geography*. Virago, London. Invaluable, meticulously researched exploration of all aspects of being female from 'organs to orgasm'. Interviews, scientific papers and a full range of contemporary theories are skilfully interwoven and presented in the most lucid and lively prose. An eye-opening delight.

Arewa, Caroline Shola. 1998. *Opening to Spirit: Contacting the Healing Power of the Chakras and Honouring African Spirituality*. Thorsons, London. A remarkably fresh angle on the traditional yogic understandings of the energy body. Arewa brings together an African feminist perspective with practical guidelines that make yogas based on the *kuṇḍalinī* model contemporary, relevant and accessible.

Armstrong, Penny and **Feldman, Sherry**. 2008 (1986). *A Midwife's Story*. Pinter and Martin, London. A first hand account of inspirational midwifery and births amongst the Amish. Full of insight and real wisdom on the power of birth.

Ashley–Farrand, Thomas. 2003. *Śakti Mantras: Tapping into the Great Goddess Energy Within*. Ballantine, New York. Mantras to the Goddess, accompanied by personal stories and explorations of the effects and applications of *śakti mantras*. Full of fascinating anecdotes, traditional stories and clear guidance based on personal experience of the use of the mantras.

Baker, Jeannine Parvati. 2001 (1974). *Prenatal Yoga and Natural Childbirth*. North Atlantic Books, Berkeley, California. Pioneering combination of a *tāntrik* approach to yoga as spiritual empowerment and a mother's perspective on pregnancy and birth.

Bernard, Theos. 1944. *Hatha Yoga*. Rider and Company, London. One of the earliest popular texts on yoga, pivotal in establishing the growth of modern postural yoga in Europe and the US.

Bhairavan, Amarananda. 2000. *Kali's Odiyya: A Shaman's True Story of Inititiation*. Nicholas Hays, York Beach, Maine. Autobiographical account of life in a Kālī-worshipping village matriarchy. Includes first hand-accounts of *tāntrik* shamanic rituals and the living power of the goddess.

Block, Francesca Lia. 2003. *Guarding the Moon: a Mother's First Year*. Harper Collins, New York. Autobiographical prose poem-cum-journal from a Los Angeles novelist. Some touching moments of insight and depth.

Bolen, Jean Shinoda. 2003. *Crones Don't Whine: Concentrated Wisdom for Juicy Women*. Conari Press/ Red Wheel/Weiser, Boston MA. A feminist approach to welcoming the wisdom of ageing by defining the thirteen qualities of a 'crone'. Practical and direct.

Bolen, Jean Shinoda. 2005. *Urgent Message from Mother: Gather the Women, Save the World*. Conari Press/Red Wheel/Weiser, San Francisco, California. Inspirational feminist call to awaken to the reality of the global ecological crisis.

Brayne, Sue. 2011. *Sex, Meaning and the Menopause*. Continuum International Publishing, London and New York. A collection of sensitive and enquiring interviews, interwoven with reflections from a psychotherapist on the nature of relationships between men and women during and after menopause.

Brizendine, Louann. 2006. *The Female Brain*. Broadway Books, New York. Fascinating neuro-psychiatric perspectives on the effects of hormonal change on women's emotional life, thought patterns and behaviours. Criticised by some for 'melodrama' and scientific inaccuracy, this is a gripping read.

Broad, William J. 2012. *The Science of Yoga: The Risks and the Rewards*. Simon and Schuster, New York. Sparkling, lively review of scientific research into yoga worldwide, criticised by some for its focus on 1970s research and absence of reference to contemporary studies.

Brooks, Douglas Renfrew. 1992. *Auspicious Wisdom: the Texts and Traditions of Srividya Śakta Tantrism in South India*. State University of New York Press, Albany, New York. A thorough, scholarly account based on detailed textual investigations by a professor of religion who has personal experience with contemporary *śākta tāntrikas*. Brooks clarifies the practices and rituals with diagrams and illustrations, and explores the complex relationship between aspects of tantrism and Brahmanical orthodoxy.

Buckley, Thomas and **Gottleid, Alma** (eds). 1992. *Blood Magic: The Anthroplogy of Menstruation*. University of California Press, London. Collection of scholarly research and an insightful introductory essay on the global spectrum of menstruation rituals and attitudes.

Burley, Mikel. 2000. *Haṭha Yoga: its Context, Theory and Practice*. Motilal Banarsidass, Delhi. Scholarly history of yoga with the additional perspectives and understandings of a practitioner. Criticised by some for its limited range of Sanskrit reference, it provides an overview of yoga in relation to Indian philosophy.

Camphausen, Rufus C. 1999. *Encyclopaedia of Sacred Sexuality: from Aphrodisiacs and Ecstasy to Yoni Worship and Zap-laṁ Yoga*. Inner Traditions, Rochester, Vermont. Fascinating illustrations and articles, with helpful indexes for tracing thematics. Accessible source of information on sexual yogas and *tantra*.

Calais-Germain, Blandine. 2003. *The Female Pelvis: Anatomy and Exercises*. Eastland Press, Seattle. Clear, elegant illustrations and explanations of the anatomy of the female pelvis. Some illuminating exploratory exercises.

Cannon, Emma. 2011. *The Baby-Making Bible, Simple Steps to Enhance your Fertility and Improve your Chances of Getting Pregnant*. Pan Macmillan, London. Sensible tips for every type of conception including the use of assisted reproductive technologies. Integrates practical guidance on nutrition, Chinese medicine and yoga.

Cannon, Emma. 2012. *You and Your Bump, Simple Steps to Pregnancy Wellbeing*. Pan Macmillan, London. Wise, integrated guidance on nutrition, yoga and health from an experienced acupuncturist.

Chia, Mantak and **Chia, Manewan**. 1986. *Healing Love Through the Tao: Cultivating Female Sexual Energy*. Healing Tao Books, Huntington, New York. The mother of many less straightforward taoist and *tāntrik* guides to the cultivation of female sexual energy: this detailed and comprehensive practical manual is clear, well illustrated and easy to follow.

Chiarelli, Pauline. 1992. *Women's Waterworks*. Neem Press, Sydney. An accessible, entertaining and effective, world best-selling guide to the function of the female bladder and pelvic muscles, written by a physiotherapist continence advisor. Available to buy direct at **www.womenswaterworks.com**

Chopra, Shambhavi Lorain. 2006. *Yoginī: Unfolding the Goddess Within*. Wisdom Tree, New Delhi. Poetic, personal and vivid encounters with a living tradition of pure *bhakti* (devotional identification) in *śākta tantra*.

Clooney, Francis X (S.J.). 2005. *Divine Mother, Blessed Mother: Hindu Goddesses and the Virgin Mary*. Oxford University Press, London. Respectful, sensitive and erudite scholarly comparison by Jesuit priest. Poetic translations of *Saundarya-Laharī* and other Sanskrit hymns to the mother explored in the light of hymns from the Marian tradition.

Collings, Jane Hardwicke. 2005. *Spinning Wheels – a Woman's Ready Reckoner: How the Cycle of the Moon, Menstruation, the Earth's Seasons and the Life Seasons Effect You on any Given Day, Helping You Understand Why You Feel the Way You Do and How to Best Go with the Flow*. Appletree House, Roberston NSW. Practical tool to understand the relationships between menstrual cycle, lunar cycle, year seasonal cycle, life season cycle: maiden, mother, maga, crone.

Connolly, Peter. 2007. *A Student's Guide to the History and Philosophy of Yoga*. Equinox, London. An accessible academic survey that sets the traditions of yogic practice in the context of Indian philosophies.

Cistele, Alison; **Vellely, Bernadette**; **Young, Josa**. 1989. *The Sanitary Protection Scandal*. Women's Environmental Network, London. Explores the global and personal hazards of the production, use and disposal of sanitary towels, tampons and babies' nappies.

Cushman, Anne. 2010. 'The Yoga of Creativity' in *Tricycle: The Buddhist Review*, Fall 2010. An elegant and emotionally intelligent exploration of the relationship between writing and the practice of yoga.

Cusk, Rachel. 2002. *A Life's Work: on Becoming a Mother*. Fourth Estate, London. Chilling, gripping and vivid account of postnatal depression. Lyrical and unputdownable.

Delaney, Janice, **Lupton, Mary Jane** and **Toth, Emily**. 1988 (1976). *The Curse: A Cultural History of Menstruation*. University of Illinois Press, Illinois. The first, ground-breaking, and now classic, feminist study of the cultural politics and anthropology of menstruation.

De Michelis, Elizabeth. 2004. *A History of Modern Yoga: Pātañjali and Western Esotericism*. Continuum, London, New York. Scholarly exposition of the development of modern yoga and its relation to the western 'New Age' movement, including a detailed study of the development of Iyengar yoga. Also includes explorations of western occultism and detailed analysis of modern western yoga classes as healing rituals of secular religion.

Devī-Māhātmya (Durgā Saptashati) English translation, text downloaded from **www.hinduism.co.za/durgā.htm** (accessed 20 December 2011).

Dinsmore-Tuli, Uma. 2002. *Yoga for Living: Feel Confident*. Dorling Kindersley, London. Clear guidance for yoga to boost self-esteem. Written for women.

Dinsmore-Tuli, Uma. 2006. *Mother's Breath: a Definitive Guide to Yoga Breathing, Sound and Awareness Practices during Pregnancy, Birth, Postnatal Recovery and Mothering*. Sitaram and Sons, London.

Dinsmore-Tuli, Uma. 2008. *Teach Yourself Yoga for Pregnancy and Birth*. Hodder Education, London. Structured around the evolution of the elements, this book offers comprehensive yoga programmes during pregnancy, birth and early postnatal recovery, including breath, hand gestures, meditations and sound work.

Doniger, Wendy. 2010. *The Hindus: an alternative history*. Oxford University Press, New York. Brilliant, staggeringly vast and packed with detail, including intriguing information about women in *tantra* and Hindu ritual. Compulsive and controversial reading.

Dupuis, Stella. 2008. *The Yogini Temples of India: In the pursuit of a Mystery*. Pilgrim's Publishing, Varanasi. Personal reflections from a pilgrimage around the *yoginī* temples of India.

Estés, Clarissa Pinkola. 1993. *Women Who Run With The Wolves*. Rider, London. A classic compendium of fairy stories, legends and tales, interpreted from a Jungian perspective to reveal the hidden powers of the wild woman.

England, Pam. 1998. *Birthing from Within: an Extra-Ordinary Guide to Childbirth*. Partera Press, New Mexico. A practical, visionary and holistic guide to childbirth that encourages the exploration of deeply held attitudes and misconceptions around pregnancy and birth through making art and self enquiry.

European Vegetarian Union (EVU). 2009. *The Ecological Consequences of Meat Consumption*. Neukirch. Available to download from **www.vegetarismus.ch/info/eoeko.htm**. A clear and well referenced exposition of the ecological arguments for vegetarianism, including statistics on the adverse effects of meat production at a personal and global level.

Farhi, Donna. 2003. *Bringing Yoga to Life: the Everyday Practice of Enlightened Living*. Harper, San Francisco. Insightful guidance from a feminine perspective on the experience of bringing yoga principles into daily life.

Farmer, Angela. 2000. *The Feminine Unfolding* (video). A spiritual biography that includes examples of Farmer's yoga practice in action. A revelation of feminine consciousness, full of insight and inspiration. See also an article by the producer of this video, Claudia Cummins, for an account of Angela Farmer's approach to yoga. **www.yogajournal.com/lifestyle/336**. For access to other video resources see **www.angela-victor.com**.

Fell, Rachel McDermott. 2001. *Singing to the Goddess: poems to Kālī and Umā from Bengal*. Oxford University Press, Oxford. Translations and commentaries on a selection of devotional poetry.

Feuerstein, Georg. 1998. *The Yoga Tradition: Its History, Literature, Philosophy and Practice*. Hohm Press. Prescott, Arizona. Survey of practices and history, including translations from key texts.

Fishman, Loren and **Saltonstall, Ellen**. 2010. *Yoga for Osteoporosis: The Complete Guide to Yoga that Builds and Preserves Strong Bones*. Norton, New York. The most detailed guide to the subject. Fascinating scientific studies and photographs as well as clear instructions including variations for osteopaenia and osteoporosis.

Flinders, Carol Lee. 1993. *Enduring Grace: Living Portraits of Seven Women Mystics*. Harper Collins e-book. Moving and perceptive reflections on the work of female Christian mystics, in the context of a feminist understanding of their spirituality.

Flinders, Carol Lee. 1998. *At the Root of this Longing: Reconciling a Spiritual Hunger and a Feminist Thirst*. Harper Collins e-book. A beautifully balanced practical, philosophical engagement with the integration of feminism and spirituality.

Flood, Gavin. 2006. *The Tantric Body: the Secret Tradition of Hindu Religion*. I. B. Taurus, London. A systematic analysis of the history and development of medieval *tantra* in relation to the practitioner's subjectivity in certain traditions. Flood focuses on the place of the physical body in *tāntrik* ritual, and although he does not write about *Śaktism*, what he says about practices that awaken an experience of divinity residing in physicality are relevant to *Śrī Vidyā* also.

Fox, Paul. 2005. 'How Popular is Yoga?' first published in *Yoga Magazine* June 2005, and downloaded 1 October 2012 from **www.corestrengthyoga.co.uk/downloads.htm**.

Foxcroft, Louise. 2010. *Hot Flushes, Cold Science: A History of the Modern Menopause*. Granta Books, London. A gripping account of the medicalisation and cultural construction of what we understand to be the menopausal experience. Compelling.

Francina, Suza. 2003. *Yoga and the Wisdom of Menopause: A Guide to Physical, Emotional and Spiritual Health at Midlife and Beyond*. Health Communications Inc., Deerfield Beach, Florida. Inspiring combination of true life stories from yoga women, and sound advice from an Iyengar yoga perspective. Especially helpful sections on yoga and perimenopausal bleeding, osteoporosis and the emotional experience of menopause.

Frawley, David. 1996 (1994). *Tantric Yoga and the Wisdom Goddesses: Spiritual Secrets of Ayurveda*. Passage Press, Salt Lake City, Utah. History, theory, practice and insights on the ten great wisdom goddesses. Includes drawings, *yantras* and *mantras*.

Frawley, David. 2008. *Inner Tantric Yoga: Working with the Universal Sakti, Secrets of Mantras, Deities and Meditation*. Lotus Press, Twin Lakes Wisconsin. Practical guidance and detailed descriptions of *mantras*, *yantras* and deities. Clear, direct and accessible instruction based on personal experience and understanding.

Friedeberger, Julie. 1996. *A Visible Wound: a Healing Journey through Breast Cancer with Practical and Spiritual Guidance for Women, their Partners and Families*. Element, Shaftesbury, Dorset. Wise and gentle reflections drawn from experience, combined with clear instructions for a healing practice.

Gaskin, Ina May. 1990 (1977). *Spiritual Midwifery*. The Book Publishing Company, Summertown, Tennessee. A classic text on the spirituality of birth, full of personal testimonials and inspiring photographs.

Gates, Janice. 2006. *Yoginī: the Power of Women in Yoga*. Mandala, San Rafael, California. An engaging combination of interviews with prominent (mostly American) *yoginīs*, biographies of influential twentieth-century *yoginīs* and an overview of the history of women in yoga.

Gendreau, Geralyn. 2006. *The Marriage of Sex and Spirit: Relationships at the Heart of Conscious Evolution*. Elite Books, Santa Rosa, California. An eclectic selection of articles from a range of US teachers and therapists, exploring different aspects of relationship and awareness. Includes articles on sacred sexuality by David Deida, Mukunda Stiles and Margot Anand.

Goswami, Shyam Sundar. 1999. *Layayoga: The Definitive Guide to the Cakras and Kundalini*. Inner Traditions, Rochester, Vermont. A masterly work of scholarship, informed by personal practice. This rich reference, on everything to do with the *cakras* and *kuṇḍalinī*, compares 282 different Sanskrit texts including *Vedic*, *Tāntrik* and *Purāṇic* sources.

Gray, Miranda. 2009 (1994). *Red Moon: Understanding and Using the Creative, Sexual and Spiritual Gifts of the Menstrual Cycle*. Dancing Eve, London. Images and words celebrating Gray's discovery of the powers of menstrual cycle awareness. Archetypal image and meditations present a cogent and beautifully spirited journey of self-discovery through the menstrual cycle.

Greer, Germaine. 1970. *The Female Eunuch*. Panther & Harper Collins, London. Up-front, passionate, and direct challenge to the patriarchy.

Greer, Germaine. 1984. *Sex and Destiny: the politics of human fertility*. Harper and Row, London. Wide-ranging survey of cultural patterns of fertility, contraception, family and sexuality. Detailed research and persuasive arguments for a global feminist awareness.

Greer, Germaine. 1992. *The Change: Women, Ageing and the Menopause*. Penguin, London. A personally inspired and thoroughly researched feminist exploration of cultural and social attitudes to menopause. Illuminating, acerbic, and full of astonishing stories and a wealth of literary and medical historical reference.

Greer, Germaine. 2007 (1999). *The Whole Woman*. Black Swan, Transworld, London. Sequel to *The Female Eunuch*, a polemical evaluation of the status of women worldwide. Passionately eloquent critique of the failings of feminism so far.

Guhyasamāja Tantra [Assembly of Secrets] Fourth-century Buddhist *tantra* that identifies women as a necessary presence for the accomplishment of *siddhis*. Made available online by Rufus Camphausen: **www.yoniversum.nl/daktexts/ttguhya.html**.

Gupta, Sanjukta. 1991. 'Women in the Saiva/Śakta Ethos' in *Roles and Rituals for Hindu Women*, ed. Julia Leslie. Motilal Banarsidas, Delhi, pp.193-209. A scholarly account of three female Saivites.

Hallinan, Joseph T. 2009. *Errornomics: Why we Make Mistakes and What We can do to Avoid Them*. Ebury Press, London. Vast span of scientific research exploring human fallibility, confusion and ignorance, including research into the effects of menstrual cycles on tip-giving.

Harper, Katherine and **Brown, Robert**. 2002. *The Roots of Tantra*. State University of New York Press, Albany New York. A broad-ranging collection of scholarly papers exploring the origins of Hindu *tantra* from many different perspectives, including art history and archaeology as well as textual explorations.

Hennezel, Marie de. 2011. *The Warmth of Our Heart Prevents our Body from Rusting: Ageing Without Growing Old*. Rodale, Berkeley, California. This is an elegant dance that balances realism and optimism, sadness and wonder. Reflections from an esteemed French psychologist with vast professional experience in palliative care for the ageing and dying.

hooks, bell. 1996. 'Contemplation and Transformation' in *Buddhist Women on the Edge*, ed. Marianne Dresser, North Atlantic Books. Intelligent, poetic feminist enquiry.

Horrigan, Bonnie. 1997. *Red Moon Passage: the Power and Wisdom of Menopause*. Thorsons, London. A collection of inspiring feminist stories from writers and teachers on women's spirituality about menopause as a spiritual quest for deep wisdom.

Hunt, Chizuko. 2010. *Yoga Practice in 21st Century Britain: The Lived Experience of Yoga Practitioners*. PhD thesis in health studies at De Montfort University. Downloaded 1 October 2012 from **www.dora.dmu.ac.uk**.

Iyengar, Geeta. 2002 (1983). *Yoga: A Gem for Women*. Timeless Books, Kootenay British Columbia. *Āsana* and *prāṇāyāma* programmes from the Iyengar yoga school for the whole of a woman's life.

Johnsen, Linda. 1994. *Daughters of the Goddess: the Women Saints of India*. Yes International, Saint Paul, Minnesota. Interviews with contemporary Indian female saints, personal reflection and philosophical considerations, including an inspiring chapter on 'Incarnating the Divine Feminine'.

Johnsen, Linda. 1999. *The Living Goddess: Reclaiming the Tradition of the Mother of the Universe*. Yes International, Saint Paul, Minnesota. An engaging and well grounded reflection on different aspects of *śākta* / goddess worship, mainly about Hindu goddesses, but ending with a fascinating exploration of western parallels.

Joshi, M. C. 2002. 'Historical and Iconographic Aspects of Śakta Tantrism' in Harper, Katherine L. and Brown, Robert R. *The Roots of Tantra*, State University of New York Press, Albany New York, pp.39–56. Traces some of the earliest evidence of *tāntrik* practice through archaeological discoveries.

Kent, Christine Ann. 2006 (2003). *Saving the Whole Woman: Natural Alternatives to Surgery for Pelvic Organ Prolapse and Urinary Incontinence*. Bridgeworks, Albuquerque, New Mexico. A radical, passionate argument against the epidemic of unnecessary and ineffective pelvic surgery, based on personal experience and medical research. Totally compelling. Includes exercises and resources.

Kinsley, David. 1987. *Hindu Goddesses: Vision of the Divine Feminine in Hindu Religious Tradition*. Motilal Banarsidas, Delhi. A detailed scholarly review of goddess forms, including a helpful chapter on the *Mahāvidyās* and a detailed appendix on goddesses in the Indus Valley Civilisation.

Kinsley, David. 1998. *The Ten Mahavidyas: Tantric Visions of the Divine Feminine*. Motilal Banarsidas, Delhi. Exhaustive and comprehensively illustrated scholarly study of the ten wisdom goddesses, exploring many perspectives on them as a group and individually.

Kissling, Elizabeth Arveda. 2006. *Capitalizing on the Curse: The Business of Menstruation*. Lynne Rienner Publishers, Boulder, Colorado. An intelligent and thought-provoking exploration of the 'rags to riches' stories of menstruation as a money-spinner and the economics of modern menstrual hygiene.

Knight, Chris. 1985. 'Menstruation as Medicine' in *Soc. Sci. Med* Vol 21, No. 6 pp 671-683. Anthropological investigation of shamanistic healing rituals. Downloaded from **www.chrisknight.co.uk/publications**.

Knight, Chris. 1987. *Menstruation and the Origins of Culture: A reconsideration of Lévi-Strauss's work on symbolism and myth*. Unpublished PhD thesis, University College London pdf downloaded from **www.chrisknight.co.uk/publications**. The original scholarship which underpins the book of the same title.

Knight, Chris. 1991. *Menstruation and the Origins of Culture*. Yale University Press, Harvard and London. Downloaded from **www.chrisknight.co.uk/publications**. A fascinating and persuasive presentation of how women's synchronous menstrual cycles are at the root of the 'human revolution'.

Lannoy, Richard. 1996. *Anandamayi: her Life and Wisdom*. Element, Shaftesbury, Dorset. Photographs and teachings of Anandamayi Ma, full of evocative archive photographs and direct quotations that capture the spirit of this remarkable spiritual teacher.

Lark, Susan M. 1996. *Heavy Menstrual Flow and Anaemia: a self-help book*. Celestial Arts, Berkeley, California. Lifestyle and nutrition pointers from a US medical doctor who offers helpful programmes and suggestions for managing and reducing menstruation pain, PMS and other menstrual difficulties.

Lark, Susan M. 1996. *Menstrual Cramps: Self-Help Book*. Celestial Arts, Berkeley, California. Practical guidance from US medic.

Lasater, Judith Hanson. 1995. *Relax and Renew: Restful Yoga for Stressful Times*. Rodmell Press, Berkeley, California. Crucial information and guidance on appropriate restorative poses for women's health.

Lasater, Judith Hanson. 2000. *Living your Yoga: Finding the Spiritual in Everyday Life*. Rodmell Press, Berkeley, California. Accessible and practical guidance from a mother and yoga teacher / writer on simple and effective ways to bring yoga practice into daily living. Realistic, down-to-earth and very feminine.

Laws, Sophie. 1990. *Issues of Blood: the Politics of Menstruation*. Macmillan, Basingstoke. Anthropological analysis from a feminist perspective of the political economic and socio-cultural structures surrounding and defining experiences of menstruation.

Leslie, Julia (ed). 1992. *Roles and Rituals for Hindu Women*. Motilal Banarsidas, Delhi. A wide-ranging collection of scholarly essays by historians and anthropologists. Of particular interest are the essays by Sanjukta Gupta qv. and by Lynn Denton on 'Varieties of Hindu Female Asceticism'.

Leslie, Julia (ed). 1996. *Myth and Mythmaking: continuous evolution in Indian tradition*. Curzon, London (Collected Papers on South Asia series). Includes a range of menstruation myths.

Lokugamage, Amali. 2001. *The Heart in the Womb: an Exploration of the Roots of Human Love and Social Cohesion*. Docamali, London. The captivating account of an obstetrician's changing perspectives on the nature and experience of pregnancy and birth: the book charts the journey from professional orthodoxy to personal discovery of the importance of acknowledging the heart in the womb.

Lucy, Janet; **Allison, Terri** and **Louden, Jennifer**. 2006. *Moon Mother, Moon Daughter: Myths and Rituals that celebrate a Girl's Coming of Age*. Publishing by the Sea, Santa Barbara, California. A beautiful, enticing and spiritually focused book that revives the ancient wisdom of coming-of-age traditions based on community and spirit. Full of stories and practical suggestions to strengthen the connection between mothers and daughters.

Lysebeth, Andre Van. 1988. *Tantra: le culte de la féminité: l'autre regard sur la vie et l'amour*. Flammarion, Lausanne. Passionate, poetic and intimate engagement with *tāntrik* philosophy and practice. Also published in English in 1995 as *Tantra, Cult of the Feminine*. Red Wheel/Weiser, York Beach ME.

Manmoyanand, Yogi. 2008. *Sivananda Buried Yoga*. O Books, Winchester, UK. Spiritual autobiography of a *yogi*, focussing on the *tāntrik* understandings revealed by enlightened masters in the Himalayas. Critiques the 'yoga for health' movement.

Marciniak, Barbara. 1992. *Bringers of the Dawn: Teachings from the Pleiadians*. Bear and Company, Rochester, Vermont. New age channelled teachings on the evolution of human consciousness, including some interesting perspectives on human sexuality.

McCall, Timothy. 2007. *Yoga as Medicine: the Yogic Prescription for Health and Healing*. Bantam, New York. Upbeat and inspiring account of yoga therapy by a US doctor and *yogi*. Helpful introduction to yoga for healing, and lots of useful general case studies, and interviews; only two specifically deal with women's health issues.

Mookerji, Ajit. 1995 (1988). *Kālī, the Feminine Force*. Thames and Hudson, London. Lavishly illustrated survey of all aspects of the goddess, including ritual, hymns and contemporary art.

Moran, Caitlin. 2011. *How to be a Woman*. Ebury Press. London. A uniquely cheeky combination of autobiographical reflection and strident feminist observations on the inequities and abuses of patriarchy. A sparkling and hilarious read.

Muscio, Inga. 2002. *Cunt: a Declaration of Independence*. Seal Press, Berkeley, California. Radical, hilarious and brilliant. The most vivid and comprehensive evaluation of how women's true sexual freedom is a force for global political change.

Naish, Francesca. 2005. *Natural Fertility: the Complete Guide to Avoiding or Achieving Conception*. Sally Milner, Sydney, Australia. Vitally important perspective on fertility and lunar cycles, optimising natural fertility, managing conception and contraception. See also **www.fertility.com.au**.

Nivedita, Sister (Bhagini). 1997. *Cradle Tales of Hinduism*. Advaita Ashrama publications department, Calcutta, India. First published in 1907, this collection of nursery stories is based on tales from Indian classics, retold for children by Sister Nivedita.

Noble, Vicki. 1991. *Shakti Woman: Feeling our Fire, Healing our World. The New Female Shamanism*. Harper One, San Francisco. A call to global and personal healing through awareness. Includes many references to yoga and *tantra*.

Noble, Vicki. 1994 (1983). *Motherpeace: A Way to the Goddess Through Myth, Art and Tarot*. Harper One, New York. Visionary feminist reinterpretation of Tarot as a tool for raising consciousness of the powers of the Goddess.

Noble, Vicki. 2007. *Archaeomythology Course Outline*. New College of California San Francisco, California. Downloaded 15 November 2011 from **www.motherpeace.com/print/Archaeomythology-Spring-2007.pdf**.

Noble, Vicki. 2011. 'Women and Yoga: Did Women Invent the Ancient Art of Yoga?' Downloaded 15 November 2011 from **www.yogahub.com/blog/women-and-yoga-by-vicki-noble**. An inspiring, personal and mother-centred view of the roots of yoga presented with verve by a leading goddess feminist.

Northrup, Christiane. 2005. *Mother-Daughter Wisdom: Creating a Legacy of Physical and Emotional Health*. Piatkus, London. Invaluable compendium and guide.

Northrup, Christiane. 2009 (1994). *Women's Bodies, Women's Wisdom: The Complete Guide to Women's Health and Well-Being*. Piatkus, London. Holistic perspective on women's health, from a conventionally trained doctor whose own practice and life have revealed the value of a 360-degree perspective on all aspects of our being to promote health and happiness.

Northrup, Christiane. 2009 (2001). *The Wisdom of Menopause: The Complete Guide to Physical and Emotional Health during the Change*. Piatkus, London. Comprehensive, inspiring and invaluable, as are all of the other titles authored by Northrup.

O'Brien, Anne. 2012. Quotations from thesis provided in personal communication with the author.

O'Brien, Paddy. 1991. *A Gentler Strength: the Yoga Book for Women*. Thorsons, London. A short, sensitive and sensible guide to yoga for all stages of a woman's life.

Odent, Michel. 2002. *The Farmer and the Obstetrician*. Free Association, London. Polemical, poetic and visionary exploration of the resonances between the industrialisation of agriculture and medicalisation of childbirth in the twentieth century. The long-term, possibly disastrous, effects of 'innovations' in both farming and birth are considered from the point of view of the consequences for the earth and human consciousness.

Odent, Michel. 2009. *The Functions of the Orgasms: the Highways to Transcendence*. Pinter and Martin, London. Radical exploration of human orgasmic experience, including breastfeeding and birth, as 'highways to transcendence' and spiritual insight. Includes reflections on the effects of rendering 'love hormones' redundant.

Odier, Daniel, trans. Clare Frock. 1997. *Tantric Quest: An Encounter with Absolute Love*. Inner Traditions, Rochester, Vermont. Spiritual autobiography and *tāntrik* philosophy presented together in a story of initiation by a female *tāntrik* guru.

Odier, Daniel. 1999. *Desire: the Tāntrik Path to Awakening*. Inner Traditions, Rochester, Vermont. *Tāntrik* philosophy and practical guidelines, including an engaging chapter with students' questions and answers, and numerous references to *tāntrik* scriptures.

Odier, Daniel, trans. Clare Frock. 2004. *Yoga Spandakarika: the Sacred Texts at the Origins of Tantra*. Inner Traditions, Rochester, Vermont. Poetic and vivid translations and extensive commentary on the *Yoga Spandakārikā*, a key text of Kashmir Shaivism, plus translations of the *Vijñāna Bhairava Tantra* and the *Song of Padmasambhava*.

Ohlig, Adelheid. 1994. *Luna Yoga: Vital Fertility and Sexuality*. Ash Tree Publishing, Woodstock, New York. Comprehensive and inspiring, full of helpful modifications and good ideas.

Oudshoorn, Nelly.1994. *Beyond the Natural Body: an Archaeology of Sex Hormones*. Routledge, London. Scholarly cultural history of the economic and scientific aspects of the development of the synthetic hormone market.

Osho. 2007. *Tantra: the Way of Acceptance*. Random House, New Delhi. Stories, photographs and an accessible presentation of Osho's perspective on the possibilities of *tantra* as a means to live in freedom.

Owen, Lara. 2009. *Her Blood is Gold*. Archive Publishing, London. An accessible and inspiring combination of anthropology of menstruation, personal testimony and pratical strategies to honour menstrual life and reduce fear and suffering around it.

Palmer, Gabrielle. 2009. *The Politics of Breastfeeding: When Breasts are Bad for Business*. Pinter and Martin, London. Radical, revealing history of how cultural and economic attitudes to breast milk impact on infant nutrition. Shocking exposé of the tools big business uses to undermine mothers' capacity to breastfeed.

Palmira, Rosemary (ed). 1990. *In the Gold of Flesh: Poems of Birth and Motherhood*. Women's Press, London. A vivid anthology of women's poems gathered in a thematic cycle: Conceiving, Forming, Labour, Birth, Newborn, Motherhood and Letting Go. A treasure trove of powerful images and experiences.

Phillips, Angela and **Rakusen, Jill**. 1989. *The New Our Bodies Ourselves: a Healthbook by and for Women* (British edition). Penguin, London. A compendium of articles, anatomy and feminist perspectives on women's health.

Placksin, Sally. 2000. *Mothering the New Mother: Women's Thoughts and Feelings after Birth*. William Morrow, New York. Super practical, encouraging guide to organising positive support for the postnatal period, including some anthropological material, lots of stories from mothers, and many helpful tips.

Pope, Alexandra. 2001. *The Wild Genie: The Healing Power of Menstruation*. Sally Milner, Sydney, Australia. Ground-breaking inspirational work on the spirituality of menstruation as the foundation of women's well-being.

Pope, Alexandra. 2001. *Walking with the Genie: The Modern Woman's Menstrual Health Kit*. Self-published. A friendly, practical no-nonsense guide to positive living for healthy menstruation.

Pope, Alexandra and **Bennett, Jane.** 2008. *The Pill: Are You Sure It's for You?* Allen and Unwin, London. Accessible, upbeat and packed with research that prompts any woman to consider the effects of the contraceptive pill from every angle.

Prakasha, Padma Aon and **Anaiya**. 2011. *Womb Wisdom: Awakening the Creative and Forgotten Powers of the Feminine*. Destiny, Rochester, Vermont. Husband and wife project rooted in esoteric meditations and visualisations. A new age approach to womb healing, with some alarmingly off-key notes: e.g. the instructions for womb breathing begins: 'Lie on your back with feet on the floor and knees bent, as if you were giving birth' (43).

Puri, Narvada. 2009. *Tears of Bliss: a Guru-Disciple Mystery*. Santosh Puri Ashram, Haridwar. The spiritual autobiography of a German woman in India. Her complete devotion to her guru, and husband Baba Santosh Puri, over a lifetime of asceticsm and service, culminating in the birth of their three children, their experiences as a spiritual family and the foundation of an *aśram* after the *guru*'s death. A moving feminine perspective on the extreme austerities of *sadhus* and the perilous path to revelation.

Radhakrishnan, S. 1996 (1953). *The Principal Upaniṣads*. Indus / Harper Collins, New Delhi. Elegant translation, meticulous and thoughtful editing, with a reflective introduction and a host of fascinating cross-cultural footnotes.

Rako, Susan. 2003. *No More Periods? The Risks of Menstrual Suppression and Other Cutting-Edge Issues about Hormones and Women's Health*. Harmony Books, New York. A comprehensive survey of scientific research and personal testimony, condensed into a slim, powerful volume. Shocking evidence of the side effects and long term health risks of menstrual suppression.

Ramaswami, Srivatsa. 2001. *Yoga for the Three Stages of Life*. Inner Traditions, Rochester, Vermont. History, personal reflections and instruction from a senior student of Krishnamacharya.

Regan, Lesley. 2001 (1997) *Miscarriage, What Every Woman Needs to Know*. Orion, London. Practical and sensitive survey of experiences from the perspective of an orthodox medic with an eye to the holistic picture of women's health.

Rele, Vasant G. 2007 (1927). *The Mysterious Kundalini: the Physical Basis of Kundalini (hatha) Yoga in Terms of Western Anatomy and Physiology*. Bharatiya Kala Prakashan, Delhi. A detailed exposition of the *cakras* and *nāḍīs* in relation to nerve plexuses and aspects of the endocrine system. Includes explanations of the *siddhis* and reflections on scientific testing of yogic feats.

Rele, Vasant G. 2000 (1931). *The Vedic Gods as Figures of Biology*. Cosmo Publications, New Delhi. A unique and fascinatingly detailed proposal to consider the Vedic gods in direct relation to aspects of human anatomy, in particular the structure of the central nervous system. Persuasive and thought-provoking.

Richardson, Diana. 2004. *Tantric Orgasm for Women*. Destiny Books, Rochester, Vermont. A practical and philosophical guide written with great openness of heart from a woman's perspective. A gem.

Riedl, Michaela. 2009. *Yoni Massage: Awakening Female Sexual Energy*. Destiny Books, Rochester, Vermont. Applied neo-*tāntrik* philosophy in the form of background and practical guidance for *yoni* massage. An inspiring and generous book, written from the practitioner's perspective, and including intimate interviews with women after receiving *yoni* massage.

Rodrigues, Dinah. 2009. *Hormone Yoga Therapy: to Reactivate Hormone Production and Eliminate the Symptoms of Menopause, TPM, Polycystic Ovaries and Infertility*. JCR Producoes, Sao Paolo. Complete programme of *āsana*, *prāṇāyāma* and meditation, with case studies.

Roy, Arundhati. 2002. 'The Greater Common Good' in *The Algebra of Infinite Justice*. Flamingo, London. pp.39-126. Roy's passionate retelling of the ecological madness of the Great Dams projects in India, in relation to the plans to dam the river Narmada, is full of detailed observation and clarity of thought.

Ruddock, Jill Shaw. 2012. *The Second Half of Our Lives*. Vermillion, London. Light-hearted but very practical guide to positive living for menopausal and postmenopausal women.

Rushdie, Salman. 1991. *Haroun and the Sea of Stories*. Penguin, London. An allegorical fantasy adventure / fairy story about language and power.

Sabatini, Sandra. 2007 (2000). *Breath: the Essence of Yoga. A Guide to Inner Stillness*. Pinter and Martin, London. Poetic reflections on the experience of breath awareness in stillness and movement. Includes classic *prāṇāyāma* practices and the application of breath awareness in *āsana*.

Samuel, Geoffrey. 2008. *The Origins of Yoga and Tantra: Indic Religions to the Thirteenth Century*. Cambridge University Press, Cambridge. A comprehensive scholarly examination of the evolution of yoga and *tantra* in historical and social contexts.

Sapolsky, Robert M. 2004. *Why Zebras Don't Get Ulcers: the Acclaimed Guide to Stress, Stress-related Diseases, and Coping*. St Martin's Griffin, New York. A brilliant review of research into human stress and what it does to us. Clear, detailed scientific explanations and oodles of footnotes.

Saraswati, Swami Muktibodhananda. 1999. *Haṭha Yoga Pradīpikā*. Bihar School of Yoga, Munger. Translation and commentary on key text of *haṭha* yoga. Practical insights and advice for the contemporary application of *haṭha* yoga techniques.

Saraswati, Swami Muktibodhananda. 1999. *Swara Yoga; the Tāntrik Science of Brain Breathing*. Bihar School of Yoga, Munger. Full of information about the flow and function of *praṇas* in the body.

Saraswati, Swami Satyadharma. 2003. *Yoga Chudamani Upanishad*. Yoga Publications Trust, Munger, Bihar. An elegant translation and comprehensive commentary including brief history of Vedic literature.

Saraswati, Swami Satyananda. 1984. *Kundalini Tantra*. Bihar School of Yoga, Munger. Classic reference on *cakra* energetics, with illustrations, practices and meditations.

Saraswati, Swami Satyananda and **Swami Muktananda**. 1992 (1977). *Nawa Yogini Tantra*. Bihar School of Yoga, Munger. The first book on yoga and women. Full of insight and helpful yoga guidance on many aspects of women's health from a Bihar School of Yoga perspective. Inspiring reference, but unreliable on guidelines during pregnancy and birth. Apart from that, everything else is trustworthy.

Saraswati, Swami Satyasangananda. 2006 (1984). *Light on the Guru and Disciple Relationship*. Yoga Publications Trust, Munger, Bihar, India. Reflections on the nature of the *guru* and the experiences of the disciple, from the perspective of one of Paramahamsa Satyananda's most devoted disciples. Also includes extracts from Satyananda's talks on the topic.

Saraswati, Swami Satyasangananda. 2003. *Srī Vijñāna Bhairava Tantra: The Ascent*. Yoga Publications Trust. Munger. Bihar, India. Transliteration, translation with perceptive and accessible (lengthy) commentary on this key text of Kashmir Shaivism.

Saraswati, Swami Satyasangananda. 2008. *Srī Saundarya-Laharī: The Descent*. Yoga Publications Trust, Munger, Bihar, India. Transliteration, translation with perceptive and accessible (lengthy) commentary on this key text of the Samaya tradition of *śakta tantra*.

Scaravelli, Vanda. 2012 (1991). *Awakening the Spine*. Pinter and Martin, London. A poetic exploration of the freedom of yoga from the perspective of one of Iyengar's most influential female yoga students.

Shaw, Eric. 2011. *A Short History of Women in Yoga*. Downloaded 15 November 2011. **www.prasanayoga.com**.

Shaw, Miranda. 1994. *Passionate Enlightenment: Women in Tantric Buddhism*. Princeton University Press, Princeton. Radical, scholarly and very detailed, this study of women teachers and practitioners of *tāntrik* Buddhism includes translations of many of the *yoginī*'s chants, and clear evidence to prove the significant presence of women in the development of key practices and philosophies of *tāntrik* Buddhism.

Shaw, Miranda. 1996. 'Wild, Wise, Passionate: Dakinis in America' in *Buddhist Women on the Edge*, ed. Marianne Dresser. North Atlantic Books, Berkeley, pp.3-12.

Shiva, Vandana. 2005. *Earth Democracy: Justice, Sustainability and Peace*. Zed Books, London. Rooted in case studies and clear observation of the Indian scene, including shocking figures on female feticide, this is a powerful, passionate and thoroughly well-grounded call to action.

Short, R V. 1976. 'The Evolution of Human Reproduction' in the *Proceedings of Royal Society* (Biological Sciences). Presentation of concepts relating to contemporary menstrual patterns in relation to women's health.

Shuttleworth, Penelope and **Redgrove, Peter**. 2005 (1978). *The Wise Wound*. Marion Boyars, London. The first literary-poetic book to address the topic of menstruation: lyrical, scholarly, fascinating and radical. An astonishing compendium of facts, figures, taboos, myths and personal reflection.

Singleton, Mark. 2010. *Yoga Body: the Origins of Modern Posture Practice*. Oxford University Press, New York. A detailed scholarly survey of the development of modern *āsana* practice in India and the West, Singleton's proposal that body-building and harmonial gymnastics have helped to shape the contemporary yoga practice has had a huge impact on current re-thinking about the history of yoga, and has prompted much debate in yoga circles worldwide.

Singleton, Mark. 2010. 'Yoga's Greater Truth' in *Yoga Journal* (November). **www.yogajournal.com/wisdom/2610?page=2.** Downloaded 15/11/11.

Singleton, Mark and **Byrne, J**. 2008. Introduction. In Singleton, M. and Byrne, J. (eds). *Yoga in the Modern World: Contemporary Perspective*. Routledge. London. Overview of the contemporary practice of yoga.

Sivananda, Radha. 2004 (1977). *Kundalini Yoga for the West*. Timeless Books, Kootenay, British Columbia. Step-by-step guide to esoteric anatomy and practices to connect with the energies of the *cakras*.

Śiva Saṁhitā. 1914. **Bahadur, Rai** and **Vasu, Srisa Candra** (trans.) Bhuvaneśvarī Ashram, Bhahdurganj. Sanskrit text, transliteration and English translation. Also available as a free download from **www.hinduebooks.blogspot.co.uk/2009/04/gheranda-samhita-treatise-on-hatha-yoga.html**.

Skolimowski, Henryk. 1994. *EcoYoga: Practice and Meditations for Walking in Beauty on the Earth*. Gaia, London. An elegant, inspiring and beautifully illustrated book, full of insights and practices for living yoga with an awareness of the broadest sense of ecology.

Sparrowe, Linda and **Walden, Patricia**. 2004. *Yoga for Healthy Bones: A Woman's Guide*. Shambhala, Boston. A sound, reassuring guide with clear instructions and photographs of āsana practice for prevention and management of osteoporosis.

Stadlen, Naomi. 2004. *What Mothers Do, Especially When It Looks Like Nothing*. Piatkus, London. Absolutely the best parenting book ever, and the only book that pregnant and postnatal mothers really need to read. A tender, wise and respectful honouring of mothering, full of mothers' own words. Affirming and encouraging.

Statistic Brain. 2011. US yoga statistics online. Downloaded 1 October 2012 from **www.statisticbrain.com/yoga-statistics**.

Stein, Elissa and **Kim, Susan**. 2009. *Flow: the Cultural Story of Menstruation*. St. Martin's Griffin, New York. Beautifully illustrated with vintage ads and product guides, this is a funny, light-hearted but thorough overview of the socio-cultural dimension of menstruation in industrial societies.

Stiles, Mukunda. 2001. *Yoga Sutras of Patanjali as interpreted by Mukunda Stiles*. Red Wheel/Weiser, San Francisco, California. Lucid, poetic and accessible translation and interpretation.

Stiles, Mukunda. 2011. *Tāntrik Yoga Secrets: Eighteen Transformational Lessons to Serenity, Radiance, and Bliss*. Red Wheel/Weiser. San Francisco, California. Heartfelt, direct and inspirational guidance.

Stone, Merlin. 1977. *When God was a Woman*. Harcourt Brace, Orlando, Florida. Landmark text in feminist history that explores Goddess worship as a global phenomenon from Paleolithic times to the Greeks and the eventual suppression of women's rites.

Stone, Michael. 2011. *Yoga for a World out of Balance: Teachings on Ethics and Social Action*. Shambhala, Boston. Clear and elegant exposition of the practical contemporary relevance of yogic ethics in everyday life, especially in relation to ecology.

Sundahl, Deborah. 2003. *Female Ejaculation and the G-Spot*. Hunter House, Alameda, California. Clear, direct and profound, this is the most comprehensive study of female ejaculation available. It considers all aspects of the experience, including practical techniques and political reasons for the suppression of information about this aspect of women's sexual expression.

Taylor, Dena and **Sumrall, Amber Coverdale**. 1991. *Women of the 14th Moon: Writings on Menopause*. The Crossing Press, Freedom, California. A broad range of short pieces from many different perspectives on menopause. Generally fascinating and strangely addictive, encompassing a huge spectrum of response that is, encouragingly, mostly positive.

Thompson, Lana. 1998. *The Wandering Womb: a Cultural History of Outrageous Beliefs about Women*. Prometheus Press, Amherst, New York. Full of archive illustrations, copious notes and wry humour in the face of some truly outrageous medical opinions and practices. This impressive little book catalogues numbers of shocking oppressions and mutilations conducted as a means to control women from medieval times to the present.

Tigunait, Pandit Rajman. 1999. *Tantra Unveiled: Seducing the Forces of Matter and Spirit*. Himalayan Institute Press, Honesdale, Pennsylvania. Reflections on aspects of *tāntrik sādhana* by the leading light of the Himalayan Institute. Includes fascinating stories from personal experience and tradition, and practical guidance on the use of *yantra*, *mantra* and other dimensions of *tāntrik* practice.

Tiwari, Maya. 1995. *Ayurveda: A Life of Balance: the Complete Guide to Ayurvedic Nutrition and Body Types with Recipes*. Healing Arts, Rochester, Vermont. Comprehensive resource for ayurvedic living including powerful chapter of food *sādhanas*.

Tiwari, Maya. 2000. *A Path of Practice: a Woman's Guide to Healing*. Ballantine Books, New York. A moving autobiographical account of deep healing from a near-death experience, and the development of a spiritual practice that nurtures the feminine and reconnects to the earth.

Tiwari, Maya. 2010. *Women's Power to Heal through Inner Medicine*. Mother OM Media, Sinking Spring, Pennsylvania. An illuminating, passionate and inspired guide to ayurvedic and yoga perspectives and techniques to reconnect with Mother Consciousness and awaken inner medicine. Philosophical reflections and clearly described practices of ritual, meditation and food medicine.

Tiwari, Maya. 2011. *Living Ahimsa Diet*. Mother OM Media, Sinking Spring, Pennsylvania. An ecological perspective on the interconnections between reverence for the earth, food *sādhana* and physical and spiritual well-being. Includes recipes and *sādhanas*.

Vishnudevananda, Swami. 1960. *The Complete Illustrated Book of Yoga*. Harmony Books, New York. One of the first comprehensive *haṭha* yoga manuals to be published directly in the west by an Indian swami.

Vostral, Sharra L. 2008. *Under Wraps: A History of Menstrual Hygiene Technology*. Lexington Books, Rowman and Littlefield, Lanham, Maryland. Scholarly techno-cultural history of the development and marketing of sanitary protection products.

Walker, Barbara G. 1983. *The Woman's Encyclopaedia of Myths and Secrets*. Harper and Row, San Francisco. A truly fascinating and staggeringly comprehensive work of inspiring feminist scholarship that sets out the evidence for the patriarchal usurpation of matrifocal, pro-menstrual spirituality, religion and culture. An invaluable reference and an extraordinary handbook for feminist debate.

Walker, Barbara G. 1985. *The Crone: Women of Age, Wisdom and Power*. Harper, San Francisco. A deeply inspiring feminist history of the roles and social significance of older women. Walker draws on anthropology and mythology to call for a revaluing of contemporary crones as a powerful force for global healing.

Walker, Barbara G. 1990. *The Essential Handbook of Women's Spirituality and Ritual*. Fair Winds Press, Gloucester, Massachusetts. A rich source of inspiration for solitary and group ceremony, meditations and rituals for all stages of women's lives.

Welch, Claudia. 2011. *Balance Your Hormones, Balance Your Life: Achieving Optimal Health and Wellness through Ayurveda, Chinese Medicine and Western Science*. Da Capo Press, a member of the Perseus Books Group, Boston, Massachusetts. The clearest and most reader-friendly account of the working of women's hormones and the relationship between stress and health. A joy to read, and full of practical, easy-to-implement guidance.

White, David Gordon. 2006 (2003). *The Kiss of the Yoginī: 'Tantric Sex' in its South Asian Contexts*. University of Chicago Press, Chicago. A brilliant, passionate and enormous scholarly masterwork. White transforms western understandings of *tantra* by bringing together a history of *tāntrik* texts, rituals, art and architecture that demonstrates the central place of *tantra* in the religious landscape of India from ancient times to the present day.

White, David Gordon. 2009. *Sinister Yogis*. University of Chicago Press. London / Chicago. A fascinating and detailed academic exploration of yoga practitioners that puts the magical wonders of the *siddhis* into historical context. Full of astonishing and vivid, juicy stories of the supernatural and sometimes sinister powers of *yogis*, this is a fabulous antidote to the nineteenth-century re-casting of yoga as a purely ascetic spiritual endeavour.

Wolf, Naomi. 1991. *The Beauty Myth: How Images of Beauty are Used Against Women*. Vintage, London. Articulate feminist critique of the beauty industry and its sphere of influence.

Wolf, Naomi. 2012. *Vagina: A New Biography*. Virago, London. Combines a personal quest with journalistic research, scientific summaries, and a US perspective on *tantra*.

Woodroffe, Sir John. 2011 (1913). *Hymns to the Goddess*. A selection of translations from the *Tantras*, *Purāṇas*, *Mahābharata* and from *Shankaracharya*. Downloaded 20 December 2011 from **www.forgottenbooks.org**.

Woodroffe, Sir John. 1927 (1918). *Śakti and Śākta: essays and addresses on the Śākta Tantrasāstra*. Ganesh and Company, Madras. A remarkable collection of densely referenced scholarly writings on *śākta tantra*. Un-indexed and so very difficult to navigate, Woodroffe's detailed defences of *tantra* reflect the deep patriarchal prudery which was endemic in Indology of the time, and which Woodroffe bravely challenged. Repays lengthy study, but utterly frustrating if you are looking for anything easily accessible.

Worth, Jennifer. 2002. *Call the Midwife: a True Story of the East End in the 1950s*. Phoenix, London. An astonishing series of birth stories celebrating the indomitable survival spirit of the women of London's poorest boroughs in the days before hospital births.

Yoga Chudamani Upanishad cf. Saraswati, Satyadharma. 2003. Yoga Publications Trust, Bihar School of Yoga, Munger. Clear translation and helpful commentary.

Yogani. 2006. *Tantra: Discovering the Power of Pre-Orgasmic Sex*. Straightforward and accessible reflections and guidance inspired by the *Vijñāna Bhairava Tantra*. AYP Enlightenment Series, AYP Publishing, Nashville Tennessee / London.

Yoni Tantra, trans. Michael Magee. 1995. Worldwide Tantra Project. Downloaded 16 December 2011 from **www.cleaves.zapto.org/news/attachments/sep2010/yoni.pdf**.

Yoginī Tantra, trans. Michael Magee. 1995. Downloaded 16 December 2011 from **www.shivashakti.com/yoginī.htm**.

PERMISSIONS

The author and publisher gratefully acknowledge the permissions granted to reproduce the copyright material in this book. Every effort has been made to trace copyright holders and to obtain their permission for the use of copyright material. The publisher apologises for any errors or omissions in the list that appears below and would be grateful to be notified of any corrections that should be incorporated in future reprints or editions of this book.

The illustration on page 19 is based on original artwork by Ingrid Andrew ('Star Web Spiral Woman', available to view on **www.yonishakti.co**).

I am grateful to Mother Maya (Maya Tiwari) for kind permission to include the *śakti mudrā* (p.151) and *mahā mulādhāra mudrā* (p.152), both of which originally appeared in *Woman's Power to Heal Through Inner Medicine*.

Appreciation and thanks are offered to Lotus Press, publishers of David Frawley's *Tāntrik Yoga and the Wisdom Goddesses*, for permission to quote extensively from his descriptions of the ten *Mahāvidyās*.

Figure 2.1 (Indus Valley Proto Siva) is reproduced courtesy of Images of India. Figure 2.2 (Indus Valley meditating figure) and Figure 2.3 (Indus Valley terracotta female figurine with infant) are copyright Harappa Archaeological Research Project/Harappa.com, and are reproduced courtesy of the Department of Archaeology and Museums, Government of Pakistan.

Many thanks to Sofya Ansari for teaching me the head-tilt *mudrā* (pp.148–9).

Gratitude to the late Mukunda Stiles, whose *taḍāsana vinyāsa* and *setu bandha vinyasa* (from *Ayurvedic Yoga Therapy*) form the basis, respectively, of the feminised swaying palm tree sequence (p.532) and the womb elevation bridge sequence (p.155–8). Mukunda's development of the Joint Freeing Series (from *Structural Yoga Therapy*) is, together with Satyananda yoga's *Pawanamuktasana* practices (from Swami Satyananda's *Asana, Prāṇāyāma, Mudrā, Bandha*), the foundation for the series for complete liberation of energy (pp.497–510).

The *yoga nidrā* practices (pp.17–21 and pp.435–59) are a creative synthesis of approaches to *yoga nidrā* devised by Swami Satyananda, Richard Miller and the Himalayan Institute.

Extracts from The Female Eunuch by Germaine Greer. Copyright © 1970 by Germaine Greer. Reprinted by permission of HarperCollins Publishers (USA).

Extracts from *Cunt, a Declaration of Independence* by Inga Muscio are reprinted by kind permission of Seal Press.

Extracts from the work of Vicki Noble are reprinted by kind permission of the author.

Extracts from *Mother-Daughter Wisdom* by Christiane Northrup are reprinted by kind permission of Piatkus, an imprint of Little, Brown Book Group.

Extracts from the unpublished thesis of Anne O'Brien are reprinted by kind permission of the author.

Extracts from *The Crone: Woman of Age, Wisdom, and Power* by Barbara G. Walker. Copyright © 1985 by Barbara G. Walker. Reprinted by permission of HarperCollins Publishers (USA).

Extracts from *Balance Your Hormones, Balance Your Life* by Claudia Welch are reprinted by kind permission of Perseus Books Group.

At the time of going to press, additional permissions had been requested from the following:

Ebury Publishing (Random House) for quotations from Caitlin Moran's *How to be a Woman*; Rider Books (Random House) for quotations from Clarissa Pinkola Estés' *Women Who Run With The Wolves*; Random House for quotations from Germaine Greer's *The Change* and *The Whole Woman*; HarperCollins publishers for quotations from Germaine Greer's *Sex and Destiny*, and Susan Rako's *No More Periods?*; Mandala Publishing for quotations from Janice Gates's *Yogini: the Power of Women in Yoga*; in addition permission has been requested from Aitken Alexander Associates to quote from the works of Germaine Greer in the UK.

APPENDIX

TEN *MAHĀVIDYĀ YANTRAS*: FOR MEDITATION AND CONTEMPLATION

APPENDIX

commentary and reflections by Nirlipta Tuli, illustrator

These colour *yantras* are painted in oil on fine linen cloth. I made these images over a period of seven years. The great project of painting all the *Mahāvidyā yantras* was a progression from the previous twenty years of making *yantras*, in particular, making dozens of Chinnamastā *yantras*.

By 1999 the home I shared with Uma was filled with Chinnamastā *yantras*. There was simply no getting away from Chinnamastā. She was everywhere. And then, following the births of our two sons, the *Mahāvidyā* plant that had been seeded when Uma bought David Frawley's book years earlier (see pp.230–1) began to bloom in both our psyches, and connect us to others who understood more about the *Mahāvidyās* than we did.

When Uma and Wendy Teasdill created the Śakti Rising retreat in 2005, the planned meditations incorporated *tratak* on the great wisdom goddess *yantras*. I was drawn into the preparations, painting huge (3ft x 3ft) oil on linen *yantras* for each of the *Mahāvidyās*. This was a vast project which I undertook (with great good-humour) sitting on the floor of our draughty conservatory in Brixton Hill surrounded by the lids of jam jars containing paints, and placing *mantras* in every brushstroke. Of course the project was so huge that it was not completed in time. On the first day of the retreat only three canvases were ready, and Uma packed the *yantras* of Kālī, Bhairavī and Chinnamastā into the roof space of our van, being careful not to smudge them because the oil paint was still wet. These *yantras* were part of the subsequent annual retreats (2009–2014) as the event metamorphosed into the Womb Wisdom retreat which Uma now co-hosts with menstrual guru Alexandra Pope.

Outside of the retreat time, for the rest of the year the *yantras* hung in our terraced house in London, so that we literally lived in a domestic temple boundaried by the *Mahāvidyā yantras* for five years, until we moved to Stroud and found homes for the goddesses on the walls of our yoga space. At the time of writing, we are still hoping that at some point in our lives we will be in a position to install all ten of the *Mahāvidyās* on the walls of a circular sacred space or 'Temple of Menstrual Enlightenment', thus creating in material reality the multi-directional psychic shield of the full set of *Mahāvidyās* as guardians of *sādhanā* (spiritual endeavour).

WHAT IS A *YANTRA*?

A *yantra* is a graphic geometric embodiment of energy. In the context of *śākta tantra*, the *Mahāvidyā yantras* are vessels that carry the qualities of the goddess with whom they are associated in a pure, abstract and concentrated form. Whereas the black and white drawings of the *Mahāvidyās* in part two represent the qualities of the goddesses, the *yantras* actually hold their energies: the *yantras* are alive with the power of the goddesses in graphic form. They are in fact considered to be the body of the goddess.

Unlike a *mandala*, which affords the artist a degree of creativity and individual expression, a *yantra* is a very specifically determined configuration of geometric forms intended to attract and manifest the energies of the deity with which it is associated.

POWER AND SYMBOLISM

The power of the *yantra* is to convey directly the energies of the entity it holds in its form and colours. For example, when we look at a *Mahāvidyā yantra* in a particular way, or with a particular intention, then we invite the power of the goddess who resides in that *yantra* to enter into us (or more correctly, to activate that aspect of her power which we already carry within us). The shape and form of the *yantra* contains her power symbolically so that her energy can literally become alive in us through our eyes.

The language of *yantra* is symbolic geometry. Downward-pointing triangles embody the descending feminine energy of Śakti, and upward-pointing triangles embody the ascending masculine consciousness of Siva. Intersections between ascending and descending triangles hold the capacity to bring Siva and Śakti together. Concentric triangles amplify the potency of individual triangles.

The square borders contain four gates to guard and provide access to the *yantra*. There is one gate on each side, so that our visual attention can travel along a route that guides us in our approach to the centre of the *yantra*, to meet the heart of the energy she holds. The very middle of the *yantra* is marked by a central spot upon which our gaze can rest. When we focus on the centre of the *yantra* we can visually enter into her – and she into us – and bring the whole of our attention within the force field of the goddess whose power is held in the *yantra*. Usually the central point of the *yantra* is in fact just a dot, but in these *Mahāvidyā yantras* the central point is an ovoid *bindu*, or *lingam*. This ovoid *bindu* is an unusual characteristic of this particular set of *yantras*, and its presence is intended to contain the seed of Siva consciousness at the heart of each *Mahāvidyā*, as an anchor, a balance and a guide.

The colours of each *yantra* are designed to express and resonate the qualities of each of the *Mahāvidyās*. Some traditions of *yantra*-making assign specific fixed colours to each goddess and others are less prescriptive. The colours of the *yantras* in *Yoni Shakti* were intuited not only as appropriate for each *yantra* but also to resonate with the functional groupings of the ten goddesses as they are interpreted in this book. The colours are also designed to operate vividly as phosphine (reverse or complementary) imagery when the after-image of the *yantra* remains on the retina after gazing with open eyes.

BASIC INSTRUCTIONS ON *TRATAK*: USING *YANTRA* FOR MEDITATION

The ritual practice of *tratak* with *yantras* is traditionally hedged about with many arcane and complex rules as to precisely when and where it should be done. The practice is worthy of a whole book of its own, but in this context, some basic instructions for one approach to *tratak* with *yantras* will suffice.

Sit comfortably with the image of the *yantra* vertically in front of you, at a level that puts the *bindu*, or central point, either directly in front of your eyes or slightly higher, or slightly lower than eye-level without having to tilt your head. All positional choices bring the *tratak* meditator into a meditative trance but in different ways, for example for some people if the eyes lift, then the *tratak* may literally be more 'uplifting' or extroverting, and if the eyes are lowered then the practice may be more introverting, or vice versa.

The distance between you and the *yantra* should enable your eyes easily to focus on the central point of the image. If you need glasses or contact lenses to focus, then you can either remove them and bring the *yantra* close enough to see clearly, or leave the glasses or lenses in place, and have the *yantra* at about arm's length.

The *yantra* should be well-illuminated without glare, for example with the light shining onto the *yantra* from the side(s). If you are using a spotlight then place it so that you cannot see the source of the light itself, because that would imprint itself on the retina. The rest of the room can be dimly lit or in darkness, and the *yantra* should be placed against a plain background so that no distracting objects interfere with the visual field.

Open your eyes and gaze into the centre of the *yantra*. Fix the gaze on the *bindu* and keep the eyes open until they start to water, or until it feels as if they need to close. You can blink once or twice, but try to keep it to a minimum. When you close the eyes after your gazing, look at the same spot which you were focused upon with your eyes open, and then focus on the image which appears in the internal gaze behind the closed eyes. It is this internal gazing at the after-image that is the most powerful part of the practice, and it should be done at minimum for the same amount of time as the open-eyed gazing, and preferably for much longer. The lengthening of the inner gaze is a skill that develops with practice, over time. It is this inner gazing which is the act of *tratak*.

Sometimes the after-image in front of the closed eyes will be very clear, sometimes it will shrink, sometimes it disintegrates or fades away, and sometimes the colours present a phosphine image with complementary colours, but other times there is a negative image with very little colour. Whatever happens to the after-image, the point of the practice is to lengthen the time of inner gazing.

MANTRA AND *YANTRA*

Traditionally, each *yantra* also has a *mantra*, or a set of sounds. The *mantras* express at an auditory level the same energy that the *yantra* embodies visually. To connect with or to activate fully the power of the goddess in the *yantra* requires both the visual and auditory forms to be present, as if the sounds of the *mantra* are the spark which detonates the charge of the *yantra*. The detonations are repeated with each repetition of the *mantra*, so cumulatively acquire increasing power.

Whilst the visual forms stand alone, and simply require that we look at them in a certain way, the *mantras* do need to be pronounced correctly, and for this reason we have chosen not to write the words for the *mantras* here in the book, but to provide audio tracks of the *mantras* to accompany each *yantra* (**www.yonishakti.co**). *Tratak* can be done silently, or whilst listening to or repeating the relevant *mantra*. *Mantra* repetition can be voiced or heard silently within the heart.

CAUTIONARY NOTE

Through the practice of *tratak* (with or without *mantra*) on the *Mahāvidyā yantras* to activate the power of the goddess energy within, it is possible to allow deep-seated *samskaras*, the results of previous karmic actions, to be released and eradicated. This can be very powerful indeed, and although it is certainly a path that can be travelled alone, it can be helpful to seek support and guidance for the journey. Workshops and mentoring on the use of the *yantras* can be accessed through **www.yonishakti.co**.

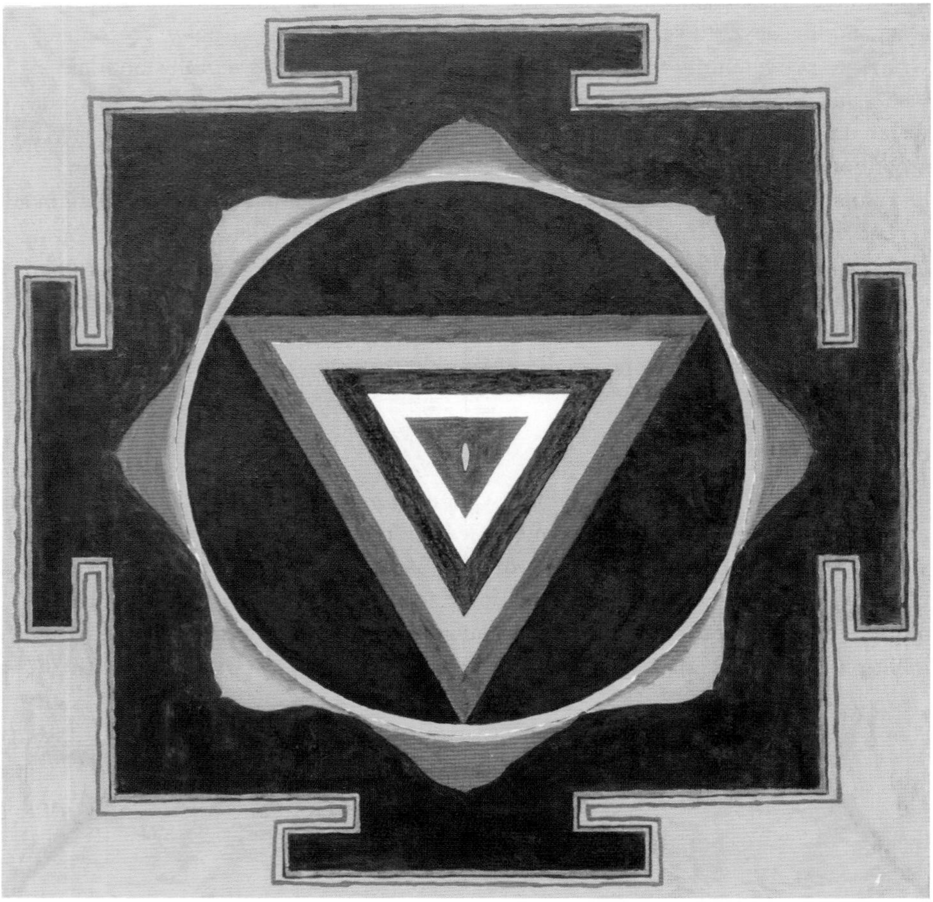

Kālī

In her role as the embodiment of change and the guardian of all cyclical wisdom, Kālī's *yantra* conveys the thunderbolt-like energy of shift and transformation. Like the *yantras* for Tārā, Chinnamastā and Bhairavī, the Kālī *yantra* is pure Śakti, with five downward-pointing triangles. The Siva consciousness is only present in the form of the *lingam bindu* in the centre of the *yantra*.

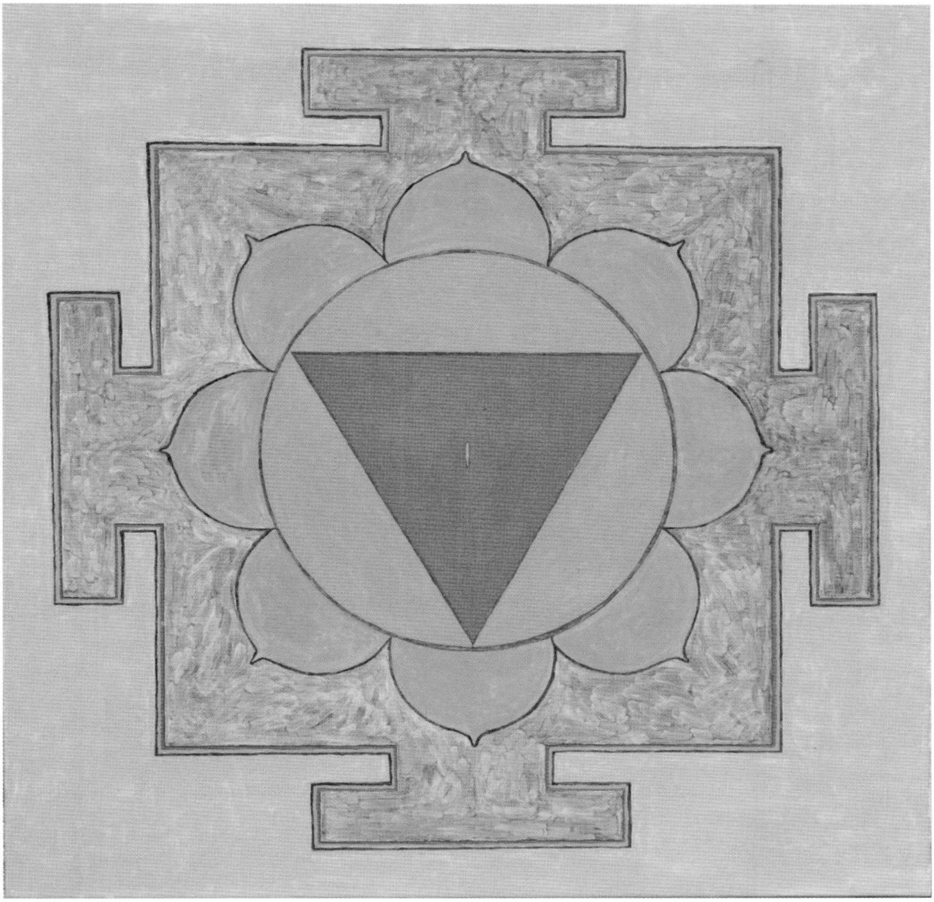

Tārā

As the 'guiding star' who carries and/or guides us through all experiences, Tārā bridges difficulties and blessings; she can be both fierce and benign. She is assigned in *Yoni Śakti* to the specific guardianship of the *maha*-cycle of menstruality, as a meta-guide for all cyclical wisdom. Like the *yantras* for Kālī, Chinnamastā and Bhairavī, the Tārā *yantra* is pure Śakti, with only a single downward-pointing triangle. The Siva consciousness is only present in the form of the *lingam bindu* in the centre of the *yantra*.

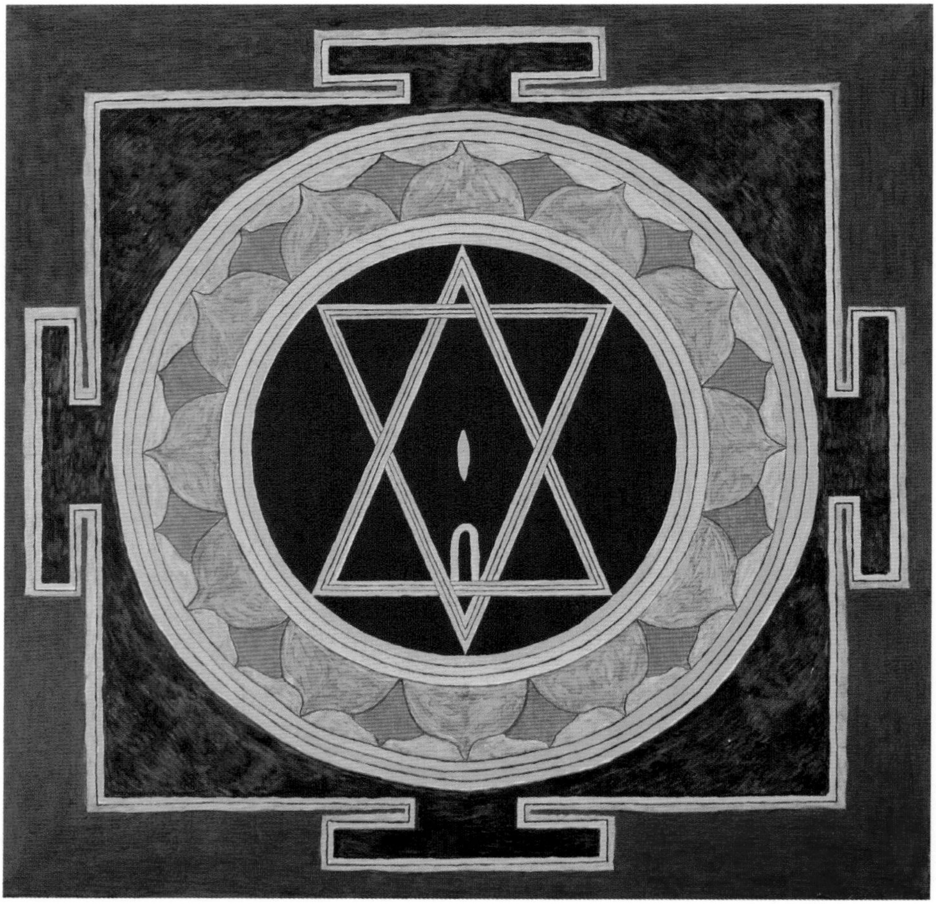

Ṣoḍasī (Tripura Sundarī)

As the eternally luscious and beautiful 'sixteen-year-old', Ṣoḍasī is the beauty of the three worlds, containing within her the immensely attractive power of innocent perfection. She is sometimes represented through the *Sri Yantra* (p.276), but also in this alternate version of the Ṣoḍasī *yantra* she holds at the base of interlocked Siva / Śakti triangles a golden *lingam* of Siva consciousness that in turn is placed within a double ring of triple circles.

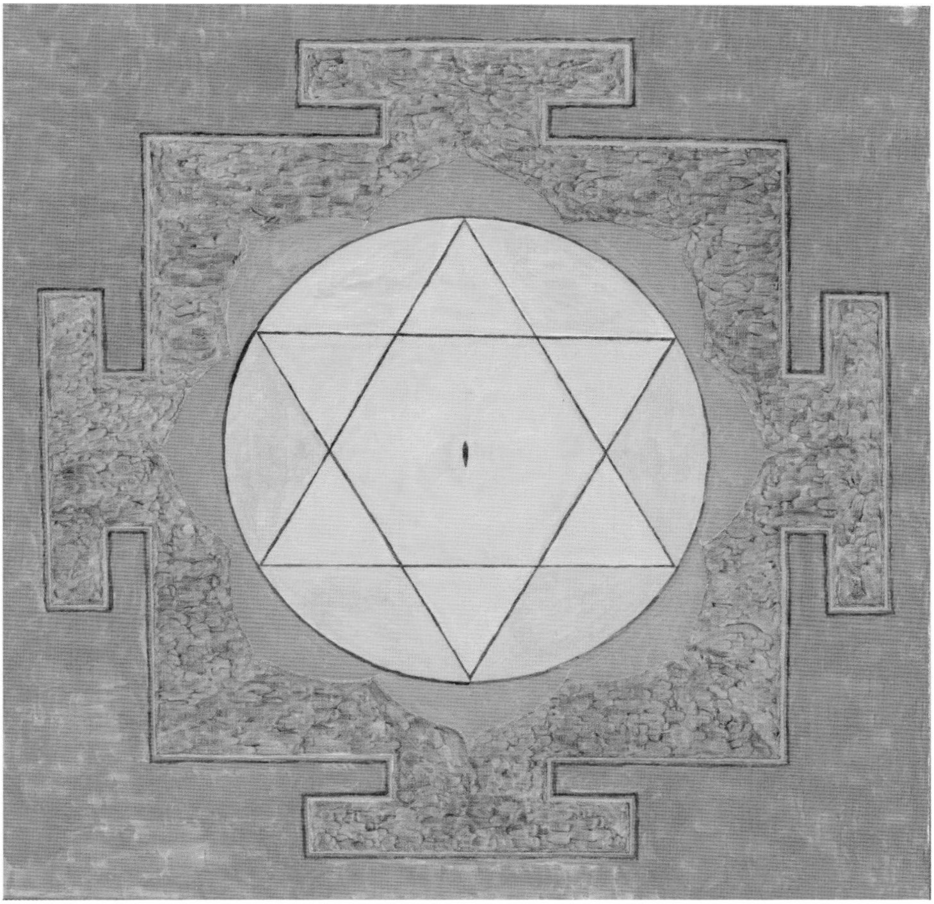

Kamalātmikā

Kamalātmikā is the rosy-hued lotus goddess of delight, who stands guardian over sexuality and sexual energy, in a direct pairing with Mataṅgi, who guards creativity. Her *yantra* presents a balance between the Siva / Śakti triangles of ascent and descent, in precisely the same geometric form as Mataṅgi and Dhūmavatī. The only differences between these three *yantras* are the colours assigned to the different segments.

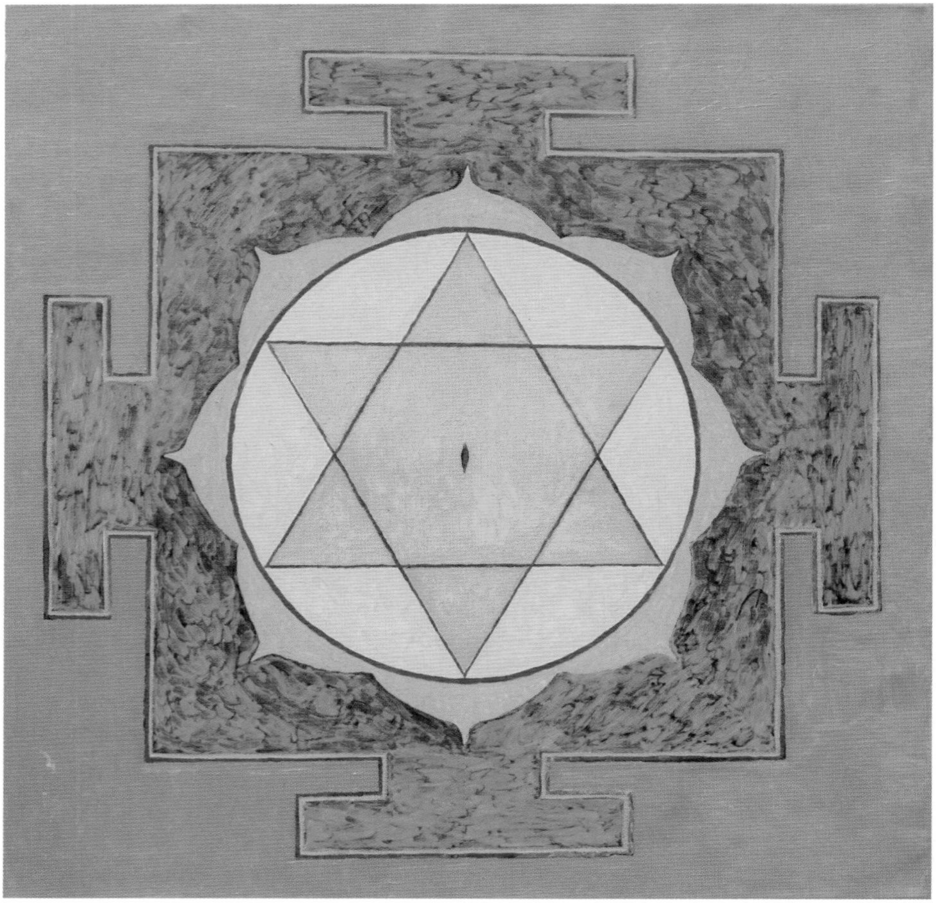

Mataṅgi

Mataṅgi is the wild outcaste poet who is appointed as the guardian of creativity, and stands in a direct pairing with Kamalātmikā, who guards sexuality. The Mataṅgi *yantra* presents a balance between the Siva / Śakti triangles of ascent and descent, in precisely the same geometric form as Kamalātmikā and Dhūmavatī. The only differences between these three *yantras* are the colours assigned to the different segments.

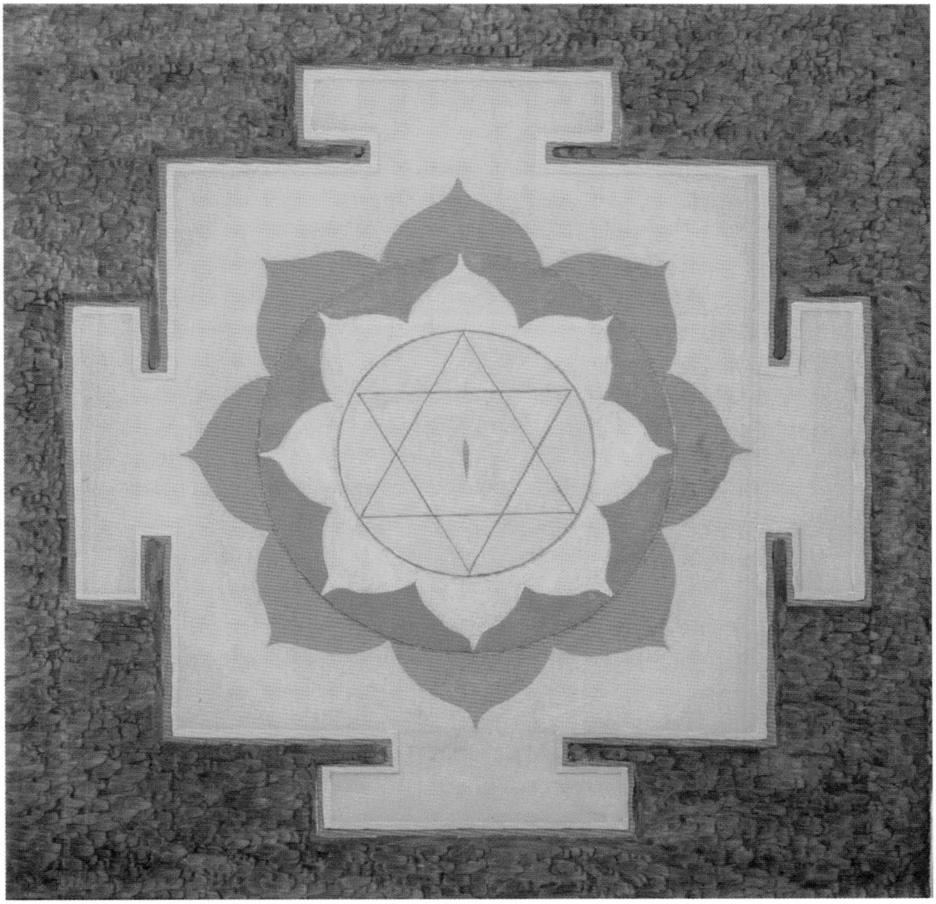

Bhuvaneśvarī

As the goddess whose body is the world, Bhuvaneśvarī is the appointed guardian for fertility, pregnancy and birth. Expansiveness and welcome are her chief qualities, and her *yantra* conveys this sense of limitless spaciousness through its double ring of lotus petals. Although, like Dhūmavatī, Mataṅgi and Kamalātmikā, she also presents a balanced (smaller) pair of Siva / Śakti ascending and descending triangles, it is only Bhuvaneśvarī's *yantra* that contains these triangles within a doubly protective and expansive pair of encircling lotus petal rings.

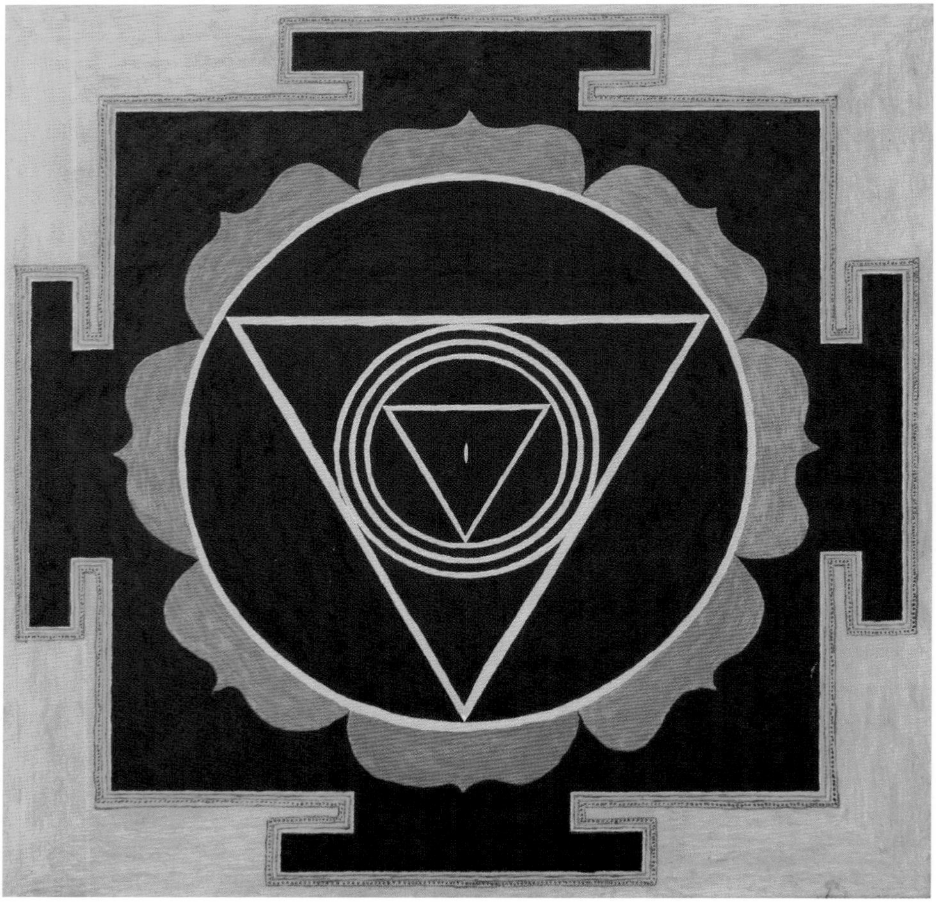

Chinnamastā

As the self-decapitated goddess who represents consciousness beyond the mind, Chinnamastā's *yantra* communicates the fierce energy of the precise moment of transformation. Like the *yantras* for Kālī, Tārā and Bhairavī, the Chinnamastā *yantra* is pure Śakti, with two concentric downward-pointing triangles. The Siva consciousness is only present in the form of the *lingam bindu* in the centre of the *yantra*.

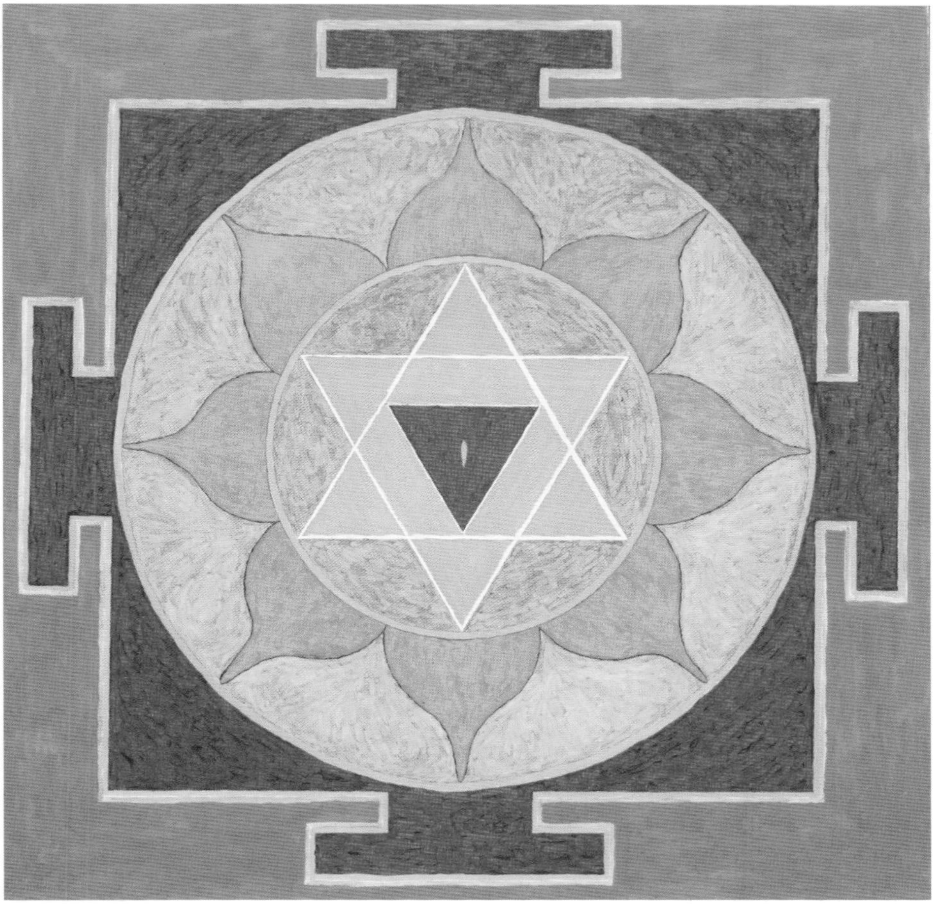

Bagalāmukhī

Standing guard over the experiences of perimenopause, Bagalāmukhī is literally the 'paralyser' with the capacity to stop us in our tracks, and to silence those who resist or attack the power of cyclical wisdom and the inevitability of change. Although, like Dhūmavatī, Kamalātmikā and Mataṅgi, her *yantra* presents a balance between the Siva / Śakti triangles of ascent and descent, in Bagalāmukhī's *yantra* an additional Śakti downward-pointing triangle is overlaid in the centre.

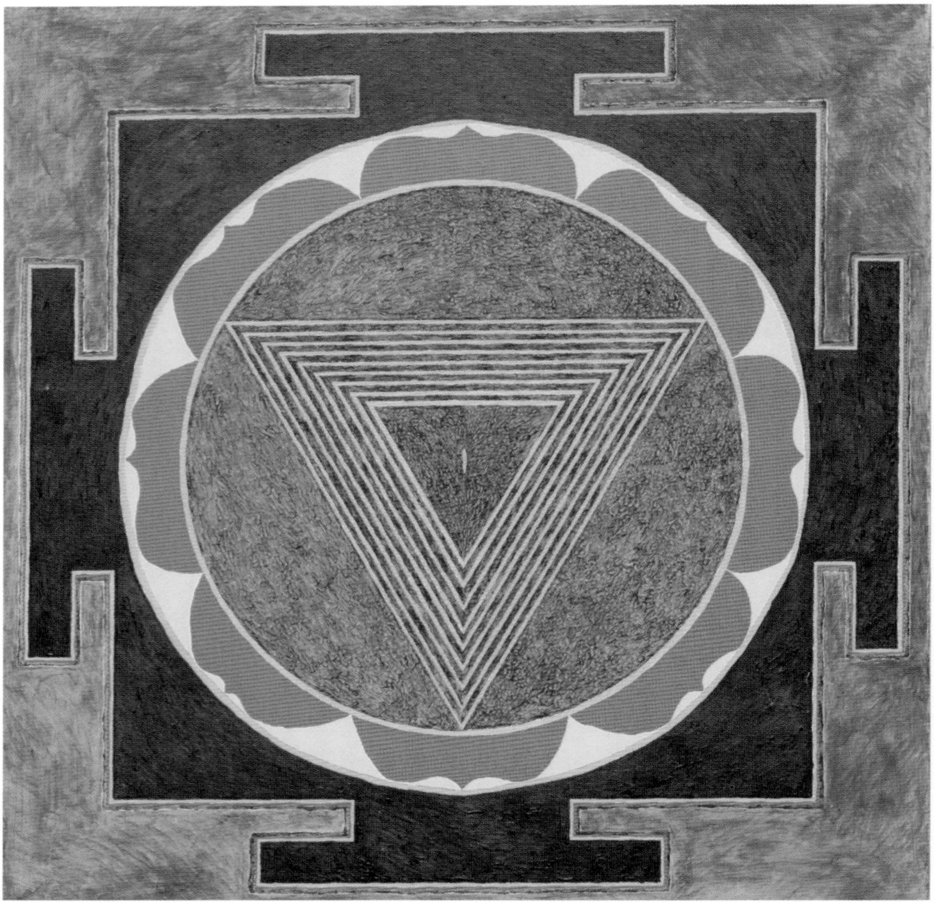

Bhairavī

As the appointed guardian for the *siddhi* of menopause, Bhairavī's warrior goddess energy conveys a fierce power to bring about necessary action and change, even in the face of resistance. She utilises the great energy of rage on behalf of the oppressed or needy, which is likened to the rage of a mother in defence of a child. Like the *yantras* for Kālī, Tārā and Chinnamastā, the Bhairavī *yantra* is pure Śakti, with nine concentric downward-pointing triangles. The Siva consciousness is only present in the form of the *lingam bindu* in the centre of the *yantra*.

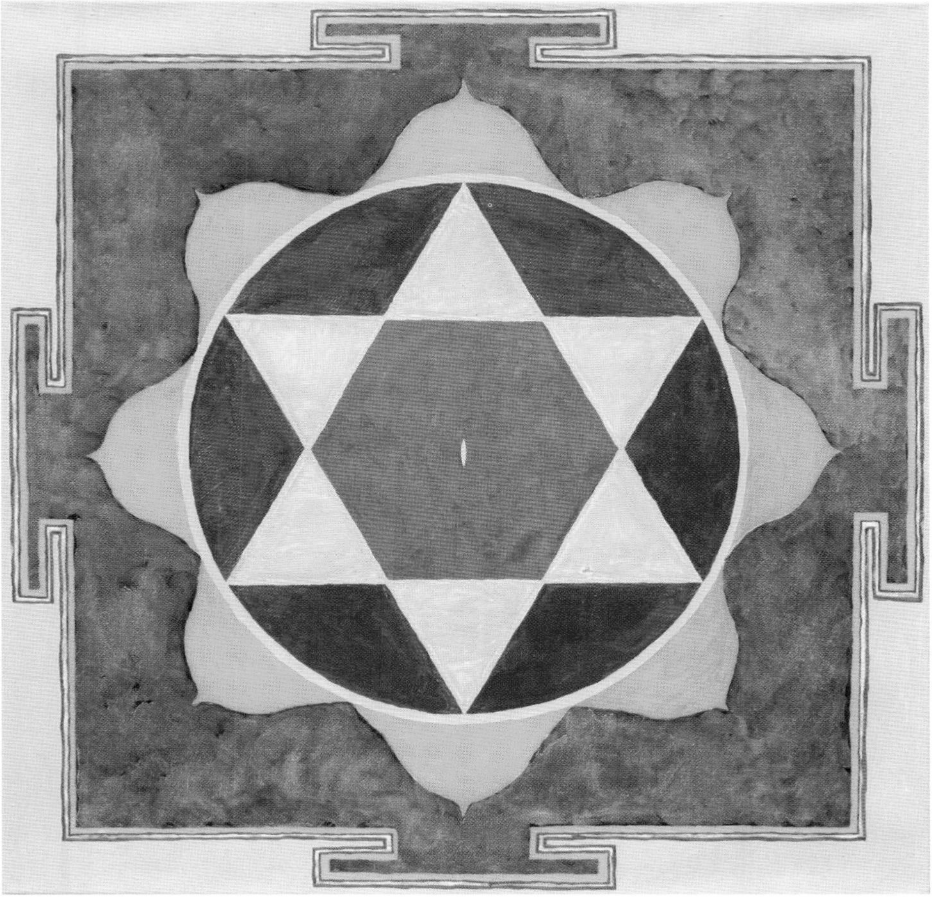

Dhūmavatī

As the grandmother goddess to all of the other Mahāvidyās, Dhūmavatī communicates the deep truth of what really matters, without baulking at the destruction, suffering and pain that such realisation may bring. The Dhūmavatī *yantra* presents a balance between the Siva / Śakti triangles of ascent and descent, in precisely the same geometric form as Kamalātmikā and Mataṅgi. The only differences between these two *yantras* and the Dhūmavatī *yantra* are the colours assigned to the different segments, and the subtly changed shapes of the outer petals.

INDEX OF THERAPEUTIC APPLICATIONS AND LIFE EXPERIENCES

The purpose of this index is to help you to identify which practices, stories and testimonies are most relevant and helpful to support your current experiences. Use this index to locate techniques that may help relieve particular difficulties, or to get further information about certain experiences or feelings. This index lists all of the experiences which are discussed in the book, so that you can search according to the nature of the experience you are having, and the page references will bring you to a place in the text where that topic is discussed and/or a supportive yoga practice is offered.

osteoporosis 66, 246, 261, 409, 423, 424
out of cycle, *see* amenorrhoea, lactational 69, 208, 368
ovaries 562, 589; polycystic 265, 66; surgical removal of, and recovery from 408
overwhelmed 265, 290, 358–9; by birthing energy 571; by love 302–3
ovulation 261–2, 270, 305, 570; and creativity 312, 316; increased earnings at 259; pains 269–70; sexual responsiveness at 284, 306; spontaneous 270; synchronous 206
oxytocin release 372; surge at orgasm 205

pain 69 233, 258, 358–9; birth *see also* labour; menstrual 106, 240, 248–9, 250, 254–6, 260, 264, 267, 279, 301, 392, 570, 599; psychic; relief 126, 351; *see also* arthritis, breastfeeding problems, grief, knee pain, mastitis, osteoporosis
painful intercourse, *see* vulvodynia
pelvic girdle pain 341
pelvic muscles 473; exercises 243–4, 364, 473, 474–7, 480–9; repair surgery, recovery from 474–7; postnatal weakness 363, 364
pelvic organs 370, 407, 480–9; dysfunction of 425; feeling 'low down' 371, 380, 390; revitalising 298, 371, 408, 480–9; shift, perimenopausal 389–90
pelvic organ prolapse 389; and sexual arousal 305; in later life 380–1, 389–90; non-surgical management 390, 407, 474–7
pelvic pain during pregnancy *see* pelvic girdle pain
pelvis, reduced mobility 285; stabilising joints 338
perimenopause 215, 377; as initiation 379–82; sexuality during 304–6; *see also* ageing, confusion, menopause, rage, regret
periods, *see* menstruation; absence of during lactation, *see* amenorrhoea
PGP *see* pelvic girdle pain
piles *see* haemorrhoids
pill, *see* contraceptive
placenta 374, 584; eating 274; ritual burying 253–3, 273–4
plastic surgery 286, 417
PMS, *see* premenstrual tension
polycystic ovaries 265, 266; *see also* ovaries
pornography, effects on sexual response 287
postnatal recovery 59, 205, 220, 345–9; and depression 370, 376; and sexuality 304; and support 354–5, 360–1; *see also* amenorrhoea (lactational), breastfeeding, exclusion, exhaustion, grief, loneliness, love, mastitis, pelvic organ prolapse
postural problems, and effects on pelvic organs 370, 425, 480–1
poverty 413
premenstrual experiences 260, 262, 312, 584; inner critic 316; tension 270, 301, 388;
pre-ovulation, vulnerability 312, 316
pregnancy 329–338; as *siddhi* 25, 117; during postnatal period, *see* Irish twins; unwanted 284, 305; yoga during 55, 59–60, 66, 70, 233, 268; *see also* anxiety, depression, insomnia, love, lower back pain, pelvic girdle pain
pregnancy losses *see* miscarriage
premature babies, care for 359, 374
procrastination 325
prolapse *see* pelvic organ prolapse
protection 62
psychic awareness, during menstruation 288, 312, 316

Q angle 372

rage 69, 670; (peri)menopausal 388, 391, 401; *see also* anger
rape 285, 570
reconnection 26, 75–78, 140, 266; need for 63, 571, 577
regret 226, 379–80, 386, 413
resentment 391, 573, 599; of menstruation 251, 257, 258, 260

sacro-iliac pain, to relieve 338, 514
self-confidence *see* confidence
self-harm 263
sex, heterosexual intercourse 297
sex, lesbian 292–3
sex, postnatally *see* postnatal recovery
sex, tantric 269, 295–7, 303
sexism, damage to women's self-confidence 315
sexual abuse *see* rape and exploitation
sexual pleasure 289–92; as healing for pelvic organ prolapse 304; enhanced by yoga practice 298–300; in relation to menstrual cycle 259–60; *see also* breast arousal, orgasm
sexuality 205, 281–9, 296–7; and creativity 262, 294, 309–11, 445; and fertility 284–5; as healing power 281, 300; and menstruation 259, 260; and yoga 298–300; *see also* birth, menopause, postnatal recovery
shame 210
sharing, need for 75–8, 120–1, 245, 287, 359, 385
sleep deprivation 339, 364, 409, 423, 586
sorrow 215, 357, 382, 413
SPD *see* pelvic girdle pain
sphincter release 300
split rectus muscles 370–1
stillbirth 346, 357–8, 365, 376, 586
stopped periods, *see* amenorrhoea
suppression 246, 313, 353; of menstrual cycle 210, 220, 254, 265, 570, 599
surrender 115, 121, 125, 132–5, 206, 226, 250–1,

INDEX OF PRACTICES

The purpose of this index is to help you to identify which practices, stories and testimonies are most relevant and helpful to support your current experiences. Use this index to locate techniques that may help relieve particular difficulties, or to get further information about certain experiences or feelings. This index lists the names (in Sanskrit and English) of all of the practices that are described in the book.

GENERAL INDEX

inner teacher, connecting with 60–61, 63–64, 75, 81–82, 276, 278, 315, 460–62
'inner yoga' 262, 267
inside out, healing from the 360, 371
instruction, yoga *see also* teachers of yoga; children present at 59, 354, 361–63; and disempowerment of women 63–75; history of 50–63; and the lineage traditions 61–63; and *paramparā* 277; UK statistics on 47–48
insurance 66
interconnection, lives as 206, 212–13
inter-generational overlaps 206, 212
intuition 211–12, 225
inversions, need for caution performing 583
invisibility, powers of 112, 116
IUCDs and yoga practice 585
Iyengar, B.K.S. 53, 56
Iyengar, Geeta 53, 91, 602
Iyengar yoga 56–58, 62, 67, 72

Jivamukti yoga 104–5
Johnsen, Linda 101
Joshi, M.C. 96, 97
joy 291, 297
justice, yoga as a force for 26, 567–581

Kālī (the black goddess): as one of ten female goddesses 218–228, 220, 225–27, 229; picture of 224; as the queen of wisdom goddesses 225–27; relation with Kamalātmikā 282; similar to Tārā 255; *yantra* 646–647; *yoga nidrā* 435–441
Kamalātmikā (the lotus goddess of delight): and cycles of women's lives 229, 281–306; as one of ten female goddesses 218–224, 227; picture of 280; relation with Kālī 282; relation with Mataṅgi 282; *yantra* 649–650; *yoga nidrā* 445–46
Kapila, Sage 180
Karaikkal Ammaiyar 105
karma yoga 50–51, 54
Kent, Christine 481, 483, 484, 492
Khalsa, Gurmukh Kaur 420
Kinsley, David 100, 219, 221, 232, 311
kirtan (devotional song) 104, 107
kissing 291
Knight, Chris 206, 573
Krishnamacharya, Tirumalai 52, 53, 54, 91
Krishnamurti 604
kuṇḍalinī yoga 61, 107, 121, 161, 292, 420

'ladies' holidays' 72
Lady Cunt Love 286
Lakśmī (goddess of wealth) 283
Lalla Ded 105–6, 107
L'am, DeAnna 245
language, use of 34–38, 89, 239
lap dancers 259
Lasater, Judith 92
Laws of Manu 97
'letting go' 139, 388
lineages, yoga: benefits of 61–63; cases of abuse in the yoga world 582, 605–9; and disempowerment 63–75, 277; history 47–60, 84–96; lack of womb awareness 582; and *paramparā* 277; potential negative effects of traditional yoga on menstruation 265–67; power and control in the lineage traditions 57, 58, 59, 61–63, 355–56, 597; and pregnancy 66; womb yoga's relationship to 603
lucid dreaming ritual 326
Lucy, Janet 245
lunar cycles 72, 77, 141, 206, 255, 270, 333
Lysebeth, Andre van 95

Magee, Mike 103
magical powers *see siddhis* (magical powers); supernatural powers
Mahādevī 105–6
Mahāvidyās (wisdom goddesses) 218–233, 282 *see also individual goddesses*
Maharshi, Ramana 230
mālā beads 561
Mallinson, Jim 86, 92
Manmoyanand, Yoga 121
manuals, yoga *see* books about yoga; texts, yoga
Marciniak, Barbara 303
Mataṅgi (the outcast poet, the utterance of the divine word): and cycles of women's lives 229, 309–27; as one of ten female goddesses 218–224, 227; picture of 308; relation with Kamalātmikā 282; *yantra* 650–51; *yoga nidrā* 445–46
MATRIKA project (Motherhood and Traditional Resources, Information, Knowledge and Action) 577
media messages: about birth 350; about older women 212, 416; about sexuality 285, 286, 289–290; vs self-awareness 232, 261
medical science: medicalisation of birth 233, 329, 333, 334, 570; and menstruation 210, 260
men: and elemental consciousness 572; experiencing female *siddhis* 118, 122; haṭha yoga as male domain (history of) 88–92, 603; involvement in yoga teaching 47–48, 57; male gratification as cultural standard for sex 285–86, 296; men gaining power through association with females 99; and menstruation 243; and the 'nine gates' 45, 90, 92, 591–94; pervasive influence on domestic sphere 313; as readers of this book 602; removal of women's sexual power 287–88
Mirābai 105
moon (lunar) cycles 72, 77, 141, 206, 255, 270, 333
moon cups 269, 577–78
moon days 72

ABOUT THE AUTHOR AND ILLUSTRATOR

Uma Dinsmore-Tuli was born in London to an Irish mother and English father in 1965, and first encountered yoga watching Thames television in 1969. She has been teaching since 1996, and training teachers and yoga therapists internationally since 2003. In 2005 she created the annual yoga and *bhakti* camp *Santosa*. She's been writing stories since 1970, spent seven years as a freelance journalist, and ten years teaching in universities before yoga become a full-time job after the publication of her first book about yoga in 2002. Her PhD is in communications, and her diploma in yoga therapy is from the Yoga Biomedical Trust. In 1986 Uma left part of her heart in County Clare, and has been returning every year to see if she can get it back. So far she's failed.

Nirlipta Tuli was born in Luton to Indian parents in 1964, and first encountered yoga in 1987 in the unlikely surroundings of HMP Blantyre House, whilst serving a custodial sentence. Having been requested by fellow inmates to teach them yoga, Nirlipta arranged for a visiting teacher to attend the prison and give classes. Upon his release, Nirlipta trained as a yoga teacher himself and has been teaching yoga since 1989, and training teachers and yoga therapists since 2010. He has a degree in art history, a masters in Indian religions, and has been painting and drawing since 1983.

In 1997 Uma and Nirlipta were instructed by Paramahamsa Satyananda to play the roles of Sitā and Rāma at their wedding at Rikhia, Jharkand in north east India. Swami Satyananda was a very present guide for the couple at this ceremony, and during the nine days of rituals and meditations surrounding it. This remarkable experience was described by Swami Satyasangananda as an 'intimate blessing', and is understood by Uma and Nirlipta to have been an initiation by Swami Satyananda into the spiritual path of family life. They feel that their work in the promotion of yoga, in particular the liberation and expansion of *yoga nidrā*, is in some small way, part of Swami Satyananda's own *saṁkalpa*, and is powered by his direct involvement in the creation of their family. Their marriage was blessed in 1998 by the late John O'Donohue at Corcomroe Abbey in Clare. Uma and Nirlipta have two sons and one daughter and they live in Stroud, UK.

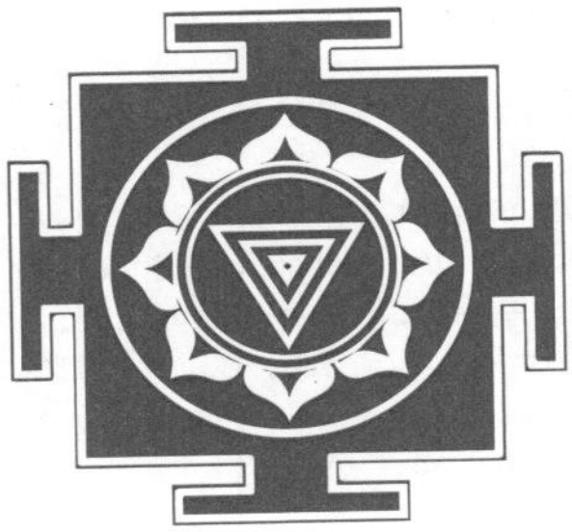

kālī kālī mahakālī
kālīke pāp hārini
dharma kām prade devi
nārāyaṇi namostute

You are Kālī, great Kālī, who removes all impurities
You grant us love to fulfill our duty –
you are the giver of both desire and dharma.
Honour, worship to you.